Recent Advances in Pharmacology

First Author & Chief Editor

Dr. Pranab Das

Second Author

Dr. Daradi Das

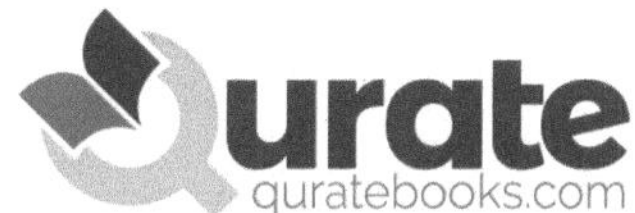

Recent Advances in Pharmacology
First Author & Chief Editor: Dr. Pranab Das
Second Author: Dr. Daradi Das

Published in 2025

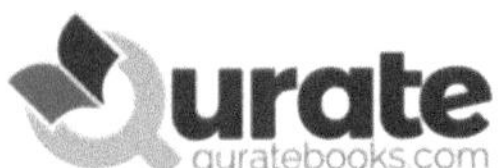

Qurate Books Pvt. Ltd.
Goa 403523, India
www.quratebooks.com
Tel: 1800-210-6527, Email: info@quratebooks.com

ISBN: 978-93-58982-16-9

Dedication

**In cherished remembrance of
my respected grandparents,
late Mr. Naresh Banik and the
late Mrs. Arati Banik,
whose blessings perpetually illuminate my path.**

**Dedicated with feelings of
love and gratitude to my parents,
Mrs. Seema Das and Mr. Prasanta Das,
for their ceaseless support, sacrifices, and steadfast belief in me.**

Author's Bio

Dr. Pranab Das

Dr. Pranab Das, M.B.B.S., M.D. (Pharmacology), is a dedicated academic and researcher, now holding the position of Senior Resident in the Department of Pharmacology at Pragjyotishpur Medical College and Hospital, Guwahati, Assam, India. He earned his M.B.B.S. degree from North Bengal Medical College and Hospital in 2019 and thereafter pursued an M.D. in Pharmacology at Silchar Medical College and Hospital, Assam.

Dr. Das has authored several original research articles published in prestigious international journals indexed in PubMed, Scopus, and, Embase and is a co-investigator in several ongoing research projects. His proficiency includes pharmaceutical utilisation research, prescription evaluation, medical prescription audit, systematic review and meta-analysis.

He has received the International Best Researcher of the Year Award, awarded by the Honourable Education Minister of Tamil Nadu, at the International Science, Technology, and Research Awards, 2024, as well as the International Outstanding Researcher Award at the International Science and Technology Awards Congress, 2025. He possesses a lifetime membership in the American Chamber of Research and serves as a peer reviewer for various prestigious international journals and book chapters.

Dr. Das has conducted numerous training sessions on Pharmacovigilance and Adverse Drug Reaction reporting at several medical institutes. He has presented at national conferences, securing third place in a national research scientific poster presentation.

His inaugural book, Recent Advances in Pharmacology, functions as a practical and comprehensive resource for postgraduate trainees, medical faculty, and undergraduate students, clarifying complex subjects with precision and therapeutic relevance.

Dr. Daradi Das

Dr. Daradi Das, M.B.B.S., M.D. (Pharmacology), is a passionate medical practitioner and scholar, presently working as a Senior Resident in the Department of Pharmacology at Pragjyotishpur Medical College, Guwahati, Assam, India.

Dr. Das, a native of Guwahati, Assam, did her primary education at St. Mary's School and attained her further secondary education at the esteemed Cotton College, Guwahati. She obtained her M.B.B.S. degree from Jorhat Medical College and subsequently her M.D. in Pharmacology from Tezpur Medical College, Assam.

Dr. Das has consistently engaged in national conferences over her academic career, presenting research papers and receiving recognition for her perceptive contributions. She has won numerous medical quiz competitions, demonstrating her keen clinical insight and extensive subject expertise.

Dr. Das, with a strong interest in pharmacological research and medical education, aims to make a significant contribution to the area by ongoing learning, clinical practice, and academic engagement.

Authors Details

First Author & Chief Editor:

Dr. Pranab Das
M.B.B.S, M.D. (Pharmacology)
Senior Resident, Department of Pharmacology
Pragjyotishpur Medical College & Hospital
Guwahati, Assam, India.

Second Author:

Dr. Daradi Das
M.B.B.S, M.D. (Pharmacology)
Senior Resident, Department of Pharmacology
Pragjyotishpur Medical College & Hospital
Guwahati, Assam, India.

Preface to the First Edition (Book Description)

Recent Advances in Pharmacology is a distinguished academic resource that comprehensively examines the innovative findings in pharmacology and contemporary medicine. This book is designed to meet the academic and clinical needs of postgraduate (M.D.) Pharmacology students, undergraduate (MBBS) students, NEET-PG/NEET-SS candidates, faculty members, and practicing clinicians, functioning as an essential resource for understanding current pharmacological developments.

In the M.D. Pharmacology curriculum, one of the four theoretical examinations only addresses recent breakthroughs in Pharmacology. This book is systematically structured to aid postgraduate students in understanding this discipline through an extensive examination of newly licensed drugs, modern therapeutic techniques, and evolving pharmacological principles. The book's distinguishing characteristic is its investigation of FDA-approved and CDSCO-approved drugs from 2021 to 2025, making it relevant for academic research and competitive assessments such as NEET-PG and NEET-SS, which often include questions about newly launched medications.

This book supports both postgraduate objectives and enhances the comprehension of MBBS students by detailing traditional and new pharmaceuticals, illuminating their mechanisms of action, clinical uses, safety profiles, and contemporary research challenges. The subject is presented in a clear and intelligible manner that facilitates comprehension for students at all levels. Each chapter concludes with a curated "Quick Bites" part, providing a comprehensive and concise overview of the significant recent developments addressed. This capability is particularly beneficial for rapid review and last-minute exam preparation, enhancing the retention of essential facts.

Recent Advances in Pharmacology, with its strong academic basis and forward-thinking viewpoint, facilitates exam preparation while enhancing a thorough understanding of the future direction of pharmacological research and drug development. This resource is vital for students, educators, and clinicians seeking to stay educated and excel in the dynamic field of pharmacology.

Acknowledments

I express my deepest gratitude to the Almighty for granting me the strength, perseverance, and guidance necessary to complete this work.

This book is lovingly dedicated to the memory of my late grandparents, Mr. Naresh Banik and Mrs. Arati Banik, whose enduring love and blessings continue to guide and inspire me each day.

I am immensely thankful to Prof. (Dr.) Hironmoy Roy, Dr. Mukundam Borah and Dr. Rohit Tigga, three exceptional mentors whose unwavering support and belief in my potential have profoundly shaped my academic journey. Prof. (Dr.) Hironmoy Roy, my undergraduate mentor, not only guided me with wisdom and care but nurtured my growth as if I was his own child. His faith in my abilities has remained a constant source of encouragement. Dr. Mukundam Borah and Dr. Rohit Tigga, my mentors during postgraduate training, has consistently demonstrated confidence in my academic pursuits and offered steadfast support. Their collective influence is foundational to my scholarly achievements and enduring passion for knowledge.

I also wish to express sincere appreciation to Prof. (Dr.) Anupam Nath Gupta, my undergraduate Pharmacology teacher during MBBS, whose passion for the subject deeply inspired me and sparked my enduring interest in pharmacology.

My heartfelt thanks to my juniors and MBBS students, whose trust and enthusiasm continually motivated me to begin and complete this book. Their curiosity and dedication reinforced the importance of sharing knowledge in a clear and practical manner.

I extend my profound appreciation to the co-author of this book, Dr. Daradi Das, for her significant contributions, including two pivotal chapters. Her collaboration, dedication, and support played a vital role in shaping this work, and I am truly grateful for her partnership in this academic endeavour.

I am profoundly honoured and deeply thankful to the esteemed academicians who so graciously agreed to pen the forewords for this book. Prof. (Dr.) Harendra Kumar Sarma, Professor and Head, Department of Pharmacology, Pragjyotishpur Medical College & Hospital, Guwahati, Assam, and Dr. Tarali Devi, Associate Professor, Department of Pharmacology, Diphu Medical College and Hospital, Diphu, Karbi Anglong, Assam, your kind consideration, encouraging words, and generous support have bestowed this work with added depth, dignity, and distinction. I remain sincerely grateful for your valuable time, trust, and guidance.

With sincere and heartfelt gratitude,

Pranab Das

Dr. Pranab Das
M.B.B.S, M.D. (Pharmacology)
Senior Resident
Department of Pharmacology
Pragjyotishpur Medical College & Hospital
Guwahati, Assam, India

Foreword

It is both a privilege and a pleasure to write the foreword for Recent Advances in Pharmacology. In an era where pharmacological science continues to evolve at an extraordinary pace, this book stands as a timely and relevant contribution bridging foundational knowledge with recent therapeutic developments. As someone involved in shaping the academic journey of students, I have witnessed Dr. Pranab Das's consistent dedication to learning, teaching, and scholarly writing. His ability to distill complex scientific information into clear, practical insights has always stood out. This volume reflects that same clarity of thought and pedagogical depth, making it a useful resource for postgraduates, undergraduates, and even practicing clinicians. The inclusion of drugs approved by regulatory authorities such as the FDA and CDSCO from 2021 to 2025 enhances its practical value, especially in the context of fast-changing therapeutic landscapes. The "Quick Bites" sections at the end of each chapter are particularly thoughtful, offering readers crisp and targeted revision tools. Dr. Pranab has always exemplified a sincere academic spirit be it through his clinical acumen, research orientation, or commitment to medical education. His contributions through this book reflect not only scholarly depth but also a genuine desire to support learners and practitioners alike. I am confident that Recent Advances in Pharmacology will serve as a dependable companion for students and educators and contribute meaningfully to clinical learning and evidence-based practice.

Anupam Nath Gupta

Prof. (Dr.) Anupam Nath Gupta
Professor and Head, Department of Pharmacology
Dean of Student's Affairs
North Bengal Medical College & Hospital
Darjeeling, West Bengal

Foreword

I feel privileged and honoured to write the foreword for this book, which is being published by Dr. Pranab Das for medical students. I am confident that it will be well appreciated by both undergraduate and postgraduate students, as well as teachers.

This book will undoubtedly serve as a valuable additional reference alongside standard textbooks, especially useful for postgraduate students in pharmacology, those in clinical disciplines, and medical practitioners. It offers focused updates on key pharmacological developments, presented in a concise and accessible format that supports both academic learning and practical application.

Given the ever-evolving landscape of drug discovery and therapeutic approaches, such a resource is timely and much needed. I am sure it will be of great help to all who seek clarity and current insight in this dynamic field.

Prof. (Dr.) Harendra Kumar Sarma
Professor and Head, Department of Pharmacology
Pragjyotishpur Medical College & Hospital
Guwahati, Assam

Foreword

It is my great pleasure to write the foreword for "Recent Advances in Pharmacology," a comprehensive and timely volume edited by Dr. Pranab Das. This book represents a significant contribution to the field of pharmacology, capturing the essence of the latest research and innovations that are transforming our understanding of therapeutics.

The chapters in this book showcase the remarkable progress being made in pharmacology, from the discovery of new molecular targets to the development of novel therapeutic strategies. Dr. Das, the bright blessed fellow in Pharmacology provides his insightful analyses of the current state of knowledge and highlight the potential implications for future research and clinical practice.

"Recent Advances in Pharmacology" is an invaluable resource for anyone seeking to stay current with the latest developments in the field. Whether you are a researcher, clinician, or student, this book will provide you with a deeper understanding of the complex interactions between drugs and biological systems.

Dr. Pranab Das is one of my very beloved jewel student with his bagful of shining achievements throughout his academic carrier, who has made me proud always. I congratulate him for such an outstanding work. I personally believe strongly that this book will be a testament to his dedication to advancing the field of pharmacology and improving human health.

Prof. (Dr.) Hironmoy Roy, MD
MHPE (M.Ed), FAIMER fellow,
MBA, PG Diploma ME, ACME
Department of Anatomy
Institute of Post Graduate Medical Education &
Research (Centre of Excellence)
Government of West Bengal

Foreword

It gives me immense pleasure and pride to contribute a few words to the book titled "Recent Advances in Pharmacology". I must appreciate Dr. Pranab Das for his initiative step in bringing out this excellent book which includes topics on recent advances in pharmacotherapeutic management of various condition, role of AI in Pharmacology, Computer-Assisted Learning (CAL), novel FDA drug approvals etc.

Learning is a perpetual journey in medical science which is ever changing in all its fields day by day. Pharmacology and Pharmacotherapeutics too have undergone significant advancements specially in the development of effective and targeted treatments including new drug delivery system and innovative therapeutic approaches. One has to keep abreast with the latest knowledge and advances taking place rapidly in medical science.

It is indeed a herculean task to bring forward such a nice educative book which will definitely be beneficial for both UG and PG students and faculties. All the chapters of this book are written in a precise up-to-date manner to ensure that they reflect the cutting-edge nature of medical knowledge.

I extend my heartiest congratulation to Dr. Pranab Das for implementing this much needed initiative of the hour. I too hope that he will continue to maintain this spirit.

My best wishes to you.

Dr. Tarali Devi
Associate Professor
Department of Pharmacology
Diphu Medical College and Hospital
Diphu, Karbi Anglong, Assam

Foreword

It is with immense pride and profound admiration that I introduce this distinguished volume, "Recent Advances in Pharmacology," authored by my exceptionally talented student, Dr. Pranab Das. In the dynamic and perpetually evolving landscape of pharmacology, maintaining currency with the latest discoveries and therapeutic innovations is not merely advantageous, but fundamentally imperative. This book stands as a compelling testament to Dr. Das's scholarly dedication, intellectual rigor, and profound insight into the cutting edge of this critical scientific discipline.

"Recent Advances in Pharmacology" transcends the scope of a mere compilation of recent findings; it represents a meticulously researched and thoughtfully presented exploration of the advancements that are fundamentally reshaping our comprehension of drug action, disease mechanisms, and the trajectory of future medical interventions. Dr. Pranab Das has navigated the inherent complexities of modern pharmacology with a clarity and depth that will undoubtedly prove invaluable to a diverse readership, ranging from established researchers and practitioners to aspiring pharmacologists and clinicians.

Throughout my tenure of teaching and mentoring Dr. Pranab, I have consistently observed in him, an unwavering commitment to scientific inquiry and a remarkable capacity for synthesizing intricate information into coherent and impactful scholarly narratives. This publication is a direct manifestation of that dedication, showcasing his significant analytical acumen and his fervent passion for contributing meaningfully to scientific discourse.

The insights offered within these pages are poised to stimulate further research, inform evidence-based clinical practice, and inspire the forthcoming generation of pharmacological breakthroughs. I possess no doubt that "Recent Advances in Pharmacology" will swiftly become an indispensable resource, firmly establishing Dr. Pranab Das as a significant and authoritative voice within the field.

I extend my sincerest congratulations to Dr. Pranab on this outstanding academic achievement and eagerly anticipate the considerable impact this book will exert upon the scientific community.

Sincerely,

Dr. Mukundam Borah
Assistant Professor
Department of Pharmacology
Gauhati Medical College, Guwahati, Assam

Foreword

The journey through postgraduate medical education is one of immense learning and transformation. At its very core lies the science of pharmacology—a discipline that is both foundational and in a state of perpetual evolution. What was considered standard therapy a decade ago may be obsolete today, replaced by innovations that were once the stuff of scientific fiction. For the aspiring specialist, keeping pace with this relentless advancement is not just an academic requirement; it is a clinical and ethical imperative.

It is in this dynamic context that Dr. Pranab Das's book,Recent Advances in Pharmacology, arrives as a much-needed and masterfully crafted resource. The sheer volume of new research, clinical trials, and therapeutic guidelines can be overwhelming for even the most diligent student. The challenge lies in separating the truly transformative "signal" from the surrounding "noise." This book accomplishes that with remarkable clarity and precision.

Dr. Pranab Das has undertaken the formidable task of curating, distilling, and presenting the most significant pharmacological developments. Instead of just listing new drugs, this book explains the "why" behind them—the novel mechanisms, the landmark trials, and the clinical contexts where they become game-changers. Each chapter serves as a lucid and authoritative guide. The content is meticulously researched and presented in a manner that bridges the gap between complex molecular mechanisms and their practical application at the patient's bedside.

This is more than a textbook for examination success; it is a companion for clinical excellence. It will empower postgraduate students to engage in informed discussions, make evidence-based therapeutic decisions, and ultimately, provide a higher standard of care.

I am confident that this work will become an indispensable part of the library of every medical postgraduate. I commend the author(s) for their dedication and scholarly contribution and wholeheartedly recommend this book to the next generation of pharmacologist who will shape the future of medicine.

Rohit Tigga

Dr. Rohit Tigga
MBBS, MD (Pharmacology)
Demonstrator
Department of Pharmacology
Silchar Medical College& Hospital, Silchar, Assam

Contents

Quick Bites

Section 1

General Pharmacology

Chapter 1

Newer Drug Delivery System

Author: Dr. Pranab Das

Introduction

Modern pharmacotherapy relies heavily on the idea of drug delivery systems (DDS), which seek to maximise therapeutic efficacy and patient compliance in addition to delivering active pharmaceutical ingredients (APIs) to target sites. Limited control over pharmacokinetics, systemic side effects, and suboptimal drug concentrations at the target site are common obstacles to traditional dosage forms, such as oral tablets, capsules, and parenteral injections.

Newer drug delivery systems (NDDS), which combine advanced materials, nanotechnology, bioengineering, and biotechnology, have become sophisticated platforms to overcome these limitations. In order to ensure low toxicity, fewer doses, and accurate targeting of diseased tissues, these systems are made to release medications in a controlled, sustained, or stimuli-responsive manner. Polymeric nanoparticles, liposomes, dendrimers, microneedles, hydrogels, transdermal patches, and implantable devices are a few well-known examples.

Historical Perspective

The invention of sustained-release tablets, which reduced the frequency of doses, marked the beginning of the evolution of drug delivery in the middle of the 20th century. But the field really took off in the 1960s when liposomes were developed, allowing medications to be encapsulated for improved bioavailability and decreased toxicity. This breakthrough was fundamental because it established the framework for targeted delivery methods and nanocarrier systems.

The pharmaceutical industry concentrated on controlled-release methods, particularly oral and transdermal routes, in the 1970s and 1980s. Injectable microspheres and implants that could release medication over weeks or months were made possible by the development of biodegradable polymers in the 1990s.

In the 21st century, the fields of material science, nanotechnology, and molecular biology came together to create systems that could target specific sites, dual-drug delivery, and respond in real time to stimuli such as temperature, pH, and enzymes. Lipid nanoparticle delivery systems are crucial, as demonstrated by the success of mRNA-based COVID-19 vaccines.

Bioengineered hydrogels, electrospun nanofibers, and microfluidics-based delivery systems for customised and disease-adapted delivery are further recent developments. In addition to supporting traditional pharmaceutical molecules, NDDS now opens the door for regenerative methods, gene editing treatments, and precision medicine.

Conventional Drug Delivery Systems

Table 1: Conventional drug delivery systems.

System	Key Features	Advantages	Disadvantages
Oral Tablets	Solid dosage form; composed of binders, disintegrants, and coatings.	Convenient and non-invasive. Stable with long shelf life. Precise dosing.	Slow onset of action. Undergoes first-pass metabolism. Not suitable for unconscious or vomiting patients.
Oral Syrups	Sugar or sweetenerbased liquid formulations that are frequently flavoured.	Easy administration for children/elderly. Quicker onset of action (due to less need of disintegration and easier dissolution in gastrointestinal juice) compared to tablets.	Less stable. Sugar content may affect diabetic patients. Bulky packaging.
Injections (Parenteral)	Administered by SC, IM, or IV route; bypasses first-pass metabolism by the gastrointestinal and hepatic system.	Rapid onset. 100% bioavailability (IV). Useful in emergencies.	Invasive and painful. Requires trained personnel. Risk of infection and pain.
Topical Creams/ Ointments	Applied directly to skin or mucous membranes; provides localized action.	Local effect with minimal systemic exposure. Avoids first-pass metabolism. Simple to use.	Limited penetration in some cases. May cause irritation or allergies. Not suitable for deep tissue infections.
Inhalers	Delivers drug directly to lungs via aerosolized particles.	Quick onset of action, especially for respiratory diseases. Lower systemic side effects.	Technique-sensitive. Limited to drugs with suitable particle size and volatility. Costly devices.

Challenges in Drug Delivery

1. **Targeting Specific Tissues:** One of the most significant challenges in drug delivery is targeting specific diseased tissues while avoiding healthy cells. In cancer treatment, for example, many chemotherapeutic agents affect not only cancer cells but also healthy tissues, leading to severe side effects. Nanoparticle-based systems have been developed to address this challenge by selectively targeting cancerous tissues through surface modifications that recognize specific receptors which are specifically expressed in cancerous cells.
2. **Overcoming Biological Barriers:** The human body has evolved to protect itself from foreign substances, making it difficult for many drugs to reach their intended site of action. Biological barriers, such as the blood-brain barrier (BBB) and intestinal epithelium, prevent many therapeutic agents from effectively reaching diseased tissues. Nanocarriers and liposomes have shown potential in overcoming these barriers by providing enhanced permeation.
3. **Ensuring Drug Stability:** Many therapeutic agents, particularly biologics, are prone to degradation in the body. Drug delivery systems like liposomes and nanoparticles can protect these agents from enzymatic degradation, prolonging their half-lives and enhancing their efficacy. However, developing stable formulations that remain active over time remains a challenge.

Types of Newer Drug Delivery Systems

1. **Nanoparticles**

   Usually ranging in size from 1 to 100 nm, nanoparticles have become an important component in the targeted delivery of medications. By delivering medications directly to diseased tissues, these systems can lessen the damage to healthy tissues. For example, cancer-cell-targeting nanoparticles can improve chemotherapy medications' selectivity and reduce their toxicity. In order to improve the efficiency of drug delivery, nanoparticles are frequently coated with ligands that bind to particular receptors on the external surface of target cells.

   Characteristics:

   - Nano-sized carriers (mostly10-100 nm or less than 1000 nm) used to deliver drugs in a targeted and controlled manner.
   - It can be polymeric, metallic, or lipid-based.

   Mechanism of Action: Targeted drug delivery through ligand-receptor interaction or passive accumulation.

   Advantages:

   - Improves bioavailability.
   - Targeted drug release – thereby increasing the efficacy and reducing the potential risk of ADRs.

   Disadvantages:

   - Complex manufacturing.
   - Potential toxicity – myelosuppression and nephrotoxicity.

   Examples and FDA Status:

   - Abraxane [Nanoparticle Albumin-bound (nab) paclitaxel] - FDA approved for metastatic breast cancer, non-small cell lung cancer (NSCLC) and pancreatic adenocarcinoma (in combination with gemcitabine).
   - Onivyde (PEGylated liposomal nanoparticle-sized formulation Irinitecan) - FDA approved for metastatic pancreatic cancer.

2. **Liposomes**

   Both hydrophilic and hydrophobic medications can be encapsulated in liposomes, which are spherical vesicles composed of phospholipids. They provide less toxicity, enhanced bioavailability, and controlled release. Compared to traditional doxorubicin, liposomal doxorubicin and other liposomal formulations have already had a major impact on oncology by lowering cardiotoxicity. Stealth liposomes, created by advances in liposome technology, are intended to elude the immune system and have an extended half-life.

   Characteristics:

   - Drugs are encapsulated in spherical vesicles called liposomes, which are made of lipid bilayers.
   - They can be unilamellar (single bilayer) or multilamellar (multiple bilayers).
   - Amphiphilic nature allows them to carry both hydrophilic and lipophilic drugs.

   Mechanism of Action: Liposomes fuse with cell membranes or undergo endocytosis to deliver the drug intracellularly.

Advantages:

- Biodegradable and biocompatible.
- Reduces toxicity [e.g. Doxil (PEGylated Doxorubicin containing liposomes) reduces doxorubicin cardiotoxicity].
- Prolonged circulation time with PEGylation.

Disadvantages:

- Stability issues.
- High production cost.

Examples and FDA Status:

- Doxil (Doxorubicin liposomal) - FDA approved for cancer therapy.
- AmBisome (Amphotericin B liposomal) - FDA approved for fungal infections.

3. **Microneedles**

A novel and minimally invasive technique for transdermal drug delivery is microneedles. Because these tiny needles can pass through the epidermis without touching nerve endings, administering drugs is painless and less uncomfortable for patients. In place of conventional injections, microneedles have been studied for the delivery of insulin, vaccines, and other biologics.

Characteristics:

- Micron-sized needles (50 to 250 micrometre in diameter) that create micro-channels in the skin to enhance drug absorption.
- Can be solid, coated, dissolving, or hollow microneedles.

Mechanism of Action: Penetrates the stratum corneum, allowing drugs to diffuse into capillaries.

Advantages:

- Minimally invasive and painless.
- Bypasses first-pass metabolism.
- Suitable for vaccines and biologics.

Disadvantages:

- Limited drug dose per application.
- Has potential for skin irritation.

Examples and FDA Status:

- Zosano's Qtrypta (Dihydroergotamine microneedle patch) - FDA approved for acute treatment of migraine.
- MicronJet (Insulin microneedles) - Under clinical trials.

4. **Implantable Devices**

Long-term, controlled, continuous drug release is possible with implanted drug delivery systems. These surgically implanted devices provide a consistent dosage of medication to a specific area of the body. The use of implantable pumps to administer insulin to diabetic patients is among the most well-known examples. In addition to lessening the inconvenience of daily injections, these devices have demonstrated promise in enhancing blood glucose control.

Characteristics:

- Devices placed under the skin or within body cavities to release drugs over an extended period.
- Can be biodegradable or non-biodegradable.

Mechanism of Action: Provides controlled drug release through diffusion, osmosis, or biodegradation.

Advantages:

- Long-term drug release.
- Improved patient compliance.

Disadvantages:

- Surgical implantation required.
- Risk of infection and device failure.

Examples and FDA Status:

- Norplant (Levonorgestrel implant) - FDA approved for contraception.
- Gliadel Wafer (Carmustine biodegradable intracranial implant) - FDA approved for brain tumours like glioblastoma.

5. **Hydrogels**

Hydrogels are cross-linked, water-swollen networks of polymers that have been studied in great detail for applications involving controlled drug release. Their ability to react to external stimuli, such as pH, temperature, or enzymes, makes them perfect for drug delivery to specific sites. Hydrogels have been applied to tissue engineering, wound healing, and regenerative medicine as growth factor carriers.

Characteristics:

- Three-dimensional networks of polymers that can retain a great deal of water.
- Can be natural (alginate, chitosan) or synthetic (polyethylene glycol).

Mechanism of Action: Release drugs via swelling and diffusion.

Advantages:

- Sustained and localized drug release.
- Biocompatibility.

Disadvantages:

- Mechanical fragility.
- Limited drug loading.

Examples and FDA Status:

- ReGel (Paclitaxel thermosensitive hydrogel) – Under clinical trials.
- HemCon bandage (Chitosan haemostatic hydrogel) - FDA approved for wound dressings and as haemostatic agents.

6. Other newer systems for delivering drugs:

Table 2: Alternative Modern Drug Delivery Systems

Newer Drug Delivery Systems	Characteristics	Mechanism of Action	Advantages	Dis-advantages	Examples & FDA-Approval Status
Occusert	Controlled drug release is provided by these ocular drug delivery systems.	The drug diffuses into the tear film from the polymer matrix.	Sustained drug release and reduces systemic side effects.	Risk of ocular irritation and difficulty in insertion and removal.	Ocusert (Pilocarpine ocular insert) - FDA approved for glaucoma treatment; inserted into the conjunctival sac. Lacrisert (Hydroxypropyl cellulose) - FDA approved for dry eye syndrome; inserted into the inferior cul-de-sac of the eye.
Trans-dermal drug delivery system (TDDS)	Avoids first-pass metabolism by applying patches to the skin to administer medications.	The drug enters the systemic circulation by diffusing through the stratum corneum of the skin.	Non-invasive and convenient and provides steady plasma levels.	Limited to lipophilic, low-molecular-weight drugs and skin irritation is possible.	Nicoderm (Nicotine transdermal patch) - FDA approved for treatment of smoking cessation. Duragesic (Fentanyl transdermal patch) - FDA approved for chronic severe pain management.
Erythro-somes	Drugs are encapsulated within red blood cells and delivered via engineered erythrocytes.	Through cell lysis or passive diffusion, the drug is gradually released from erythrocytes.	Long circulation half-life and reduced immune response mediated destruction of the drug delivery system.	Complex preparation and risk of haemolysis is there.	Still under research; not yet FDA-approved.
Micelles	Micelles are colloidal structures that self-assemble in aqueous solutions in amphiphilic environment. The lipophilic medications are encapsulated in a hydrophobic core, whereas the hydrophilic shell keeps the micelle structure intact.	Improved solubility and passive aiming is achieved through the enhanced permeability and retention (EPR) pheno-menon.	Solubili-zation of poorly soluble drugs and provides targeted drug delivery.	Limited drug loading capacity and also shows some stability concerns.	Genexol-PM (Paclitaxel micelles) – Not FDA-approved, but approved in South Korea for metastatic breast cancer and non-small cell lung cancer (NSCLC). SP1049C (Doxorubicin micelle) - Under clinical trials for advanced oesophageal and gastric cancers.

Future Directions

1. **Gene Therapy and Nanocarriers:** The potential for combining gene therapy with nanocarrier systems opens a new frontier in drug delivery. Nanocarriers such as viral vectors, liposomes, and dendrimers can introduce genetic material into cells, perhaps providing treatments for hereditary illnesses. Ongoing research in this field aims to improve the targeting and efficiency of gene delivery.

2. **Personalized Drug Delivery:** Advances in genomics and proteomics are paving the way for personalized drug delivery systems. These technologies will allow for the development of patient-specific therapies and drug delivery systems tailored to individual genetic profiles. This shift towards the promise of individualized medicine and the pledge of maximizing the effectiveness of medications while reducing their negative effects.

3. **Artificial Intelligence in Drug Delivery:** Machine learning algorithms and artificial intelligence (AI) are being used to forecast drug interactions, optimize formulations, and design new drug delivery systems. AI can simulate drug interactions with biological systems, allowing for the development of more efficient medication delivery platforms. This integration AI's role in medicine development is expected to significantly and drastically cut down on the time and expense needed to introduce novel treatments to the market.

Conclusion

The field of drug delivery systems are undergoing rapid change, with new platforms for therapeutic intervention being developed, thanks in substantial part to the advancements in biotechnology, nanotechnology, and biomaterials. Newer drug delivery systems promise to overcome the shortcomings of conventional approaches and provide patients with safer, more accurate, and more efficient solutions to their issues and concerns as research in this field continues to grow. With the potential to improve patient outcomes and fundamentally alter how we treat illnesses, the future of medicine rests in the ongoing development of these technologies.

References

1. Zahednezhad F, Allahyari S, Sarfraz M, Zakeri-Milani P, Feyzizadeh M, Valizadeh H. Liposomal drug delivery systems for organ-specific cancer targeting: early promises, subsequent problems, and recent breakthroughs. Expert Opinion on Drug Delivery. 2024 Sep 1;21(9):1363-84.
2. Ghosal K, Pani A, Chowdhury T, Kundu A, Thomas S. Multi-vesicular liposome and its applications: a novel chemically modified approach for drug delivery application. Mini Reviews in Medicinal Chemistry. 2024 Jan 1;24(1):26-38.
3. Elumalai K, Srinivasan S, Shanmugam A. Review of the efficacy of nanoparticle-based drug delivery systems for cancer treatment. Biomedical Technology. 2024 Mar 1;5:109-22.
4. Wang X, Mao K, Zhang X, Zhang Y, Yang YG, Sun T. Red blood cell derived nanocarrier drug delivery system: A promising strategy for tumor therapy. Interdisciplinary Medicine. 2024 Jul;2(3):e20240014.
5. Dave S, Shriyan D, Gujjar P. Newer drug delivery systems in anesthesia. Journal of Anaesthesiology Clinical Pharmacology. 2017 Apr 1;33(2):157-63.
6. Huang Q, Zeng Y, Qiu Y, Zou J, Li F, Liu X, Nezamzadeh-Ejhieh A, Song H, Liu J. Applications and prospects of new transdermal drug delivery system based on metal-organic frameworks for diabetic wound healing. Dyes and Pigments. 2024 Mar 1;222:11186.
7. Langer R. New methods of drug delivery. Science. 1990 Sep 28;249(4976):1527-33.
8. Li C, Wang J, Wang Y, Gao H, Wei G, Huang Y, Yu H, Gan Y, Wang Y, Mei L, Chen H. Recent progress in drug delivery. Acta pharmaceutica sinica B. 2019 Nov 1;9(6):1145-62.
9. Davoodi P, Lee LY, Xu Q, Sunil V, Sun Y, Soh S, Wang CH. Drug delivery systems for programmed and on-demand release. Advanced drug delivery reviews. 2018 Jul 1;132:104-38.
10. Lv Y, Li W, Liao W, Jiang H, Liu Y, Cao J, Lu W, Feng Y. Nano-drug delivery systems based on natural products. Int J Nanomedicine. 2024;19:541–569.
11. Akbarzadeh A, Rezaei-Sadabady R, Davaran S, Joo SW, Zarghami N, Hanifehpour Y, Samiei M, Kouhi M, Nejati-Koshki K. Liposomal drug delivery systems: An update review. Biotechnol Adv. 2013;31(6):593–606.

12. Mohammadnia A, Ranjbar R, Nazari M. An overview of microneedle applications, materials, and fabrication methods. J Pharm Innov. 2022;17:1199–212.
13. Robinson DH, Mauger JW. Drug delivery systems. American journal of hospital pharmacy. 1991 Oct 1;48(10_suppl):S14-23.
14. Lavan DA, McGuire T, Langer R. Small-scale systems for in vivo drug delivery. Nature biotechnology. 2003 Oct 1;21(10):1184-91.
15. Tiwari G, Tiwari R, Sriwastawa B, Bhati L, Pandey S, Pandey P, Bannerjee SK. Drug delivery systems: An updated review. International journal of pharmaceutical investigation. 2012 Jan;2(1):2.
16. Sanjay ST, Zhou W, Dou M, Tavakoli H, Ma L, Xu F, Li X. Recent advances of controlled drug delivery using microfluidic platforms. Advanced drug delivery reviews. 2018 Mar 15;128:3-28.
17. Allen TM, Cullis PR. Drug delivery systems: entering the mainstream. Science. 2004 Mar 19;303(5665):1818-22.
18. Katzung BG, Vanderah TW. *Basic & Clinical Pharmacology*. 15th ed. New York: McGraw Hill; 2021.
19. Gupta M. Implantable Drug Delivery Systems. Kanpur: C.S.J.M. University; 2021. Available from: https://gyansanchay.csjmu.ac.in/wp-content/uploads/2021/11/Implantable-Drug-Delivery-Systems-Lecture.pdf.
20. Mitchell MJ, Jain RK, Langer R. Engineering and physical sciences in oncology: challenges and opportunities. Nat Rev Mater. 2017;2(1):17071.
21. Brunton LL, Knollmann BC, Hilal-Dandan R. *Goodman & Gilman's: The Pharmacological Basis of Therapeutics*. 13th ed. New York: McGraw Hill; 2018.
22. Torchilin VP. Micellar nanocarriers: pharmaceutical perspectives. Pharmaceutical research. 2007 Jan;24:1-6.
23. Petros RA, DeSimone JM. Strategies in the design of nanoparticles for therapeutic applications. Nature reviews Drug discovery. 2010 Aug;9(8):615-27.
24. Sercombe L, Veerati T, Moheimani F, Wu SY, Sood AK, Hua S. Advances and challenges of liposome assisted drug delivery. Frontiers in pharmacology. 2015 Dec 1;6:286.
25. Prausnitz MR, Langer R. Transdermal drug delivery. Nature biotechnology. 2008 Nov;26(11):1261-8.
26. Ita KB. Transdermal drug delivery: Progress and challenges. Journal of Drug Delivery Science and Technology. 2014 Jan 1;24(3):245-50.
27. Kim YC, Park JH, Prausnitz MR. Microneedles for drug and vaccine delivery. Advanced drug delivery reviews. 2012 Nov 1;64(14):1547-68.
28. Sill TJ, Von Recum HA. Electrospinning: applications in drug delivery and tissue engineering. Biomaterials. 2008 May 1;29(13):1989-2006.
29. Liechty WB, Kryscio DR, Slaughter BV, Peppas NA. Polymers for drug delivery systems. Annual review of chemical and biomolecular engineering. 2010 Jul 15;1(1):149-73.
30. Allen LV, Popovich NG, Ansel HC. Ansel's pharmaceutical dosage forms and drug delivery systems. 9th ed. Philadelphia: Lippincott Williams & Wilkins; 2011.
31. Krpetic Z, Miah A, Arrigo R. Nanomaterials Targeting Red Blood Cells: Implications for Drug Delivery and Biosensing. Biosensors and Nanotheranostics. 2025 Apr 16;4(1):1-8.
32. Yang J, Shi X, Kuang Y, Wei R, Feng L, Chen J, Wu X. Cell-nanocarrier drug delivery system: a promising strategy for cancer therapy. Drug delivery and translational research. 2024 Mar;14(3):581-96.
33. Paiva MT, Kishima JO, Silva JB, Mantovan J, Colodi FG, Mali S. Crosslinking methods in polysaccharide-based hydrogels for drug delivery systems. Biomedical Materials & Devices. 2024 Mar;2(1):288-306.

Chapter 2

Gene Therapy

Author: Dr. Pranab Das

Introduction

Gene therapy is an advanced medical technique designed to treat or prevent diseases by altering the genetic information within a patient's cells. It offers potential for treating genetic illnesses, specific malignancies, and viral infections by rectifying malfunctioning genes, substituting absent genes, or incorporating new genes to amplify therapeutic outcomes.

In the last ten years, advancements in genetic engineering methods, including CRISPR-Cas9, zinc finger nucleases (ZFNs), and viral vector delivery systems, have markedly enhanced the accuracy and safety of gene therapy. Originally conceived in the 1970s, the inaugural approved gene therapy study in humans occurred in 1990, addressing a kid with severe combined immunodeficiency (SCID). Since that time, the area has advanced swiftly, with multiple FDA-approved gene treatments now accessible for ailments such as spinal muscular atrophy (SMA), inherited retinal diseases, and haematologic disorders. This chapter examines the concepts, classifications, sequential methodologies, applications, benefits, and constraints of gene therapy, highlighting recent developments and future possibilities.

Definition

According to the US FDA, gene therapy is a technique that modifies a person's genes to treat or cure disease. Gene therapies can work by several mechanisms:

- Replacing a disease-causing gene with a healthy copy of the gene.
- Inactivating a disease-causing gene that is not functioning properly.
- Introducing a new or modified gene into the body to help treat a disease.

Gene therapy products are being studied to treat diseases including cancer, genetic diseases, and infectious diseases.

Vectors

There are a variety of types of gene therapy vectors and gene therapy techniques, including:

- **Plasmid DNA:** Circular DNA molecules can be genetically engineered to carry therapeutic genes into human cells.
- **Viral vectors:** Viruses have a natural ability to deliver genetic material into cells, and therefore some gene therapy products are derived from viruses. Once viruses have been modified to remove their ability to cause infectious disease, these modified viruses can be used as vectors (vehicles) to carry therapeutic genes into human cells.
- **Bacterial vectors:** Bacteria can be modified to prevent them from causing infectious disease and then used as vectors (vehicles) to carry therapeutic genes into human tissues.

- **Human gene editing technology:** The goals of gene editing are to disrupt harmful genes or to repair mutated genes.
- **Patient-derived cellular gene therapy products:** Cells are removed from the patient, genetically modified (often using a viral vector) and then returned back to the patient.

Principles of Gene Therapy

Gene therapy operates on the principle of genetic modification, which can be achieved in three main ways:

1. **Gene Replacement:** Replacing a mutated gene with a functional copy.
2. **Gene Inactivation:** Silencing or editing a defective gene that causes disease.
3. **Gene Addition:** Introducing a new gene to help combat disease (e.g. adding genes to stimulate immune responses in cancer therapy).

Types of Gene Therapy

Gene therapy is categorized based on target cells and modification approaches:

A. Based on Target Cells

Table 1: Categories of gene therapy according to target cells.

Type	Description	Applications
Germline Gene Therapy	Modifies genes in sperm, eggs, or embryos, passing changes to future generations.	Used in experimental settings for inherited genetic disorders like cystic fibrosis and muscular dystrophy.
Somatic Gene Therapy	Alters non-reproductive cells, affecting only the treated individual.	Used in FDA-approved therapies for cancers, spinal muscular atrophy (SMA), haemophilia, and sickle cell disease.

B. Based on Gene Modification Method

Table 2: Categories of gene therapy according to gene modification techniques.

Type	Description	Examples
Ex Vivo Gene Therapy	Cells are extracted from the patient, genetically modified in a lab, and reintroduced.	CAR-T cell therapy for leukaemia, ex vivo therapy for β-thalassemia.
In Vivo Gene Therapy	The therapeutic gene is directly delivered into the patient's body via a vector.	AAV-based therapies for retinal disorders, muscular dystrophy.

Procedure of Gene Therapy

The process of gene therapy involves multiple precise steps to ensure safety, effectiveness, and minimal adverse effects.

1. **Identification of the Target Gene**
   - Scientists determine the defective or missing gene causing the disease.
   - Genetic sequencing techniques like Whole Genome Sequencing (WGS) are used.
   - If a gene is overactive, scientists aim to silence or modify its activity.

2. **Selection of the Gene Delivery Method**

   The method of delivering the therapeutic gene is crucial for treatment success. Two main categories exist:

A. **Viral Vectors (Most Common)**
   1. Adeno-Associated Virus (AAV) – Used in Luxturna for eye diseases.
   2. Lentivirus – Used for CAR-T cell therapy in leukaemia.
   3. Retrovirus – Used in early gene therapy trials.

B. **Non-Viral Methods (Experimental/undergoing trial)**
   1. CRISPR-Cas9 – Direct gene editing at the DNA level.
   2. Liposomes – Nanoparticles carrying genetic material.
   3. Electroporation – Uses electrical pulses to introduce genes into cells.

3. **Gene Insertion or Modification**
   - The therapeutic gene is integrated into the patient's DNA.
   - Gene expression levels are monitored to ensure stable function.

4. **Monitoring and Evaluation**
   - Blood samples, imaging, and biomarker studies help to assess gene activity.
   - Patients are observed for immune system reactions.

5. **Follow-up and Safety Assessment**
   - Long-term monitoring for tumour formation or genetic mutations.
   - Some patients require multiple gene therapy doses for sustained effects.

Applications of Gene Therapy

Gene therapy has transformed modern medicine, offering potential cures for previously untreatable diseases. Below are major applications:

A. **Genetic Disorders**
   1. Spinal Muscular Atrophy (SMA) – FDA-approved Zolgensma (AAV vector-based therapy).
   2. Haemophilia A & B – Gene therapy is in Phase 3 clinical trials to introduce functional clotting factor genes.
   3. Sickle Cell Disease – Casgevy and Lyfgenia (CRISPR-based therapy) were FDA-approved in 2023.

B. **Cancer Therapy**
   1. CAR-T Cell Therapy – Uses gene-modified T-cells to attack cancer cells (FDA-approved Kymriah, Yescarta).
   2. Oncolytic Viral Therapy – Genetically engineered viruses target tumours (T-VEC for melanoma).

C. **Neurological Disorders**
   1. Huntington's Disease – Early-stage clinical trials using RNA-based gene therapy.
   2. Parkinson's Disease – Gene therapy aims to restore dopamine production.

D. **Eye Diseases**
   1. Inherited Retinal Dystrophy – FDA-approved Luxturna delivers a functional RPE65 gene to restore vision.

E. **Infectious Diseases**
    1. HIV Gene Editing – CRISPR-based gene therapy aims to eliminate latent HIV reservoirs.

Advantages of Gene Therapy

Gene therapy offers advantages that traditional treatments cannot match:

1. Potential to cure genetic diseases by addressing the root cause.
2. One-time treatment for some disorders (e.g. Zolgensma for SMA).
3. Reduced dependency on lifelong medications (e.g. haemophilia gene therapy).
4. Personalized medicine – Tailored therapy for individual genetic profiles.
5. Minimal side effects compared to chemotherapy or radiation therapy.

Limitations of Gene Therapy

Despite its benefits, gene therapy faces several limitations:

1. High Cost – Gene therapy treatments can cost over $1 million per patient (e.g. Zolgensma = $2.1 million).
2. Immune Response Issues – Some patients develop immune rejection to viral vectors.
3. Limited Long-Term Data – Most gene therapies are new, and long-term effects are not fully understood.
4. Ethical Concerns – Germline gene editing is controversial and banned in most countries.
5. Accessibility Issues – Not all countries have access to gene therapy treatments.

Conclusion

Gene therapy represents a significant achievement in contemporary medicine, providing prospective treatments and cures for genetic abnormalities, malignancies, and chronic illnesses. Gene therapy addresses diseases at their fundamental origin by altering or substituting faulty genes, rather than simply alleviating symptoms. In the past twenty years, swift progress in gene editing technologies, viral vector delivery methods, and regulatory approvals has resulted in multiple FDA-approved gene treatments and ongoing clinical trials for various disorders.

References

1. World Health Organization. *WHO Report on Gene Therapy and Global Ethics.* Geneva: WHO; 2023.
2. Santos L. The Global Governance of Human Genome Editing and the World Health Organization Framework. In Governance of Human Gene Editing and Transhumanism: Tasks for Today's Bioethics 2025 Jan 10 (pp. 3-13). Cham: Springer Nature Switzerland.
3. Sharma R. Innovative genoceuticals in human gene therapy solutions: challenges and safe clinical trials of orphan gene therapy products. Current Gene Therapy. 2024 Feb 1;24(1):46-72.
4. Puzzo F, Kay MA. The deLIVERed promises of gene therapy: past, present and future of liver-directed gene therapy. Molecular Therapy. 2025 Mar 27.
5. Rehman SU. Advancement in Gene therapy: Current and Future of Gene Therapy. Kashmir Journal of Science. 2025 Mar 17;4(01).
6. Butt MH, Zaman M, Ahmad A, Khan R, Mallhi TH, Hasan MM, Khan YH, Hafeez S, Massoud EE, Rahman MH, Cavalu S. Appraisal for the potential of viral and nonviral vectors in gene therapy: A review. Genes. 2022 Jul 30;13(8):1370.
7. Arjmand B, Larijani B, Sheikh Hosseini M, Payab M, Gilany K, Goodarzi P, Parhizkar Roudsari P, Amanollahi Baharvand M, Hoseini Mohammadi NS. The horizon of gene therapy in modern medicine: advances and challenges. Cell Biology and Translational Medicine, Volume 8: Stem Cells in Regenerative Medicine. 2020:33-64.
8. National Institutes of Health. Gene therapy for neurological disorders [Internet]. *ClinicalTrials.gov;* 2024 [cited 2025 Mar 23]. Available from: https://clinicaltrials.gov.

9. U.S. Food & Drug Administration. FDA gene therapy approval reports [Internet]. *FDA.gov*; 2023 [cited 2025 Mar 23]. Available from: https://www.fda.gov.
10. Dunbar CE, High KA, Joung JK, et al. Gene therapy comes of age. *Science*. 2018;359(6372):175–80.
11. Ball J, Bradley A, Le A, Tisdale JF, Uchida N. Current and future treatments for sickle cell disease-from hematopoietic stem cell transplantation to in vivo gene therapy. Molecular Therapy. 2025 Mar 12.
12. Vajiram & Ravi. Gene therapy: Concept, types, applications, and challenges [Internet]. New Delhi: Vajiram and Ravi; c2025 [cited 2025 May 9]. Available from: https://vajiramandravi.com/upsc-exam/gene-therapy/.
13. Liu Z, Zhang H, Jia H, Wang H, Huang Z, Tang Y, Wang Z, Hu J, Zhao X, Li T, Sun X. The clinical safety landscape for ocular AAV gene therapies: a systematic review and meta-analysis. iScience. 2025 Mar 22.

Chapter 3

Stem Cell Therapy

Author: Dr. Pranab Das

Introduction

One of the most revolutionary developments in contemporary regenerative medicine and therapeutic pharmacology is stem cell therapy. This therapeutic approach captures the special biological properties of stem cells, specifically their ability to self-renew and differentiate into various specialised cell types, and is characterised by its potential to replace, repair, or regenerate damaged tissues and organs. Stem cell-based therapies are opening the door to a new era of individualised and curative treatment approaches ranging from neurological disorders and cardiovascular diseases to autoimmune conditions and cancers.

But even with its promise, stem cell therapy has many ethical, legal, and scientific obstacles to overcome. These include the difficulty of controlling cell differentiation in vivo, tumourigenicity, and immune rejection risks. With new developments in cell reprogramming, biomaterials, and 3D bioprinting, as well as ongoing clinical trials, the field is growing quickly and may one day be able to treat diseases that were thought to be incurable.

Historical Perspective

Stem cell research began with the discovery of haematopoietic stem cells (HSCs) in the 1960s, which transformed bone marrow transplantation as a treatment for haematological malignancies. Since that time, the field has quickly expanded to encompass a variety of stem cell types, each with unique biological potentials and therapeutic implications, including adult (somatic) stem cells, induced pluripotent stem cells (iPSCs), and embryonic stem cells (ESCs). Stem cell therapy now has the potential to replace damaged or lost cells as well as be used for tissue engineering, gene therapy, and medication delivery.

Definition

Stem cells are used to regenerate, repair, or replace tissues that have been damaged due to injury, disease, or aging. These cells are either obtained through autologous means from the patient's own body or donated by another individual (allogeneic).

Different Kinds of Stem Cells

1. **Embryonic Stem Cells (ESCs):** Since ESCs are pluripotent, they can differentiate into any type of cell and are derived from early-stage embryos. However, they also carry the risk of immunological rejection and ethical issues, which limits their widespread use.

2. **Adult Stem Cells (ASCs):** ASCs are multi-potent cells that can differentiate into only specific cell types. They are found in specific tissues like bone marrow and fat. Leukaemia and cardiovascular disorders have been treated with them.

3. **Induced Pluripotent Stem Cells (iPSCs):** Adult cells that have undergone genetic reprogramming to regain their pluripotency are known as iPSCs. By using the patient's own cells for therapy, this technology bypasses ethical issues and provides a customised therapeutic approach.

Mechanism of Action

Stem cells can restore function through several mechanisms:

- **Differentiation into specialized cells:** Stem cells have the capacity to develop into specialised cells and can take the place of damaged tissues' cells, such as cardiomyocytes or brain neurones.
- **Secretion of bioactive molecules:** By reducing inflammation, extending cell life, and stimulating endogenous cells to repair damaged tissues, these cells have the ability to release specific bioactive molecules that can aid in cellular or tissue repair.
- **Modulation of immune responses:** Certain stem cells encourage the host immune response to lessen inflammation and autoimmune reactions, improve the lifespan of immune cells, and reduce inflammation.

Procedure of Stem Cell Treatment

The procedure for different stem cell therapies area based on the disease being treated and the type of stem cells used. However, the general steps are as follows:

1. **Patient Evaluation & Pre-Treatment Assessment**
   - **Medical History & Diagnosis:** To ascertain the patient's eligibility for stem cell therapy, a comprehensive medical evaluation is conducted.
   - **Imaging & Lab Tests:** To identify the eligible patients, MRIs, CT scans, blood tests, and tissue biopsies may be performed.
2. **Stem Cell Sourcing & Processing**
   - Types of Stem Cells Used:
     1. **Autologous Stem Cells:** These are extracted from the patient's own blood, adipose tissue, or bone marrow.
     2. **Allogeneic Stem Cells:** These are collected from a donor and include adult stem cell banks or umbilical cord blood.
     3. **Induced Pluripotent Stem Cells (iPSCs):** Mature cells that have been reprogrammed so as to function similarly to ESCs.
     4. **Embryonic Stem Cells (ESCs):** Because of ethical concerns, embryonic stem cells (ESCs), which are derived from blastocysts, are not as frequently used.
   - **Processing & Purification:** To improve therapeutic outcomes, the gathered stem cells are purified, processed, and occasionally genetically altered. They are grown or cultivated in specialised bioreactors to produce the necessary quantity of cells (Figure 1).

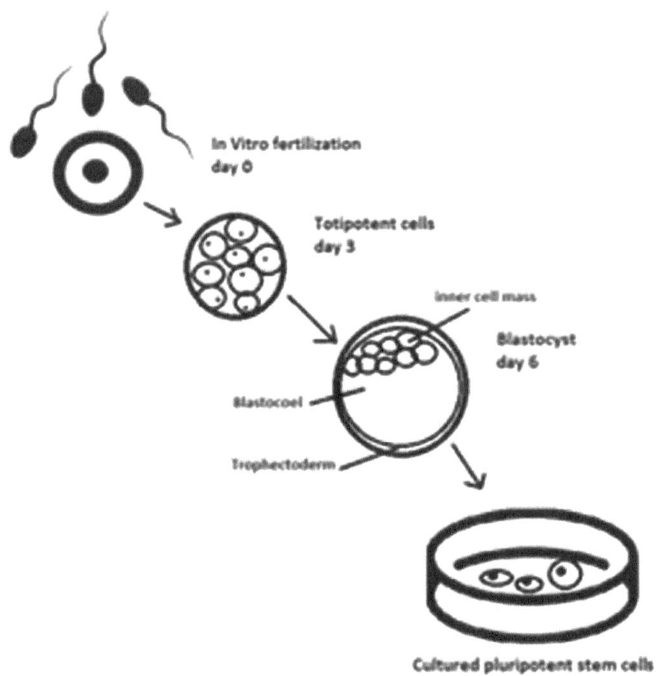

Figure 1: Simplified overview of how cultured pluripotent stem cells are developed in the lab (Source: Zakrzewski W et al.).

3. **Stem Cell Delivery & Administration**
   - **Route of Administration:**
     1. **Intravenous (IV) Infusion:** Used for systemic stem cell delivery for diseases such as cancer, heart disease, and autoimmune disorders. For example, haematopoietic stem cell transplantation (HSCT) for lymphoma or leukaemia.
     2. **Intra-arterial Injection:** Injection into a specific artery supplying the target organ.
     3. **Intrathecal/Intra-ventricular Injection:** Directly the stem cells are introduced into cerebrospinal fluid for neurological conditions (e.g. spinal cord injury, ALS).
     4. **Direct Tissue Injection:** Stem cells injected into damaged organs (e.g. heart, cartilage, joints). E.g.: Intra-cardiac injection directly into heart muscle in heart failure and cardiomyopathies.
     5. **Implantation via Scaffold:** Stem cells embedded in 3D biomaterials for organ regeneration.
4. **Post-Treatment Monitoring & Follow-Up**
   - **Monitoring for Adverse Reactions:** Patients are closely monitored for immune rejection, infection, or tumour formation.
   - **Follow-Up Imaging & Biomarker Testing:** MRI, PET scans, and blood tests are required to track the therapeutic efficacy.

Advantages of Stem Cell Therapy

A. **Regenerative & Healing Potential**
   - **Tissue Repair & Regeneration:** Stem cells replenish injured or diseased cells in organs.
   - **Neuroprotection:** Used to aid in the healing process following spinal cord injuries, Parkinson's disease, and stroke.

B. **Minimal Invasive Procedures**

- **Avoids Surgery in Certain Situations:** Many applications involve IV infusions or direct injections, reducing surgical risks.

C. **Immunomodulation & Anti-Inflammatory Effects**

- Used to treat autoimmune diseases, such as Crohn's disease and multiple sclerosis.

D. **Personalization & Long-Term Benefits**

- **Autologous Therapy Reduces Rejection Risk:** Using the patient's own cells, autologous therapy lowers the risk of rejection.
- iPSCs allows disease modelling & drug testing.

Recent Advances in Stem Cell-Based Treatments

1. **Mesenchymal Stem Cells (MSCs):** Multipotent mesenchymal stem cells have the ability to develop into various sorts of cells, such as osteocytes, adipocytes, and chondrocytes. They are frequently sourced from the bone marrow or adipose tissue and are being investigated for their potential to treat inflammatory conditions, autoimmune disorders, and tissue injuries. MSCs can modulate the immune system, which reduce inflammation and encourages the healing of tissue. Clinical trials have demonstrated their potential in the treatment of ailments like graft-versus-host disease (GVHD), Crohn's disease, and myocardial infarction.
2. **Induced Pluripotent Stem Cells (iPSCs):** iPSCs have garnered significant attention in the past few years as they offer the possibility of patient-specific therapy. By means of somatic cell reprogramming into a state of pluripotency, iPSCs can develop into any kind of cell, making them ideal candidates for personalized regenerative medicine. Studies have demonstrated their efficacy in autoimmune diseases, drug screening, and potentially treating neurodegenerative conditions such amyotrophic lateral sclerosis (ALS) and Parkinson's disease.
3. **Neural Stem Cells (NSCs):** It is possible for neural stem cells (NSCs) to differentiate into neurones, astrocytes, and oligodendrocytes. These cells are being explored for their potential to treat neurodegenerative diseases, like Parkinson's and Alzheimer's disease. Preclinical studies have shown that NSCs can replace lost neurons, promote neuroprotection, and enhance recovery in animal models of central nervous system injuries.
4. **Hematopoietic Stem Cells (HSCs):** The function of haematopoietic stem cells is to generate all types of blood cells and have been used in the treatment of bone marrow transplants, blood disorders like leukaemia, lymphoma, and aplastic anaemia. Recent research has expanded the use of HSCs in gene therapy approaches to treat genetic diseases like sickle cell anaemia and thalassemia, offering curative potential.

FDA-Approved Stem Cell Therapies

A. **Approved Hematopoietic Stem Cell Therapies:**

- Haematopoietic stem cell transplantation (HSCT) is used to treat genetic disorders and blood cancers. Products that have been approved are as follows:
    1. **Strimvelis:** Ex-vivo gene-modified stem cell therapy for ADA-SCID (severe immunodeficiency) – EMA-approved (not FDA-approved).
    2. **LentiGlobin (Bluebird Bio):** β-thalassemia and sickle cell disease can be treated with gene-modified stem cells called LentiGlobin (Bluebird Bio).
    3. **Zynteglo:** Gene-modified autologous stem cell therapy – Transfusion-dependent β-thalassemia is treated with gene-modified autologous stem cell therapy.

B. **FDA-Approved Mesenchymal Stem Cell (MSC) Therapies:**
   - **Remestemcel-L (Ryoncil):** Paediatric acute graft-versus-host disease (GVHD) is treated with allogenic mesenchymal stem cell therapy.

C. **Induced Pluripotent Stem Cell (iPSC) Therapies:**
   - Clinical trials are ongoing for heart failure, Parkinson's disease, and macular degeneration.

Challenges in Stem Cell Therapy

1. **Ethical Concerns:** The use of embryonic stem cells (ESCs) has raised ethical debates surrounding the destruction of embryos. However, with the development of iPSCs, which do not require embryos, these concerns have been mitigated to some extent. Nonetheless, ethical considerations continue to impact public perception and regulatory policies surrounding stem cell research.
2. **Immune Rejection:** Allogeneic stem cell transplants, where the donor and recipient are not the same, can lead to immune rejection, where the body detects the transplanted cells as foreign cells and mounts an immune response. This pose a significant challenge in therapies using ESCs and allogeneic iPSCs. Autologous stem cell therapy (where the patient's own cells are used) minimizes this risk but may not always be feasible.
3. **Tumourigenicity:** One of the major risks associated with stem cell therapy, particularly with ESCs and iPSCs, is the potential for uncontrolled growth, leading to the formation of tumours known as teratomas. Careful monitoring of differentiation processes and pre-clinical testing is essential to mitigate this risk in clinical applications.
4. **Regulatory and Clinical Hurdles:** Stem cell therapies face significant regulatory challenges, as ensuring the safety, efficacy, and ethical standards of these treatments is complex. Clinical trials are required to demonstrate that stem cell treatments are both secure and efficient, but these trials are often expensive and time-consuming. Regulatory agencies like the FDA and EMA are working to establish clear guidelines for the approval of stem cell-based therapies.

Future Directions

1. **Gene-Editing Technologies with Stem Cells:** CRISPR-Cas9 and other gene-editing tools have revolutionized the potential of stem cell therapy. Gene editing can correct genetic defects at the source, making it possible to create patient-specific, genetically corrected iPSCs. These edited cells could be used to treat a variety of hereditary illnesses, such as sickle cell disease, cystic fibrosis, and muscular dystrophy.
2. **Bioengineering and Tissue Regeneration:** The integration of stem cell therapy with bioengineering technologies has the capacity to transform tissue regeneration. Researchers are developing 3D scaffolds and bioprinting techniques to produce organs and tissues that are functioning in the lab, which could eventually be used in transplantation donors and reduce transplant rejection.
3. **Stem Cells in Aging and Longevity:** As knowledge of stem cell biology advances, the potential of stem cells to combat aging is being investigated by researchers. Stem cells are essential for tissue regeneration and repair, and the depletion of stem cell function over time contributes to the aging process. Therapies that rejuvenate or replace aging stem cells hold promise for treating age-related diseases and potentially extending lifespan.

Conclusion

Modern regenerative medicine, which holds new promise for the treatment of a wide range of diseases, from diabetes and heart disease to neurodegenerative disorders, is led by stem cell therapy. Despite its promise, the field of stem cell therapy faces challenges with immunological rejection, tumourigenicity, and moral and ethical quandaries. But these obstacles are being quickly overcome by developments in gene editing, bioengineering, and personalised medicine, opening the door to safer and more effective stem cell-based treatments. As more research is ongoing, stem cell therapy is showing promise in transforming healthcare and providing treatments for diseases that were previously incurable.

References

1. Mei R, Wan Z, Yang C, Shen X, Wang R, Zhang H, Yang R, Li J, Song Y, Su H. Advances and clinical challenges of mesenchymal stem cell therapy. Frontiers in Immunology. 2024 Jul 19;15:1421854.
2. Ghoneim MA, Gabr MM, El-Halawani SM, Refaie AF. Current status of stem cell therapy for type 1 diabetes: a critique and a prospective consideration. Stem Cell Research & Therapy. 2024 Jan 29;15(1):23.
3. Rahimi Darehbagh R, Seyedoshohadaei SA, Ramezani R, Rezaei N. Stem cell therapies for neurological disorders: current progress, challenges, and future perspectives. European Journal of Medical Research. 2024 Jul 25;29(1):386.
4. Abusalah MA, Abd Rahman EN, Choudhary OP. Evolving trends in stem cell therapy: an emerging and promising approach against various diseases. International Journal of Surgery. 2024 Nov 1;110(11):6862-8.
5. Maguire G. Stem cell therapy without the cells. Communicative & integrative biology. 2013 Nov 9;6(6):e26631.
6. Herberts CA, Kwa MS, Hermsen HP. Risk factors in the development of stem cell therapy. Journal of translational medicine. 2011 Dec;9:1-4.
7. Mirzaei H, Sahebkar A, Sichani LS, Moridikia A, Nazari S, Sadri Nahand J, Salehi H, Stenvang J, Masoudifar A, Mirzaei HR, Jaafari MR. Therapeutic application of multipotent stem cells. Journal of cellular physiology. 2018 Apr;233(4):2815-23.
8. Thomas ED, Lochte Jr HL, Lu WC, Ferrebee JW. Intravenous infusion of bone marrow in patients receiving radiation and chemotherapy. New England Journal of Medicine. 1957 Sep 12;257(11):491-6.
9. Rani M, Kumar S, Rizvi MM. Role of stem cells in cancer therapeutics. In: Tiwari R, Mishra V, editors. Handbook of research on advancements in cancer therapeutics. Hershey (PA): IGI Global; 2021:467–85.
10. Arno A, Smith AH, Blit PH, Shehab MA, Gauglitz GG, Jeschke MG. Stem cell therapy: a new treatment for burns?. Pharmaceuticals. 2011 Oct 21;4(10):1355-80.
11. Alexander MS, Casar JC, Motohashi N. Stem cell differentiation and therapeutic use. Stem Cells International. 2015 Aug 4;2015:308128.
12. Zakrzewski W, Dobrzyński M, Szymonowicz M, Rybak Z. Stem cells: past, present, and future. Stem Cell Res Ther. 2019;10:68.
13. Oh IH, Kim DW. Three-dimensional approach to stem cell therapy. Journal of Korean Medical Science. 2002 Apr 1;17(2):151-60.
14. Mousaei Ghasroldasht M, Seok J, Park HS, Liakath Ali FB, Al-Hendy A. Stem cell therapy: from idea to clinical practice. International journal of molecular sciences. 2022 Mar 5;23(5):2850.
15. Takahashi K, Yamanaka S. Induction of pluripotent stem cells from mouse embryonic and adult fibroblast cultures by defined factors. cell. 2006 Aug 25;126(4):663-76.
16. Zakrzewski W, Dobrzyński M, Szymonowicz M, Rybak Z. Stem cells: past, present, and future. Stem cell research & therapy. 2019 Dec;10:1-22.
17. Huang L, Fu C, Xiong F, He C, Wei Q. Stem cell therapy for spinal cord injury. Cell transplantation. 2021 Feb 4;30:0963689721989266.
18. Volarevic V, Markovic BS, Gazdic M, Volarevic A, Jovicic N, Arsenijevic N, Armstrong L, Djonov V, Lako M, Stojkovic M. Ethical and safety issues of stem cell-based therapy. International journal of medical sciences. 2018 Jan 1;15(1):36.
19. Yanamandra B, Chan A, Ip G, Liu A, Pedraza X, Matos EX. Bridging the Gap: Regenerative Medicines and the Future of Personalized Treatment and Research.
20. Cardoso BA, Neparidze N. Two decades of targeted therapies in hematology: new targets and novel combinations. Frontiers in Hematology. 2025 Jan 24;4:1548984.
21. Jarrell D, Vereide D, Arnold C, Murphey M, Yingst A, Koning R, Perdue N, Romanov A, Busch C, Slukvin I, Crisman R. A Synthetic Receptor Enables Breakthrough Scale Manufacturing of iPSC-Derived CD19-CAR Cell Therapies for Hematologic and Autoimmune Diseases. Blood. 2024 Nov 5;144:148.
22. Sun M, Li M, Hu M, Fan Y, Liu Y, Sun J, Zhang J. Fully Bioactive Nanodrugs: Stem Cell-Derived Exosomes Engineered with Biomacromolecules to Treat CCl4-and Extreme Hepatectomy-Induced Acute Liver Failure. ACS nano. 2024 Dec 3;18(50):33907-21.

Section 2

Autonomic Nervous System

Chapter 4

Recent Advances in the Management of Glaucoma

Author: Dr. Pranab Das

Introduction

Glaucoma is a group of progressive optic neuropathies characterized by structural changes in the optic nerve head and corresponding irreversible visual field loss. Often associated with elevated intraocular pressure (IOP) as a major modifiable risk factor, glaucoma is one of the leading causes of blindness worldwide. The number of individuals affected by glaucoma continues to rise with an aging population, highlighting the need for more effective and targeted therapies.

Although numerous treatment modalities—pharmacological, laser, and surgical—have been developed to manage glaucoma, preventing disease progression remains challenging for several reasons. First, many patients are asymptomatic in early stages, thereby, delaying diagnosis and intervention. Second, adherence to often complex eye drop regimens can be suboptimal. Third, IOP reduction alone may not fully halt the disease in all patients, suggesting that additional mechanisms, such as ocular blood flow and neuroprotective factors, also influence disease progression. Recognizing these gaps, recent research efforts have emphasized developing novel pharmacotherapies, innovative drug delivery systems, and treatments that address neuroprotection. This chapter provides an overview of glaucoma's definition and classification, outlines conventional medications, and highlights the latest advances in drug therapies and management strategies that offer promise for improved outcomes.

Historical Perspective

The therapeutic landscape for glaucoma has significantly progressed over the last century, driven by advancements in pharmacology and an enhanced understanding of intraocular pressure (IOP) regulation. In the early 19th century, Sir William Bowman first linked elevated intraocular pressure with optic nerve damage, thereby establishing the foundation for pressure-lowering interventions. The 20th century marked the advent of modern pharmacotherapy, initiated by the introduction of pilocarpine in the 1870s, which emerged as the first widely utilised miotic for the reduction of intraocular pressure (IOP). Subsequently, carbonic anhydrase inhibitors emerged in the 1950s, with acetazolamide establishing itself as a fundamental component of oral glaucoma treatment. In 1978, Dr. Thomas Zimmerman introduced timolol, a non-selective beta-blocker, which significantly transformed topical treatment through its efficacy in reducing aqueous humour production. The 1990s marked a significant advancement with the introduction of latanoprost, a prostaglandin analogue created by Dr. Carl Bito, which led to a clinical preference for once-daily, highly effective therapies that improved uveoscleral outflow.

In the following decades, selective alpha-2 agonists such as brimonidine were developed, along with fixed-dose combinations designed to enhance adherence. The recent introduction of rho kinase (ROCK) inhibitors, including netarsudil, and nitric oxide-donating prostaglandin analogues such as latanoprostenebunod, signifies advancements in pharmacological approaches aimed at new outflow pathways. The changing treatment paradigm demonstrates a continuous focus on neuroprotection, individualised therapy, and long-term disease management, paving the way for advancements in gene therapy and sustained drug delivery systems in the near future.

Definition

Glaucoma is broadly defined as a progressive optic neuropathy with characteristic structural and functional damage to the optic nerve head and resultant visual field defects. Elevated intraocular pressure is a critical risk factor, but it is not the sole determinant—some patients develop glaucomatous changes even with "normal" IOP levels (normal-tension glaucoma), while others tolerate higher pressures without evident nerve damage (ocular hypertension). Nonetheless, lowering IOP remains the only proven modifiable approach to slow disease progression across all major types of glaucoma.

Types of Glaucoma

While there are multiple forms of glaucoma, the two primary categories are:

1. **Primary Open-Angle Glaucoma (POAG):**
   - The most common type, particularly in older adults.
   - Characterized by a wide and open anterior chamber angle but with increased resistance to aqueous humour outflow or enhanced aqueous humour secretion, typically at the trabecular meshwork.
   - Risk factors include elevated IOP, older age, positive family history, African or Hispanic ethnicity, and thinner central corneal thickness.
2. **Angle-Closure Glaucoma (ACG)**
   - Occurs when the iris bows forward, blocking or narrowing the trabecular meshwork outflow pathway.
   - May present acutely (acute angle closure) with a rapid rise in IOP, ocular pain, red eye, and blurry vision—a true ophthalmic emergency—or more chronically.
   - Management often involves laser peripheral iridotomy, in addition to pharmacotherapy, to relieve pupillary block.

Beyond these categories, there are secondary glaucoma (e.g. pseudo-exfoliation, uveitis, neovascular) resulting from underlying aetiologies, as well as developmental glaucoma occurring in children. Regardless of the subtype, long-term control of IOP is central to prevents optic nerve damage and preserving sight.

Brief Note on Conventional Medications

For decades, IOP-lowering therapies have been the bedrock of glaucoma management. Traditional pharmacological classes, summarized below, aim to either reduce aqueous humour production or enhance its outflow through various routes.

Table 1: Concise overview of standard pharmacological interventions for glaucoma management.

Drug Class / Drug Names	Mechanism of Action	Adverse Drug Reactions	Uses
Prostaglandin (PGF2-alpha) Analogues (e.g. Latanoprost, Bimatoprost)	Increase uveoscleral outflow of aqueous humour, significantly lowering IOP.	Conjunctival hyperaemia, eyelash growth, iris pigmentation changes.	First-line therapy for open-angle glaucoma.
Beta-Blockers (e.g. Timolol)	Decrease aqueous humour production by blocking beta-adrenergic receptors in the ciliary epithelium.	Systemic absorption can cause bradycardia, respiratory effects, local irritation.	Primary open-angle glaucoma (POAG).
Alpha-2 Agonists (e.g. Brimonidine)	Decrease aqueous humour production and increase uveoscleral outflow.	Local allergy, dry mouth, fatigue, possible systemic hypotension (if gets absorbed from nasolacrimal duct).	Short-term IOP control in glaucoma and post-surgical IOP reduction.
Carbonic Anhydrase Inhibitors (e.g. Dorzolamide, Acetazolamide)	Inhibit carbonic anhydrase, reducing bicarbonate formation and thus aqueous humour secretion.	Metallic taste, paraesthesia, GI upset, possible metabolic acidosis (oral).	Adjunct therapy in glaucoma. Acetazolamide for acute angle-closure glaucoma.
Cholinergic Agonists (e.g. Pilocarpine)	Constrict the pupil, pulling on trabecular meshwork to increase aqueous outflow.	Miosis, accommodative spasm, brow ache, reduced night vision.	Acute angle-closure glaucoma. Used if other treatments fail in POAG.
Fixed-Dose Combinations (e.g. Timolol + Dorzolamide)	Combine mechanisms (decreasing production + improving outflow) for synergistic effect, simplifying regimens.	Side effects from individual components; improved compliance as compared to separate drops.	Primary open-angle glaucoma (POAG) and also in acute angle-closure glaucoma.

Although these agents are effective for many patients, challenges persist: some require multiple daily doses, which can hamper adherence; others may cause local or systemic side effects; and certain patients exhibit progressive disease despite seemingly adequate IOP control. These limitations have spurred the search for novel or adjunctive therapies, new delivery systems, and potential neuroprotective agents beyond simple IOP control.

Newer Drugs / Recent Advances

Recent advances in glaucoma pharmacotherapy reflect a multifaceted approach like refining IOP reduction, enhancing drug delivery, and exploring neuroprotection of retinal ganglion cells. The following are some notable developments:

1. Netarsudil

Introduction: Netarsudil is a Rho kinase (ROCK) inhibitor, used to lower IOP in primary open-angle glaucoma (POAG) and ocular hypertension (OHT). It enhances aqueous humour outflow, improving trabecular function and reducing episcleral venous pressure.

Clinical Trial Phase / FDA-Approval: FDA-approved for POAG and OHT under the brand name Rhopressa. Evaluated in ROCKET-1 and ROCKET-2 clinical trials, demonstrating significant IOP reduction.

Mechanism of Action:

a. Enhancement of Trabecular Meshwork Outflow

The trabecular meshwork serves as the principal drainage route for aqueous humour. ROCK inhibition results in diminished phosphorylation of myosin light chain (MLC), hence decreasing actomyosin contractility in trabecular meshwork cells. This leads to the relaxation and dilation of the trabecular meshwork fibres, enhancing the meshwork's porosity. The relaxed trabecular meshwork results in the expansion of Schlemm's canal endothelial cells, hence diminishing resistance to aqueous humour outflow. Netarsudil also reduces extracellular matrix protein deposition (e.g., fibronectin, laminin), hence enhancing the permeability of the trabecular meshwork. Research indicates that ROCK inhibitors interfere with the actin cytoskeleton and reduce cellular stiffness, hence promoting aqueous humour flow through the trabecular meshwork. This represents a significant advantage over prostaglandin analogues, which predominantly function through the uveoscleral route.

b. Reduction of Episcleral Venous Pressure (EVP)

EVP is a significant factor influencing IOP. ROCK inhibition diminishes vascular smooth muscle contraction by obstructing MLC phosphorylation, resulting in the dilation of episcleral veins. This leads to a decrease in episcleral venous resistance, promoting the drainage of aqueous humour into the systemic circulation. By dilating the episcleral veins, netarsudil reduces the back pressure against which aqueous humour exits the eye, thereby augmenting outflow. This distinctive process is not affected by any other glaucoma medications.

c. Decreased Aqueous Humour Production

Netarsudil partly works by blocking the norepinephrine transporter (NET), which normally clears norepinephrine from nerve endings. When NET is inhibited, norepinephrine stays outside the nerve cells for a longer time and continues stimulating beta-adrenergic receptors in the ciliary body of the eye. Normally, stimulating these receptors increases the production of aqueous humour, the fluid inside the front of the eye. However, when receptors are exposed to constant stimulation over time, they can become less sensitive, a process known as receptor desensitization. As the receptors respond less actively, the production of aqueous humour can slightly decrease. This small reduction in fluid production adds to the overall effect of lowering eye pressure. However, the primary action of netarsudil is through Rho kinase (ROCK) inhibition, which relaxes the eye's drainage tissues and helps fluid flow out more easily. Therefore, while NET inhibition provides a minor additional benefit by slightly reducing fluid formation, the major pressure-lowering effect comes from improving fluid outflow via ROCK inhibition.

Key Pharmacokinetic Parameters: It is administered topically in eye as 0.02% ophthalmic solution. Systemic absorption is minimal, thereby, reducing systemic side effects. Peak concentration in aqueous humour is achieved approximately 1 hour after administration. It is metabolized by esterases in the eye, forming an active metabolite, AR-13503 and is eliminated primarily via renal excretion as inactive metabolites.

Adverse Drug Reactions: Conjunctival hyperaemia (most common), corneal verticillata (asymptomatic corneal deposits), mild eye irritation, pain, and blurred vision.

Uses: First-line or adjunct therapy in primary open angle glaucoma and ocular hypertension.

Dose: 0.02% ophthalmic solution, one drop once daily in the evening (topical).

2. Latanoprostene Bunod (LBN)

Introduction: Latanoprostenebunod (LBN) is a novel prostaglandin analogue (PGA) that donates nitric oxide (NO) to enhance trabecular meshwork outflow, providing dual-action IOP reduction.

Clinical Trial Phase / FDA-Approval: FDA-approved under the brand name Vyzulta. Studied in VOYAGER and APOLLO trials, showing superior IOP-lowering efficacy over latanoprost.

Mechanism of Action:

a. Dual IOP-Lowering Mechanism

1. **Prostaglandin F2α (PGF2α) Receptor Activation - Increased Uveoscleral Outflow**
   - Latanoprostenebunod (LBN) is metabolized in the eye into latanoprost acid, which activates prostaglandin F2α (PGF2α) receptors in the ciliary muscle.
   - This increases uveoscleral outflow, a well-established mechanism seen in latanoprost and other prostaglandin analogues.
2. **Nitric Oxide-Mediated Trabecular Meshwork Relaxation - Increased Trabecular Outflow**
   - LBN releases nitric oxide (NO), which activates soluble guanylate cyclase (sGC) in the trabecular meshwork.
   - NO binds to sGC, increasing cyclic GMP (cGMP) levels, which leads to activation of protein kinase G (PKG).
   - PKG then reduces actin cytoskeleton tension in trabecular meshwork cells, causing relaxation and increased permeability.
   - This mechanism lowers intraocular pressure more effectively than prostaglandin analogues alone.

b. Reduction of Episcleral Venous Pressure (EVP)

- NO also dilates episcleral veins, which reduces EVP, thereby facilitating aqueous humour production,further lowering IOP.
- This provides an additional IOP-lowering mechanism beyond traditional prostaglandins.

c. Neuroprotective Potential

- Nitric oxide has been shown to protect retinal ganglion cells (RGCs) from ischemic damage, suggesting potential neuroprotective effects of LBN.

Key Pharmacokinetic Parameters: It is administered topically in eye as 0.024% solution, once daily. It shows rapid corneal penetration. It is hydrolysed to latanoprost acid and nitric oxide. LBN is metabolized in the cornea into two active compounds: Latanoprost acid, which increases uveoscleral outflow and Nitric oxide (NO), which enhances trabecular meshwork outflow and reduces episcleral venous pressure (EVP). It is highly localized to the anterior chamber, with minimal systemic absorption. Latanoprost acid is metabolized by the liver, while NO exerts its effect locally. Plasma half-life is 4-6 hours. Metabolites are excreted out in urine.

Adverse Drug Reactions: Conjunctival hyperaemia, eyelash growth, iris pigmentation changes and macular oedema.

Uses: First-line IOP-lowering agent for primary open angle glaucoma and ocular hypertension.

Dose: 0.024% ophthalmic solution, one drop once daily in the evening (topical).

3. Sustained-Release Bimatoprost Implant

Introduction: Bimatoprost SR (sustained-release) is a biodegradable implant designed for long-term prostaglandin therapy, reducing the need for daily eye drops.

Clinical Trial Phase/FDA-Approval: FDA-approved under the brand name Durysta. Evaluated in ARTEMIS trials, showing prolonged IOP control for up to 6 months.

Mechanism of Action:

a. Prostaglandin F2α Analogue Activation - Increased Uveoscleral Outflow

- Bimatoprost is a prodrug converted into bimatoprost free acid in the ciliary body.
- This activates prostaglandin F2α (FP) receptors, leading to remodelling of the extracellular matrix (ECM) in the ciliary muscle.
- Bimatoprost stimulates MMP-2 and MMP-9, which break down collagen and ECM proteins, increasing the space for aqueous humour drainage.
- By reducing ECM stiffness, bimatoprost enhances fluid egress through the ciliary muscle, an additional drainage route.
- This results in increased aqueous humour outflow via the uveoscleral pathway, effectively lowering IOP.

b. Biodegradable Implant Ensures Sustained Drug Release

- The implant is composed of a biodegradable polymer (NOVADUR™), which slowly releases bimatoprost over 4–6 months.
- This eliminates the need for daily eye drops and ensures continuous IOP reduction.

Key Pharmacokinetic Parameters: It is administered as a single intracameral implant placed in the anterior chamber of the eye. The implant ensures sustained drug release over 4–6 months, ensuring continuous IOP reduction. Peak intraocular concentration (Cmax) is reached within hours after implantation. Bimatoprost is converted into its active free acid in the ciliary body, where it increases aqueous outflow. It is metabolized by corneal and aqueous humour esterases into inactive metabolites.

Adverse Drug Reactions: Conjunctival hyperaemia, mild eye irritation, foreign body sensation and corneal endothelial cell loss.

Uses: Long-term primary open angle glaucoma (POAG) and ocular hypertension (OHT) treatment.

Dose: 10 mcg intracameral implant, administered once every 4–6 months.

4. Travoprost Punctal Plug Delivery (TP-PPL)

Introduction: Travoprost is the isopropyl ester of prostaglandin F2 alpha in which the pentyl group is replaced by a 3- (trifluoromethyl) phenoxymethyl group. Travoprostpunctal plug delivery is a sustained-release travoprost system, eliminating the need for daily eye drops.

Clinical Trial Phase / FDA-Approval: Phase III trials ongoing for POAG and OHT.

Mechanism of Action:

a. Prostaglandin F2α Receptor Activation - Increased Aqueous Outflow

- Travoprost is a prodrug that undergoes hydrolysis to form travoprost free acid, which binds to prostaglandin F2α (FP) receptors in the ciliary muscle.

- This leads to extracellular matrix (ECM) remodelling and relaxation of the ciliary muscle, increasing uveoscleral outflow of aqueous humour.
- This mechanism results in IOP reduction by 6-8 mmHg.

b. Sustained Drug Release via Punctal Plug Technology

- The punctal plug is made of a biodegradable hydrogel that expands upon insertion into the lacrimal punctum.
- It slowly releases travoprost into the tear film, allowing continuous drug absorption through the cornea and conjunctiva.
- This eliminates the need for daily eye drops, reducing fluctuations in drug concentration and improving adherence.

c. Enhanced Bioavailability Compared to Topical Drops

- Avoids first-pass metabolism through the nasolacrimal duct, enhancing ocular bioavailability.
- Reduces systemic side effects associated with topical prostaglandins.

Key Pharmacokinetic Parameters: It is administered as a punctal plug inserted into the lacrimal punctum, which gradually releases travoprost into the tear film. Travoprost is absorbed through the cornea and conjunctiva, avoiding first-pass metabolism. Peak concentration (Cmax) is achieved within hours after insertion. It is highly localized to the anterior chamber, with minimal systemic absorption. Travoprost prodrug is hydrolysed into travoprost free acid, its active form. It is metabolized by corneal esterases and cleared through aqueous humour drainage. Elimination half-life is 45–60 days, supporting sustained IOP control.

Adverse Drug Reactions: Conjunctival hyperaemia, punctal plug displacement, mild eye irritation and corneal epithelial defects.

Uses: Long-term IOP control in non-adherent primary open angle glaucoma patients.

Dose: 500 mcg to 1000 mcg twice daily (topical).

5. Trabodenoson

Introduction: Trabodenoson is a selective adenosine A1 receptor agonist that enhances trabecular meshwork outflow.

Clinical Trial Phase / FDA-Approval: Phase III trials completed; further studies needed.

Mechanism of Action:

a. Activation of Adenosine A1 Receptors - Increased Trabecular Meshwork Outflow

- Trabodenoson is a selective A1 adenosine receptor agonist that stimulates endothelial nitric oxide synthase (eNOS).
- This leads to cyclic AMP (cAMP) upregulation, promoting extracellular matrix (ECM) remodelling in the trabecular meshwork (TM).
- A1 receptor activation increases MMP-2 and MMP-3 expression, which degrades ECM proteins in the trabecular meshwork and Schlemm's canal, lowering outflow resistance.
- A1 receptor activation reduces transforming growth factor-beta (TGF-β) signalling, which is known to cause fibrotic ECM deposition in glaucoma.

- This results in reduced trabecular resistance, allowing for enhanced aqueous humour drainage.

b. Sustained Drug Release via Punctal Plug Technology

- The punctal plug is inserted into the lacrimal punctum, releasing trabodenoson continuously into the tear film.
- The drug is absorbed through the conjunctiva and cornea, reducing IOP without requiring daily drops.
- Advantages:
  I. Longer duration of action (≥90 days).
  II. Eliminates compliance issues associated with topical drops.

c. Additional Neuroprotective Effects

- Trabodenoson has potential neuroprotective properties due to its effects on mitochondrial function and oxidative stress reduction.
- This may slow retinal ganglion cell (RGC) loss, making it a potential disease-modifying therapy.

Key Pharmacokinetic Parameters: It is administered as a punctal plug inserted into the lacrimal punctum, allowing continuous drug release into the tear film. Trabodenoson is absorbed through the conjunctiva and cornea, reaching the anterior chamber. Peak intraocular concentration (Cmax) is achieved within hours after insertion. It is highly localized to the anterior chamber, minimizing systemic exposure. It is metabolized by ocular enzymes into inactive metabolites. It is cleared via aqueous humour outflow, with minimal systemic elimination. Elimination half-life is 45–60 days, supporting long-acting IOP control.

Adverse Drug Reactions: Mild conjunctival hyperaemia, foreign body sensation and blurred vision.

Uses: Under investigation for primary open angle glaucoma and ocular hypertension.

Dose: 15 mcg travoprost per plug, placed in lower punctum, delivering medication over up to 90 days (investigational dose).

6. Other recent advances in the treatment of glaucoma:

Table 2: Recent advancements in glaucoma therapy.

Drug / Strategy	Mechanism of Action	Clinical Trial Phase / Status	Adverse Reactions	Distinctive / Salient Features
Selective Laser Trabeculoplasty (SLT)	Non-pharmacological, but of note in recent paradigms; stimulates trabecular meshwork cells to improve outflow.	Used as first-line or adjunct.	Mild ocular discomfort, transient IOP spike, inflammation.	Can reduce medication burden; sometimes as effective as eye drops in early POAG.
ROCK/NET Inhibitors (e.g. Roclatan® = Netarsudil + Latanoprost)	Combination of ROCK inhibition (improved trabecular meshwork outflow) and prostaglandin analogue effect (increased uveoscleral outflow).	Approved in some countries.	Similar tonetarsudil: hyperaemia, mild ocular discomfort.	Potential for superior IOP reduction compared to monotherapy; synergy of dual mechanisms.
Neuroprotective Agents (e.g. Citicoline, Memantine, Brimonidine)	Various mechanisms: stabilize retinal ganglion cells, reduce excitotoxicity and improve mitochondrial function.	Trials ongoing/ off-label use in some countries.	Vary by agent; some systemic, some ocular side effects.	Aimed at halting glaucomatous optic neuropathy progression beyond IOP-lowering alone.

Conclusion

Glaucoma is a multifactorial disease primarily managed by lowering intraocular pressure (IOP) to slow vision loss. While traditional agents like prostaglandin analogues and beta-blockers remain essential, newer therapies—such as Rho kinase inhibitors, nitric oxide donors, and sustained-release delivery systems—offer improved outflow and adherence. The growing emphasis on neuroprotection reflects the need to preserve vision beyond IOP control, with agents like brimonidine and investigational options such as citicoline and gene therapy showing potential. Personalized treatment strategies that combine established and emerging therapies are now central to care. Despite challenges like adherence and cost, advances in pharmacology and drug delivery continue to expand the possibilities for preserving vision and improving quality of life in glaucoma patients.

References

1. Schuster AK, Erb C, Hoffmann EM, Dietlein T, Pfeiffer N. The diagnosis and treatment of glaucoma. Deutsches Ärzteblatt International. 2020 Mar 27;117(13):225.
2. Musa I, Bansal S, Kaleem MA. Barriers to care in the treatment of glaucoma: socioeconomic elements that impact the diagnosis, treatment, and outcomes in glaucoma patients. Current Ophthalmology Reports. 2022 Sep;10(3):85-90.
3. Mincione F, Nocentini A, Supuran CT. Advances in the discovery of novel agents for the treatment of glaucoma. Expert Opinion on Drug Discovery. 2021 Oct 3;16(10):1209-25.
4. Asrani S, Civan MM, et al. New therapeutic targets in the treatment of glaucoma. Ophthalmology. 2019;126(1):S44–S55.
5. Al-Humimat G, Marashdeh I, Daradkeh D, Kooner K. Investigational Rho kinase inhibitors for the treatment of glaucoma. Journal of Experimental Pharmacology. 2021 Feb 25:197-212.
6. Quigley HA, Broman AT. The number of people with glaucoma worldwide in 2010 and 2020. British journal of ophthalmology. 2006 Mar 1;90(3):262-7.
7. Heijl A, Leske MC, Bengtsson B, Hyman L, Bengtsson B, Hussein M, Early Manifest Glaucoma Trial Group. Reduction of intraocular pressure and glaucoma progression: results from the Early Manifest Glaucoma Trial. Archives of ophthalmology. 2002 Oct 1;120(10):1268-79.
8. Weinreb RN, Aung T, Medeiros FA. The pathophysiology and treatment of glaucoma: a review. Jama. 2014 May 14;311(18):1901-11.
9. Kass MA, Heuer DK, Higginbotham EJ, Johnson CA, Keltner JL, Miller JP, Parrish RK, Wilson MR, Gordon MO, Ocular Hypertension Treatment Study Group. The Ocular Hypertension Treatment Study: a randomized trial determines that topical ocular hypotensive medication delays or prevents the onset of primary open-angle glaucoma. Archives of ophthalmology. 2002 Jun 1;120(6):701-13.
10. Serle JB, Katz LJ, McLaurin E, Heah T, Ramirez-Davis N, Usner DW, Novack GD, Kopczynski CC. Two phase 3 clinical trials comparing the safety and efficacy of netarsudil to timolol in patients with elevated intraocular pressure: rho kinase elevated IOP treatment trial 1 and 2 (ROCKET-1 and ROCKET-2). American journal of ophthalmology. 2018 Feb 1;186:116-27.
11. Lewis RA, Christie WC, Day DG, Craven ER, Walters T, Bejanian M, Lee SS, Goodkin ML, Zhang J, Whitcup SM, Robinson MR. Bimatoprost sustained-release implants for glaucoma therapy: 6-month results from a phase I/II clinical trial. American journal of ophthalmology. 2017 Mar 1;175:137-47.
12. Asrani S, Robin AL, Serle JB, Lewis RA, Usner DW, Kopczynski CC, Heah T, Ackerman SL, Alpern LM, Bashford K, Bluestein EC. Netarsudil/latanoprost fixed-dose combination for elevated intraocular pressure: three-month data from a randomized phase 3 trial. American journal of ophthalmology. 2019 Nov 1;207:248-57.
13. Yin H, Kanasty RL, Eltoukhy AA, Vegas AJ, Dorkin JR, Anderson DG. Non-viral vectors for gene-based therapy. Nat Rev Genet. 2014;15(8):541–55.
14. Weinreb RN, Robinson MR, Dibas M, Stamer WD. Matrix metalloproteinases and glaucoma treatment. J OculPharmacol Ther. 2020;36(2):71–86.
15. Weinreb RN, Khaw PT. Primary open-angle glaucoma. The lancet. 2004 May 22;363(9422):1711-20.
16. Hoy SM. Latanoprostenebunod ophthalmic solution 0.024%: a review in open-angle glaucoma and ocular hypertension. Drugs. 2018 May;78:773-80.
17. Weinreb RN, Liebmann JM, Martin KR, Kaufman PL, Vittitow JL. Latanoprostenebunod 0.024% in subjects with open-angle glaucoma or ocular hypertension: pooled phase 3 study findings. Journal of glaucoma. 2018 Jan 1;27(1):7-15.
18. Shaikh O, Kuziez L, Saeedi OJ, Abbasian J, Elhusseiny AM. Topical Netarsudil in Childhood Glaucoma: A Systematic Review. Current Eye Research. 2025 Jan 3:1-6.
19. Soltani G, Shalaby WS, Razeghinejad R. Latanoprostenebunod: the first nitric oxide-donating antiglaucoma medication. Medical Gas Research. 2025 Jun 1;15(2):220-7.

20. Tan SS, Wong TT. Drug delivery systems in glaucoma–Current innovations and future perspectives. Asia-Pacific Journal of Ophthalmology. 2025 Mar 1;14(2):100163.
21. Mann E, Kammer JA, Sawhney G, An J, Werts EC, Vera V, Rivas M, Lai H, Sonparote S, Craven ER. Prospective 18-Month Study of Bimatoprost Intracameral Implant in Patients with Open-Angle Glaucoma or Ocular Hypertension in US Clinical Practice. Drugs. 2025 Feb 13:1-8.

Chapter 5

Recent Advances in the Treatment of Myasthenia Gravis

Author: Dr. Pranab Das

Introduction

Myasthenia gravis (MG) is a neuromuscular condition predominantly distinguished by muscular weakness and fatigue. While the illness often manifests in maturity, symptoms may emerge at any age. The disorder may be confined to certain muscle groups, notably the ocular muscles (ocular myasthenia), or may progress to a more generalised form (generalised myasthenia gravis), affecting many muscle groups. Individuals with myasthenia gravis typically exhibit eyelid weakness and drooping (ptosis); ocular muscle weakness, leading to double vision (diplopia); and pronounced muscle exhaustion after exertion. Common additional signs encompass facial muscle weakness, impaired speaking (dysarthria), difficulties with chewing and swallowing (dysphagia), and proximal limb paralysis affecting the upper arms and legs.

Furthermore, approximately 10% of affected patients may experience potentially life-threatening consequences resulting from significant involvement of the respiratory muscles (myasthenic crisis). Myasthenia gravis is caused by an aberrant immune response in which the body's immune system (i.e., antibodies) erroneously targets and progressively damages specific receptors in muscles that receive nerve signals (antibody-mediated autoimmune response). Treatments encompass pharmaceuticals including anticholinesterase agents, immunosuppressive agents, and efgartigimod, as well as procedures such as plasmapheresis, antibody infusions, and thymectomy.

Historical Perspective

Over the past century, the treatment options for myasthenia gravis (MG), an autoimmune neuromuscular disease marked by varying muscle weakness, have steadily changed. Physostigmine was the first pharmacological breakthrough in the 1930s. Neostigmine and pyridostigmine, acetylcholinesterase inhibitors, were then developed to alleviate symptoms by improving neuromuscular transmission. Dr. Mary Walker and later Simpson and Nastuk established the autoimmune basis of MG in the 1950s by showing that MG was associated with antibodies against the acetylcholine receptor (AChR), which laid the groundwork for immunosuppressive treatment.

A major development that provided efficient long-term immunosuppression was the introduction of corticosteroids and azathioprine in the 1960s and 1970s. Mycophenolate mofetil and cyclosporine were then used, which enhanced steroid-sparing alternatives. In contrast, thymectomy has been demonstrated to considerably improve outcomes in patients with AChR antibody-positive generalised MG, especially following the historic MGTX trial. Myasthenic crisis and exacerbations can now be treated quickly and temporarily with plasma exchange and intravenous immunoglobulin (IVIG).

Targeted biologic therapies have entered a new era in recent decades. In 2017, the REGAIN trial led to the approval of eculizumab, a monoclonal antibody against complement protein C5, for treatment-refractory generalised MG. Newer complement inhibitors such as ravulizumab have been developed to build on this. Neonatal Fc receptor (FcRn) inhibitors, like efgartigimod and rozanolixizumab, which lower circulating IgG auto antibodies and were authorised for generalised MG in 2021 and 2023, respectively, represent another advancement. These treatments, which offer quicker, more effective, and more tolerable symptom control, represent a substantial shift in MG treatment towards precision immunomodulation and customised care.

Definition

Myasthenia gravis (MG) is an autoimmune neuromuscular illness defined by an antibody-mediated assault on acetylcholine receptors (AChR) or muscle-specific kinase (MuSK) at the neuromuscular junction, resulting in muscle weakening and tiredness.

Types

1. Classification Based on Clinical Presentation

A. Ocular Myasthenia Gravis (OMG):

- Weakness limited to the eye muscles, causing drooping eyelids (ptosis) and double vision (diplopia).
- Accounts for 15% of MG cases, but some may progress to generalized MG.

B. Generalized Myasthenia Gravis (GMG):

- Affects multiple muscle groups, including limbs, respiratory muscles, and bulbar muscles (involved in swallowing and speech).
- Subdivided into mild (II), moderate (III), and severe (IV) based on severity.

2. Classification Based on Age of Onset

A. Early-onset MG (EOMG):

- Symptoms appear before the age of 50.
- More common in females and often associated with thymic hyperplasia.

B. Late-onset MG (LOMG):

- Symptoms appear after the age of 50.
- More common in males and frequently associated with thymoma.

3. Classification Based on Antibody Presence

A. AChR-antibody positive MG:

- Most common type (85% of cases).
- Autoantibodies target acetylcholine receptors at the neuromuscular junction.

B. MuSK-antibody positive MG:

- Less common (5-10% of cases).
- Autoantibodies target muscle-specific kinase (MuSK), leading to more severe bulbar and respiratory symptoms.

C. LRP4-antibody positive MG:

- A rarer subtype where antibodies attack the low-density lipoprotein receptor-related protein 4 (LRP4).

D. Seronegative MG:

- Cases where no known antibodies are detected but clinical symptoms confirm MG.

4. Congenital Myasthenic Syndromes (CMS)

- Unlike autoimmune MG, CMS is caused by genetic mutations affecting neuromuscular transmission.
- Symptoms start in infancy or early childhood.
- Treated differently from autoimmune MG.

Brief Note on Conventional Medicines

The following table provides a detailed pharmacological overview of conventional drugs used in MG treatment.

Table 1: Concise overview of conventional medications utilised in the management of myasthenia gravis.

Drug Name /Drug Class	Mechanism of Action	Adverse Drug Reactions	Uses
Pyridostigmine (Acetylcholinesterase Inhibitor)	Pyridostigmine inhibits acetylcholinesterase (AChE), the enzyme responsible for breaking down acetylcholine (ACh) in the synaptic cleft. By preventing ACh degradation, it increases ACh availability at the neuromuscular junction, thereby enhancing muscle contraction. Unlike neostigmine, pyridostigmine has a longer half-life and fewer muscarinic side effects.	Cholinergic crisis (excess ACh: salivation, bradycardia, muscle fasciculations), gastrointestinal disturbances (nausea, diarrhoea, abdominal cramps), blurred vision, sweating, and excessive secretions.	First-line symptomatic treatment for MG. Used in all forms of MG, including ocular and generalized MG.
Neostigmine (Acetylcholinesterase Inhibitor)	Similar to pyridostigmine, neostigmine inhibits AChE, but it has a shorter duration of action. It enhances neuromuscular transmission, improving muscle strength in MG. However, it has stronger muscarinic effects than pyridostigmine.	Excessive salivation, sweating, lacrimation, bradycardia and hypotension, abdominal cramps, diarrhoea, nausea, cholinergic crisis in high doses.	Alternative to pyridostigmine; used in acute MG exacerbations or when pyridostigmine is ineffective.
Prednisone (Corticosteroid, Immunosuppressant)	Prednisone is a glucocorticoid that suppresses the immune response by inhibiting T-cell activation and reducing autoantibody production against the acetylcholine receptor (AChR). It lowers inflammation and immune-mediated damage at the neuromuscular junction.	Weight gain, hyperglycaemia, hypertension, osteoporosis, cataracts, mood changes, increased risk of infections due to immunosuppression.	Used in moderate to severe MG cases when AChE inhibitors alone are insufficient. Helps in long-term immune suppression.
Azathioprine (Immunosuppressant)	Azathioprine is a purine synthesis inhibitor that interferes with DNA replication in rapidly dividing immune cells (T and B lymphocytes). This leads to reduced autoantibody production, helping in long-term immune suppression in MG patients.	Bone marrow suppression (leukopenia, anaemia), hepatotoxicity (elevated liver enzymes, hepatitis), increased infection risk.	Used as a steroid-sparing agent to reduce corticosteroid dependence in chronic MG.

Newer Drugs / Recent Advances

The expansion of precision medicine has led to the development of a wide range of innovative therapies for myasthenia gravis. Below is some of the most influential and recent classes of newer drugs:

1. Rozanolixizumab

Introduction: Rozanolixizumab is a humanised monoclonal antibody (IgG4) that specifically targets the neonatal Fc receptor (FcRn). It has been formulated for the management of autoimmune disorders in which pathogenic autoantibodies are implicated. It is predominantly utilised for the treatment of generalised myasthenia gravis (gMG), especially in individuals who test positive for acetylcholine receptor (AChR) or muscle-specific kinase (MuSK) autoantibodies.

Clinical Trial Phase / FDA-Approval: FDA-approved in 2023 for the treatment of gMG in adults with AChR or MuSK autoantibodies. The endorsement was predicated on clinical enhancements in MG-ADL (Myasthenia Gravis - Activities of Daily Living) scores relative to placebo.

Mechanism of Action: Rozanolixizumab is a humanised monoclonal antibody of the IgG4 subclass that targets the neonatal Fc receptor (FcRn). It aims to diminish circulating pathogenic IgG autoantibodies, rendering it a promising therapeutic option for autoimmune neuromuscular disorders such as generalised myasthenia gravis (gMG) and chronic inflammatory demyelinating polyneuropathy (CIDP).

1. **FcRn-Mediated IgG Recycling**
   - FcRn is a transmembrane receptor expressed in endothelial cells, monocytes, and hematopoietic tissues.
   - It binds to IgG at low pH (6.0) within endosomes, preventing lysosomal degradation and allowing IgG recycling back into circulation.
   - This mechanism prolongs IgG half-life (21 days).
2. **Rozanolixizumab Blocks FcRn-IgG Interaction**
   - Rozanolixizumab binds with high affinity to FcRn, preventing IgG from interacting with the receptor.
   - This inhibition disrupts IgG recycling, leading to accelerated lysosomal degradation.
   - As a result, total circulating IgG, including pathogenic IgG autoantibodies (e.g. anti-AChR and anti-MuSK in gMG), is significantly reduced.
3. **Rapid Clearance of Autoantibodies**
   - Within 2-3 weeks of therapy, IgG levels drop by 60-80%, reducing autoimmune-mediated damage at neuromuscular junctions.
   - Lower autoantibody levels improve neuromuscular transmission, reduce symptom severity, and enhance muscle strength.
4. **Potential Synergy with Other Immunotherapies**
   - Rozanolixizumab may enhance the efficacy of other immunosuppressive drugs by depleting autoantibodies more effectively.
   - Combination therapy with complement inhibitors (e.g. eculizumab, ravulizumab) or plasma exchange may further improve outcomes.

Key Pharmacokinetic Parameters: Rozanolixizumab demonstrates dose-dependent, non-linear pharmacokinetics attributable to FcRn saturation. It is delivered subcutaneously (s.c.) at a dosage of 7 mg/kg or 10 mg/kg on a weekly basis. The volume of distribution (4-5 L) indicates that it is distributed into the extracellular fluid compartment. It does not considerably penetrate the blood-brain barrier, rendering it suitable for peripheral autoimmune disorders. Rozanolixizumab, a monoclonal antibody, is subject to proteolytic degradation into amino acids through lysosomal mechanisms. It does not engage in CYP450 metabolism, hence diminishing the dangers of drug-drug interactions. Excretion largely occurs through reticuloendothelial breakdown, with negligible renal clearance.

Adverse Drug Reactions: Headache, injection-site reactions, increased risk of infections, hypersensitivity reactions and nausea.

Uses: Generalized Myasthenia Gravis (FDA-approved indication) and under investigation for chronic inflammatory demyelinating polyneuropathy (CIDP) (Phase III trial).

Dose: 7 mg/kg subcutaneously once weekly for 6 weeks.

2. Zilucoplan

Introduction: Zilucoplan (brand name ZILBRYSQ®) is a small-molecule macrocyclic peptide that inhibits complement C5, and it is created by UCB Pharma. It is licensed by the FDA for the treatment of generalised myasthenia gravis (gMG) in adult patients possessing anti-acetylcholine receptor (AChR) antibodies. In contrast to intravenous (i.v.) complement inhibitors such as eculizumab and ravulizumab, zilucoplan is delivered subcutaneously (s.c.), providing a more convenient and self-administered therapeutic alternative.

Clinical Trial Phase / FDA-Approval: FDA-approved in 2023 for generalized myasthenia gravis (gMG) in AChR antibody-positive patients.

Mechanism of Action: Zilucoplan is a unique macrocyclic peptide that inhibits complement C5 by obstructing its cleavage, hence averting the development of the membrane attack complex (MAC).

1. **Complement Activation in gMG**
   - In generalized myasthenia gravis (gMG), autoantibodies target the acetylcholine receptor (AChR) at the neuromuscular junction, activating the classical complement pathway.
   - This leads to the cleavage of complement protein C5 into C5a and C5b by C5 convertase.
   - C5b binds to C6, C7, C8, and C9 to form the MAC, leading to neuromuscular damage, inflammation, and muscle weakness.
2. **Zilucoplan Inhibits C5 Cleavage & MAC Formation**
   - Zilucoplan binds directly to C5, preventing its cleavage into C5a and C5b.
   - This inhibits C5a-mediated pro-inflammatory effects and C5b-MAC-induced neuromuscular destruction.
3. **Competitive Inhibition of C5b6 Formation**
   - Unlike eculizumab, which binds only to C5, zilucoplan also prevents C5b from interacting with C6, further blocking C5b6 formation and MAC assembly.
4. **Selective Complement Blockade Without Broad Immunosuppression**
   - Unlike traditional immunosuppressants (e.g. corticosteroids, azathioprine), zilucoplan preserves early complement function (C3, C4) while selectively inhibiting terminal complement activation.
   - This reduces neuromuscular damage without compromising overall immune defense.

Key Pharmacokinetic Parameters: Zilucoplan exhibits linear pharmacokinetics with dose-proportional exposure, supporting once-daily subcutaneous administration. Volume of distribution (5-6 L) suggests that it primarily remains in the extracellular space. It does not cross the blood-brain barrier (BBB), making it ideal for peripheral autoimmune diseases. As a peptide-based drug, zilucoplan is metabolized via proteolytic degradation. No CYP450 enzyme involvement, reducing drug-drug interaction risks. Excreted primarily through proteolysis, with minimal renal clearance.

Adverse Drug Reactions: Injection-site reactions, headache, increased risk of infections, nausea and fatigue.

Uses: FDA-approved for generalized myasthenia gravis and under investigation for neuromyelitis optica spectrum disorder (NMOSD) (Phase II).

Dose: 0.3 mg/kg subcutaneously once daily.

3. Efgartigimod

Introduction: Efgartigimod is an antagonist of the neonatal Fc receptor (FcRn) created by argenx for the treatment of generalised myasthenia gravis (gMG) and chronic inflammatory demyelinating polyneuropathy (CIDP). This is a human IgG1-derived Fc fragment designed to diminish harmful IgG autoantibodies, rendering it a potential treatment for IgG-mediated autoimmune disorders. Efgartigimod gained its initial FDA approval in 2021 for generalised myasthenia gravis (gMG) and subsequently obtained FDA approval for chronic inflammatory demyelinating polyneuropathy (CIDP) in 2024. It is offered in two formulations: intravenous (i.v.) infusion and subcutaneous (s.c.) injection.

Clinical Trial Phase / FDA-Approval: FDA-approved for adult patients with AChR antibody-positive generalized myasthenia gravis. Also approved (2024) for chronic inflammatory demyelinating polyneuropathy (CIDP) in adults.

Mechanism of Action: Efgartigimod is a human IgG1-derived Fc fragment specifically designed to interact with the neonatal Fc receptor (FcRn). It specifically inhibits FcRn-mediated IgG recycling, resulting in a swift decrease in harmful IgG autoantibodies, so establishing it as a crucial treatment for IgG-mediated autoimmune disorders such as generalised myasthenia gravis (gMG) and chronic inflammatory demyelinating polyneuropathy (CIDP).

1. **FcRn-Mediated IgG Recycling**
   - FcRn, a membrane-bound receptor, is expressed in endothelial cells, monocytes, and hematopoietic tissues.
   - Normally, IgG binds to FcRn at low pH (6.0) in endosomes, preventing degradation and allowing IgG recycling back into circulation.
   - This process extends IgG half-life (21 days) and contributes to IgG homeostasis.
2. **Efgartigimod Blocks FcRn-IgG Interaction**
   - Efgartigimod competes with endogenous IgG for FcRn binding due to its higher affinity at acidic pH.
   - This prevents IgG from being recycled, causing autoantibody degradation in lysosomes.
   - As a result, total IgG levels (including pathogenic IgG autoantibodies) are significantly reduced (60-75%).
3. **Rapid Clearance of Autoantibodies**
   - Pathogenic IgG autoantibodies (e.g. anti-AChR, anti-MuSK in gMG, and anti-GM1 in CIDP) are depleted within 2-3 weeks.
   - Lower autoantibody levels improve neuromuscular transmission and immune-mediated neuropathies.

4. **Preserves Other Immunoglobulin Functions**
   - Unlike broad-spectrum immunosuppressants, efgartigimod does not affect IgA, IgM, or complement pathways, preserving other immune functions.

Key Pharmacokinetic Parameters: Efgartigimod demonstrates linear, dose-proportional pharmacokinetics, with a half-life prolonged due to FcRn binding affinity. It is administered via intravenous infusion (10 mg/kg) every four weeks or as a subcutaneous injection (efgartigimod alfa + hyaluronidase for expedited absorption). It does not penetrate the blood-brain barrier (BBB), rendering it appropriate for peripheral autoimmune disorders. Efgartigimod, as a recombinant Fc fragment, is subject to proteolytic breakdown into amino acids. It does not undergo CYP450 metabolism, hence minimising the danger of drug-drug interactions.

Adverse Drug Reactions: Headache, injection-site reactions, increased infection risk and hypersensitivity reactions.

Uses: FDA-approved for B-ALL and diffuse large B-cell lymphoma (DLBCL).

Dose: 10 mg/kg IV once weekly for 4 weeks (1 cycle).

4. Ravulizumab

Introduction: Ravulizumab (brand name Ultomiris®) is a monoclonal antibody (mAb) that targets complement component C5, created by Alexion Pharmaceuticals. It is a prolonged-acting successor to eculizumab (Soliris®), engineered to deliver persistent C5 inhibition with a longer dose schedule.

Clinical trial phase / FDA-Approval: FDA-approved (2022) for generalised myasthenia gravis and FDA approved (2024) for Neuromyelitis Optica Spectrum Disorder (NMOSD).

Mechanism of action: Ravulizumab is a humanized monoclonal antibody (IgG2/4) that selectively inhibits complement component C5. It is designed to provide longer-lasting inhibition compared to eculizumab, offering sustained suppression of complement-mediated haemolysis and inflammation.

1. **Complement System Activation in Diseases**
   - In complement-mediated disorders like paroxysmal nocturnal haemoglobinuria (PNH), atypical haemolytic uremic syndrome (aHUS), and generalized myasthenia gravis (gMG), an overactive complement system damages host cells.
   - Activation of C5 by C5 convertase leads to the generation of C5a (a potent pro-inflammatory molecule) and C5b, which triggers membrane attack complex (MAC) formation (C5b-9), leading to cell lysis and inflammation.
2. **Ravulizumab Inhibits C5 Cleavage**
   - Ravulizumab binds specifically to C5, blocking its cleavage into C5a and C5b.
   - This prevents C5b-9 MAC formation, protecting host cells from complement-mediated destruction.
3. **Prevention of Haemolysis & Tissue Damage**
   - In PNH, ravulizumab prevents the destruction of red blood cells (RBCs) by MAC, reducing haemolysis.
   - In aHUS, it prevents endothelial damage and thrombosis caused by uncontrolled complement activation.
   - In gMG, it reduces neuromuscular inflammation, preventing symptom exacerbation.

4. **Enhanced Half-Life Through Fc Engineering**
   - Ravulizumab was designed with two amino acid substitutions in the Fc region, increasing IgG recycling via the neonatal Fc receptor (FcRn).
   - This modification extends its half-life, allowing dosing every 8 weeks compared to every 2 weeks for eculizumab.

Key Pharmacokinetic Parameters: Ravulizumab exhibits linear, dose-proportional pharmacokinetics with a long elimination half-life, allowing infrequent dosing (every 8 weeks). Peak plasma concentration (Tmax) is achieved within 30 minutes to 2 hours post-infusion. As a monoclonal antibody, it is degraded by proteolysis in the reticuloendothelial system. No CYP450 involvement in metabolism, making drug-drug interactions unlikely. Clearance occurs primarily via Fc receptor-mediated endocytosis and lysosomal degradation.

Adverse Drug Reactions: Increased risk of meningococcal infections, infusion-related reactions, upper respiratory tract infections and headache.

Uses: The FDA has granted approval for Paroxysmal Nocturnal Haemoglobinuria (PNH), Atypical Haemolytic Uremic Syndrome (aHUS), Generalised Myasthenia Gravis (gMG), and Neuromyelitis Optica Spectrum Disorder (NMOSD).

Dose: Initial intravenous dosage on Day 1: 2400 mg for patients weighing ≥40 to <60 kg; 2700 mg for those weighing ≥60 to <100 kg; 3000 mg for individuals weighing ≥100 kg. Initiation of maintenance dosage two weeks post-loading. 3000–3600 mg, contingent upon weight, administered intravenously every 8 weeks.

5. Batoclimab

Introduction: Batoclimab, or IMVT-1401, is a fully humanised monoclonal antibody targeting the neonatal Fc receptor (FcRn), developed by Immunovant, Inc. for the treatment of IgG-mediated autoimmune disorders, such as generalised myasthenia gravis (gMG), thyroid eye disease (TED), and chronic inflammatory demyelinating polyneuropathy (CIDP). Batoclimab increases the destruction of pathogenic IgG autoantibodies, which are responsible for disease progression in myasthenia gravis (MG) and other autoimmune illnesses, by inhibiting FcRn. Batoclimab has not yet obtained FDA approval and is presently undergoing Phase 3 clinical trials for generalised Myasthenia Gravis (gMG) and Chronic Inflammatory Demyelinating Polyneuropathy (CIDP).

Clinical trial phase / FDA-Approval: Phase III trial for generalised myasthenia gravis and CIDP.

Mechanism of action: Batoclimab (IMVT-1401) is a fully humanised monoclonal antibody (mAb) that selectively inhibits the neonatal Fc receptor (FcRn). This inhibition results in the accelerated degradation of pathogenic IgG autoantibodies, making it a promising therapy for IgG-mediated autoimmune diseases, including generalized myasthenia gravis (gMG), thyroid eye disease (TED), and chronic inflammatory demyelinating polyneuropathy (CIDP).

1. **IgG Recycling and FcRn Function**
   - FcRn is responsible for recycling IgG antibodies in endothelial and hematopoietic cells.
   - Normally, IgG is taken up into endosomes, where FcRn binds it at low pH (6.0), preventing degradation and allowing its recycling into circulation.
   - This extends the half-life of IgG (21 days), leading to prolonged immune responses in autoimmune diseases.

2. **Batoclimab Disrupts FcRn-IgG Binding**
   - Batoclimab binds with high affinity to the IgG-binding site on FcRn, blocking FcRn-mediated IgG recycling.
   - This prevents IgG from being transported back into circulation, resulting in rapid IgG degradation in lysosomes.
3. **Reduction of Pathogenic IgG Autoantibodies**
   - Since autoimmune diseases like gMG, TED, and CIDP are driven by pathogenic IgG, reducing total IgG directly lowers the autoantibody burden.
   - Studies have shown 65-75% reduction in IgG levels with batoclimab treatment, leading to symptom improvement in autoimmune disorders.
4. **Selective IgG Reduction Without Affecting Other Immune Functions**
   - Unlike broad-spectrum immunosuppressants, batoclimab does not affect IgA, IgM, or complement pathways, preserving innate immunity.
   - This targeted approach minimizes infection risks compared to corticosteroids or traditional immunosuppressants.

Key Pharmacokinetic Parameters: Batoclimab exhibits linear pharmacokinetics with dose-dependent IgG suppression, making it a candidate for weekly or biweekly dosing. It remains primarily in circulation, targeting FcRn-expressing endothelial cells. As a monoclonal antibody, batoclimab undergoes proteolytic degradation into amino acids. It is not metabolized by the cytochrome P450 (CYP450) system, reducing drug-drug interaction risks. It is primarily cleared via lysosomal degradation and reticuloendothelial system processing.

Adverse Drug Reactions: Dyslipidaemia, injection-site reactions, headache and mild GI upset.

Uses: Undergoing Phase III trials for generalized myasthenia gravis and CIDP.

Dose: 680 mg subcutaneously once weekly (trial dosing).

6. Other recent advances in treatment of myasthenia gravis

Table 2: Recent advancements in the medical management of myasthenia gravis.

Intervention / Treatment	Principle	Procedure	Adverse Effects	Uses
Plasma Exchange (PLEX)	Removes circulating autoantibodies and immune complexes.	Blood is drawn, plasma is replaced with albumin/saline, and RBCs are reinfused.	Hypotension, infection risk, bleeding, allergic reactions.	Used in myasthenic crisis or severe exacerbations.
Intravenous Immunoglobulin (IVIG)	Neutralizes pathogenic autoantibodies and modulates immune response.	IV infusion of high-dose IgG from pooled donors.	Headache, fever, thrombosis, renal dysfunction.	Used for rapid symptom control in myasthenic crisis and refractory MG.

Autologous Hematopoietic Stem Cell Transplantation (AHSCT)	Autologous CD34+ hematopoietic stem cells (HSCs) are reinfused into the patient after the immune system is ablated. These stem cells differentiate into new, self-tolerant immune cells, reducing autoimmunity.	High-dose immunosuppression followed by reinfusion of patient's own stem cells.	Severe immunosuppression, infections, secondary malignancies.	Investigational therapy for severe, refractory MG.
Neuromodulation (Transcranial Magnetic Stimulation - TMS &Vagus Nerve Stimulation - VNS)	Alters cortical excitability to improve neuromuscular transmission.	Non-invasive brain or vagus nerve stimulation using electrical pulses.	Mild headache, dizziness, discomfort at stimulation site.	Under research for MG symptom modulation and fatigue reduction.

Conclusion

With the development of targeted therapies that specifically alter the immune system, the landscape of treatment for generalised myasthenia gravis (gMG) has changed dramatically. Newer FcRn inhibitors (efgartigimod, rozanolixizumab), complement inhibitors (ravulizumab, zilucoplan), and experimental treatments (batoclimab) provide more accurate, durable, and practical treatment choices. These treatments have reduced the need for broad-spectrum immunosuppressants while improving quality of life and symptom control. To improve MG management even more, future studies will concentrate on combination therapies, oral formulations, and long-term safety. Current non-pharmacological developments in the management of myasthenia gravis provide targeted immune modulation and symptom relief, even though pharmaceutical treatments are still the gold standard. While PLEX, IVIG, and thymectomy are proven procedures, AHSCT and neuromodulation techniques are promising experimental treatments. Long-term effectiveness, safety, and patient-specific therapy optimisation will be the main topics of future research.

References

1. Varlas V, Borş RG, Baroş A, Cîrstoiu MM, Frîncu F, Carp-Velişcu A, Mehedinţu C. Myasthenia gravis in pregnancy–a multidisciplinary approach. Obstetricăşi Ginecologie. 2022 Apr 1;70(2).
2. Sánchez-Tejerina D, Sotoca J, Llaurado A, López-Diego V, Juntas-Morales R, Salvado M. New targeted agents in myasthenia gravis and future therapeutic strategies. Journal of Clinical Medicine. 2022 Oct 28;11(21):6394.
3. Alfaidi N, Karmastaji S, Matic A, Bril V. FcRn inhibitor therapies in neurologic diseases. CNS drugs. 2024 Jun;38(6):425-41.
4. Costa L, Fernandes C. Zilucoplan: A Newly Approved Macrocyclic Peptide for Treatment of Anti-Acetylcholine Receptor Positive Myasthenia Gravis. Drugs and Drug Candidates. 2024 Mar 27;3(2):311-27.
5. Menon D, Bril V. Pharmacotherapy of generalized myasthenia gravis with special emphasis on newer biologicals. Drugs. 2022 Jun;82(8):865-87.
6. Uysal SP, Morren JA. Promising therapies for the treatment of myasthenia gravis. Expert Opinion on Pharmacotherapy. 2024 Mar 3;25(4):395-408.
7. Ma C, Liu D, Wang B, Yang Y, Zhu R. Advancements and prospects of novel biologicals for myasthenia gravis: toward personalized treatment based on autoantibody specificities. Frontiers in pharmacology. 2024 May 27;15:1370411.
8. Dalakas MC. Role of complement, anti-complement therapeutics, and other targeted immunotherapies in myasthenia gravis. Expert Review of Clinical Immunology. 2022 Jul 3;18(7):691-701.

9. Crisafulli S, Boccanegra B, Carollo M, Bottani E, Mantuano P, Trifirò G, De Luca A. Myasthenia gravis treatment: from old drugs to innovative therapies with a glimpse into the future. CNS drugs. 2024 Jan;38(1):15-32.
10. Schneider-Gold C, Gilhus NE. Advances and challenges in the treatment of myasthenia gravis. Therapeutic advances in neurological disorders. 2021 Dec;14:17562864211065406.
11. Cavalcante P, Mantegazza R, Antozzi C. Targeting autoimmune mechanisms by precision medicine in Myasthenia Gravis. Frontiers in immunology. 2024 Jun 6;15:1404191.
12. Li X, Chen J, Wang Y, Zheng S, Wan K, Liu X. Registered trials on novel therapies for myasthenia gravis: a cross-sectional study on Clinical Trials. gov. Scientific reports. 2024 Jan 24;14(1):2067.
13. RCEMLearning. Myasthenia Gravis: Basic Science and Pathophysiology [Internet]. London: Royal College of Emergency Medicine; [cited 2025 May 9]. Available from: https://www.rcemlearning.org/modules/myasthenia-gravis/lessons/basic-science-and-pathophysiology-47/.
14. Gusovsky Chevalier AV, Lin CC, Kerber K, Reynolds EL, Callaghan BC, Burke JF. Cost Trends of New-To-Market Neurologic Medications: An Insurance Claims Database Analysis. Neurology. 2025 Mar 25;104(6):e213428.
15. Antozzi C, Guptill J, Bril V, Gamez J, Meuth SG, Nowak RJ, Quan D, Sevilla T, Jouvin MH, Jin J, Karcher K. Safety and efficacy of nipocalimab in patients with generalized myasthenia gravis: results from the randomized phase 2 vivacity-MG study. Neurology. 2024 Jan 23;102(2):e207937.
16. Barnett C, Tabasinejad R, Bril V. Current pharmacotherapeutic options for myasthenia gravis. Expert Opinion on Pharmacotherapy. 2019 Dec 12;20(18):2295-303.
17. Gilhus NE, Verschuuren JJ. Myasthenia gravis: subgroup classification and therapeutic strategies. The Lancet Neurology. 2015 Oct 1;14(10):1023-36.
18. Vakrakou AG, Karachaliou E, Chroni E, Zouvelou V, Tzanetakos D, Salakou S, Papadopoulou M, Tzartos S, Voumvourakis K, Kilidireas C, Giannopoulos S. Immunotherapies in MuSK-positive Myasthenia Gravis; an IgG4 antibody-mediated disease. Frontiers in Immunology. 2023 Jul 26;14:1212757.
19. Ramanathan S, Ryan CS, Baker SK. Novel therapies and emerging interventions for MG. *Nat Rev Neurol*.2023;19(4):221-235.
20. Berenbaum F. Targeted therapies in osteoarthritis: a systematic review of the trials on www. clinicaltrials. gov. Best Practice & Research Clinical Rheumatology. 2010 Feb 1;24(1):107-19.

Section 3

Central Nervous System

Chapter 6

Recent Advances in General Anaesthesia

Author: Dr. Pranab Das

Introduction

General anaesthesia (GA) is fundamental to contemporary surgical practice, facilitating safe and painless treatments across all specialities. In recent decades, the discipline has advanced swiftly, propelled by breakthroughs in pharmacology, molecular biology, monitoring technologies, and patient safety. The objectives of general anaesthesia—hypnosis, analgesia, amnesia, and muscle relaxation—are now attained with greater precision, reduced undesirable effects, and expedited recovery.

Recent advancements encompass target-controlled infusion systems, ultra-short-acting drugs such as remimazolam, closed-loop feedback systems, and depth-of-anaesthesia monitoring utilising EEG-derived indices like the Bispectral Index (BIS). These advancements seek to customise anaesthetic depth for each individual, thereby reducing issues such as intraoperative awareness and protracted recovery. There is an increasing focus on multimodal anaesthesia to diminish dependence on opioids, hence alleviating the dangers of postoperative nausea, ileus, and long-term dependency.

Historical Perspective

William T.G. Morton's successful demonstration of ether anaesthesia in 1846 marked the beginning of general anaesthesia in the middle of the 19th century. This crucial event marked the beginning of a new era in surgery, turning it from a dangerous and agonising procedure into a more controlled and compassionate one. Despite early worries about toxicity and mortality, ether, nitrous oxide, and chloroform were introduced into clinical practice in later decades.

In the 20th century, intravenous anaesthetics—most notably thiopental in the 1930s and ketamine and propofol later—replaced volatile agents. By enhancing gas exchange and airway safety, the mid-1900s saw the development of the endotracheal tube and positive pressure ventilation, which further transformed anaesthesia.

Guedel's classification of anaesthesia stages, which offered a methodical framework to evaluate anaesthetic depth, was a significant historical turning point. The development of opioids and neuromuscular blocking agents allowed for longer and more intricate surgeries. Computer-assisted delivery systems, capnography, and pulse oximetry have significantly improved safety in recent decades.

The history of general anaesthesia shows a striking shift from empirical approaches to evidence-based, mechanically driven care, from crude ether masks to highly advanced automated anaesthesia workstations.

Definition

General anaesthesia is a medically induced state of unconsciousness, accompanied by analgesia, amnesia, and muscle relaxation. It is achieved using a combination of intravenous and inhalational anaesthetic agents, often administered along with adjuncts like muscle relaxants and opioids to provide a comprehensive anaesthetic effect.

Types of General Anaesthesia

1. **Inhalational Anaesthesia:** In order to induce and maintain anaesthesia, volatile anaesthetics such as desflurane and sevoflurane are administered via inhalational route.
2. **Intravenous Anaesthesia:** Anaesthesia is induced by intravenous administration of medications such as propofol, ketamine, and etomidate; these are frequently used in conjunction with inhalational agents for maintenance.
3. **Total Intravenous Anaesthesia (TIVA):** This approach completely avoids the use of inhaled medications by utilising only intravenous agents, such as propofol and remifentanil, to both induce and maintain anaesthesia.

The stages of GA is illustrated in Figure 1.

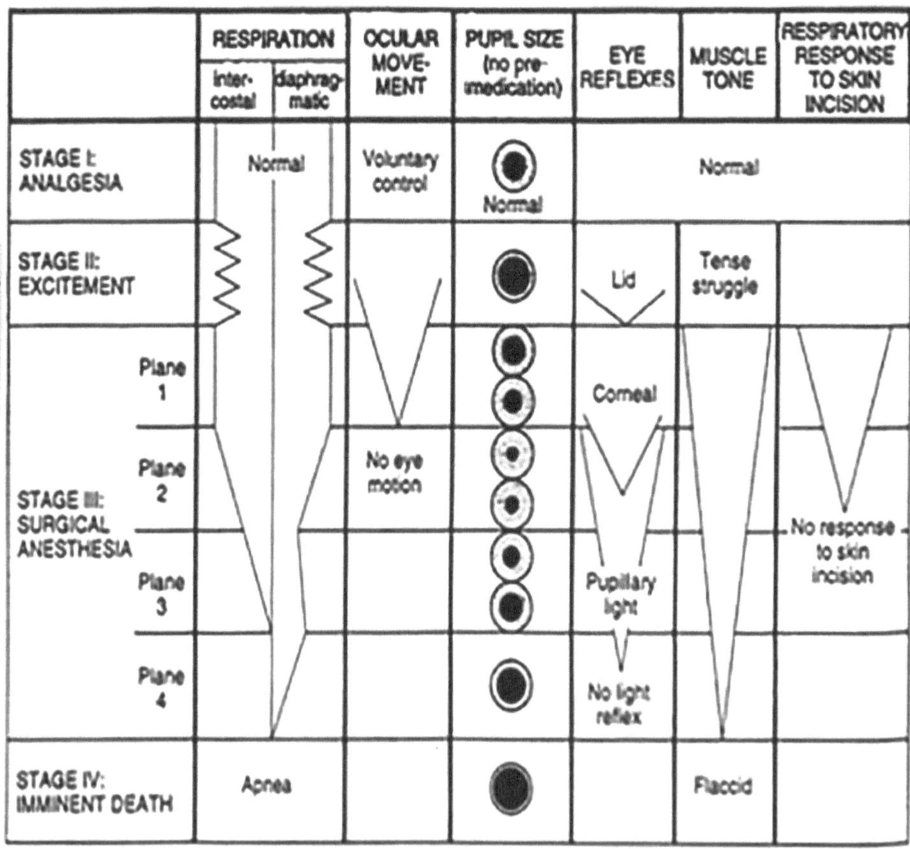

Figure 1: Stages of General Anaesthesia (Source: Hagar H. General anesthesia).

Conventional Anaesthetic Agents

Table 1: Traditional anaesthetic agents.

Type	Drug Names	Mechanism of Action	Key Features	Adverse Drug Reactions (ADRs)	Indications
Inhalational	Halothane	Potentiates GABA-A receptor activity and reduces excitatory neurotransmission by NMDA receptor inhibition.	Highly potent, smooth induction, slow recovery, sensitizes myocardium to catecholamines.	Hepatotoxicity (Halothane hepatitis), malignant hyperthermia, hypotension, arrhythmias.	Induction and maintenance of general anaesthesia (limited use due to hepatotoxicity).
	Isoflurane	Enhances GABA-A receptor function and reduces neuronal excitability by NMDA receptor inhibition.	Less arrhythmogenic, maintains cardiac output.	Respiratory depression, hypotension, pungency (airway irritation).	Maintenance of general anaesthesia.
	Sevoflurane	Potentiates GABA-A receptor activity and hyperpolarizes neurons.	Low pungency, rapid induction and recovery.	Nephrotoxicity (due to fluoride metabolites), hypotension.	Induction and maintenance of anaesthesia, preferred in paediatric cases.
	Nitrous oxide (N2O)	Antagonizes NMDA receptors, causing analgesia and sedation.	Strong analgesic, weak anaesthetic, second gas effect.	Diffusion hypoxia, expansion of air cavities (contraindicated in pneumothorax).	Used in combination with other anaesthetics for analgesia.
Intravenous	Thiopental	Prolongs the duration of opening of chloride channels in GABA-A receptors - Chloride channel complex causing rapid CNS depression.	Ultra-short acting, highly lipophilic.	Respiratory depression, hypotension, accumulation in adipose tissue prolongs recovery, laryngospasm.	Induction of anaesthesia and short surgical procedures.
	Propofol	Potentiates GABA-A receptors.	Anti-emetic properties, rapid clearance, rapid onset and recovery.	Hypotension, respiratory depression, bradycardia, propofol infusion syndrome.	Induction and maintenance of anaesthesia and ICU sedation.
	Etomidate	Enhances GABAergic neurotransmission with minimal cardiovascular effects.	Hemody-namically stable, no analgesic effect.	Adrenocortical suppression, myoclonus, nausea & vomiting.	Induction of anaesthesia in hemodynamically unstable patients.
	Ketamine	NMDA receptor antagonist produces dissociative anaesthesia and analgesia.	Hypertension, hallucinations, emergence reactions (vivid dreams, hallucinations, delusions).	Preserves airway reflexes, increases sympathetic tone.	Induction of anaesthesia and analgesia in trauma/emergency settings.

Newer Anaesthetic Agents and Their Current Status:

1. Ciprofol

Introduction: Haisco Pharmaceutical Group Co., Ltd. (Chengdu, China) developed ciprofol (HSK3486), which received Chinese approval in 2020.

Clinical Trial Phase / FDA-Approval: After a priority review, the China National Medical Products Administration (NMPA) approved ciprofol on December 15, 2020, for use as a sedative during gastrointestinal endoscopy. Ciprofol was later authorised for bronchoscopy and for the induction, maintenance, and sedation in general anaesthesia. A new use of ciprofol for sedation in critical care was recently authorised by the NMPA.

Mechanism of Action: Ciprofol, like propofol, is a direct agonist of the GABA-A receptor and a positive allosteric modulator. Ciprofol competitively binds to butylbicyclophosphorothionate and t-butylbicycloorthobenzoate residues in the chloride channels of GABA-A receptors of GABA-A receptor chloride channel complex in the brain and induces chloride influx. By elevating intracellular chloride concentration it induces hyperpolarisation of nerve cell membranes, resulting in sedative and anaesthetic actions.

Key Pharmacokinetic Parameters: It has a swiftonset of action, reaching peak plasma concentration within minutes. It has a short half-life, allowing for quick recovery post-sedation. It is primarily metabolized in liver, involving CYP enzymes, leading to production of inactive metabolites. It undergoes renal and biliary clearance, with no significant accumulation upon repeated dosing.

Adverse Drug Reactions: Respiratory depression, bradycardia, hypotension and arrythmia.

Uses: In China, ciprofol is currently approved for use in sedation and anaesthesia during non-tracheal intubation procedures, as well as for the induction and maintenance of general anaesthesia and sedation in intensive care units.

Dose: 0.4–0.5 mg/kg IV for induction; 0.2–0.3 mg/kg/h IV for maintenance.

2. Remimazolam

Introduction: A novel benzodiazepine used for intravenous sedation, Remimazolam (CNS7056) is distinguished by its incredibly brief duration of action. It was recently approved for use in general anaesthesia and procedural sedation.

Clinical Trial Phase / FDA-Approval: Approved in a number of nations (China, Japan, and the USA); phase 3 research is still underway in a number of other countries.In 2020, the FDA approved it.

Mechanism of Action: Remimazolam exhibits a strong affinity for the benzodiazepine site on GABA-A receptors in the brain, which is situated at the interface of alpha (α) and gamma (γ) subunits. After binding to the benzodiazepine binding site, it increases the frequency of chloride channel opening which ultimately leads to the elevation of intracellular chloride ion concentration, resulting in membrane hyperpolarisation and the inhibition of neuronal action potential conduction leading to sedation and anaesthesia. Remimazolam was noted to exhibit slightly greater potency at the α1-containing subtypes compared to midazolam. The α1-containing subtypes of GABA-A are significant as they are believed to mediate sedation and amnesia.

Key Pharmacokinetic Parameters: The onset of action is rapid, with peak plasma concentration reaching within 1 to 3 minutes. In contrast to its parent compound, midazolam, remimazolam is not metabolised by cytochrome P-450 isozymes. The ester moiety of remimazolam serves as a substrate for non-specific tissue esterase enzymes, allowing for metabolism independent of any specific organ. This may render it a valuable therapeutic option for individuals with hepatic or renal impairment. Five significant metabolites were characterised, comprising three phase I metabolites (resulting from oxidation, reduction, and hydrolysis of the parent drug) and two phase II metabolites (resulting from conjugation of the drug or its metabolites with another molecule). Carboxylesterase enzymes play a crucial role in the metabolism of remimazolam and are located in the cytosol and rough endoplasmic reticulum of tissues. The elimination half-life is approximately 7 to 13 minutes.

Adverse Drug Reactions: Headache, drowsiness, hypotension and involuntary movements.

Uses: Applications include inducing and maintaining general anaesthesia and sedation in the intensive care unit, as well as providing sedation during endoscopic procedures (upper gastrointestinal endoscopy, colonoscopy, and bronchoscopy).

Dose: 6–12 mg/kg/h IV (induction); 1–2 mg/kg/h (maintenance).

3. Sugammadex

Introduction: Sugammadex is a modified gamma-cyclodextrin that is used to reverse the effects of vecuronium and rocuronium, two steroidal non-depolarizing neuromuscular blocking agents. In the recovery room, residual neuromuscular blockade is estimated to occur in about 30 to 60% of the time after surgery. Hypoxia, weakness of the supralaryngeal muscles resulting in upper airway obstruction, problems with swallowing, and an increased risk of aspiration are all linked to low-level of neuromuscular blockade. Sugammadex considerably reduces the possibility of residual neuromuscular paralysis and speeds up the rate at which neuromuscular blockade is reversed.

Clinical Trial Phase / FDA-Approval: FDA-approved drug.

Mechanism of Action: Sugammadex has a core sufficiently large to accommodate the aminosteroid non-depolarizing neuromuscular blocking drugs (NMBDs), rocuronium and vecuronium. Upon entry into the core of sugammadex, rocuronium and vecuronium undergoes non-covalent hydrophobic interactions which stabilises the NMBD-sugammadex complex, resulting in the formation of water-soluble inclusion complexes which are ultimately excreted and removed out through urine. The association constant for the sugammadex-rocuronium inclusion complex is notably high. A higher association constant indicates a greater affinity between molecules. Therefore, when rocuronium binds to sugammadex, it is regarded as irreversibly fixed. The association constant of the sugammadex-vecuronium complex is three times lower than that of the sugammadex-rocuronium complex.

Sugammadex reverses neuromuscular blockade through the encapsulation of free neuromuscular blocking drugs in plasma. This reduces the plasma concentration of free NMBD, establishing a concentration gradient between the muscle tissue compartment and plasma. As a result, free neuromuscular blocking drugs (NMBD) transportoccurs from the muscle tissue compartment to the plasma. These NMBD are again encapsulated by plasma sugammadex, which sustains a lower concentration of free NMBD in the plasma and the cycle is repeated. As a result, the concentration of NMBD at the nicotinic acetylcholine receptor in the neuromuscular junction decreases rapidly. This facilitates the resumption of neuromuscular activity. Sugammadex does not inhibit acetylcholinesterase, unlike traditional reversal agents like neostigmine; thus, the co-administration of an antimuscarinic drug, such as glycopyrrolate, is not required.

Key Pharmacokinetic Parameters: Immediate reversal of neuromuscular blockade occurs typically within 1–3 minutes. Sugammadex exhibits a volume of distribution ranging from 11 to 14 litres, an elimination half-life of approximately two hours, and a clearance rate of 88 ml/min. Sugammadex undergoes no metabolism and is primarily excreted unchanged by the kidneys, with over 90% eliminated renally within 24 hours. Plasma half-life is approximately of 2 hours.

Adverse Drug Reactions: Nausea, vomiting, headache, bradycardia, QT prolongation, itching and dysgeusia.

Uses: To offset the effects of muscle relaxants such as vecuronium and rocuronium. It is administered as a single intravenous injection.

Dose: 2 mg/kg IV (moderate neuromuscular block); 4 mg/kg IV (deep neuromuscular block); 16 mg/kg IV (immediate reversal after high-dose rocuronium).

4. Dexmedetomidine:

Introduction: It is a highly selective a2-adrenergic receptor (AR) agonist with a reasonably high ratio of α2/α 1-activity, but it does not cause respiratory depression, which makes it a safe and effective adjunct in a variety of therapeutic applications.

Clinical Trial Phase / FDA-Approval: FDA-approved drug.

Mechanism of Action: Dexmedetomidine is an alpha agonist with sympatholytic, hypnotic, analgesic, sedative, and anxiolytic effects. These effects are caused by agonizing (stimulating) the brainstem's alpha-2 receptors, which are the pre-synaptic auto-receptors, which upon stimulation, prevents norepinephrine from being released form central sympathetic neurones thereby reducing central sympathetic outflow. Compared to alpha-1 receptors, it has a 1600 to 1 selectivity for alpha-2 receptors. Dexmedetomidine's potential to lengthen the duration of a peripheral nerve block is not entirely understood, however it is thought to be a perineural mechanism rather than a systemic or central mechanism, which seems to do so by inhibiting the cation current.

Key Pharmacokinetic Parameters: Onset of Action is within 5–10 minutes after i.v. administration. It is rapidly dispersed throughout tissues and removed by the liver. Plasma half-life is of 1.5 to 2 hours approximately.

Adverse Drug Reactions: Bradycardia, hypertension, and hypotension are the three most common adverse effects of dexmedetomidine. Bradycardia and hypotension are brought on by presynaptic alpha receptor stimulation, which reduces central sympathetic outflow and norepinephrine release.

Uses: Dexmedetomidine's FDA-approved uses include peri-procedural (or peri-operative) sedation of non-intubated patients and sedation of intubated and mechanically ventilated patients in the intensive care unit (ICU). Over time, off-label uses have expanded to include treating alcohol withdrawal, preventing and treating delirium, treating insomnia in the intensive care unit, and offering additional analgesia. Dexmedetomidine has also been used in peripheral nerve blocks to prolong the duration of analgesia.

Dose: Initial dosage: 1 µg/kg administered over 10 minutes; maintenance dosage: 0.2–0.7 µg/kg/hour.

5. Cyclopropyl-Methoxycarbonyl Metomidate (CPMM):

Introduction: The "soft" etomidate analogue cyclopropyl-methoxycarbonyl metomidate (CPMM) is presently being researched as a propofol substitute for the induction and maintenance of anaesthesia. It is known as a "soft" etomidate analogue as it shows a rapid onset and offset of action, metabolised quickly into inactive metabolites and etomidate inhibits 11β-hydroxylase which causes adrenocortical suppression, but due to the rapid clearance of CPPM, the risk of adrenocortical suppression with CPPM is low.

Clinical Trial Phase / FDA-Approval: Currently in Phase I of clinical trial.

Mechanism of Action: It is a selective GABA-A receptor positive modulator, which enhances the inhibitory effects of the neurotransmitter GABA, leading to sedation and anaesthesia.

Key Pharmacokinetic Parameters: Rapid onset, with peak anaesthetic effects observed within 30–60 seconds after i.v. administration. CPMM is hydrolysed by esterases into ethanol and a pharmacologically inactive metabolite called CPM-acid. CPMM has a quick clearance rate and a modest volume of distribution.

Adverse Drug Reactions: Involuntary movements, hypotension, injection-site pain, nausea and vomiting.

Uses: Currently under Phase I clinical trial as a substitute to propofol for anaesthetic induction and maintenance.

Dose: Still under evaluation.

6. Other Recent Advances in General Anaesthesia

a. **Depth of Anaesthesia Monitoring:** Innovations in monitoring systems, such as entropy monitoring and the Bispectral Index (BIS), allow anaesthesiologists to assess the depth of anaesthesia and adjust drug dosages accordingly. These technologies improve patient safety by minimizing the risks of awareness during surgery (intraoperative awareness) and optimizing drug administration to prevent excessive anaesthetic exposure, which can lead to longer recovery times.

b. **Target-Controlled Infusion (TCI):** Target-based infusion systems enable the precise delivery of intravenous anaesthetic agents, maintaining a stable concentration of drugs in the blood or at the site of action. This system is particularly useful in total intravenous anaesthesia (TIVA), where it can optimize dosing, reduce drug wastage, and provide smoother induction and maintenance of anaesthesia. TCI systems are designed to adjust the infusion rate based on variables unique to each patient, like weight, age, and overall health, improving both the efficiency and safety of anaesthesia administration.

c. **Perioperative Opioid-Sparing Strategies:** With the growing concerns about opioid-related side effects and the risk of dependency, there has been a focus on opioid-sparing techniques in anaesthesia. Multimodal anaesthesia, which reduces the use of opioids before and after surgery by combining non-opioid analgesics such as acetaminophen, nonsteroidal anti-inflammatory medications (NSAIDs) and regional anaesthesia procedures (such as nerve blocks). Additionally, newer agents like dexmedetomidine are gaining popularity for their ability to provide analgesia and sedation without causing respiratory depression which is commonly associated with opioids.

d. **Pharmacogenomics in Anaesthesia:** Pharmacogenomics is playing an emerging role in anaesthesia, offering insights into how genetic factors influence individual responses to anaesthetic agents. By understanding genetic variations that affect drug metabolism and receptor sensitivity, anaesthesiologists can tailor anaesthetic regimens to each patient's genetic profile, improving efficacy and reducing the risk of adverse effects. For example, individuals with variants in the butyrylcholinesterase gene may have prolonged paralysis when exposed to succinylcholine, necessitating alternative agents.

Challenges in General Anaesthesia

1. **Postoperative Nausea and Vomiting (PONV):** PONV is still among the most prevalent complications of general anaesthesia, affecting up to 30-40% of patients. The development of newer antiemetic agents, such as aprepitant, which is an antagonist of the neurokinin-1 (NK1) receptor, has improved the management of PONV in high-risk patients. Combining these agents with standard antiemetics like ondansetron has led to more effective prevention and treatment of this distressing side effect.
2. **Enhanced Recovery After Surgery (ERAS) Protocols:** ERAS procedures/protocols are supported by evidence strategies designed to enhance perioperative care, lower recovery time, and enhance the outcome for patients. These protocols include recommendations for anaesthetic management, such

as the use of short-acting agents, opioid-sparing techniques, and early mobilization of patient, all of which contribute to faster recovery and reduced hospital stays.

3. **Awareness during Surgery:** Intraoperative awareness, though rare, is a serious complication that can occur when patients regain consciousness during surgery. Depth of anaesthesia monitoring tools like BIS and entropy monitoring have greatly reduced the incidence of this phenomenon by providing feedback on a patient's state of consciousness in real time. However, continued research is necessary to minimize the awareness risk, especially in high-risk populations such as trauma and cardiac surgery patients.

4. **Long-Term Cognitive Effects:** Postoperative cognitive dysfunction (POCD) is a concern, particularly in patients who are from geriatric age-group, undergoing general anaesthesia. Research on neuroprotective strategies, such as minimizing anaesthetic exposure and using neuroprotective agents, is ongoing to mitigate the risk of long-term cognitive impairment following surgery.

Future Directions in General Anaesthesia

1. **Neuroprotective Anaesthesia:** With increasing evidence linking general anaesthesia to postoperative cognitive dysfunction (POCD) in elderly patients, neuroprotective strategies are being developed. Agents like xenon, an inert gas with neuroprotective properties, are being explored for their ability to provide anaesthesia without the neurotoxic effects associated with traditional agents. Xenon has shown promise in protecting brain cells from ischemic injury and reducing the risk of POCD in animal models.

2. **Nanotechnology in Anaesthesia:** The anaesthetic applications of nanotechnology delivery of drugs are a promising area of research. Nano-formulations of anaesthetic agents could allow for more precise targeting of drug action, improving both the efficacy and safety of anaesthesia. Additionally, nanoparticles can be designed to deliver anaesthetics in a regulated way, potentially reducing the dosage required and minimizing side effects.

Conclusion

The goals of recent developments in general anaesthesia have been to decrease complications like postoperative cognitive dysfunction, opioid dependency, and PONV, as well as to optimise drug delivery and improve patient safety. Anaesthesia practice has been completely transformed by the creation of new anaesthetic agents such as remimazolam and dexmedetomidine, as well as advancements in drug delivery and monitoring technologies. The combination of pharmacogenomics, nanotechnology, and neuroprotective techniques holds promise for improving the efficacy and safety of general anaesthesia in the years to come as research advances.

References

1. Karunarathna I, Bandara S, Jayawardana A, De Alvis K, Gunasena P, Gunathilake S, Hapuarachchi T. Newer advancements in neuroanaesthesia and neurocritical care.
2. Weibel S, Schaefer MS, Raj D, Rücker G, Pace NL, Schlesinger T, Meybohm P, Kienbaum P, Eberhart LH, Kranke P. Drugs for preventing postoperative nausea and vomiting in adults after general anaesthesia: an abridged Cochrane network meta-analysis. Anaesthesia. 2021 Jul;76(7):962-73.
3. Kissin I. Components of general anesthesia: history of the concept transformation. Anesthesia& Analgesia. 2023 Sep 1;137(3):702-7.
4. Robinson DH, Toledo AH. Historical development of modern anesthesia. Journal of Investigative Surgery. 2012 May 22;25(3):141-9.
5. Hagar H. General anesthesia [Internet]. Riyadh: King Saud University Medical Sciences Campus; 2018 [cited 2025 May 9]. Available from: https://ksumsc.com/download_center/Archive/2nd/438/1-%20Neuropsychiatry%20block/Male%20group/Pharmacology/General%20anesthesia-2018-ishfaq.pdf.

6. Hemmings HC, Akabas MH, Goldstein PA, Trudell JR, Orser BA, Harrison NL. Emerging molecular mechanisms of general anesthetic action. Trends in pharmacological sciences. 2005 Oct 1;26(10):503-10.
7. Mayhew D, Mendonca V, Murthy BV. A review of ASA physical status–historical perspectives and modern developments. Anaesthesia. 2019 Mar;74(3):373-9.
8. Giovannitti Jr JA, Thoms SM, Crawford JJ. Alpha-2 adrenergic receptor agonists: a review of current clinical applications. Anesthesia progress. 2015;62(1):31.
9. Franks NP. Molecular targets underlying general anaesthesia. British journal of pharmacology. 2006 Jan;147(S1):S72-81.
10. Waugaman WR, Foster SD. New advances in anesthesia. Nursing Clinics of North America. 1991 Jun 1;26(2):451-61.
11. Gupta B, Sahay N, Vinod K, Sandhu K, Basireddy HR, Mudiganti RK. Recent advances in system management, decision support systems, artificial intelligence and computing in anaesthesia. Indian Journal of Anaesthesia. 2023 Jan 1;67(1):146-51.
12. Townsend DR. Recent Advances in Anaesthesia and Intensive Care–Volume 24: Jeremy N. Cashman, R. Michael Grounds. Cambridge University Press, 2007, 250 pp., ISBN 978-0-521-70649-0.
13. Seger C, Cannesson M. Recent advances in the technology of anesthesia. F1000Research. 2020 May 18;9:F1000-aculty.
14. Mahmoud M, Mason KP. Recent advances in intravenous anesthesia and anesthetics. F1000Research. 2018 Apr 17;7:F1000-aculty.
15. Li J, Wang X, Liu J, Wang X, Li X, Wang Y, Ouyang W, Li J, Yao S, Zhu Z, Guo Q. Comparison of ciprofol (HSK3486) versus propofol for the induction of deep sedation during gastroscopy and colonoscopy procedures: A multi-centre, non-inferiority, randomized, controlled phase 3 clinical trial. Basic & Clinical Pharmacology & Toxicology. 2022 Aug;131(2):138-48.
16. Hudaib M, Malik H, Zakir SJ, Rabbani S, Gnanendran D, Syed AR, Suri NF, Khan J, Iqbal A, Hussain N, Abdullah M. Efficacy and safety of ciprofol versus propofol for induction and maintenance of general anesthesia: a systematic review and meta-analysis. Journal of Anesthesia, Analgesia and Critical Care. 2024 Apr 11;4(1):25.
17. Hu Q, Liu X, Wen C, Li D, Lei X. Remimazolam: an updated review of a new sedative and anaesthetic. Drug Design, Development and Therapy. 2022 Jan 1:3957-74.
18. Noor N, Legendre R, Cloutet A, Chitneni A, Varrassi G, Kaye AD. A comprehensive review of remimazolam for sedation. Health psychology research. 2021 Jun 11;9(1):24514.
19. Zhang Y, Jiang Y, Lei Q, Li C, Jin SA, Wang Q, Huang Y, Li Y, Hong Y, Wang S, Lin H. Phase III clinical trial comparing the efficacy and safety of adamgammadex with sugammadex for reversal of rocuronium-induced neuromuscular block. British Journal of Anaesthesia. 2024 Jan 1;132(1):45-52.
20. World Federation of Societies of Anaesthesiologists (WFSA). An overview of sugammadex: pharmacokinetics and efficacy. *WFSA* [Internet]. Available from: https://resources.wfsahq.org/atotw/an-overview-of-sugammadex/.
21. Grewal A. Dexmedetomidine: new avenues. Journal of Anaesthesiology clinical pharmacology. 2011 Jul 1;27(3):297-302.
22. Reel B, Maani CV. Dexmedetomidine. [Updated 2023 May 1]. In: StatPearls [Internet]. Treasure Island (FL): StatPearls Publishing; 2025 Jan-. Available from: https://www.ncbi.nlm.nih.gov/books/NBK513303/.
23. Ge R, Pejo E, Gallin H, Jeffrey S, Cotten JF, Raines DE. The pharmacology of cyclopropyl-methoxycarbonyl metomidate: a comparison with propofol. AnesthAnalg. 2014 Mar;118(3):563-7.
24. Zhou J, Wang L, Zhong Z, Yuan L, Huang J, Zou P, Cao X, Peng D, Liao B, Zeng J. Pharmacological mechanism and clinical application of ciprofol. Frontiers in Pharmacology. 2025 Mar 25;16:1572112.
25. Xin Y, Lu P, Guan S, Si S, Sun R, Xia W, Xu H. Efficacy and Safety of Remimazolam in Short Endoscopic Procedures: A Systematic Review and Meta-Analysis. Medicina. 2025 Mar 5;61(3):453.
26. Nissen KD, Moos CM, Wolf A, Strøm T. Paediatric sedation with intranasal dexmedetomidine: Protocol for a systematic review and meta-analysis. PloS one. 2025 Jan 13;20(1):e0317406.
27. Philip AB, Brohan J, Goudra B. The Role of GABA Receptors in Anesthesia and Sedation: An Updated Review. CNS drugs. 2025 Jan;39(1):39-54.
28. Kaye AD, Villafarra EA, Everett ES, Ware EE, Mashaw SA, Brouillette WD, Elder CG, Moss T, Muiznieks L, Herron E, Ahmadzadeh S. Safety and efficacy of sugammadex in management of patients with myasthenia gravis undergoing general anesthesia: A systematic review. Heliyon. 2025 Jan 8.

Chapter 7

Newer Sedatives and Hypnotics

Author: Dr. Pranab Das

Introduction

Pharmacological substances called sedatives and hypnotics are mainly used to cause drowsiness, lower anxiety, and encourage sleep. Depending on the dosage and agent, these substances can produce a range of effects from anxiolysis to general anaesthesia by altering neurotransmission in the central nervous system (CNS). Barbiturates, benzodiazepines, non-benzodiazepine hypnotics (like Z-drugs), and more recent medications like remimazolam are the most widely used classes.

The difference between a hypnotic and a sedative is primarily functional: hypnotics help induce and sustain sleep, whereas sedatives calm the patient and lessen excitement. However, depending on the dosage, many medications display both characteristics. As pharmacology advances, more attention is being paid to short-acting, receptor-specific drugs that have lower dependence risk, better safety margins, and fewer side effects. The advent of drugs such as orexin receptor antagonists and dexmedetomidine (α2-agonist) marks the transition to mechanism-specific treatments in CNS modulation.

Historical Perspective

Sedatives and hypnotics have an extensive documented history that mirrors the development of CNS pharmacotherapy as a whole. Due to their calming properties, herbal remedies like opium, henbane, and mandrake root were used as sedatives as early as ancient civilisations. Despite their toxicity, the synthesis of chloral hydrate and bromides during the 19th century marked a turning point in the development of sedative-hypnotics.

Barbiturates, such as barbital, were introduced in 1903 and revolutionised sedation and sleep induction. They were used for decades until overdose and addiction problems led to the search for safer alternatives. Barbiturates were rapidly replaced in the majority of indications by benzodiazepines, particularly diazepam and chlordiazepoxide, which offered a better safety profile and a wider therapeutic window. The 1960s marked the beginning of this era.

Recent developments in sedative agents like remimazolam and non-benzodiazepine hypnotics like zolpidem and zaleplon demonstrate the continued improvement of molecular targets like the GABA-A receptor subunits. The goals of these advancements are to lessen residual sedation, dependence potential, and cognitive impairment.

In CNS drug development, the history of sedatives and hypnotics, from plant-based traditional remedies to receptor-selective synthetic compounds, serves as an example of striking a balance between therapeutic benefit and pharmacovigilance.

Definition

Sedatives are drugs that subdues excitement, while hypnotics are employed to induce and maintain sleep. Higher dosages of sedatives usually result in hypnotic effects, so the difference between sedatives and hypnotics frequently depends on the dosage.

Types of Sedatives and Hypnotics

1. **Benzodiazepines:** Benzodiazepines are widely used for their sedative, muscle relaxant, and anxiolytic effects. They work by enhancing the effects of the neurotransmitter gamma-aminobutyric acid (GABA) at the GABA-A receptor (GABA facilitator).
2. **Non-BenzodiazepineGABA-A Agonists (Z-drugs):** Z-drugs include medications such as eszopiclone, zolpidem, and zaleplon. Although they are selective for specific GABA-A receptor subtypes (alpha-1 subunit containing receptor subtype), they function similarly to benzodiazepines and mainly induce sleep without having any discernible anxiolytic or anticonvulsant effects.
3. **Melatonin Receptor Agonists:** Ramelteon is a selective agonist of the melatonin receptors MT1 and MT2, which regulates the sleep-wake cycle and aids in the treatment of insomnia, particularly in patients who have trouble falling asleep.
4. **Orexin Receptor Antagonists:** A novel class of hypnotics known as orexin receptor antagonists blocks the orexin system, which is essential for wakefulness. Lemborexant and suvorexant are two medications that provide a novel way to encourage sleep, especially in individuals who suffer from insomnia.

Conventional Sedatives and Hypnotics

Table 1: Classical Sedatives and Hypnotics.

Drug Class	Drug Names	Mechanism of Action	Adverse Drug Reactions	Uses	Key Features
Barbiturates	Thiopental	Increases the duration of Cl- channel opening and acts a GABA-mimetic at higher doses.	CNS, CVS & respiratory depression, hangover is common.	As a sedative, hypnotic in insomnia, induction of anaesthesia (no longer used now).	Thiopental is ultra-short acting, shows redistribution & highly lipophilic.
Benzodia-zepines	Clonazepam, Diazepam, Lorazepam, Midazolam	Increases the frequency of Cl- channel opening. Acts as GABA-facilitator.	Amnesia, hypotension, bradycardia, headache, daytime somnolence.	Sedative & hypnotic in insomnia, anxiety disorders, depression, pre-medication for anaesthesia.	Short-acting, water-soluble, strong amnesic effect, less tolerance & dependence as compared to barbiturates.
Z-compounds	Zolpidem, Zopiclone, Zaleplon	Positive allosteric modulator of GABA-A receptor.	Neuropsychiatric symptoms, anterograde amnesia.	Short-term or transient insomnia, jet lag.	Non-addictive, improves sleep onset &less distortion of sleep architecture.

Melatonin receptor agonist	Melatonin, Ramelteon	Activates MT1 & MT2 receptor: Shifts timing of circadian rhythm & induces sleep.	Dizziness, Fatigue, Endocrine disturbances.	Short-term or transient insomnia, jet lag.	Less risk of dependence & tolerance.

Newer Sedatives and Hypnotics

1. Dual orexin receptor antagonist (DORA):

Introduction: DORA includes medications such as Lemborexant, Daridorexant, and Suvorexant. The first of its kind to be approved as a dual orexin receptor antagonist (DORA) for the treatment of insomnia is suvorexant.

Clinical Trial Phase / FDA-Approval:

Suvorexant: Received FDA-Approval in 2014 under the brand name Belsomra.

Lemborexant: Approved by the FDA in 2019 under the brand name Dayvigo.

Daridorexant: The newest in this class, approved in 2022 under the brand name Quviviq.

Mechanism of Action: Lateral hypothalamus secrete orexins, which are excitatory neurotransmitters. These orexins activates orexin receptors (OX1R and OX2R) which are situated in tuberomammillary histaminergic neurons. Stimulation of these receptors releases histamine, which is the key bioactive molecule to maintain wakefulness. Suvorexant decreases alertness and promotes sleep by inhibiting these G-protein coupled orexin receptors (OX1R and OX2R), which prevent orexin from stimulating histaminergic neurons.

Key Pharmacokinetic Parameters:

Table 2: Critical pharmacokinetic characteristics of DORA.

Parameter	Suvorexant	Lemborexant	Daridorexant
Action commencement	30 min	15-30 min	30-60 min
Half-life	12 hours	17-19 hours	8 hours
Metabolism	CYP3A4	CYP3A4	CYP3A4
Elimination	Faeces (major), Urine (minor)	Faeces (major), Urine (minor)	Faeces (major), Urine (minor)
Plasma Protein binding	99%	94%	99%

Adverse Drug Reactions: Abnormal thinking, behavioural changes, somnolence, headache, hypnagogic hallucinations, and sleep paralysis.

Uses: Treatment for chronic insomnia.

Dose: Lemborexant: 5–10 mg orally at bedtime; Daridorexant: 25–50 mg orally at bedtime; Suvorexant: 10–20 mg orally at bedtime.

2. Remimazolam

Introduction: Remimazolam is a benzodiazepine class of sedative which is used in the treatment of insomnia, a condition characterized by difficulty in getting asleep and/or remaining awake at night.

Clinical Trial Phase / FDA-Approval: Approved in several countries (Japan, China, USA); ongoing Phase 3 clinical trials for insomnia. FDA-approved on 2020 for procedural sedation in adults undergoing invasive procedures.

Mechanism of Action: Remimazolam exhibits a strong affinity for the benzodiazepine site on GABA-A receptors in the brain, which is situated at the interface of alpha (α) and gamma (γ) subunits. After binding to the benzodiazepine binding site, it increases the frequency of chloride channel opening which ultimately leads to the elevation of intracellular chloride ion concentration, resulting in membrane hyperpolarisation and the inhibition of neuronal action potential conduction leading to sedation. Remimazolam was noted to exhibit slightly greater potency at the α1-containing subtypes compared to midazolam. The α1-containing subtypes of GABA-A are significant as they are believed to mediate sedation and amnesia.

Key Pharmacokinetic Parameters: The onset of action is rapid, with peak plasma concentration reaching within 1 to 3 minutes. In contrast to its parent compound, midazolam, remimazolam is not metabolised by cytochrome P-450 isozymes. The ester moiety of remimazolam serves as a substrate for non-specific tissue esterase enzymes, allowing for metabolism independent of any specific organ. This may render it a valuable therapeutic option for individuals with hepatic or renal impairment. Five significant metabolites were characterised, comprising three phase I metabolites (resulting from oxidation, reduction, and hydrolysis of the parent drug) and two phase II metabolites (resulting from conjugation of the drug or its metabolites with another molecule). Carboxylesterase enzymes play a crucial role in the metabolism of remimazolam and are located in the cytosol and rough endoplasmic reticulum of tissues. The elimination half-life is approximately 7 to 13 minutes.

Adverse Drug Reactions: Headache, drowsiness, hypotension and involuntary movements.

Uses: ICU sedation, general anaesthesia induction and maintenance, and endoscopy (upper GI endoscopy, colonoscopy, and bronchoscopy) sedation.

Dose: Initial bolus: 5 mg i.v. over 1 minute followed by supplemental dose of 2.5 mg i.v. every 2 minutes as needed.

3. Zuranolone

Introduction: Zuranolone, also known as Sage 217, is a new antidepressant that has sedative properties. Unlike benzodiazepines, this neurosteroid, an orally-active allopregnanolone, acts as a positive allosteric modulator of the γ-aminobutyric acid (GABA) receptor.

Clinical Trial Phase / FDA-Approval: FDA-approved in 2023 for the treatment of postpartum depression under the brand name Zurzuvae and is also in Phase III trials for its use as sedative in many countries.

Mechanism of Action: The neuroactive steroid zuranolone modulates the GABA-A receptors (both synaptically and extrasynaptically) in a positive allosteric manner. It binds to a non-benzodiazepine location on the receptor to increase the GABA-A receptor gated chloride channel conductance both synaptically and extrasynaptically. This increases the chloride conductance which ultimately leads to increased chloride influx in the neurones, leading to hyperpolarization of neurones and reduced neuronal excitability leading to sedation.

Key Pharmacokinetic Parameters: Peak zuranolone concentrations occurs five to six hours after oral dosing (Tmax). Fatty meal increases its oral bioavailability. Plasma protein binding is 99%. It is excreted in both urine and faeces. Plasma t1/2 is 19-24 hours.

Adverse Drug Reactions: Drowsiness, dizziness, diarrhoea, mild cognitive impairment, and tiredness.

Uses: FDA-approved for treatment of postpartum depression and also undergoing clinical trials as sedative.

Dose: 30–50 mg orally once daily.

4. Agomelatine

Introduction: The structures of agomelatine and melatonin are similar. Because it is a potent agonist at melatonin receptors and an antagonist at serotonin-2C (5-HT2C) receptors, agomelatine is used to treat depression. It has sedative qualities as well.

Clinical Trial Phase / FDA-Approval: Currently in phase III clinical trial in several countries and approved for use (Phase IV trial) in Australia for treatment of depression. EMA approved for treatment of depression. Currently in early phases (Phase 1) of clinical trial as sedative.

Mechanism of Action: Agomelatine, a new antidepressant, acts as an antagonist at serotonin (5-HT2C) receptors and an agonist at melatonin receptors (MT1 and MT2). By acting on MT1 and MT2 receptors it acts as sedative by inducing sleep (MT1 receptor action) and also by shifting the timing of circadian rhythm (MT2 receptor action). 5-HT2C receptors are present in the GABA interneurons at raphe nucleus. 5-HT (serotonin) released from serotonergic neurones of raphe nucleus stimulates these 5-HT2C receptors at GABA interneurons - stimulates GABA interneurons - releases GABA - GABA inhibits dopaminergic neurones & nor-adrenergic neurones of pre-frontal cortex - decreases DA (Dopamine) and NA (Noradrenaline) release within the prefrontal brain. Agomelatine by inhibiting the 5-HT2C receptors inhibits GABA interneurons and rises NA and DA release in the prefrontal cortex.

Key Pharmacokinetic Parameters: Oral bioavailability is less than 5%. Plasma protein binding 95%. It is biotransformed in liver by CYP1A2 (major), CYP2C9 and CYP2C19 (minor) enzymes. Plasma half-life is about 1-2 hours.

Adverse Drug Reactions: Headache, nausea, dizziness and hepatotoxicity.

Uses: Agomelatine is indicated to treat major depressive episodes with insomnia in adults.

Dose: 25–50 mg orally at bedtime.

5. Tasimelteon

Introduction: Non-24-Hour Sleep-Wake Disorder (N24HSWD) can be treated with Tasimelteon, a selective dual melatonin receptor agonist. This disorder, which frequently affects blind people who are unable to perceive light, is frequently characterized by spells of daytime sleepiness and sleeplessness at night. Lack of light stimulation lengthens the 24-hour circadian cycle in blind people, which can result in more delayed sleep onset. Tasimelteon has been demonstrated to enhance sleep by resynchronizing the circadian cycle through its "non-photic" method, which involves activating melatonin receptors MT1 and MT2 in the brain's suprachiasmatic nucleus. The FDA designated tasimelteon an orphan medicine, making it the only medication currently licensed for the treatment of N24HSWD.

Clinical Trial Phase / FDA-Approval: FDA-approved for Non-24-Hour Sleep-Wake Disorder (N24HSWD).

Mechanism of Action: Tasimelteon works by selectively activating both the MT1 and MT2 melatonin receptors in the supra-chiasmatic nucleus (SCN) of hypothalamus, thereby helps in inducing sleep (MT1 receptor action) and regulating circadian rhythm (MT2 receptor action).

Key Pharmacokinetic Parameters: About 90% of tasimelteon is bonded to plasma proteins. Tasimelteon undergoes extensive metabolism in liver. Tasimelteon is mostly broken down by oxidation at several locations and oxidative dealkylation, which opens the dihydrofuran ring and then undergoes additional oxidation to produce a carboxylic acid. The two main isozymes involved in tasimelteon metabolism are CYP1A2 and CYP3A4. The primary phase II metabolic pathway is phenolic glucuronidation. It is mainly excreted in urine.

Adverse Drug Reactions: Headache, hepatotoxicity, nightmares or unusual dreams.

Uses: Tasimelteon oral capsules are prescribed to adults with non-24 hour sleep-wake disorder and to individuals aged 16 and above with Smith-Magenis Syndrome who have nighttime sleep difficulties. Tasimelteon oral suspension is recommended for the treatment of Smith-Magenis syndrome patients aged 3 to 15 who have overnight sleep problems.

Dose: 20 mg orally ODHS.

Challenges and Limitations of Traditional Sedatives

1. **Dependence and Tolerance:** One of the significant limitations of traditional sedatives, particularly benzodiazepines, is how long-term use leads to tolerance and dependence. Patients often require increasing doses to accomplish the same sedative effect, which can lead to drug abuse and withdrawal symptoms upon discontinuation. Newer agents, such as orexin receptor antagonists, offer an alternative with a decreased chance of dependency.

2. **Cognitive Impairment:** Many sedative-hypnotics, especially benzodiazepines, are connected to cognitive impairments, particularly among senior citizens. These impairments can include memory problems, confusion, and even an increased risk of dementia with prolonged use. The newer drugs, such as Lemborexant and Daridorexant, have been designed to minimize these cognitive side effects while maintaining their sedative efficacy.

3. **Residual Daytime Sleepiness:** Another common issue with sedatives and hypnotics is the lingering sedative effects the next day, which can impair daytime functioning and increase the risk of accidents, particularly in tasks that require alertness like driving. Agents like Daridorexant, with their shorter half-lives, aim to reduce next-day sedation while maintaining effectiveness during the night.

Future Directions in Sedative and Hypnotic Research

1. **Neurosteroid Modulators:** Neurosteroids, which modulate GABAergic activity in the brain, are a new class of sedative-hypnotics being explored. Drugs like ganaxolone are currently under investigation for their potential use in both epilepsy and sleep disorders. These agents have shown promise in reducing neural excitability while maintaining a favourable profile of side effects in contrast to traditional GABA-A agonists.

2. **Personalized Sedative Therapy:** Advances in pharmacogenomics are clearing the path for personalized methods for sedative therapy. Genetic variations that influence drug metabolism, such as polymorphisms in the cytochrome P450 enzyme family, can significantly impact an individual's response to sedatives and hypnotics. Understanding these genetic differences could lead to more individualized treatment regimens that maximize efficacy and minimize side effects.

Conclusion

A significant advancement in the treatment of anxiety and insomnia has been made with the creation of more recent sedatives and hypnotics. Many of the drawbacks of conventional sedatives, such as dependence, cognitive impairment, and residual daytime sleepiness, are addressed by these medications, which target novel pathways like the orexin system and introduce agents with faster onset and shorter half-lives. Future sedative-hypnotic treatments might provide even more individualised, secure, and efficient choices for patients as research advances, especially for those with underlying mental health issues or chronic sleep disorders.

References

1. Sneyd JR, Gambus PL, Rigby-Jones AE. Current status of perioperative hypnotics, role of benzodiazepines, and the case for remimazolam: a narrative review. British Journal of Anaesthesia. 2021 Jul 1;127(1):41-55.
2. Philip AB, Brohan J, Goudra B. The Role of GABA Receptors in Anesthesia and Sedation: An Updated Review. CNS drugs. 2025 Jan;39(1):39-54.
3. Shan W, Gao S, Ai M, Lan H, Duan G, Dong X, Xu Q, Wu Y, Wu J. The efficacy and safety of remimazolam besylate, ciprofol, and propofol during hysteroscopy. Frontiers in Pharmacology. 2025 Jan 8;15:1427755.
4. DeMartino C, Fleiss N. Premedication for Neonatal Intubation. Neonatal Airway Management. 2025 Jan 25:195-220.
5. Mihic SJ, Harris RA. Hypnotics and sedatives. In: Brunton LL, Chabner BA, Knollmann BC, editors. Goodman & Gilman's The Pharmacological Basis of Therapeutics. 12th ed. New York: McGraw-Hill; 2011. p. 457–89.
6. López-Muñoz F, Ucha-Udabe R, Alamo C. The history of barbiturates a century after their clinical introduction. Neuropsychiatric disease and treatment. 2005 Dec 1;1(4):329-43.
7. Vinkers CH, Olivier B. Mechanisms underlying tolerance after long-term benzodiazepine use: a future for subtype-selective GABAA receptor modulators? Adv Pharmacol Sci. 2012;2012:416864.
8. Meyer RE, Fish R. Pharmacology of injectable anesthetics, sedatives, and tranquilizers. In: Veterinary pharmacology and therapeutics. 8th ed. Ames: Wiley-Blackwell; 2008. p. 19–46.
9. Stahl SM. Mechanism of action of suvorexant. CNS Spectr. 2016;21(3):215–8.
10. Byatt C, Volans G. ABC of poisoning. Sedative and hypnotic drugs. British Medical Journal (Clinical research ed.). 1984 Nov 3;289(6453):1214.
11. Arnaout B, Petrakis IL. Sedative-hypnotics and anxiolytics. Addiction Medicine: Science and Practice. 2011:511-23.
12. Khouzam HR, Jackson S. Orexin receptor antagonists: alternative treatment of primary insomnia. Clin Psychol Ment Health Care. 2022;3(1):1–8. Available from: https://aditum.org/images/currentissue/1650263467Modified_Galley_Proof.pdf.
13. Ciraulo DA, Oldham M. Chapter Sixteen—Sedative Hypnotics. The Effects of Drug Abuse on the Human Nervous System (eds. Madras, B & Kuhar, M). 2014:499-532.
14. Sanger DJ. The pharmacology and mechanisms of action of new generation, non-benzodiazepine hypnotic agents. CNS drugs. 2004 Nov;18(Suppl 1):9-15.
15. Santos C, Olmedo RE, Kim J. Sedative-hypnotic drug withdrawal syndrome: recognition and treatment [digest]. Emergency medicine practice. 2017 Mar 22;19(3 Suppl Points & Pearls):S1-2.
16. Naveed M, Li LD, Sheng G, Du ZW, Zhou YP, Nan S, Zhu MY, Zhang J, Zhou QG. Agomelatine: an astounding sui-generis antidepressant? Curr Neuropharmacol. 2022;15(7):19.
17. Sukys-Claudino L, Moraes WA, Tufik S, Poyares D. The newer sedative-hypnotics. Brazilian Journal of Psychiatry. 2010;32:288-93.
18. Kaufmann CN, Spira AP, Depp CA, Mojtabai R. Continuing versus new prescriptions for sedative-hypnotic medications: United States, 2005–2012. American journal of public health. 2016 Nov;106(11):2019-25.
19. Clayton AH, Lasser R, Nandy I, Sankoh AJ, Jonas J, Kanes SJ. Zuranolone in major depressive disorder: results from MOUNTAIN—a phase 3, multicenter, double-blind, randomized, placebo-controlled trial. The Journal of Clinical Psychiatry. 2023 Feb 20;84(2):45750.
20. Millan MJ. Agomelatine for the treatment of generalized anxiety disorder: focus on its distinctive mechanism of action. Therapeutic Advances in Psychopharmacology. 2022 Jun;12:20451253221105128.
21. Dhillon S, Clarke M. Tasimelteon: first global approval. Drugs. 2014 Mar;74:505-11.
22. Kripke DF. Is suvorexant a better choice than alternative hypnotics?. F1000Research. 2015 Aug 3;4:456.
23. Hu Q, Liu X, Wen C, Li D, Lei X. Remimazolam: an updated review of a new sedative and anaesthetic. Drug Design, Development and Therapy. 2022 Jan 1:3957-74.
24. Noor N, Legendre R, Cloutet A, Chitneni A, Varrassi G, Kaye AD. A comprehensive review of remimazolam for sedation. Health psychology research. 2021 Jun 11;9(1):24514.
25. FDA Approves First Oral Treatment for Postpartum Depression. *FDA News Release*. 2023. Available from: https://www.fda.gov/news-events/press-announcements/fda-approves-first-oral-treatment-postpartum-depression.
26. Gahr M, Freudenmann RW, Connemann BJ, Hiemke C, Schönfeldt-Lecuona C. Agomelatine and hepatotoxicity: implications of cumulated data derived from spontaneous reports of adverse drug reactions. Pharmacopsychiatry. 2013 Sep;46(6):214-20.
27. Polymeropoulos CM, Mohrman MA, Keefe MS, Brzezynski JL, Wang J, Prokosch LS, Polymeropoulos VM, Xiao C, Birznieks G, Polymeropoulos MH. Efficacy of Tasimelteon (HETLIOZ®) in the Treatment of Jet Lag Disorder Evaluated in an 8-h Phase Advance Model; a Multicenter, Randomized, Double-Blind, Placebo-Controlled Trial. Front Neurol. 2020 Jul 9;11:611.

28. Ngomana C, Komape KD, Bronkhorst E. A review on holistic and pharmacological management of insomnia. SA Pharmaceutical Journal. 2025 Jan 1;92(1):11-6.
29. Yamamoto T, Inoue T, Kishimoto N, Seo K. Safety and efficacy of remimazolam in sedation dentistry: a scoping review. Journal of Dental Anesthesia and Pain Medicine. 2025 Jan 22;25(1):15.
30. Kargar A, Fetratjoo DH, Moattar R, Tarki A, Golsokhan A, Pouyan N, Amjadi-Goojgi Z, Mostafaei H, Kakeri F, Zendehbad AS, Lima BS. Efficacy of Add-on Agomelatine on Agitation, Aggression, and Neuroprotection in Alzheimer's Disease: A Randomized, Blinded, Controlled Trial. The American Journal of Geriatric Psychiatry. 2025 Mar 20.
31. Fallon JM, Hashemaghaie M, Peterson CE, Tran D, Wu SR, Valdes JM, Pedicini NM, Adams ME, Soltis M, Mansour W, Wright MC. Protocol and design of the REPOSE study: a double-blinded, randomised, placebo-controlled trial to evaluate the efficacy of suvorexant to improve postoperative sleep and reduce delirium severity in older patients undergoing non-cardiac surgery. BMJ open. 2025 Mar 1;15(3):e091099.

Chapter 8

Newer Antiepileptics

Author: Dr. Pranab Das

Introduction

Approximately 50 million people worldwide suffer from epilepsy, which continues to be one of the most prevalent chronic neurological disorders. Nearly 30% of patients still have drug-resistant epilepsy in spite of the extensive range of antiepileptic drugs (AEDs). The continuous development and approval of more recent AEDs, which aim to reduce pharmacokinetic variability and drug interactions while enhancing seizure control, tolerability, and quality of life, has been fuelled by this therapeutic gap.

The more recent AEDs, like lacosamide, perampanel, brivaracetam, cenobamate, and eslicarbazepine acetate, have a variety of modes of action, such as SV2A synaptic vesicle protein binding, AMPA receptor antagonism, and control of voltage-gated sodium channels. Some of these medications are also being investigated for their broad-spectrum efficacy and neuroprotective potential in addition to their use as monotherapy and adjunctive treatments.

Historical Perspective

Potassium bromide was first used in antiepileptic medication therapy in the middle of the 19th century. The first truly effective AED (anti-epileptic drug), phenobarbital, was introduced in 1912. Phenytoin, carbamazepine, valproic acid, and ethosuximide were among the few first-generation AEDs that dominated epilepsy treatment for a large portion of the 20th century.

Nevertheless, these early medications frequently had complex pharmacokinetics, limited therapeutic indices, and severe side effects, particularly when used in polytherapy regimens. In response, the 1990s saw a revolution in the pharmacology of epilepsy with the introduction of a number of second-generation AEDs, including levetiracetam, topiramate, and lamotrigine, all of which had improved safety profiles and fewer drug-drug interactions.

More recently, developments in biological systems, such as, neuroimaging, and molecular genetics have transformed the discovery of AEDs, enabling a move away from chance finds and towards target-based development. The therapeutic objective has not changed in spite of these advancements: seizure freedom without systemic or cognitive side effects.

Definition

Antiepileptic drugs (AEDs) are drugs for seizure control, which subdues seizure by stabilizing neuronal activity, often by modulating ion channels or neurotransmitter brain systems. The objective of AED therapy is to prevent abnormal neuronal firing that leads to seizures without causing significant sedation or cognitive impairment.

Types of Antiepileptic Drugs (AEDs)

1. **Sodium Channel Blockers:** By blocking voltage-gated sodium channels, which prevent neurones from firing repeatedly, these AEDs lower neuronal excitability. Phenytoin and carbamazepine are two examples.
2. **Calcium Channel Modulators:** By modifying calcium channels, these substances lower the release of excitatory neurotransmitters and stabilise neuronal activity. For instance, ethosuximide is used to treat absence seizures.
3. **GABAergic Drugs:** These medications increase neuronal inhibition and decrease excitability by enhancing the brain's natural gamma-aminobutyric acid (GABA) inhibitory effects. Barbiturates and benzodiazepines are classic examples.
4. **Glutamate Receptor Modulators:** These medications lessen excessive neuronal activity that causes seizures by blocking excitatory glutamate neurotransmission. Examples include Felbamate and Topiramate.

Conventional Antiepileptic Drugs

Table 1: Standard Antiepileptic Medications.

Drug Class	Drug Name	Mechanism of Action	Adverse Drug Reactions	Indications
Sodium channel blockers	Phenytoin	Stabilizes neuronal membranes by blocking voltage-gated sodium channels and preventing rapid repetitive firing.	Gingival hyperplasia, hirsutism, ataxia, nystagmus, osteoporosis.	Focal seizures, generalized tonic-clonicseizures, status epilepticus.
	Carbama-zepine		Diplopia, ataxia, hyponatremia (SIADH), agranulocytosis.	Focal seizures, generalized tonic-clonic seizures, trigeminal neuralgia.
	Lamotrigine		Skin rash (Stevens-Johnson Syndrome), diplopia.	Generalized seizures, focal seizures.
Calcium channel modulator	Ethosuxi-mide	Blocks the thalamus's T-type calcium channels.	GI distress, fatigue, hiccups.	Absence seizures.
	Gabapentin	Inhibits presynaptic voltage-gated calcium channels, reducing excitatory neurotransmitter release.	Dizziness, ataxia, peripheral oedema.	Focal seizures, neuropathic pain.
GABAergic Enhancers	Pheno-barbital	Enhances GABA-A receptor activity, prolonging chloride channel opening.	Sedation, cognitive impairment, dependence.	Generalized seizures, status epilepticus.
	Clonazepam	Benzodiazepine increases the frequency of GABA-A receptor activity.	Sedation, tolerance, dependence.	Absence seizures, myoclonic seizures.
	Valproate	Increases GABA synthesis, inhibits sodium channels and T-type calcium channels.	Hepatotoxicity, weight gain, teratogenicity (neural tube defects).	Generalized seizures, absence seizures, bipolar disorder, migraine prophylaxis.

Glutamate Inhibitors	Topiramate	Blocks AMPA receptors and enhances GABAergic transmission.	Cognitive impairment, kidney stones, weight loss.	Focal and generalized seizures, migraine prophylaxis.

Newer Antiepileptic Drugs (AEDs)

1. Brivaracetam

Introduction: Brivaracetam is an anticonvulsant that works by attaching itself to the brain's synaptic vesicle glycoprotein 2A (SV2A) and is used to treat partial-onset seizures.

Clinical Trial Phase / FDA-Approval: FDA-approved drug, under the brand name Briviact.

Mechanism of Action: Brivaracetam has a high affinity for SV2A and binds to it. SV2A regulates neurotransmitter release via synaptic vesicle exocytosis - increased excitatory neurotransmitter release - causes neuronal excitotoxicity - contribute to epileptogenesis. Brivaracetam binds to SV2A with 15 to 30 times higher affinity than levetiracetam and modulates vesicle fusion with axon terminal membrane and thereby modulates neurotransmitter release - decreased excitatory neurotransmitter release - anti-epileptogenic action. Another recognized mechanism of brivaracetam's anti-epileptogenic activity is its inhibition of Na^+ channels.

Key Pharmacokinetic Parameters: It is rapidly absorbed, with an oral bioavailability of 100%, and weak plasma binding of less than 20%. Brivaracetam levels in saliva and plasma have a strong correlation, and the volume of distribution is somewhat less than that of bodily water. It undergoes significant metabolism, mostly due to amidase hydrolysis of the acetamide group to the carboxylic acid metabolite. It is primarily excreted in urine.

Adverse Drug Reactions: Changes in mood or behaviour, problems with coordination, or unusual tiredness or weakness, drowsiness and dizziness.

Uses: Used as a supplemental treatment for patients 16 years of age or older who have partial-onset seizures.

Dose: 50 mg/day (25 mg BID or 50 mg once daily).

2. Perampanel

Introduction: Perampanel is a selective, non-competitive antagonist of AMPA receptors. AMPA receptors mediate excitatory glutamate neurotransmission. It offers the benefit of once-daily dosage for both focal seizures and generalized tonic-clonic seizures. Nevertheless, it has been linked to psychological adverse effects, such as aggression and irritability.

Clinical Trial Phase / FDA-Approval: FDA-approved drug, approved under the brand name Fycompa.

Mechanism of Action: Perampanel is a new non-competitive selective antagonist at the postsynaptic ionotropic alpha-amino-3-hydroxy-5-methyl-4-isoxazolepropionic acid (AMPA) glutamate receptor. Although glutamate is a well-known excitatory neurotransmitter in the neurological system, it is unclear how exactly perampanel prevents epilepsy in people. Antagonism of AMPA receptors has been shown to help prevent the onset and progression of seizures and may reduce the overstimulation of excitatory neurones in the central nervous system, which in turn may have anticonvulsant effects. Additionally, AMPA receptor antagonists may prevent the death of neurones.

Key Pharmacokinetic Parameters: Rapid and complete absorption (100% oral bioavailability) having a very low first-pass metabolism. 95% bound to plasma proteins. Cytochrome P450 (CYP) 3A4/5, CYP1A2, and

CYP2B6 mediate the extensive oxidation and subsequent glucuronidation of perampanel. Perampanel has a half-life of roughly 105 hours.

Adverse Drug Reactions: Dizziness, fatigue, headache, ataxia, falls (especially in elderly patients), somnolence and irritability.

Uses: Perampanel is approved for the treatment of partial-onset seizures in patients with epilepsy who are four years of age or older, with or without secondary generalised seizures. It can also be taken as a supplementary therapy to treat primary generalised tonic-clonic seizures in epileptics aged 12 years and above.

Dose: 2 mg once daily at bedtime.

3. Eslicarbazepine Acetate

Introduction: Eslicarbazepine (ESL) is a prodrug of carbamazepine, which blocks sodium channels that are voltage-gated. It is primarily used for focal seizures and has a better tolerability profile than carbamazepine, with a decreased chance of negative consequences like hyponatremia. Eslicarbazepine is also metabolized less extensively by the liver, which may reduce drug-drug interactions.

Clinical Trial Phase / FDA-Approval: FDA-approved drug (approved under the brand name Aptiom).

Mechanism of Action: ESL specifically enhances the slow inactivation of voltage-gated sodium channels (VGSC), in hyperactive neurones, hence diminishing neuronal excitability and action potential discharge. Eslicarbazepine preferentially binds to the inactivated state of the sodium channel, rather than the resting state. It stabilises the channel in the slow-inactivated state, inhibiting its transition to the resting or open state. This diminishes the quantity of accessible channels for reopening, resulting in fewer action potentials and reduced neuronal activity. In contrast to medications such as carbamazepine, which primarily focus on rapid inactivation, ESL preserves typical neural activity, as normal firing does not significantly induce slow inactivation, thereby it specifically targets hyperactive neurones, which experience frequent depolarisations leading to increased delayed inactivation and mitigates cognitive and motor adverse effects often associated with older sodium channel blockers. Lastly, Cav3.2 T-type Ca2+ channels are inhibited by ESL. In mice, it has been demonstrated that blocking these channels reduces spontaneous seizures and eliminates the neuropathological indicators of chronic epilepsy. The capacity of ESL to prevent seizures is improved by blocking these epileptogenic channels.

Key Pharmacokinetic Parameters: About 94% of administered eslicarbazepine is bioavailable, and 30% of it is bound to human plasma proteins. In the CSF fluid, it has an effective half-life of 20 to 24 hours. Two to three hours after oral administration, the drug achieves its peak plasma concentration, and four to five days later, it enters a steady state in the plasma. It is primarily excreted via urine.

Adverse Drug Reactions: The most common side effects include headache, fatigue, dizziness, and diplopia. There may also be nausea, vomiting, impaired vision, and somnolence.

Uses: Eslicarbazepine acetate is a safe and efficient option for treating partial-onset seizures as an adjuvant or monotherapy. Because it can be taken once daily, interacts with fewer drugs, and has fewer side effects, eslicarbazepine acetate is better than its predecessors, carbamazepine and oxcarbazepine.

Dose: 400 mg once daily.

4. Lacosamide

Introduction: Lacosamide is a novel AED that improves or enhances slow inactivation of voltage-gated sodium channel without influencing fast inactivation, a mechanism distinct from other sodium channel blockers. This selective effect reduces the likelihood of side effects associated with sodium channel modulation. Lacosamide is authorized to treat adult focal seizures and has demonstrated a good safety and tolerability profile.

Clinical Trial Phase / FDA-Approval: FDA-approved drug (approved under the Vimpat brand).

Mechanism of Action: Lacosamide stabilizes hyperexcitable neuronal membranes and inhibits recurrent neuronal firing by selectively enhancing the slow inactivation of voltage-gated sodium channels, thereby delaying their return to their active state. This reduces repetitive neuronal firing without significantly affecting normal physiological activity. It may also interact with collapsin response mediator protein-2. The rapid component of voltage-gated sodium currents is unaffected by lacosamide, unlike traditional sodium channel blockers.

Key Pharmacokinetic Parameters: Following oral treatment, lacosamide is fully absorbed with very little first-pass effect. It has a high bioavailability (about 100%). The rate and degree of absorption are unaffected by food. O-desmethyl lacosamide, a significant, pharmacologically inactive metabolite in humans, is produced when CYP3A4, CYP2C9, and CYP2C19 metabolize lacosamide. Mostly it is eliminated by urine.

Adverse Drug Reactions: Dizziness, nausea, cardiac conduction defects, tremors, blurred vision and confusion.

Uses: Children and adults with partial-onset seizures are treated with lacosamide in the US and Europe. In Canada, it is only allowed for use by adults. It can also be used as an adjuvant medication to treat primary generalised tonic-clonic seizures in patients aged four and up. Extended-release capsules of Lacosamide are used to treat partial-onset seizures in adults and children weighing at least 50 kg.

Dose: 50 mg BID.

5. Ganaxolone

Introduction: Ganaxolone is a neuroactive steroid and a new antiepileptic drug, chemically analogous to allopregnanolone, intended to augment GABAergic inhibition without exhibiting hormonal effects. It is specifically utilised for uncommon genetic epilepsies.

Clinical Trial Phase / FDA-Approval: In 2022, the FDA approved ganaxolone under the brand name Ztalmy to treat seizures associated with CDKL5 deficiency disorder (CDD) in children ages 2 years and up. It consequently became the first drug approved for this uncommon condition. Prior to being approved, it underwent successful Phase 3 trials (Marigold Study).

Mechanism of Action: Ganaxolone is a positive allosteric modulator of the GABA-A receptor, binding specifically to a neurosteroid site on both synaptic and extrasynaptic receptors. It hyperpolarises neurones by augmenting GABA-induced chloride inflow, hence diminishing neuronal excitability. Its effect on extrasynaptic GABA-A δ-subunit-containing receptors provides prolonged tonic inhibition, which may be particularly significant in hereditary epilepsies. Significantly, ganaxolone does not interact with hormone receptors, so circumventing the endocrine side effects associated with endogenous neurosteroids.

Key Pharmacokinetic Parameters: The drug ganaxolone is taken orally. It shows moderate bioavailability and undergoes extensive metabolism in the liver, mainly through CYP3A4. Plasma half-life is approximately 34 to 38 hours. The extended half-life facilitates dosing three times a day in clinical practice. Plasma peak concentrations occur approximately 1 to 2 hours after administration. It shows high degree of plasma protein binding. It is mainly eliminated through faeces, with a lesser amount excreted in urine.

Adverse Drug Reactions: Typical dose-related adverse effects include somnolence, dizziness, fatigue, diarrhoea and gait disturbances.

Uses: Ganaxolone is approved for the treatment of CDKL5 deficiency, a severe and uncommon form of developmental and epileptic encephalopathy (DEE). Additionally, it is being studied for status epilepticus, fragile X syndrome, and Lennox-Gastaut syndrome.

Dose: 63 mg/kg/day.

6. Other recently approved drugs:

A. Cannabidiol (CBD)

The FDA has approved a specific, purified form of cannabidiol (CBD) called Epidiolex, to treat uncommon types of epilepsy, such as Dravet syndrome and Lennox-Gastaut syndrome in patients of more than or equal to 2 years of age. Its exact mechanism is not entirely known, although it is believed to include the modulation of multiple receptors, including TRPV1 and GPR55, and the inhibition of adenosine reuptake. CBD represents a novel treatment choice for those suffering from drug-resistant epilepsy, particularly in paediatric populations.

Recent Advances in the Management of Status Epilepticus

Status epilepticus is an emergency medical condition characterised by persistent seizure lasting five minutes or longer, or by two or more seizures occurring without complete recovery of consciousness in between. Prompt treatment is essential to prevent permanent neurological damage. Traditional treatment involves the use of benzodiazepines, followed by second-line AEDs like phenytoin or valproate if the seizures persist. Recent advances in SE management focus on new AEDs, improved protocols for treatment escalation, and the development of non-invasive options.

1. **Intranasal and Buccal Midazolam:** The use of non-invasive routes of benzodiazepine administration has been a significant advance in SE management. Intranasal and buccal midazolam provide rapid seizure control without the need for intravenous access, making them ideal for pre-hospital and emergency use. These formulations have been shown to be as effective as intravenous diazepam for terminating seizures and offer the advantage of easier administration in non-clinical settings.
2. **Ketamine in Refractory Status Epilepticus (RSE):** Ketamine, an antagonist of the NMDA receptor, has gained attention for its use in refractory status epilepticus (RSE), where seizures are unresponsive to conventional treatments. Ketamine's neuroprotective properties, combined with its ability to block excitotoxicity via NMDA receptor inhibition, make it a valuable option in RSE or refractory status epilepticus. Studies have shown that ketamine can be effective in controlling seizures when traditional AEDs fail, offering hope in difficult-to-treat cases.
3. **Lacosamide in Status Epilepticus:** Lacosamide has also been studied for use in SE, particularly in cases where first- and second-line treatments are ineffective. Its novel mechanism of action, enhancing slow sodium channel inactivation, makes it a promising option for managing both focal and generalized SE. Early administration of Lacosamide in the treatment protocol has been connected to with improved outcomes and less danger of progression to RSE or refractory status epileptics.

Recent Advances in Status Epilepticus (SE) Management

Table 2: Recent Developments in the Management of Status Epilepticus (SE).

Treatment	Mechanism of Action	Clinical Use	Salient Features
Intranasal Midazolam	GABA-A receptor agonist	Pre-hospital SE management	Non-invasive, rapid onset
Ketamine	NMDA receptor antagonist	Refractory status epilepticus (RSE)	Effective in RSE, shows neuroprotective effects
Lacosamide	Enhances slow sodium channel inactivation	Early SE management	Reduces progression to refractory SE

Challenges and Limitations of Newer AEDs

1. **Cost and Accessibility:** While newer AEDs often offer better tolerability and fewer side effects, they are generally more expensive than traditional options, which may limit accessibility for some patients, especially in low-income settings. The high cost of cannabidiol, for example, can be prohibitive for families managing paediatric epilepsy.
2. **Side Effects and Drug Interactions:** Although many newer AEDs are associated with fewer side effects than older drugs, they are not without risks. Perampanel, for instance, has been linked to psychiatric side effects, which can be severe in some patients. Careful monitoring and dose adjustments are essential to mitigate these risks.
3. **Efficacy in Drug-Resistant Epilepsy:** Despite the development of newer AEDs, drug-resistant epilepsy remains a significant challenge. For patients who do not respond to multiple AEDs, surgical interventions, such as vagus nerve stimulation or resective surgery, may still be necessary. The search for more effective treatments for drug-resistant epilepsy continues to be a key focus of epilepsy research.

Conclusion

The therapeutic options for managing epilepsy have vastly increased with the development of more recent antiepileptic drugs, especially for patients with drug-resistant forms of the condition. Agents that offer new improved safety profiles and modes of action, such as brivaracetam, perampanel, and cannabidiol, represent significant advancements in the field. The use of ketamine and intranasal midazolam, two recent developments in the treatment of status epilepticus, has improved our capacity to treat acute seizures in emergency situations. Nevertheless, issues with medication costs, adverse effects, and treatment resistance still exist, underscoring the necessity of ongoing study and development in the treatment of epilepsy.

References

1. Onyekere C, Smart S. Seizure Alert: An Interdisciplinary Protocol for the Timely Administration of Anti-epileptic Medication in the Setting of Status Epilepticus (P7-3.005). InNeurology 2025 Apr 8 (Vol. 104, No. 7_Supplement_1, p. 5775). Hagerstown, MD: Lippincott Williams & Wilkins.
2. Nivitha M, Narayanan J, Chitra V. A review on the cognitive impairment caused by anti-epileptics and their management.
3. ALSaeedy M, Hasan A, Al-Adhreai A, Alrabie A, Qaba H, Mashrah A, Öncü-Kaya EM. An overview of liquid chromatographic methods for analyzing new generation anti-epileptic drugs. Journal of Liquid Chromatography & Related Technologies. 2022 May 9;45(5-8):66-83.
4. Löscher W, Schmidt D. Modern antiepileptic drug development has failed to deliver: ways out of the current dilemma. Epilepsia. 2011;52(4):657–78.
5. Bialer M, White HS. Key factors in the discovery and development of new antiepileptic drugs. Nat Rev Drug Discov. 2010;9(1):68–82.

6. Perucca E, French J, Bialer M. Development of new antiepileptic drugs: challenges, incentives, and recent advances. The lancet neurology. 2007 Sep 1;6(9):793-804.
7. French JA, Gazzola DM. New generation antiepileptic drugs: what do they offer in terms of improved tolerability and safety?. Therapeutic advances in drug safety. 2011 Aug;2(4):141-58.
8. White HS. Preclinical development of antiepileptic drugs: past, present, and future directions. Epilepsia. 2003 Sep;44:2-8.
9. Brodie MJ. Antiepileptic drug therapy the story so far. Seizure. 2010 Dec 1;19(10):650-5.
10. Sánchez-Villalobos JM, Aledo-Serrano Á, Villegas-Martínez I, Shaikh MF, Alcaraz M. Epilepsy treatment in neuro-oncology: a rationale for drug choice in common clinical scenarios. Front Pharmacol. 2022;13:991244.
11. Rho JM, White HS. Brief history of anti-seizure drug development. Epilepsia open. 2018 Dec;3:114-9.
12. Manford M. Recent advances in epilepsy. Journal of neurology. 2017 Aug;264(8):1811-24.
13. Beuchat I, Novy J, Rossetti AO. Newer antiepileptic drugs for status epilepticus in adults: What's the evidence?. CNS drugs. 2018 Mar;32:259-67.
14. Trinka E, Brigo F, Shorvon S. Recent advances in status epilepticus. Curr Opin Neurol. 2016;29(2):189-98.
15. Trinka E, Kälviäinen R. 25 years of advances in the definition, classification and treatment of status epilepticus. Seizure. 2017 Jan 1;44:65-73.
16. Jaques L, Rossetti AO. Newer antiepileptic drugs in the treatment of status epilepticus: impact on prognosis. Epilepsy &Behavior. 2012 May 1;24(1):70-3.
17. Kapur J. Status epilepticus and seizures. Current Opinion in Critical Care. 1998 Apr 1;4(2):83-8.
18. Ernst LD, Boudreau EA. Recent advances in epilepsy management. Current Opinion in Anesthesiology. 2016 Oct 1;29(5):558-62.
19. Fatuzzo D, Novy J, Rossetti AO. Use of newer antiepileptic drugs and prognosis in adults with status epilepticus: comparison between 2009 and 2017. Epilepsia. 2018 Jul;59(7):e98-102.
20. Klein P, Diaz A, Gasalla T, Whitesides J. A review of the pharmacology and clinical efficacy of brivaracetam. Clinical pharmacology: advances and applications. 2018 Jan 19:1-22.
21. Raedler LA. Fycompa (perampanel hydrate) receives expanded indication for primary generalized tonic-clonic seizures. American Health & Drug Benefits. 2016 Mar;9(Spec Feature):88.
22. Greenwood J, Valdes J. Perampanel (Fycompa): a review of clinical efficacy and safety in epilepsy. Pharmacy and Therapeutics. 2016 Nov;41(11):683.
23. Galiana GL, Gauthier AC, Mattson RH. Eslicarbazepine acetate: a new improvement on a classic drug family for the treatment of partial-onset seizures. Drugs in R&D. 2017 Sep;17:329-39.
24. Beydoun A, D'Souza J, Hebert D, Doty P. Lacosamide: pharmacology, mechanisms of action and pooled efficacy and safety data in partial-onset seizures. Expert review of neurotherapeutics. 2009 Jan 1;9(1):33-42.
25. Rang HP, Ritter JM, Flower RJ, Henderson G. *Rang & Dale's Pharmacology*. 9th ed. Elsevier; 2020.
26. Brunton LL, Hilal-Dandan R, Knollmann BC. *Goodman & Gilman's The Pharmacological Basis of Therapeutics*. 13th ed. New York: McGraw-Hill Education; 2018.
27. Knupp KG, Mowrey W, Tollerson D, Wusthoff CJ, Du W, Laux LC, et al. Randomized trial of ganaxolone in CDKL5 deficiency disorder. Epilepsia. 2021;62(9):2158–70.
28. U.S. Food and Drug Administration. Ztalmy (ganaxolone) prescribing information [Internet]. Silver Spring (MD): FDA; 2022 [cited 2025 Apr 4]. Available from: https://www.accessdata.fda.gov/drugsatfda_docs/label/2022/215600s000lbl.pdf.

Chapter 9

RecentAdvancesin the Management of Parkinsonism

Author: Dr. Pranab Das

Introduction

The hallmarks of Parkinson's disease (PD), a progressive neurodegenerative illness, include bradykinesia, rigidity, resting tremor, and postural instability. These symptoms arise from a lack of dopamine in the striatal pathways caused by the degeneration of dopaminergic neurones in the substantia nigra pars compacta. The cornerstone of managing Parkinson's disease (PD) is still pharmacological intervention, which aims to control both motor and non-motor symptoms, modulate non-dopaminergic systems, and restore dopaminergic tone.

Current anti-parkinsonian medications target different dopaminergic pathway points. The best symptomatic treatment is still levodopa, frequently in combination with peripheral dopa-decarboxylase inhibitors (like carbidopa). Nevertheless, dyskinesias and motor fluctuations are linked to long-term levodopa use. Adjunctive medications have been developed to address these problems, including glutamate antagonists (e.g., amantadine), catechol-O-methyltransferase (COMT) inhibitors, monoamine oxidase-B (MAO-B) inhibitors, and dopamine agonists. More recent medications such as opicapone, istradefylline, and safinamide are aiding in the improvement of patient outcomes and therapy.

Historical Perspective

Anticholinergic drugs, such as belladonna alkaloids, were empirically used to treat tremors in the 19th century, which is when anti-parkinsonian pharmacotherapy first emerged. However, Ehringer and Hornykiewicz's discovery of the pathophysiological role of dopamine in Parkinson's disease in the 1950s and 1960s marked the beginning of the therapeutic revolution. Levodopa therapy was introduced in 1967 as a result of this ground-breaking discovery, revolutionising the treatment of Parkinson's disease and continuing to be the gold standard today.

The development of dopamine agonists (such as pramipexole and bromocriptine) in later decades offered substitutes or supplements to levodopa and assisted in delaying motor complications. The 1990s saw the development of COMT inhibitors (entacapone, tolcapone) and MAO-B inhibitors (selegiline, rasagiline), which increased the half-life of levodopa and further enhanced dopaminergic action.

In order to treat levodopa-induced dyskinesias and motor fluctuations, more recent developments have focused on non-dopaminergic pathways, such as glutamatergic, adenosinergic, and serotonergic systems. The shift from symptomatic relief to disease-modifying approaches is also reflected in research into gene therapy, neuroprotective drugs, and continuous infusion systems.

The transition from belladonna extracts to receptor-specific modulators demonstrates an impressive development influenced by advances in patient-centered care, medication design, and neuroscience.

Definition

The American Psychological Association (APA) defines Parkinson's disease (PD) as a progressive neurodegenerative disorder that impairs the brain's dopamine-producing neurones, resulting in movement problems such as tremors, rigidity, and bradykinesia. Although Parkinson's disease is the most prevalent cause of Parkinsonism, identical symptoms can also be caused by other disorders such as progressive supranuclear palsy (PSP) and multiple system atrophy (MSA).

Types of Parkinsonism

1. **Primary Parkinsonism (Parkinson's Disease):** This is the most prevalent and typical form of the illness, characterised by the progressive death of dopamine-producing neurones in the brain.
2. **Secondary Parkinsonism:** Parkinsonism induced by additional elements, like drugs, toxins, or head trauma.
3. **Atypical Parkinsonism:** Includes disorders like progressive supranuclear palsy (PSP) and multiple system atrophy (MSA), which resemble Parkinson's disease but progress more quickly and have more non-motor symptoms.

Conventional Treatments for Parkinsonism

Table 1: Standard interventions for Parkinsonism.

Drug Class	Drug Name	Pharmacokinetics	Adverse Drug Reaction	Indications
Dopamine precursor	Levodopa	High first pass metabolism in g.i.t. mucosa & liver. About 1% of administered Levodopa enters the brain. Plasma t1/2 is 1-2 hours.	Nausea, vomiting, postural hypotension, cardiac arrhythmia, exacerbation of angina, dyskinesia, depression, hallucination.	The preferred drug and still the first line of treatment for Parkinson's disease is levodopa.
Peripheral DOPA decarboxylase inhibitor	Carbidopa	Levodopa's plasma t1/2 is prolonged. Systemic concentration of dopamine is reduced – nausea & vomiting is minimized.	Involuntary movements & behavioural abnormalities may be more pronounced. Excessive day time sleepiness may occur.	Currently, levodopa is practically used along with dopa decarboxylase inhibitor.
Dopaminergic agonist	Pramipexole	Twice as potent as ropinirole, but comparable in efficacy & tolerability.	Nausea, dizziness, hallucination, postural hypotension, behavioural abnormalities like impulsive shopping, betting, gambling.	Used as a monotherapy in early cases & along with levodopa in advanced cases.
MAO-B inhibitors	Selegiline	Partly metabolised by liver into amphetamine which sometimes causes insomnia & agitation. It interacts with Pethidine, SSRIs, etc.	Nausea, postural hypotension, insomnia, accentuation of levodopa induced involuntary movements.	Used along with levodopa +/- carbidopa.

COMT inhibitors	Entacapone	Entacapone acts only in the periphery. Duration of action - 2 hrs.	Nausea, vomiting, diarrhoea, dyskinesia, postural hypotension, hallucinations.	Useful for managing motor fluctuations ("wearing off" effect) in patients taking levodopa. Prolongs levodopa effect & allows levodopa dose to be reduced.
Central anticholinergics	Trihexyphenidyl	Rapidly absorbed for g.i.t. Onset of action is within 1 hr. Duration of action is 6-12 hrs.	Dry mouth, constipation, hypotension, and urinary retention.	Drug of choice for drug-induced Parkinsonism.

Recent Advances in Pharmacotherapy

1. Liposome based targeting of Dopamine to the brain:

It is currently in pre-clinical phase of clinical trials. The diacylglycerol moiety of the liposomes is connected by a linker to a five-amino acid peptide derived from amyloid precursor protein (APP), which is recognized by particular BBB transporter(s) and receptor(s). Drugs can be delivered into the brain through the blood-brain barrier thanks to this liposomal mechanism. In a mouse model of Parkinson's disease (PD), the brain-directed liposomal system was employed. When liposomes loaded with dopamine (DA) were administered intraperitoneally (IP), there was a positive association between the liposomal DA dose and the behavioural effects in mice treated with hemi-parkinsonian amphetamine. The ideal dopamine (DA) dose was 60 µg/kg. Compared to standard dosages of the DA precursor levodopa (in the mg/kg range), this is a much lower dose. Mice treated with amphetamine showed a considerable rise in striatal DA within 5 minutes after receiving IP injections of APP-targeted liposomes loaded with a DA dosage of 800 µg/kg. A significant DA release from the liposomal drug delivery is shown by the increase in striatal DA content that lasted for at least three hours after administration. Neither the liver nor the heart showed any increase in DA content. Rats and guinea pigs also showed comparable increases in striatal DA. The APP-targeted liposomal DA delivery technology allows substances to pass across the blood-brain barrier and could be used to treat Parkinson's disease and other brain disorders.

Dose: Not yet clinically standardized.

2. Safinamide

Introduction: A more recent medication called safinamide acts as a selective inhibitor of monoamine oxidase B (MAO-B). It is distinct from other anti-Parkinson's drugs due to its dual mechanism, which provides both dopaminergic and non-dopaminergic effects. In the later stages of the disease, safinamide is used as an adjuvant to levodopa to help regulate motor irregularities. Safinamide is a useful adjunct to Parkinson's treatment since clinical studies have demonstrated that it decreases "off" time without exacerbating dyskinesias.

Clinical Trial Phase / FDA-Approval: FDA-approved medication. It received approval under the Xadago brand.

Mechanism of Action: Safinamide is a reversible selective inhibitor of MAO-B. In comparison to rasagiline, which is 203 times more selective for MAO-B, and selegiline, which is 127 times more selective for MAO-B, safinamide has roughly 1,000 times greater selectivity for MAO-B over MAO-A. By inhibiting the MAO-B enzyme, predominantly expressed in brain tissues, it elevates dopamine levels in the striatum by reducing its degradation mediated by the MAO-B enzyme. Consequently, while safinamide should not be used together with other MAO inhibitors or sympathomimetic agents, the "cheese reaction" has not been demonstrated in phase IV trials, and theoretically, the associated risk is much reduced. Safinamide is distinctive since it not only inhibits MAO-B but also obstructs voltage-gated sodium and N-type calcium channels, hence altering glutamate release and exhibiting effects akin to the NMDA receptor antagonism of amantadine. Furthermore, its pharmacological profile suggests it may influence the metabolism of biogenic amines beyond dopamine. Consequently, it has been suggested that safinamide may alleviate non-motor symptoms of Parkinson's disease (PD), including melancholy, apathy, and cognitive function (perhaps via enhancing attentiveness, analogous to the effects reported in patients with other NMDA receptor antagonists). It has been investigated and has potential in alleviating pain syndromes in people with Parkinson's disease (PD) due to its influence on dopamine, sodium, and calcium channels. Finally, data suggests that safinamide exhibits neuroprotective properties attributed to its ion channel blockade and MAO-B inhibition, observed in both in vitro and in vivo studies (animal models).

Key Pharmacokinetic Parameters: It is quickly absorbed, reaching its peak concentration (Cmax) two to four hours after consumption. Food has no influence on its absorption, and the first-pass effect is minimal. Just 5% of safinamide is eliminated unaltered through the urine, and its elimination half-life is roughly around 20–26 hours. Compared to the half-lives of the other MAO-B inhibitors, this is noticeably longer. Three processes lead to metabolism of the drug: oxidation of safinamide or safinamide acid (to N-dealkylated acid), oxidative breakage of the ether link (to O-debenzylated safinamide), and amide hydrolytic oxidation (to safinamide acid). These metabolites don't have any pharmacological activity.

Adverse Drug Reactions: Nausea, dyskinesia, insomnia and orthostatic hypotension.

Uses: The FDA and European Commission approved safinamide as an adjunct therapy to levodopa for patients with advanced Parkinson's disease experiencing motor fluctuations, either as a standalone treatment or in combination with other Parkinson's disease medications.

Dose: 50–100 mg once daily orally.

3. IRX4204

Introduction: IRX4204 is a second-generation RXR agonist currently being assessed in studies focused on the treatment of non-small cell lung cancer and Parkinson's disease.

Clinical Trial Phase / FDA-approval: Currently in phase I/II trial.

Mechanism of Action: Selectively activates RXR-Nurr 1 receptor complex. It crosses BBB, activates Nurr 1 receptor (orphan receptor), which oversees the maintenance & survival of dopaminergic neurons.

Activation of Nurr 1 receptor:

1. Promotes TH gene transcription - Increase in TH+ neurons.
2. Activates Ret & subsequent signalling pathway - Increase dopaminergic neuron survival.
3. Inhibits NF-kB pro-inflammatory pathway - Decreases neuroinflammation.
4. Regulates mitochondrial reproduction & regulation of mitochondrial function.

Key Pharmacokinetic Parameters: IRX4204 is well absorbed and has pharmacokinetics consistent with once per day oral dosing to humans.

Adverse Drug Reactions: Nausea, diarrhea, hypersensitivity and possible hepatotoxicity.

Uses: Currently in phase I/II study for Parkinson's disease treatment.

Dose: 1-5 mg/day (in clinical trials).

4. Prasinezumab

Introduction: Prasinezumab, an investigational humanised monoclonal immunoglobulin G1 antibody, targeting an epitope located at the carboxyl terminus of human alpha-synuclein.

Clinical Trial Phase / FDA-Approval: Currently in Phase II (IIb) trial (PASADENA trial).

Mechanism of Action: It exhibits a robust affinity and avidity for human aggregated alpha-synuclein. Preclinical pharmacological evaluations were performed on two transgenic mouse lines, Line D and Line 61, exhibiting alpha-synuclein aggregation disorders to evaluate the efficacy and potency of the murine variant of prasinezumab (9E4). During a period of five to six months, the mice were administered prasinezumab (9E4) by weekly intraperitoneal injections. They exhibited enhanced cognitive and motor functions, reduced gliosis, less neuronal and synaptic loss, and decreased intraneuronal accumulation of alpha-synuclein disease, as seen by alpha-synuclein inclusions in cortical and subcortical areas. Preclinical data indicate a potential role of the lysosomal route, while the principal mechanism of action of prasinezumab is proposed to be the suppression of cell-to-cell transmission of alpha-synuclein by the extracellular neutralisation of alpha-synuclein aggregates.

Key Pharmacokinetic Parameters: It is administered intravenously. It shows linear pharmacokinetics within the therapeutic range used in Parkinson's trials. Plasma t1/2 is approximately about 18-28 days. It is mainly eliminated by bile.

Adverse Drug Reactions: Undergoing ADR evaluation in ongoing clinical trials.

Uses: Early Parkinson's disease.

Dose: 1500–4500 mg IV every 4 weeks.

5. Istradefylline

Introduction: Istradefylline is a selective antagonist of adenosine A2A receptors that modulates dopaminergic activity by blocking the inhibitory effects of adenosine on dopamine D2 receptors. It is approved in conjunction with levodopa to treat "off" episodes. Studies show that istradefylline can significantly reduce "off" time, especially in individuals with motor irregularities in spite of optimized dopaminergic therapy.

Clinical Trial Phase / FDA-Approval: Approved by FDA under the brand name Nourianz.

Mechanism of Action: It is believed that istradefylline works by antagonizing the adenosine A2A receptor to provide its antiparkinsonian effects. It is uncertain how elevated expression of these receptors in the striatum or substantia nigra (SN) relates to the pathophysiology of Parkinson's disease. Adenosine stimulates the A2A receptors on indirect pathway neurones by binding to them, thereby activating Gs protein signalling - this increases cAMP generation – which increases GABA release from striatal neurones, thereby reducing motor activity and thalamus inhibition. Dopamine shortage already overactivates the indirect pathway in Parkinson's disease, hence aggravating bradykinesia and stiffness. On indirect pathway neurones, istradefylline is a selective antagonist of the adenosine A2A receptors. It results in decreased A2A receptor activation - decreased cAMP production - reduced GABA release from striatal neurones - less thalamic inhibition and more thalamocortical excitation - improved movement.

Key Pharmacokinetic Parameters: It is administered orally and peak plasma levels are achieved in 4 hours. Plasma protein binding is 98%. The active 4'-O-monodesmethyl istradefylline (M1) is the main metabolite detected in urine. The primary metabolizers of istradefylline are CYP1A1, CYP3A4, and CYP3A5. CYP1A2, CYP2B6, CYP2C8, CYP2C9, CYP2C18, and CYP2D6 also have a role in istradefylline metabolism. Istradefylline has a terminal elimination half-life of 64–69 hours.

Adverse Drug Reactions: Dyskinesia, dizziness, nausea, hallucinations, insomnia and constipation.

Uses: Approved by the FDA to lessen motor fluctuations as an additional treatment for Parkinson's disease.

Dose: 20–40 mg once daily orally.

6. Drugs in Phase IV trial & FDA-approved drugs:

a. **Inhaled Levodopa:** In 2018, the FDA authorised inhaled Levodopa powder. Inhaled Levodopa is utilised in conjunction with oral Levodopa/Carbidopa therapy to manage OFF periods. Adverse effects include cough, upper respiratory tract infection, discoloured sputum, and nausea. It is offered in a 42 mg Levodopa inhalation cartridge. Dosage - 84 milligrams inhaled up to five times day.

b. **Scored Levodopa/Carbidopa tablet:** A novel scored tablet comprising Carbidopa/Levodopa 6.25/25 mg in each segment for precise dosing was introduced in 2021. Each tablet consists of four parts that can be detached and ingested individually. It is offered as a Carbidopa/Levodopa pill of 25/100 mg. Dosage - 1 pill three times per day.

c. **Sublingual Apomorphine:** One of the strong dopamine agonist is apomorphine. It was utilized as a rescue treatment for OFF episodes and has been accessible as a subcutaneous (s.c.) injection since 2004. There are certain inherent difficulties in using the s.c. injection. –

   1. Assembly of medication
   2. Supervised dose titration
   3. Side effects like nausea, injection site pain & reactions.
   4. This makes it difficult to self-administer.

In May 2020, FDA approved sublingual apomorphine for the treatment of OFF episodes. It is available as 10, 15, 20, 25 & 30 mg sublingual film. Dose – 10-30 mg upto 5 times a day (>2 hrs apart), concomitant anti-emetic should be started 3 days before the initiation of therapy.

d. **Opicapone:** Levodopa/Carbidopa is administered in conjunction with COMT inhibitors to extend the duration of Levodopa's efficacy. Entacapone and tolcapone, both inhibitors of catechol-O-methyltransferase (COMT), have been utilised for an extended period. Nonetheless, owing to its significant and fatal hepatotoxicity, tolcapone is no longer widely utilised. The utilisation of entacapone is similarly constrained, due to its repeated daily dose regimen. Opicapone received FDA approval in 2020 and was determined to be preferable to the aforementioned two medications due to its reduced hepatotoxicity potential. It is administered orally once each day. It is offered in a 50 mg tablet form. Dose – 50 mg once day; 25 mg once daily for moderate hepatic impairment. Adverse effects include dyskinesia, diarrhoea, and hypotension.

e. **Extended-release Amantadine:** Amantadine functions as an antagonist of NMDA receptors. An extended-release version of amantadine hydrochloride was licensed in 2018 as an adjuvant treatment for OFF episodes in levodopa-induced Parkinson's disease (PD). It is available in 129 mg, 193 mg, and 258 mg tablets. Dosage - 129 milligrams each morning. Adverse effect notably are hallucinations, vertigo, xerostomia, and constipation.

Recent Advances in Non-Pharmacological Treatment

1. **Deep Brain Stimulation (DBS):** Patients with severe Parkinson's disease are now routinely treated with deep brain stimulation who do not adequately respond to medication. Electrodes are surgically inserted into particular brain areas during DBS, such as the globus pallidus or the subthalamic nucleus (STN) or Globus Pallidus interna (GPi), to modulate abnormal brain activity. DBS has been demonstrated to enhance quality of life, lessen the need for medication, and improve motor symptoms in patients with PD. Recent advances in DBS technology include directional leads that allow for more precise targeting of stimulation thereby reducing its side effects.
2. **Focused Ultrasound (FUS):** Without requiring surgery, focused ultrasound targets and destroys particular regions of brain tissue using high-intensity sound waves. FUS is being investigated for different neurodegenerative diseases and has demonstrated potential in treating tremor-dominant Parkinson's disease. Unlike DBS, focused ultrasound does not require the implantation of electrodes, offering a less invasive option for patients with movement disorders.
3. **Gene Therapy:** Gene therapy is a new area in the treatment of Parkinson's disease, focusing on delivering genes that can restore or protect dopaminergic neurons. One promising approach is the delivery of genes that are involved in for enzymes like tyrosine hydroxylase and aromatic L-amino acid decarboxylase that are involved in the production of dopamine. Early-phase clinical Parkinson's disease gene therapy trials have shown potential in slowing disease progression and improving motor problems, although further study is required before these therapies become widely available.

Non-Pharmacological Advances

Table 2: Non-Pharmacological Innovations in the Management of Parkinsonism.

Treatment	Mechanism of Action	Clinical Use	Salient Features
Deep Brain Stimulation (DBS)	Modulates abnormal brain activity	Advanced Parkinson's disease	Reduces medication needs, improves motor symptoms
Focused Ultrasound (FUS)	Destroys targeted brain tissue via sound waves	Tremor-dominant Parkinson's	Non-invasive, does not require implants
Gene Therapy	Restores or protects dopaminergic neurons	Early clinical trials for Parkinson's disease	Potential to slow disease progression

Challenges in Parkinsonism Management

1. **Motor Complications:** Although very successful, long-term levodopa treatment has motor side effects including dyskinesias and motor fluctuations ("on-off" phenomenon). Although newer pharmacotherapies like safinamide and istradefylline help to reduce these complications.
2. **Non-Motor Symptoms:** Parkinson's disease consists of non-motor symptoms in addition to a motor condition, including depression, cognitive decline, and autonomic dysfunction. While treatments like DBS help to manage motor symptoms, addressing non-motor symptoms remains a critical unmet need in PD management.
3. **Disease Progression:** Despite symptomatic treatment, this neurodegenerative condition known as Parkinson's disease has no cure. While recent advances, including gene therapy, offer hope for neuroprotection, however, stopping or slowing down the advancement of illness or disease progression remains a major obstacle in the field of PD management.

Future Directions in Parkinsonism Research

1. **Neuroprotective Therapies:** The creation of neuroprotective treatments which are able to stop or slow down Parkinson's disease's advancement is a major goal of current research. Agents targeting mitochondrial dysfunction, oxidative stress, and inflammation are being investigated for their potential to protect neurons from degeneration.
2. **Stem Cell Therapy:** Stem cell therapy offers the potential to replace lost dopaminergic neurons in patients with Parkinson's disease. Clinical trials are ongoing to determine the safety and efficacy of stem cell-based treatments for neurodegeneration, with early results showing promise in restoring motor function.

Conclusion

With the advent of newer pharmacotherapies, non-pharmacological treatments, and emerging technologies, the management of Parkinsonism is transforming. Novel approaches to treating motor symptoms are offered by medications like safinamide, opicapone, and istradefylline. Meanwhile, patients with drug-resistant Parkinson's disease may benefit from advancements like deep brain stimulation and focused ultrasonic waves. Nevertheless, there are still difficulties in controlling non-motor symptoms and the course of the illness. Treatments for Parkinsonism may change in the future thanks to ongoing research into gene therapy, neuroprotection, and stem cell therapies.

References

1. Wal A, Wal P, Vig H, Jain NK, Rathore S, Krishnan K, Srivastava A. Treatment of Parkinson's Disease: Current Treatments and Recent Therapeutic Developments. Current Drug Discovery Technologies. 2023 Sep 1;20(5):54-70.
2. Mizuno Y. Definition and classification of Parkinsonian drugs. InNeuroPsychopharmacotherapy 2022 Nov 5 (pp. 2823-2852). Cham: Springer International Publishing.
3. Papagiouvannis G, Theodosis-Nobelos P, Rekka EA. A Review on Therapeutic Strategies against Parkinson's Disease: Current Trends and Future Perspectives. Mini-Reviews in Medicinal Chemistry. 2025 Feb;25(2):96-111.
4. Goetz CG. The history of Parkinson's disease: early clinical descriptions and neurological therapies. Cold Spring Harbor perspectives in medicine. 2011 Sep 1;1(1):a008862.
5. Fahn S. The history of dopamine and levodopa in the treatment of Parkinson's disease. Movement disorders: official journal of the Movement Disorder Society. 2008;23(S3):S497-508.
6. Clarke CE. Has drug therapy changed the natural history of Parkinson's disease?. Journal of neurology. 2010 Nov;257(Suppl 2):262-7.
7. Rascol O, Fabbri M, Poewe W. Amantadine in the treatment of Parkinson's disease and other movement disorders. The Lancet Neurology. 2021 Dec 1;20(12):1048-56.
8. Kempster P, Ma A. Parkinson's disease, dopaminergic drugs and the plant world. Frontiers in pharmacology. 2022 Sep 5;13:970714.
9. Deuschl G, de Bie RM. New therapeutic developments for Parkinson disease. Nature Reviews Neurology. 2019 Feb;15(2):68-9.
10. Astradsson A, Cooper O, Vinuela A, Isacson O. Recent advances in cell-based therapy for Parkinson disease. Neurosurgical Focus. 2008 Mar 1;24(3-4):E6.
11. Fleischhacker WW, Brooks DJ, Tolosa E. Advances in the pharmacological management of Parkinson disease. Springer Vienna; 2003.
12. Schapira AH, Agid Y, Barone P, Jenner P, Lemke MR, Poewe W, Rascol O, Reichmann H, Tolosa E. Perspectives on recent advances in the understanding and treatment of Parkinson's disease. European journal of neurology. 2009 Oct;16(10):1090-9.
13. Baweja GS, Gupta S, Kumar B, Patel P. Recent updates on structural insights of MAO-B inhibitors: a review on target-based approach. Mol Divers. 2023;28(3):1823–45.
14. Singh N, Pillay V, Choonara YE. Advances in the treatment of Parkinson's disease. Progress in neurobiology. 2007 Jan 1;81(1):29-44.
15. Oertel WH. Recent advances in treating Parkinson's disease. F1000Research. 2017 Mar 13;6:260.
16. Stoker T, Barker R. Recent developments in the treatment of Parkinson's disease. F1000Res. 2020;9.
17. Dhall R, Kreitzman DL. Advances in levodopa therapy for Parkinson disease: review of RYTARY (carbidopa and levodopa) clinical efficacy and safety. Neurology. 2016 Apr 5;86(14_supplement_1):S13-24.

18. Antonini A, Moro E, Godeiro C, Reichmann H. Medical and surgical management of advanced Parkinson's disease. Movement Disorders. 2018 Jul;33(6):900-8.
19. Kahana M, Weizman A, Gabay M, Loboda Y, Segal-Gavish H, Gavish A, Barhum Y, Offen D, Finberg J, Allon N, Gavish M. Liposome-based targeting of dopamine to the brain: a novel approach for the treatment of Parkinson's disease. Mol Psychiatry. 2021 Jun;26(6):2626-32.
20. Bette S, Shpiner DS, Singer C, Moore H. Safinamide in the management of patients with Parkinson's disease not stabilized on levodopa: a review of the current clinical evidence. Ther Clin Risk Manag. 2018 Sep 18;14:1737-45.
21. Sanders M, Medicetty S, Chandraratna R. IRX4204: A Clinical Stage, Potent, and Highly Selective RXR Agonist Compound Is Brain Penetrant, and Promotes Differentiation of Oligodendrocyte Precursor Cells (OPCs) In Vitro (I7-2.001). Neurology. 2014 Apr 8;82(10_supplement):I7-2.
22. Zhang CL, Han QW, Chen NH, Yuan YH. Research on developing drugs for Parkinson's disease. Brain research bulletin. 2021 Mar 1;168:100-9.
23. Wang J, Bi W, Zhao W, Varghese M, Koch RJ, Walker RH, Chandraratna RA, Sanders ME, Janesick A, Blumberg B, Ward L. Selective brain penetrable Nurr1 transactivator for treating Parkinson's disease. Oncotarget. 2016 Feb 4;7(7):7469.
24. Pagano G, Boess FG, Taylor KI, Ricci B, Mollenhauer B, Poewe W, Boulay A, Anzures-Cabrera J, Vogt A, Marchesi M, Post A. A phase II study to evaluate the safety and efficacy of prasinezumab in early Parkinson's disease (PASADENA): rationale, design, and baseline data. Frontiers in neurology. 2021 Oct 1;12:705407.
25. Schenk DB, Koller M, Ness DK, Griffith SG, Grundman M, Zago W, Soto J, Atiee G, Ostrowitzki S, Kinney GG. First-in-human assessment of PRX002, an anti-α-synuclein monoclonal antibody, in healthy volunteers. Mov Disord. 2017 Feb;32(2):211-8.
26. Cummins L, Cates ME. Istradefylline: A novel agent in the treatment of "off" episodes associated with levodopa/carbidopa use in Parkinson disease. Ment Health Clin. 2022 Jan 21;12(1):32-6.
27. Torres-Yaghi Y, Qian J, Cummings H, Shimoda H, Ito S, Batson S, Mitchell S, Pagan F. Comparative Safety of Istradefylline Among Parkinson Disease Adjunctive Therapies: A Systematic Review and Meta-analysis of Randomized Controlled Studies. Clinical Neuropharmacology. 2025 Jan 1;48(1):7-12.
28. Xiao B, Tan EK. Prasinezumab slows motor progression in Parkinsons disease: beyond the clinical data. npj Parkinson's Disease. 2025 Feb 19;11(1):31.
29. Asvos X, El Mubarak MA, Karampelas T, Rampias T, Tamvakopoulos C, Sivolapenko GB, Papakyriakou A, Topouzis S, Vassilatis DK, Fokas D. BRF110, an Orally Active Nurr1-RXRα-Selective Rexinoid, Enhances BDNF Expression without Elevating Triglycerides. Journal of Medicinal Chemistry. 2025 Feb 13.
30. Tan Y, Wei Q, Xu P, Tao E, Wang L, Cattaneo C, Shang H, Chen S. Comparing the efficacy and safety of safinamide with rasagiline in China Parkinson's disease patients with a matching adjusted indirect comparison. Scientific Reports. 2025 Mar 26;15(1):10502.

Chapter 10

Newer Antipsychotics

Author: Dr. Pranab Das

Introduction

Antipsychotic drugs are crucial for treating bipolar disorder, schizoaffective disorders, schizophrenia, and other psychotic conditions. Second-generation (atypical) antipsychotics with wider therapeutic profiles and better tolerability were developed in response to the drawbacks of first-generation (typical) antipsychotics, specifically extrapyramidal side effects (EPS), tardive dyskinesia, and hyperprolactinemia.

Aripiprazole, lurasidone, cariprazine, brexpiprazole, and lumateperone are some of the more recent atypical antipsychotics that have been on the market since the 1990s and are always evolving. These substances frequently have effects on glutamatergic or muscarinic pathways, serotonin 5-HT2A antagonism, and dopamine D2 partial agonism. Their creation represents a paradigm shift towards multimodal neuroreceptor targeting to treat negative and cognitive symptoms, which are frequently intractable with older medications, in addition to positive symptoms.

Historical Perspective

A turning point in psychopharmacology was the discovery of chlorpromazine in 1952, which ushered in the era of pharmacological treatment of psychosis. The calming effects of chlorpromazine, which was first created as an antihistaminic, established the basis for dopamine antagonism as a therapeutic principle. This was later validated by medications such as haloperidol.

However, the search for safer alternatives was prompted by the fact that first-generation antipsychotics (FGAs) were mainly effective for positive symptoms (such as delusions and hallucinations) and frequently caused severe motor side effects. Second-generation antipsychotics (SGAs), which combined antipsychotic efficacy with a lower incidence of EPS, were made possible by the approval of clozapine in the 1970s, despite early worries about agranulocytosis.

SGAs, such as quetiapine, olanzapine, and risperidone, rapidly expanded in the 1990s and 2000s. Third-generation antipsychotics, like aripiprazole, which improved efficacy and safety by introducing the idea of dopamine partial agonism, came after these. In order to more successfully treat resistant and cognitive symptoms of schizophrenia, current research investigates novel targets like glutamatergic modulation and trace amine-associated receptors (TAAR1).

Definition

Antipsychotics are medications used to manage psychosis, primarily by targeting dopamine pathways in the brain, though many newer agents also act on serotonin and other neurotransmitter systems. First-generation (typical) and second-generation (atypical) antipsychotics are two main groups of antipsychotics.

Types of Antipsychotics

1. **First-Generation Antipsychotics (FGAs):** FGAs primarily act as dopamine D2 receptor antagonists, which is why they are frequently referred to as conventional antipsychotics. Chlorpromazine and haloperidol are two examples of such drugs. These drugs have a high risk of tardive dyskinesia and extrapyramidal symptoms (EPS), even though they provide relief from positive symptoms of schizophrenia.
2. **Second-Generation Antipsychotics (SGAs):** SGAs, also referred to as atypical antipsychotics, work on serotonin 5-HT2A and dopamine D2 receptors, providing a more well-rounded treatment that reduces the risk of EPS while easing both positive and negative symptoms of psychosis. Olanzapine, risperidone, and quetiapine are a few examples.

Conventional Antipsychotics (First Generation Antipsychotics)

Mechanism of Action (D2 Antagonism):

1. Mesolimbic/Mesostriatal Dopamine Pathway:

The mesolimbic/mesostriatal dopamine pathway is overactive in schizophrenia – increased dopamine (DA) release in the synapse – leading to positive symptoms of schizophrenia (delusions, hallucinations). First-generation antipsychotics block the D2 receptors and thereby decrease the positive effects of schizophrenia.

But, because D2 receptors are blocked in the mesolimbic area, which is the area for motivation and reward, there is a risk of the development of secondary negative symptoms (apathy, anhedonia) of schizophrenia as side-effect.

2. Mesocortical Dopamine pathway:

In schizophrenia, mesocortical dopamine pathway becomes hypoactive – decrease dopamine release in pre-frontal cortex (PFC) – leads to the appearance of cognitive symptoms (loss of memory and concentration), negative symptoms (loss of interest, apathy) and affective symptoms (mania, hypomania, depression). So, first generation antipsychotics (D2 antagonists) further decreases the dopamine action in the PFC - worsens negative symptoms of schizophrenia.

3. Tuberoinfundibular pathway:

D2 antagonist decreases dopamine release in pituitary lactotrophs (as dopamine normally inhibits prolactin release) – so, decrease in dopamine release causes consequent increase in prolactin release – hyperprolactinaemia occurs as side-effect.

4. Nigrostriatal pathway (NSP):

D2 antagonist – decreases DA action in nigrostriatal pathway by causing blockade of D2 receptors in NSP – leads to Drug induced Parkinsonism (DIP). On chronic use of FGAs, there occurs chronic blockade of D2 receptors ultimately leading to reflex upregulation of D2 receptors in NSP – increase DA action in NSP – Tardive dyskinesia (hyperkinetic motor condition).

Table 1: Information regarding first-generation antipsychotic medications.

First Generation Anti-psychotics (FGAs)	Receptor Antagonism	Side-effect Profile				
		Extrapyramidal	Sedative	Hypotensive	Anti-emetic	Weight gain
Chlorpromazine	D2, D3, alpha-1, H1	+++	+++	+++	++	+++
Fluphenazine	D2, D3, alpha-1, H1, 5-HT7	+++	+	+	+++	+/-
Haloperidol	D2, D3, alpha-1, H1	+++	+	+	+++	-
Trifluoperazine	D2, D3, alpha-1, H1	++	+	++	+	-
Perphenazine	D2, D3, alpha-1	++	+	++	+	-

Newer Antipsychotics (Second generation antipsychotics or SGAs)

Mechanism of Action:

Newer antipsychotics have multiple mechanism of actions which causes increased efficacy and decreased toxicity. Apart from D2 antagonism they have the following other mechanisms:

1. 5-HT2A antagonism:

Serotonin (5-HT) stimulates 5-HT2A receptors present in the glutamatergicneurones in pre-frontal cortex (PFC) – increase glutamate release – released glutamate stimulates dopaminergic neurones in emotional striatum – increase dopamine (DA) release in emotional striatum. In schizophrenia, this pathway becomes hyperactive, resulting in increase in DA release in emotional striatum – positive symptoms of schizophrenia. Hence, by 5-HT2A antagonism – there is decrease in DA release in emotional striatum – relieves positive symptoms.

5-HT stimulates 5-HT2A receptors in glutamatergicneurones in PFC – increase glutamate release – stimulates GABA interneurons – increase GABA release in motor striatum – GABA inhibits DA neurones in motor striatum – decrease DA release in motor striatum. In schizophrenia, hyperactivity of this pathway occurs, which leads to deficiency of DA in motor striatum – drug-induced parkinsonism (DIP). Hence, 5-HT2A antagonists reduces the risk of DIP.

5-HT stimulates 5-HT2A receptors present in glutamatergicneurons in PFC – increase glutamate release – glutamate thus released stimulates GABA interneurons in PFC – increase GABA release – GABA inhibits DA neurones in PFC – decrease DA release in PFC. In schizophrenia, hyperactivity of this pathway occurs, resulting in severe deficiency of DA in PFC, which leads to negative and cognitive symptoms of schizophrenia. 5-HT2A antagonist thereby increases DA release in PFC thereby reducing cognitive and negative symptoms of schizophrenia.

5-HT – Stimulates 5-HT2A receptors in pituitary lactotrophs – stimulates prolactin release. Hence, 5-HT2A antagonist decreases prolactin release and does not cause hyperprolactinaemia.

2. D2 partial agonism:

D2 partial agonism produces submaximal D2 response without producing side-effects of D2 antagonists - antipsychotic effect is perceived without any hyperprolactinaemia.

3. 5-HT1A partial agonism:

5-HT - stimulates 5-HT1A receptors present in glutamatergic neurons in substantia nigra (SN) - increase glutamate release - glutamate stimulates GABA interneurons - increase GABA release - GABA inhibits DA neurones in motor striatum - decrease DA release in motor striatum - DIP. Hence, 5-HT1A partial agonist increases DA release in motor striatum - reduces DIP.

5-HT stimulates 5-HT1A receptors in glutamatergicneurones of Ventral Tegmental Area (VTA) - increase glutamate release - glutamate stimulates GABA interneurons - increase GABA release - GABA inhibits DA neurones in PFC - decrease DA release in PFC - negative, cognitive and affective symptoms of schizophrenia. 5-HT1A partial agonist - Stimulates glutamatergicneurones submaximally thereby reducing glutamate release - Reducing the activation of GABA interneurons - improvement of negative, cognitive and affective symptoms of schizophrenia.

Some salient features about newer antipsychotics:

1. Cariprazine

Introduction: Cariprazine is an atypical antipsychotic and a piperazine derivative initially developed in Hungary. It functions as a partial agonist at central dopamine D2, dopamine D3, and serotonin 5-HT1A receptors, while acting as an antagonist at serotonin 5-HT2A receptors. Cariprazine has been studied in several mental conditions, including schizophrenia, bipolar disorder, and major depressive disorder.

Clinical Trial Phase / FDA-Approval: Cariprazine received its initial clearance in the United States (FDA approval) under the trade name Vraylar and was subsequently authorised by Health Canada in April 2022 for the treatment of schizophrenia, bipolar I disorder, and as an adjunctive therapy for major depressive disorder (MDD).

Key Pharmacokinetic Parameters: Cariprazine and its major active metabolites are highly bound (91 to 97%) to plasma proteins. Cariprazine is extensively metabolized by CYP3A4 and, to a lesser extent, by CYP2D6 to form two major metabolites, desmethylcariprazine (DCAR) and didesmethylcariprazine (DDCAR). Both DCAR and DDCAR are pharmacologically active metabolites. Mainly excreted by faeces (63%) and partly by urine (21%).

Adverse Drug Reaction: Akathisia, nausea, insomnia and sedation. It has a favourable side-effect profile with minimal sedation and a lower risk of weight gain compared to other SGAs.

Uses: It is presently utilised for the treatment of schizophrenia, manic episodes, depressive illness, and episodes associated with bipolar I disorder.

Dose: 1.5–6 mg once daily orally.

2. Lumateperone

Introduction: Lumateperone is an innovative antipsychotic that influences serotonin, dopamine, and glutamate systems. The compound exhibits a distinct mechanism of action, functioning as an antagonist at serotonin 5-HT2A receptors, a partial agonist at presynaptic dopamine D2 receptors, and a postsynaptic D2 antagonist. Lumateperone has received approval for the treatment of schizophrenia and is currently under investigation for its efficacy in bipolar depression. The safety profile is favourable, characterised by a low incidence of weight gain and minimal metabolic side effects.

Clinical Trial Phase / FDA-Approval: FDA-approved for schizophrenia treatment under brand name Caplyta.

Key Pharmacokinetic Parameters: Lumateperoneis able to permeate multidrug resistance protein 1 (MDR1) and is very lipophilic at a pH of 7.4 (biological pH of intestinal lumen), which are characteristics that allow the antipsychotic to be absorbed in the small intestine and the blood brain barrier. Lumateperone is approximately 97.4% plasma protein bound. Lumateperone is extensively metabolized. The carbonyl side chain is reduced by ketone reductase to produce the primary active metabolite. It is mainly excreted by faeces and partly by urine.

Adverse Drug Reactions: Drowsiness, dizziness, nausea, seizures and hypotension.

Uses: Used to manage both positive and negative symptoms of schizophrenia.

Dose: 42 mg once daily orally.

3. Brexpiprazole

Introduction: Brexpiprazole is classified as an atypical antipsychotic, functioning as a novel D2 dopamine and serotonin 5-HT1A partial agonist, as well as a 5-HT2A antagonist. It is therefore referred to as a serotonin-dopamine activity modulator (SDAM). It exhibits a strong affinity for serotonin, dopamine, and alpha (α)-adrenergic receptors. Brexpiprazole, while structurally akin to aripiprazole, exhibits distinct binding affinities for dopamine and serotonin receptors. Brexpiprazole exhibits a reduced potential for partial agonist-mediated adverse effects, such as extrapyramidal symptoms, in comparison to aripiprazole. This difference is attributed to brexpiprazole's lower intrinsic activity at the D2 receptor. It exhibits heightened antagonism at the 5-HT2A receptors.

Clinical Trial Phase / FDA-Approval: Brexpiprazole received FDA approval under the brand name Rexulti.

Key Pharmacokinetic Parameters: Peak concentration is achieved in 4 hours. Brexpiprazole is 99% bound to plasma proteins, mainly serum albumin and α1-acid glycoprotein. Brexpiprazole is mainly metabolized by CYP3A4 and CYP2D6. Brexpiprazole and its major metabolite, DM-3411, were the predominant drug moieties in the systemic circulation. The terminal elimination half-life of brexpiprazole and its major metabolite, DM-3411, were 91 hours and 86 hours, respectively. It is primarily excreted via faeces.

Adverse Drug Reactions: Akathisia, weight gain, constipation, fatigue and somnolence.

Uses: Used in the treatment of schizophrenia; agitation associated with dementia due to Alzheimer's disease; and as an adjunct in the treatment of major depressive disorder.

Dose: 1–4 mg/ day orally.

4. Pimavanserin

Introduction: Pimavanserin is a selective serotonin inverse agonist at 5-HT2A receptors and is used for the treatment of Parkinson's disease psychosis. Unlike most antipsychotics, pimavanserin does not directly affect dopamine receptors, making it an ideal choice for the control of psychosis in Parkinson's disease patients, where dopamine blockade could worsen motor symptoms. Pimavanserin is also being investigated for usage in Alzheimer 's-related psychosis and schizophrenia.

Clinical Trial Phase / FDA-approval: Approved by the FDA under the brand name Nuplazid.

Key Pharmacokinetic Parameters: In human plasma, pimavanserin is rather protein-bound (95%). Mostly metabolised CYP3A4 and CYP3A5 hepatic cytochrome enzymes, Pimavanserin also metabolises CYP2J2, CYP2D6, and other cytochrome and flavin-containing monooxygenase enzymes in less degree. Plasma half-life is around 57 hours. Mainly excreted in faeces.

Adverse Drug Reactions: Peripheral oedema, confusion, nausea, constipation and gait disturbances.

Uses: Pimavanserin is a medication utilised to manage and mitigate the hallucinations and delusions associated with Parkinson's disease psychosis.

Dose: 34 mg once daily orally.

5. Aripiprazole Lauroxil

Introduction: Aripiprazole lauroxil is an injectable formulation of aripiprazole that offers long-acting, extended-release properties. This design aims to reduce the frequency of administration and enhance medication adherence among patients with schizophrenia. The drug is administered every four to six weeks, offering the advantages of aripiprazole's partial agonistic action at dopamine D2 and 5-HT1A receptors and acts as an antagonist at 5-HT2A receptors without requiring daily dosing. This extended-release formulation mitigates the risk of relapse associated with non-adherence, a prevalent issue in the management of schizophrenia.

Clinical Trial Phase / FDA-Approval: The FDA approved aripiprazole lauroxil under the brand name Aristada.

Key Pharmacokinetic Parameters: At therapeutic dosages, serum protein binding of aripiprazole and its main metabolite is >99% where they are mostly bound to albumin. Via esterases, ariprazolelauroxil is hydroxylated to produce N-hydroxymethyl-aripiprazole which undergoes a fast, nonenzymatic spontaneous cleavage, sometimes known as water-mediated hydrolysis. Hepatic CYP3A4 and CYP2D6 further metabolize ariprazole to produce dehydro-ariprazole, with little pharmacological action.

Adverse Drug Reactions: Akathisia, injection site reactions (pain, redness, swelling), sedation and weight gain.

Uses: Ariprazolelauroxil is prescribed to treat psychotic diseases including schizophrenia.

Dose: 441–1064 mg IM every 4–8 weeks.

Recent Advances in the Management of Schizophrenia

1. **Personalized Medicine and Pharmacogenomics:** Among the most important developments in antipsychotic treatment recently is the application of pharmacogenomic testing to personalize therapy. Pharmacogenomics studies how genetic variations influence a patient's response to medications, letting doctors customize medicines according to personal genetic profiles. Variations in genes coding for enzymes engaged in drug metabolism (e.g. CYP2D6) can affect how patients metabolises antipsychotic drugs, influencing both efficacy and side effects. This method reduces trial-and-error, hence improves treatment outcomes and optimizing drug dosages.
2. **Long-Acting Injectable Antipsychotics (LAIs):** Long-acting injectable antipsychotics are increasingly being used to improve adherence and prevent relapse in patients with schizophrenia. In addition to aripiprazole lauroxil, other long-acting formulations such as risperidone microspheres and paliperidone palmitate provide extended-release dosing, reducing the frequency of injections to once

a month or longer. LAIs are particularly useful in patients with poor adherence, ensuring consistent plasma levels of the medication and lowering of the relapse risk.

3. **Cognitive Enhancers:** Negative symptoms and cognitive impairment remain significant challenges in schizophrenia treatment. Recent research focuses on cognitive enhancers that targets neurotransmitter systems beyond dopamine, thereby lowering the relapse risk. Drugs like d-cycloserine and sarcosine, which enhance NMDA receptor function, are being investigated as adjuncts to antipsychotic therapy to improve cognitive deficits in schizophrenia.

Challenges in Antipsychotic Therapy

1. **Metabolic Side Effects:** Despite the advances in antipsychotic therapy, adverse metabolic effects, including weight gain, diabetes, and dyslipidaemia, remain a significant concern, particularly with some SGAs like olanzapine. Newer agents like lumateperone and brexpiprazole aim to reduce these metabolic risks, but long-term safety data are still needed to confirm these benefits.

2. **Treatment Resistance:** About 20–30% of people with schizophrenia are said to be treatment-resistant, that is, they do not react sufficiently to conventional antipsychotic medication. Although clozapine is still the gold standard for treatment-resistant schizophrenia, its usage is restricted because of agranulocytosis risk and regular blood testing requirements. Research into novel agents, including glutamate modulators and cannabinoid receptor antagonists, is ongoing to address treatment resistance.

3. **Adherence:** Non-adherence to medication remains one of the biggest challenges in managing schizophrenia, leading to relapse and hospitalization. Long-acting injectables like aripiprazole lauroxil provide a solution to this problem, offering sustained drug release and reducing the burden of daily medication adherence.

Future Directions in Antipsychotic Research

1. **Third-Generation Antipsychotics:** Third-generation antipsychotics, like cariprazine and brexpiprazole, represent a fresh class of drugs acting as partial agonists at dopamine D2 receptors. These medications seek to adjust dopamine levels rather than fully blocking it, reducing the risk of side effects like EPS while maintaining its efficacy in treating psychosis. Future research will likely focus on refining this mechanism to improve cognitive and negative symptoms.

2. **Gene Therapy and Neuroinflammation:** Emerging research into the role of neuroinflammation in schizophrenia suggests that targeting inflammatory pathways may offer new therapeutic options. Gene therapy approaches that modulate neuroinflammatory genes or reduce oxidative stress in the brain are being explored as potential treatments for schizophrenia's psychosis and cognitive impairment.

Conclusion

With improved efficacy and a decreased risk of side effects, the treatment options for psychotic disorders have expanded with the introduction of more recent antipsychotics like cariprazine, brexpiprazole, and lumateperone. The accuracy and efficacy of antipsychotic treatment are continuously being improved by advancements in pharmacogenomics, long-acting injectables, and cognitive enhancers. However, issues like adherence, treatment resistance, and metabolic side effects continue to be major areas of focus for further study. The next generation of antipsychotic treatments may benefit from the continued investigation of novel mechanisms, such as glutamate modulation and neuroinflammation.

References

1. Grace AA, Uliana DL. Insights into the mechanism of action of antipsychotic drugs derived from animal models: standard of care versus novel targets. International Journal of Molecular Sciences. 2023 Jan;24(15):12374.
2. De Bartolomeis A, Barone A, Begni V, Riva MA. Present and future antipsychotic drugs: A systematic review of the putative mechanisms of action for efficacy and a critical appraisal under a translational perspective. Pharmacological research. 2022 Feb 1;176:106078.
3. Meyer JM. How antipsychotics work in schizophrenia: a primer on mechanisms. CNS spectrums. 2025 Jan;30(1):e6.
4. Kane JM, Correll CU. Past and present progress in the pharmacologic treatment of schizophrenia. The Journal of clinical psychiatry. 2010 Sep 15;71(9):13909.
5. Weston-Green K. Antipsychotic drug development: from historical evidence to fresh perspectives. Frontiers in Psychiatry. 2022 Jun 16;13:903156.
6. Kapur S, Mamo D. Half a century of antipsychotics and still a central role for dopamine D2 receptors. Progress in Neuro-Psychopharmacology and Biological Psychiatry. 2003 Oct 1;27(7):1081-90.
7. López-Muñoz F, Shen WW, D'ocon P, Romero A, Álamo C. A history of the pharmacological treatment of bipolar disorder. International journal of molecular sciences. 2018 Jul 23;19(7):2143.
8. Millan MJ, Goodwin GM, Meyer-Lindenberg A, Ögren SO. Learning from the past and looking to the future: emerging perspectives for improving the treatment of psychiatric disorders. European Neuropsychopharmacology. 2015 May 1;25(5):599-656.
9. Gründer G, Hippius H, Carlsson A. The'atypicality'of antipsychotics: a concept re-examined and re-defined. Nature Reviews Drug Discovery. 2009 Mar;8(3):197-202.
10. Carpenter WT, Koenig JI. The evolution of drug development in schizophrenia: past issues and future opportunities. Neuropsychopharmacology. 2008 Aug;33(9):2061-79.
11. PsychDB. Antipsychotics: mechanism, types, potency, and monitoring [Internet]. PsychDB; [cited 2025 May 9]. Available from: https://www.psychdb.com/meds/antipsychotics/home
12. Lacro J, Eastham J, Jeste D, Lohr J. Newer antipsychotics and antidepressants for elderly people. Curr Opin Psychiatry. 1996;9:290-3.
13. Mortimer AM. Newer and older antipsychotics: A comparative review of appropriate use. CNS Drugs. 1994 Nov;2(5):381-96.
14. Barnes TR, Joyce EM. Antipsychotic drug treatment: recent advances. Current Opinion in Psychiatry. 2001 Jan 1;14(1):25-37.
15. Spina E, Scordo MG. Newer antipsychotics: comparative review of drug interactions. Expert Review of Neurotherapeutics. 2001 Nov 1;1(2):171-82.
16. Gardner DM, Baldessarini RJ, Waraich P. Modern antipsychotic drugs: a critical overview. Cmaj. 2005 Jun 21;172(13):1703-11.
17. Spina E, De Leon J. Metabolic drug interactions with newer antipsychotics: a comparative review. Basic & clinical pharmacology & toxicology. 2007 Jan;100(1):4-22.
18. Littrell KH, Littrell SH. Emerging applications of newer antipsychotic agents in specific patient populations. Journal of the American Psychiatric Nurses Association. 1998 Aug 1;4(4):S42-52.
19. Smith DC. Are Newer Antipsychotics Better?. Ethical Human Sciences and Services. 2001;3(1):61-2.
20. Stahl SM. Stahl's Essential Psychopharmacology: Neuroscientific Basis and Practical Applications. 5th ed. Cambridge: Cambridge University Press; 2021.
21. Pastrana MA, Flores JC, Rothschild AJ. Challenges in the Treatment of Psychotic Bipolar Depression. Journal of Clinical Psychopharmacology. 2024 Jul 1;44(4):407-12.
22. Eaves S, Rey JA. Brexpiprazole (Rexulti): A New Monotherapy for Schizophrenia and Adjunctive Therapy for Major Depressive Disorder. P T. 2016 Jul;41(7):418-22.
23. National Center for Biotechnology Information (NCBI). Brexpiprazole: Mechanism and Clinical Uses. *NCBI Bookshelf* [Internet]. Available from: https://www.ncbi.nlm.nih.gov/books/NBK557712/.
24. Raedler LA. Aripiprazole Lauroxil (Aristada): Long-Acting Atypical Antipsychotic Injection Approved for the Treatment of Patients with Schizophrenia. Am Health Drug Benefits. 2016 Mar;9(Spec Feature):40-3.
25. Liu D, Zhang X, Xu H. Post-marketing safety of pimavanserin: a real-world pharmacovigilance study based on the FDA adverse event reporting system (FAERS). Expert Opinion on Drug Safety. 2025 Jan 30.
26. Citrome L, Correll CU, Cutler AJ, Dunbar M, Hoberg AR, Hopkinson C, Mattingly GW, McGrory JA, Rege B, Weiden PJ, McDonnell D. Aripiprazole Lauroxil: Development and Evidence-Based Review of a Long-Acting Injectable Atypical Antipsychotic for the Treatment of Schizophrenia. Neuropsychiatric Disease and Treatment. 2025 Dec 31:575-96.
27. Ward C, Milovančević MP, Kohegyi E, Hefting N, Aurang C, Chen D, Larsen KG, Hobart M, Correll CU. Efficacy and safety of brexpiprazole in adolescents with schizophrenia: a multicountry, randomised, double-blind, placebo-controlled, phase 3 trial with an active reference. The Lancet Psychiatry. 2025 Apr 7.
28. Cuomo A, Forleo GB, Ghodhbane T, Johnsen J, Montejo AL, Oliveira CV, Pillinger T, Ramos-Quiroga JA, Samara M, Seerden PH, Thomas Stoeckl T. Physical illness in schizophrenia and the role of tolerability in antipsychotic selection: an expert consensus with a focus on cariprazine. Annals of General Psychiatry. 2025 Dec;24(1):1-0.

Chapter 11

Newer Antidepressants

Author: Dr. Pranab Das

Introduction

Depression is a common mental health problem impacting millions of people internationally. A large class of psychotropic drugs known as antidepressants is mainly used to treat major depressive disorder (MDD), anxiety disorders, and a variety of other neurological and psychiatric disorders. They work by altering neurotransmitters in the brain, particularly dopamine (DA), norepinephrine (NE), and serotonin (5-HT), which are involved in mood regulation, emotion processing, and thought processes.

The pharmacological landscape of antidepressants has changed dramatically, with next-generation agents—specifically, selective serotonin reuptake inhibitors (SSRIs) and serotonin-norepinephrine reuptake inhibitors (SNRIs)—progressively replacing first-generation medications like monoamine oxidase inhibitors (MAOIs) and tricyclic antidepressants (TCAs). These more recent agents have better adherence, safety profiles, and tolerability. More recently, rapid-acting and multimodal antidepressants have entered clinical practice through novel mechanisms like melatonergic agonism (e.g., agomelatine), NMDA receptor antagonism (e.g., ketamine, esketamine), and GABAergic modulation (e.g., zuranolone).

Historical Perspective

Accidental clinical observations made in the middle of the 20th century are a major part of the history of antidepressant medication development. The discovery that the antitubercular medication isoniazid and its derivative iproniazid improved mood in the 1950s led to the identification of monoamine oxidase inhibition as a possible antidepressant mechanism. Imipramine, which was first created as an antipsychotic, was later found to have strong antidepressant effects, establishing the monoaminergic theory of depression.

TCAs and MAOIs, which were effective but also linked to significant side effects and overdose risks, were made possible by these early discoveries. The first SSRI, fluoxetine, was introduced in the 1980s, redefining the way depression was treated by providing a safer and more tolerable substitute. This sparked a surge of second-generation antidepressants, which transformed mental health treatment worldwide.

Since the 2000s, ketamine and esketamine have been developed as rapid-acting antidepressants as a result of research into non-monoaminergic targets, such as the glutamatergic system. These medications have demonstrated potential in treating suicidal thoughts and treatment-resistant depression (TRD), conditions that traditional therapies were unable to address.

Antidepressants have evolved from simple serendipitous beginnings to complex neuropharmacology, reflecting the scientific effort to identify the neurobiological causes of mood disorders.

Definition

Antidepressants are medications used to alleviate the symptoms of depression by modifying chemical imbalances in the brain, particularly those involving serotonin, norepinephrine, and dopamine. Newer antidepressants seek to overcome both the limitations of older drugs (such as delayed onset and adverse drug effects) and target previously unexplored pathways like glutamate signalling.

Types of Antidepressants

1. **Selective Serotonin Reuptake Inhibitors (SSRIs):** SSRIs, which include fluoxetine and sertraline, are the most often prescribed antidepressants. They increase serotonin's availability in the synaptic cleft by blocking its reuptake by the neurones.
2. **Serotonin-Norepinephrine Reuptake Inhibitors (SNRIs):** SNRIs, like venlafaxine and duloxetine, increase serotonin and norepinephrine levels, offering a more in-depth approach to treating the symptoms of depression.
3. **Atypical Antidepressants:** Alternative mechanisms to conventional SSRIs and SNRIs are provided by medications such as bupropion, which primarily affects dopamine and norepinephrine, and mirtazapine, which has dual action on serotonin and norepinephrine receptors.

Conventional Antidepressants

Table 1: Traditional antidepressant pharmacotherapies.

Drug Class	Drug Names	Mechanism of Action	Adverse Drug Reactions
SSRIs	Fluoxetine, Sertraline, Fluvoxamine, Escitalopram	Blocks SERT (Serotonin reuptake transporter) in axons of serotonergic neurones - increase 5-HT concentration in synapse.	Headache, sexual dysfunction, insomnia and nausea.
SNRIs	Venlafaxine, Desvenlafaxine, Duloxetine	Blocks both SERT and NET (norepinephrine transporter) in axons of serotonergic and nor-adrenergic neurones - increases concentration of 5-HT, NA (nor-adrenaline) and DA (dopamine) in several areas of brain including pre-frontal cortex (PFC).	Similar to SSRIs but better tolerated.
Atypical antidepressants	Bupropion	Blocks NET and DAT (Dopamine transporter) - increases NA and DA concentration in PFC.	Dry mouth, nausea, constipation, sweating and headache.

Newer Antidepressant Drugs

1. Esketamine

Introduction: Esketamine, a ketamine derivative, is an expeditiously acting antidepressant sanctioned for treatment-resistant depression (TRD). Administered as a nasal spray, esketamine specifically targets the glutamatergic system by functioning as an NMDA receptor antagonist, leading to a fast antidepressant effect—typically within hours. Esketamine signifies a transformative advancement in the treatment of depression, particularly for patients unresponsive to conventional therapy.

Clinical Trial Phase / FDA-Approval: Esketamine, marketed by Janssen Pharmaceuticals under the brand name Spravato, was approved by the FDA as a nasal spray medication for major depression that is resistant to treatment (TRD).

Mechanism of Action: Esketamine, the S-enantiomer of racemic ketamine, is a non-competitive antagonist of the N-methyl-D-aspartate (NMDA) receptor, an ionotropic glutamate receptor. It binds to the allosteric site (not the glutamate binding site) and blocks the receptor. Receptor blockade leads to decrease calcium influx in the GABAergic interneurons in the pre-frontal cortex (PFC) - reduced GABA release - removal of inhibitor response of GABA on glutamatergicor excitatory neurons - increased glutamate release. Since NMDA receptors are blocked, hence the released glutamate now binds to the available AMPA receptors - AMPA receptor stimulation - promotes BDNF - promotes synaptic growth - ultimately contributing to rapid and sustained antidepressant effects.

Key Pharmacokinetic Parameters: Due to the fact that this drug is administered via nasal spray, absorption is rapid. The mean absolute bioavailability is approximately 48% after esketamine nasal spray administration. The time to achieve peak esketamine plasma concentration is 20 to 40 minutes after the last nasal spray of esketamine. Esketamine is mainly metabolized to the noresketamine metabolite by cytochrome P450 (CYP) enzymes like CYP2B6 and CYP3A4, and to a lesser extent, CYP2C9 and CYP2C19. It is mainly excreted by urine.

Adverse Drug Reactions: Sleepiness, dizziness, dissociation, and nausea.

Uses: Esketamine is suggested, in conjunction with an oral antidepressant, for the management of treatment-resistant depression in adults. It is also suggested for the management of depressive symptoms in people with major depressive disorder exhibiting acute suicidal ideation or conduct.

Dose: 56 mg or 84 mg intranasally twice/week for 4 weeks, then weekly/biweekly maintenance.

2. Brexanolone

Introduction: Brexanolone is a synthetic version of allopregnanolone, a neuroactive steroid that modulates GABA-A receptors. It is specifically approved for the treatment of postpartum depression, a condition that affects new mothers and can have significant impacts on both the mother and child. Brexanolone works rapidly, often within 48 hours, providing a fast-acting option for severe postpartum depression. However, its administration requires a continuous 60-hour intravenous infusion in a controlled healthcare setting.

Clinical Trial Phase / FDA-Approval: FDA-approved drug. Approved in 2019 under the brand name Zulresso.

Mechanism of Action: The mechanism of action of brexanolone is not fully known. Brexanolone is an aqueous formulation of allopregnanolone. Allopregnanolone is a major metabolite of progesterone. Levels of allopregnanolone continue to rise with progesterone during pregnancy, with the highest levels in the third trimester. Allopregnanolone is a potent, endogenous neuroactive steroid that modulates neuronal excitability through positive allosteric modulation on the synaptic (minor site of action) and extrasynaptic (major site of action) GABA-A receptors. GABA-A receptors are ligand-gated chloride channels that serve as the primary inhibitory neurotransmitter receptors in the brain. Brexanolone does not interact with the GABA binding site; instead, it binds to a distinct neurosteroid binding site on the receptor. It augments GABA-A receptor function by elevating both channel opening frequency and duration, hence potentiating GABA-induced inhibition. Augmented GABAergic inhibition results in decreased hyperactivity in brain regions such as the amygdala and hypothalamus, stabilisation of mood-related circuits, and prompt relaxing and anxiolytic effects. The extrasynaptic GABA-A receptors possess δ-subunits, differentiating them from conventional synaptic receptors. They mediate tonic inhibition rather than phasic. Brexanolone preferentially enhances tonic inhibition, which is especially important for mood and stress regulation.

Key Pharmacokinetic Parameters: Brexanolone has a 9-hour elimination half-life and is well bound to plasma proteins (99%) after injection. Since brexanolone is mostly metabolized by extra-hepatic, non-CYP routes through glucuronidation, sulfation, and keto-reduction, hepatic impairment does not require a dosage modification. The majority of excretion occurs in urine.

Adverse Drug Reactions: The most frequent side effects linked to brexanolone include hot flashes, xerostomia, sedation/somnolence, disorientation, and loss of consciousness.

Uses: Postpartum depression.

Dose: 90 µg/kg/hr continuous IV infusion over 60 hours.

3. Agomelatine

Introduction: Melatonin and agomelatine share structural similarities. Agomelatine is used to treat depression because it is a strong agonist at melatonin receptors and an antagonist at serotonin-2C (5-HT2C) receptors. It also has sedative properties.

Clinical Trial Phase / FDA-Approval: Completed phase III clinical trial in several countries and approved for use in Europe and Australia.

Mechanism of Action: Agomelatine, a new antidepressant, acts as an antagonist at serotonin (5-HT2C) receptors and an agonist at melatonin receptors (MT1 and MT2). By acting on MT1 and MT2 receptors it acts as sedative by inducing sleep (MT1 receptor action) and by shifting the timing of circadian rhythm (MT2 receptor action). 5-HT2C receptors are present in the GABA interneurons at raphe nucleus. 5-HT released from serotonergic neurones of raphe nucleus stimulates these 5-HT2C receptors at GABA interneurons – stimulates GABA interneurons – releases GABA – GABA inhibits dopaminergic neurones & noradrenergic neurones of pre-frontal cortex – decreases DA (Dopamine) and NA (Noradrenaline) release in the prefrontal cortex. Agomelatine, by inhibiting the 5-HT2C receptors, inhibits GABA interneurons and increases NA and DA release in the pre-frontal cortex.

Key Pharmacokinetic Parameters: Bio availability is less than 5%. It is metabolised in liver by CYP1A2 and exhibits 95% plasma protein binding. Plasma half-life is around 2 hours. It is excreted mainly in urine.

Adverse Drug Reactions: Headache, nausea, dizziness and hepatotoxicity.

Uses: Adult major depressive episodes can be treated with agomelatine.

Dose: 25–50 mg once daily at bedtime.

4. Vortioxetine

Introduction: Vortioxetine is a multimodal antidepressant that inhibits the serotonin transporter and acts as both a partial agonist and antagonist at several serotonin receptors. This medicine is a great option for patients with depression-related cognitive impairment, as it is thought to enhance mood and cognition. Vortioxetine successfully mitigates cognitive symptoms of depression, such as impaired concentration and memory, in addition to its antidepressant properties.

Clinical Trial Phase / FDA-Approval: FDA-approved drug (approved under the brand name Brintellix/ Trintellix).

Mechanism of Action: The exact mechanism of action of vortioxetine is unknown. Due to its strong affinity for the serotonin transporter (SERT), vortioxetine blocks SERT, which raises serotonin (5-HT) in synapses. Vortioxetine acts as a partial agonist at the 5-HT1A presynaptic autoreceptors and an partial agonist/ antagonist at the 5-HT1B/1D receptor – ultimately removing the negative regulation of 5-HT release and thereby increasing the concentrations of 5-HT in the synapse. Antagonistic action at the 5-HT7 receptor is thought to enhance the effects of SERT inhibition. The control of nausea and vomiting is more directly linked to antagonistic interactions at the 5-HT3 receptor (Figure 2).

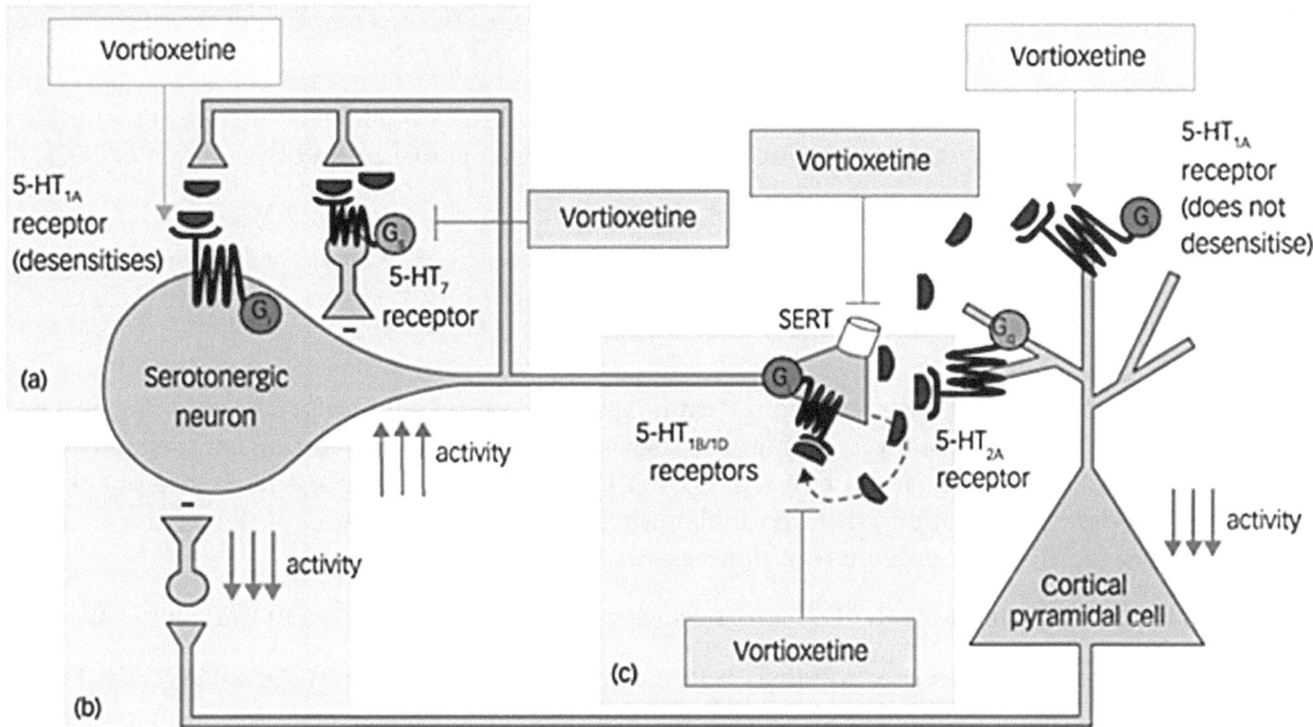

Figure 2: Vortioxetine enhances serotonin signalling in the brain through a combination of actions that modulate the serotonergic system. It targets neurons in the dorsal raphe nucleus (DRN), which send serotonin to distant regions like the cortex. In this context, serotonin is represented as semicircles in diagrams, and the effects of vortioxetine on neuronal activity are typically illustrated using arrows. Primarily, vortioxetine increases serotonin levels by inhibiting the serotonin transporter (SERT), preventing the reuptake of serotonin into the presynaptic neuron and thereby maintaining higher levels in the synaptic cleft. Additionally, it disrupts three important feedback mechanisms that normally limit serotonin release:

1. Autoregulatory feedback in the DRN: Serotonin usually inhibits its own release through two pathways – 5-HT1A receptors on the serotonergic neuron's own axon branches and 5-HT7 receptors on local inhibitory interneurons. Vortioxetine activates 5-HT1A receptors on DRN neurons (leading to desensitization over time) and blocks 5-HT7 receptors on interneurons. This action disables both limbs of the self-regulating feedback loop, allowing sustained serotonin release.

2. Cortical feedback loop: Cortical pyramidal neurons typically express both 5-HT1A and 5-HT2A receptors and can inhibit serotonin output by activating interneurons that project back to the DRN. Vortioxetine stimulates post-synaptic 5-HT1A receptors in the cortex, which do not desensitize, thereby reducing pyramidal cell activity and weakening this retrograde inhibition.

3. Presynaptic autoreceptor inhibition: 5-HT1B and 5-HT1D receptors normally act as brakes on serotonin release in response to its presence in the synapse. Vortioxetine blocks these receptors, effectively removing this final inhibitory mechanism and enabling prolonged serotonin release.

By simultaneously increasing serotonin levels and disabling the natural inhibitory checkpoints, vortioxetine achieves a robust and sustained enhancement of serotonergic transmission (Source: Alexander et al.)

Key Pharmacokinetic Parameters: It's bioavailability after oral administration is 75%. CYP2D6, CYP3A4/5, CYP2C19, CYP2C9, CYP2A6, CYP2C8, and CYP2B6 are the main enzymes involved in the extensive metabolism of vortioxetine. This is followed by glucuronic acid conjugation. Vortioxetine's principal inactive metabolite, the carboxylic acid metabolite, is produced by the primary enzyme, CYP2D6. It is 98% plasma protein bound and mainly excreted in urine.

Adverse Drug Reactions: The most prevalent adverse effects include cephalalgia, vertigo, xerostomia, and nausea. Serious side effects included pancreatitis, an increased risk of suicide, and hypertensive crisis.

Uses: Vortioxetine is indicated for the treatment of major depressive disorder (MDD).

Dose: 10–20 mg once daily.

5. Vilazodone

Introduction: Vilazodone is a SPARI (Serotonin Partial Agonist Reuptake Inhibitor), functioning as a partial agonist at the serotonin 5-HT1A autoreceptor and as a serotonin reuptake inhibitor. In contrast to traditional SSRIs, this combination facilitates rapid antidepressant effects while reducing the incidence of sexual side effects. It is an advantageous option for individuals pursuing prompt alleviation of depressive symptoms, as it operates more rapidly than previous antidepressants.

Clinical Trial Phase / FDA-Approval: FDA-approved drug (Approved under the brand name Viibryd).

Mechanism of Action: Vilazodone, sometimes referred to as SPARI (Serotonin Partial Agonist Reuptake Inhibitor), combines SERT inhibition with partial agonism of 5-HT1A autoreceptors. Compared to SSRIs alone, vilazodone raises brain 5-HT levels more quickly and significantly because:

1. SERT inhibition in axon terminals - leads to decrease in 5-HT reuptake - increase 5-HT release in synapse.

2. 5-HT1A partial agonists are a type of "artificial serotonin" that are: selective for presynaptic somatodendritic 5-HT1A autoreceptors - stimulation of 5-HT1A autoreceptor leads to decreased 5-HT release. But on chronic use there is continuous stimulation of 5-HT1A autoreceptor - desensitization & downregulation of 5-HT1A autoreceptor - removal of restriction in 5-HT release - increase 5-HT release in synapse.

Because of both above mechanism (SERT inhibition + 5-HT1A partial agonism) - Faster downregulation of these 5-HT1A autoreceptors occurs than SSRI alone. Also, 5-HT1A partial agonism occurs immediately at postsynaptic 5-HT1A receptors - increase 5-HT release (as normally post-synaptic 5-HT1A receptors stimulation - increase in 5-HT release).

Key Pharmacokinetic Parameters: It is 96–99% plasma protein bound. Vilazodone is metabolized extensively by the hepatic CYP3A4 enzyme. It's dose should be reduced to 20 mg/ day with concomitant use of any potent CYP3A4 inhibitors, that is, erythromycin, amiodarone, protease inhibitors, or ketoconazole. Vilazodone's activity is primarily due to the parent drug and there are no active metabolites. Plasma half-life is around 25 hours. It is excreted mainly in urine.

Adverse Drug Reactions: Less incidence of side-effects as compared to SSRIs. ADRs includes headache, nausea, vomiting and diarrhoea.

Uses: Vilazodone is approved for treatment of major depressive disorder.

Dose: 10 mg once daily for starting 7 days, then 20–40 mg daily.

Recent Advances in the Management of Depression

1. **Glutamatergic Modulation:** Traditional antidepressants primarily target monoamine neurotransmitters (serotonin, dopamine, norepinephrine). However, recent research highlights the role of the glutamatergic system in depression. Esketamine's rapid action through NMDA receptor antagonism is a testament to the growing interest in glutamate modulation. This approach opens the door to developing faster-acting antidepressants, particularly for patients with TRD.
2. **Neurosteroids:** Brexanolone represents a novel class of antidepressants that modulate GABAergic neurotransmission through neurosteroids. It offers a rapid therapeutic effect, particularly in postpartum depression, where quick intervention is critical for both maternal and infant health. Neurosteroids like brexanolone provide a promising new avenue for treating severe forms of depression.
3. **Pharmacogenomics in Antidepressant Therapy:** The integration of pharmacogenomic testing in antidepressant therapy is helping clinicians personalize treatment plans. Genetic variations in enzymes, such as CYP2D6 and CYP2C19, which metabolize antidepressants, can influence drug efficacy and tolerability. By identifying genetic markers, clinicians can modify antidepressant dosages to fit the particular needs of each patient, lowering the possibility of side effects and improving treatment outcomes.

Challenges in Antidepressant Therapy

1. **Delayed Onset of Action:** The delayed beginning of action of conventional antidepressant medication is one of its main problems, with many SSRIs and SNRIs taking weeks to achieve full efficacy. The advent of rapid-acting agents like esketamine and brexanolone represents a major leap forward, though access to these treatments can be limited due to cost and the need for administration in specialized healthcare settings.
2. **Treatment Resistance:** Approximately one-third of depressed patients don't react to standard antidepressant treatments. For these patients, treatment-resistant depression (TRD) presents a major therapeutic challenge. Esketamine and other drugs targeting novel pathways provide new hope for TRD, though ongoing research is needed to identify more effective, accessible treatments.
3. **Side Effects:** Although newer antidepressants tend to have better side-effect profiles than those of older medications, issues like sexual dysfunction (SSRIs) and sedation (neurosteroids) still persist. Finding treatments that offer rapid relief with minimal side effects continues to be a problem in the field of psychopharmacology.

Future Directions in Antidepressant Research

1. **Triple Reuptake Inhibitors (TRIs):** Triple reuptake inhibitors target serotonin, norepinephrine, and dopamine simultaneously, offering a broader spectrum of action compared to SSRIs and SNRIs. Early clinical trials have shown that TRIs may provide faster relief of depressive symptoms, with maybe fewer adverse effects associated with weight gain and sexual problems. To evaluate their long-term safety and effectiveness, more studies are being conducted.
2. **Psychedelic-Assisted Therapy:** The potential of psychedelics like MDMA and psilocybin is being studied to treat depression, particularly in cases of TRD. These substances appear to promote neuroplasticity and increase connectivity between the parts of the brain that control mood. Early studies suggest that psychedelic-assisted therapy, when administered under medical supervision, could offer long-lasting relief after just a few sessions.
3. **Inflammation and Depression:** Inflammation may contribute to the onset of depression, according to mounting data. The potential of anti-inflammatory drugs, including COX-2 inhibitors, to reduce depression symptoms is being investigated, especially in individuals with high inflammatory markers.

This is a new method of treating a group of individuals who might not react to traditional treatments that only target neurotransmitters.

Conclusion

The field of antidepressant therapy is changing as novel drugs like agomelatine, brexanolone, and esketamine are being introduced, increasing the number of depression treatment options. These medications are useful additions to the therapeutic toolbox because they provide novel mechanisms of action, quicker onset, and enhanced tolerability, especially for patients with treatment-resistant depression. A new era in individualised and quick-acting treatments for depression is heralded by the combination of neurosteroid-based therapies, glutamatergic modulation, and pharmacogenomics. Treatment resistance, delayed access to new drugs, and the continuous search for antidepressants with fewer adverse effects are some of the obstacles that still exist.

References

1. Sharma K, Sundriyal A, Loshali A, Agrawal M, Krishna CG, Singh Y. Mechanism of action of antidepressants. InHow Synthetic Drugs Work 2023 Jan 1 (pp. 255-273). Academic Press.
2. Kornhuber J, Gulbins E. New molecular targets for antidepressant drugs. Pharmaceuticals. 2021 Sep 2;14(9):894.
3. Chen T, Cheng L, Ma J, Yuan J, Pi C, Xiong L, Chen J, Liu H, Tang J, Zhong Y, Zhang X. Molecular mechanisms of rapid-acting antidepressants: New perspectives for developing antidepressants. Pharmacological research. 2023 Aug 1;194:106837.
4. López-Muñoz F, Alamo C. Monoaminergic neurotransmission: the history of the discovery of antidepressants from 1950s until today. Current pharmaceutical design. 2009 May 1;15(14):1563-86.
5. Hillhouse TM, Porter JH. A brief history of the development of antidepressant drugs: from monoamines to glutamate. Experimental and clinical psychopharmacology. 2015 Feb;23(1):1.
6. De Bodinat C, Guardiola-Lemaitre B, Mocaër E, Renard P, Muñoz C, Millan MJ. Agomelatine, the first melatonergic antidepressant: discovery, characterization and development. Nature reviews Drug discovery. 2010 Aug;9(8):628-42.
7. Hashimoto K. Rapid-acting antidepressant ketamine, its metabolites and other candidates: A historical overview and future perspective. Psychiatry Clin Neurosci. 2019;73(9):613–27.
8. Spina E, Trifirò G, Caraci F. Clinically significant drug interactions with newer antidepressants. CNS drugs. 2012 Jan;26:39-67.
9. Carvalho A, Sharma M, Brunoni A, Vieta E, Fava G. The safety, tolerability and risks associated with the use of newer generation antidepressant drugs: A critical review of the literature. PsychotherPsychosom. 2016;85:270-288.
10. Ahmed N, Albishi F, Khan S, Alsayegh A, Stip E, Makhoul S. Management of treatment-resistant depression with esketamine nasal spray: clinical questions for daily practice in Gulf Cooperation Council countries. Middle East Curr Psychiatry. 2023;30.
11. Hatcher S, Arroll B. Newer antidepressants for the treatment of depression in adults. BMJ. 2012 Jan 19;344.
12. arko J. Antidepressants, old and new: a review of their adverse effects and toxicity in overdose. Emergency Medicine Clinics of North America. 2000 Nov 1;18(4):637-54.
13. Stahl SM. Stahl's Essential Psychopharmacology: Neuroscientific Basis and Practical Applications. 5th ed. Cambridge: Cambridge University Press; 2021.
14. Zelek-Molik A, Litwa E. Trends in research on novel antidepressant treatments. Frontiers in Pharmacology. 2025 Jan 27;16:1544795.
15. Jóźwiak-Bębenista M, Sokołowska P, Wiktorowska-Owczarek A, Kowalczyk E, Sienkiewicz M. Ketamine–A New Antidepressant Drug with Anti-Inflammatory Properties. The Journal of Pharmacology and Experimental Therapeutics. 2024 Jan 1;388(1):134-44.
16. Wang SM, Han C, Lee SJ, Patkar A, Masand P, Pae CU. Vilazodone for the treatment of major depressive disorder: focusing on its clinical studies and mechanism of action. Psychiatry Investig. 2015;12(2):155–63.
17. Ślifirski G, Król M, Turło J. 5-HT receptors and the development of new antidepressants. International journal of molecular sciences. 2021 Aug 20;22(16):9015.
18. Turner EH, Cipriani A, Furukawa TA, Salanti G, de Vries YA. Selective publication of antidepressant trials and its influence on apparent efficacy: Updated comparisons and meta-analyses of newer versus older trials. PLoS medicine. 2022 Jan 19;19(1):e1003886.
19. Hetrick SE, McKenzie JE, Bailey AP, Sharma V, Moller CI, Badcock PB, Cox GR, Merry SN, Meader N. New generation antidepressants for depression in children and adolescents: a network meta-analysis. Cochrane Database of Systematic Reviews. 2021(5).
20. Alexander, Laith & Young, Allan. (2022). Recent Advances in the Psychopharmacology of Major Depressive Disorder. BJPsych Advances. 29. 1-14. 10.1192/bja.2022.14.

21. Gonda X, Dome P, Neill JC, Tarazi FI. Novel antidepressant drugs: Beyond monoamine targets. CNS spectrums. 2023 Feb;28(1):6-15.
22. De Oliveira Costa J, Gillies MB, Schaffer AL, Peiris D, Zoega H, Pearson SA. Changes in antidepressant use in Australia: a nationwide analysis (2015–2021). Australian & New Zealand Journal of Psychiatry. 2023 Jan;57(1):49-57.
23. Almeida FB, Pinna G, Barros HM. The role of HPA axis and allopregnanolone on the neurobiology of major depressive disorders and PTSD. International journal of molecular sciences. 2021 May 23;22(11):5495.
24. Epperson CN, Rubinow DR, Meltzer-Brody S, Deligiannidis KM, Riesenberg R, Krystal AD, Bankole K, Huang MY, Li H, Brown C, Kanes SJ. Effect of brexanolone on depressive symptoms, anxiety, and insomnia in women with postpartum depression: Pooled analyses from 3 double-blind, randomized, placebo-controlled clinical trials in the HUMMINGBIRD clinical program. Journal of Affective Disorders. 2023 Jan 1;320:353-9.
25. Chauhan M, Parry R, Bobo WV. Vilazodone for major depression in adults: pharmacological profile and an updated review for clinical practice. Neuropsychiatric Disease and Treatment. 2022 Jun 14;18:1175.
26. Yang X, Fang S, Lyu W, Hu Y, Xu H, Jiang X, Zhao Y, Zhang Y, Li J, Kuang W. Vortioxetine for depression in adults: A systematic review and dose–response meta-analysis of randomized controlled trials. Psychiatry and Clinical Neurosciences. 2024 Sep;78(9):536-45.
27. Ju Y, Ou W, Chen H, Yang L, Long Y, Liang H, Xi Z, Huang M, Chen W, Lv G, Shao F. Agomelatine as adjunctive therapy with SSRIs or SNRIs for major depressive disorder: a multicentre, double-blind, randomized, placebo-controlled trial. BMC medicine. 2025 Mar 5;23(1):137.

Chapter 12

Recent Advances in the Management of Alzheimer's Disease

Author: Dr. Pranab Das

Introduction

Alzheimer's disease (AD) is a progressive neurological disorder predominantly impacting older individuals, with Alzheimer-type dementia representing its most prevalent manifestation. Characterised by amnesia, disorientation, linguistic challenges, and compromised problem-solving abilities, Alzheimer's disease ultimately hinders fundamental daily activities and profoundly affects both patients and carers. As worldwide populations age, the incidence of Alzheimer's disease has increased significantly, prompting major scientific endeavours to create effective medicines that extend beyond symptom care and seek to prevent or halt disease development.

Recent advancements have enhanced comprehension of the disease's fundamental underpinnings, encompassing the functions of amyloid-beta plaques, hyperphosphorylated tau tangles, neuroinflammation, oxidative stress, vascular impairment, and synaptic degeneration. These findings have highlighted the necessity for comprehensive therapeutic approaches that simultaneously address several biological pathways. This chapter delineates the pathology of Alzheimer's disease, summarises traditional therapeutic strategies, and emphasises novel interventions that show potential for enhancing patient outcomes.

Historical Perspective

The journey of Alzheimer's disease (AD) management spans over a century, beginning with Alois Alzheimer's (year 1906) description of the disorder's hallmark neuropathological features: amyloid plaques and neurofibrillary tangles. However, clinical treatment remained elusive for decades, limited to symptomatic and behavioural interventions.

It wasn't until the 1990s that pharmacological management began to take shape, with the approval of cholinesterase inhibitors such as donepezil, rivastigmine, and galantamine, which aim to enhance cholinergic neurotransmission. These were followed by memantine, an NMDA receptor antagonist, approved in 2003 for moderate-to-severe AD. These therapies provided only modest symptomatic benefits and no disease modification, reflecting the therapeutic limitations of early approaches.

The 2000s marked a shift toward understanding Alzheimer's as a proteinopathy, characterized by amyloid-β accumulation, tau hyperphosphorylation, and neuroinflammation. This understanding spurred development of disease-modifying therapies (DMTs), particularly anti-amyloid monoclonal antibodies. The controversial approval of aducanumab by the FDA in 2021 and subsequent approval of lecanemab and donanemab represented watershed moments in AD therapy, despite debates over clinical efficacy and cost.

Simultaneously, advances in biomarker science—including CSF analysis, PET imaging, and plasma assays—enabled earlier and more accurate diagnosis, even at the preclinical stage. These tools, combined with digital health platforms and AI-driven diagnostics, are transforming the landscape from reactive care to preventive and precision medicine.

The evolution of Alzheimer's disease management reflects a broader shift from symptom control to targeted pathophysiological intervention. Although challenges remain, particularly in terms of access and efficacy, these milestones offer cautious optimism for altering the course of the disease.

Definition

The chronic neurodegenerative disease known as Alzheimer's disease is characterised by aberrant tau protein tangle and amyloid-beta plaque deposition in the brain, along with a decline in cognitive abilities, particularly in the areas of memory, language, and executive function. Alzheimer's disease is typically inherited and is often associated with advanced age, though it can also strike younger people. The diagnosis is made by clinical assessment, neuroimaging, and, in certain cases, advanced biomarker analysis.

Types

The current understanding of Alzheimer's disease subtypes is derived from genetic factors and when symptoms first appear. Hence researchers divide it into these main types:

- **Early-onset Alzheimer's disease (EOAD):** Close to 10% of Alzheimer's disease cases in people have an early onset before the age of 65 years. These cases are named early-onset Alzheimer's disease or EOAD. Genetic mutations found in the genes PSEN1, PSEN2 or APP leads to its development.
- **Late-onset Alzheimer's disease (LOAD):** Late-onset Alzheimer's disease (LOAD) represents the majority of this condition because it develops in patients above 65 years of age. The inheritance of Apolipoprotein E (APOE) ε4 allele increases LOAD risk but medical professionals consider this factor to be predominantly a risk factor and not the real cause.

Each person's Alzheimer's disease follows different paths in terms of progression because their underlying Aβ plaques and tau tangle pathology does not result in similar manifestations. Recent research indicates that Alzheimer's presents various pathophysiological substances among patients leading to conditions such as vascular dementia and Lewy body pathology which prove challenging to diagnose and treat.

Brief Note on Conventional Medicines

The treatment plans for Alzheimer's disease exist to enhance and normalize cognitive functioning and preserved daily functionality. Medical treatments available for Alzheimer's disease provide symptomatic help coupled with a brief delay of brain deterioration while offering no cure for the disease progression. The standard medical treatments employed for Alzheimer's disease include the following approach:

Table 1: Concise overview of conventional medications utilised in the management of Alzheimer's Disease.

Drug Class (Drug names)	Mechanism of Action	Common Dosage Forms	Usual Side Effects
Cholinesterase Inhibitors (e.g. galantamine, rivastigmine, and donepezil)	Preventing acetylcholine from being broken down, thereby enhancing cholinergic neurotransmission in the brain.	Oral tablets, transdermal patches (Rivastigmine).	Nausea, vomiting, diarrhoea, bradycardia, muscle cramps.
NMDA Receptor Antagonist (e.g. Memantine)	Modulates the glutamatergic system by blocking NMDA receptors, preventing excitotoxicity from excess glutamate.	Oral tablets, oral solution.	Dizziness, headache, constipation, confusion.
Combination Therapy (e.g. Donepezil + Memantine)	Combines cholinesterase inhibition with NMDA receptor blockade for a potentially additive symptomatic effect.	Oral tablets (fixed-dose combination).	Similar to the above, though side effects may accumulate or may add up.
Symptomatic Treatments (e.g. Antidepressants, Antipsychotics)	Manage neuropsychiatric symptoms like depression, agitation, or psychosis.	Oral tablets, oral solutions.	Sedation, extrapyramidal symptoms, weight gain, metabolic changes.

The medications provide temporary protection against cognitive deterioration but fail to stop or reverse Alzheimer's pathological neural damages in brain tissue. The treatment adherence process becomes difficult due to drug side effects together with existing medical conditions and cognitive impairment deficits that require multidisciplinary care and caregiver assistance as essential patient care elements.

Newer Drugs / Recent Advances

The advances in Alzheimer's disease treatment have grown better because medical staff understand the multifaceted pathophysiology of the disease including amyloid-beta roles and effects of tau pathology and neuroinflammation alongside synaptic dysfunction. Modern biomarkers and advanced imaging methods now enhance drug development by allowing healthcare providers to perform better patient classification and direct their interventions more specifically. Some promising newer therapies are being investigated as well as recently receiving approval based on the data presented below. New developments in Alzheimer's research may rapidly change the status of these compounds according to clinical trial results.

1. Lecanemab

Introduction: Scientists developed Lecanemab as a humanised monoclonal antibody intended to target soluble amyloid-beta (Aβ) protofibrils. Experts agree that disease progression in Alzheimer's disease depends on these structures. The regulatory body (FDA) granted the approval of Lecanemab after Biogen and Eisai developed it together in 2023 through the accelerated approval pathway.

Clinical Trial Phase / FDA-Approval: Lecanemab has completed Phase III trials (CLARITY-AD study) and received FDA-Approval in 2023 for early Alzheimer's disease (AD) patients.

Mechanism of Action: Lecanemab works by binding to soluble amyloid-beta (Aβ) protofibrils and stopping them from aggregating into insoluble amyloid plaques. It is a monoclonal antibody. The process entails:

1. **Selective Targeting of Soluble Protofibrils**
   - Unlike other monoclonal antibodies that bind to aggregated plaques, Lecanemab specifically binds to soluble Aβ protofibrils (early toxic oligomers).
   - These protofibrils are more neurotoxic than mature plaques and play a crucial role in synaptic dysfunction.
2. **Microglia-Mediated Phagocytosis**
   - Once Lecanemab binds to protofibrils, it triggers microglia activation, leading to enhanced phagocytosis and clearance of Aβ.
3. **Reduced Aβ Deposition and Plaque Formation**
   - By removing protofibrils, Lecanemab prevents the formation of mature amyloid plaques.
   - This leads to lower brain amyloid levels, which correlates with slowed cognitive decline.
4. **Minimization of Neuroinflammation**
   - Aβ accumulation causes chronic neuroinflammation, which contributes to neuronal damage.
   - Lecanemab's clearance of protofibrils reduces this inflammatory response.

Key Pharmacokinetic Parameters: Across clinically investigated doses, lecanemab shows dose-proportional serum concentrations and linear pharmacokinetics. With an approximate half-life of seven days, it is administered intravenously and can be dosed every two weeks. Since the medication is mostly eliminated by reticuloendothelial catabolism of IgG antibodies, it exhibits little hepatic metabolism. After a few weeks of dosing, steady-state levels are usually reached, and fibrinogen has been found to be a significant plasma protein binding partner that may affect the distribution and removal of the protein. Lecanemab supports fixed dosing regimens for the majority of patients due to its low interpatient variability in exposure.

Adverse Drug Reactions: Amyloid-related imaging abnormalities (ARIA) like microhaemorrhages, hyperkalaemia, headache, infusion-related reactions, and increased risk of cerebral oedema.

Uses: Mild cognitive impairment (MCI), early-stage Alzheimer's disease (Phase III trial).

Dose: 10 mg/kg IV every 2 weeks.

2. Donanemab

Introduction: Donanemab is an anti-amyloid monoclonal antibody targeting modified Aβ species. It has been effective in decreasing cognitive decline and lowering the load of amyloid plaque.

Clinical Trial Phase / FDA-Approval: Currently in Phase III clinical trials (TRAILBLAZER-ALZ 2 study) and awaiting regulatory approval.

Mechanism of Action: Donanemab is an IgG1 monoclonal antibody targeting N-terminal pyroglutamate-modified Aβ (N3pE Aβ), which is more aggregation-prone. It works via:

1. **Selective Binding to Pyroglutamate Aβ**
   - Pyroglutamate-modified Aβ is a highly neurotoxic and aggregation-prone species found in mature plaques.
   - Donanemab selectively binds to these toxic forms, enhancing their clearance.
2. **Microglia Activation and Phagocytosis**
   - The Fc region of Donanemab interacts with microglial Fc receptors, leading to phagocytosis of Aβ.
   - This facilitates plaque clearance and reduces amyloid burden.

3. **Reduction of Tau Pathology**
   - By removing amyloid plaques, Donanemab indirectly lowers tau hyperphosphorylation.
   - This helps to preserve neuronal integrity and slows disease progression.

Key Pharmacokinetic Parameters: Due to its big size this medication has restricted ability to pass through the blood-brain barrier. Plasma half-life is 8-10 days. The medication gets administered as an intravenous (IV) injection and undergoes reticuloendothelial degradation metabolism. Monoclonal antibody degradation pathways destroy and eliminate this component in the human body.

Adverse Drug Reactions: ARIA (brain swelling and microhaemorrhages), flu-like symptoms and infusion reactions.

Uses: Alzheimer's disease that is mild to moderate (Phase III study).

Dose: 700 mg IV Q2W for 3 doses, then 1400 mg Q4W (The expanded form of Q2W is "Quaque 2 Weeks" & Q4W means "Quaque 4 Weeks", which means every 2 weeks and every 4 weeks respectively).

3. Blarcamesine (ANAVEX 2-73)

Introduction: Blarcamesine is a sigma-1 receptor agonist with potential neuroprotective and anti-inflammatory properties. It modulates cellular homeostasis and enhances neuronal survival.

Clinical Trial Phase/FDA-Approval: Phase IIb/III trials completed, showing promising results for cognitive stabilization.

Mechanism of Action: Blarcamesine is a sigma-1 receptor (S1R) agonist, providing neuroprotection, anti-inflammatory effects and cognitive enhancement through:

1. **Modulation of S1R Activity**
   - The sigma-1 receptor is a molecular chaperone located in the endoplasmic reticulum (ER) and mitochondria-associated membranes (MAMs).
   - Activation of S1R regulates calcium homeostasis, ER stress response, and mitochondrial function.
2. **Reduction in Oxidative Stress and Apoptosis**
   - Blarcamesine reduces reactive oxygen species (ROS) and mitochondrial dysfunction.
   - This protects neurons from oxidative stress-induced apoptosis.
3. **Enhancement of Synaptic Plasticity**
   - Blarcamesine enhances synaptic transmission by modulating NMDA receptor activity.
   - This improves learning and memory functions.
4. **Regulation of Tau Phosphorylation**
   - By reducing ER stress and inflammation, tau hyperphosphorylation is suppressed, preventing neurofibrillary tangle formation.

Key Pharmacokinetic Parameters: It exhibits good oral bioavailability, though exact percentage values are still under investigation. The plasma half-life is roughly around 20 hours. The route of administration is oral. It is metabolised in liver (CYP450 enzymes) and is mainly eliminated via hepatic pathways, with minimal renal clearance.

Adverse Drug Reactions: Dizziness, fatigue, neuropsychiatric adverse effects (anxiety and agitation) and gastrointestinal disturbances.

Uses: Neurodegenerative illnesses like Alzheimer's and mild cognitive impairment in Parkinson's disease (Phase IIb/III trials).

Dose: 30–50 mg/day orally.

4. GV-971 (Sodium Oligomannate)

Introduction: China now approves GV-971 which originated from marine polysaccharides as a treatment for mild-to-moderate Alzheimer's disease (AD). The medication activates gut microbiota functions which decreases brain inflammation.

Clinical Trial Phase / FDA-Approval: Approved in China; currently in Phase III trials in Europe and the United States.

Mechanism of Action: GV-971 is an oligosaccharide derived from marine algae that exerts anti-inflammatory and anti-amyloid effects via gut-brain axis modulation.

1. **Regulation of Gut Microbiota**
   - GV-971 modifies gut microbiome composition, reducing pro-inflammatory bacteria.
   - This decreases systemic and central nervous system (CNS) inflammation.
2. **Inhibition of Aβ Aggregation**
   - GV-971 directly binds to Aβ monomers and oligomers, preventing their aggregation into plaques.
3. **Reduction of Neuroinflammation**
   - Aβ accumulation triggers microglial activation and cytokine release.
   - GV-971 reduces the manufacturing of inflammatory cytokines (TNF-α, IL-1β, and IL-6), protecting neurons.

Key Pharmacokinetic Parameters: Orally administered with good oral absorption. The predicted bioavailability reaches between 30–40%. This drug remains hydrophilic which restrains its ability to pass the blood-brain barrier, yet it influences gut microbiota levels indirectly. The plasma half-life exists at about 14 hours. Metabolism occurs minimally within the liver before its removal through the urine and stools.

Adverse Drug Reactions: Diarrhoea, nausea, headache, and mild allergic reactions.

Uses: Alzheimer's disease (mild to moderate severity).

Dose: 450 mg orally twice daily.

5. Simufilam

Introduction: Simufilam is a medication with tiny molecules that restores the structure of filamin A (FLNA), an intracellular protein involved in neuroinflammation and tau pathology.

Clinical Trial Phase / FDA-Approval: Currently in Phase III trials.

Mechanism of Action: Simufilam is a small molecule targeting Filamin A (FLNA), a cytoskeletal protein involved in Aβ signalling and tau aggregation.

1. **Restoration of FLNA Function**
   - In AD, Aβ disrupts FLNA, causing tau hyperphosphorylation and synaptic dysfunction.
   - Simufilam restores FLNA structure, improving neuronal stability.

2. **Reduction of Neuroinflammation**
   - Simufilam blocks Aβ-FLNA interactions, reducing inflammatory cytokine release from microglia.
3. **Enhancement of Synaptic Function**
   - By stabilizing FLNA, Simufilam restores NMDA receptor function, improving cognition.

Key Pharmacokinetic Parameters: Orally administered drug with good oral bioavailability. Plasma half-life is 16 hours. The drug transitions efficiently through the blood-brain barrier because of its oil-absorbing properties. This drug requires liver (CYP3A4) enzyme metabolism before it leaves the body by renal elimination routes and faecal excretion processes.

Adverse Drug Reactions: Fatigue, headache, mild gastrointestinal discomfort and QT prolongation.

Uses: The pharmaceutical application targeting mild to moderate Alzheimer's disease continues in Phase III clinical trials (Phase III study).

Dose: 100–300 mg orally BID.

6. Gantenerumab

Introduction: Gantenerumab represents a completely human IgG1 monoclonal antibody for AD which targets aggregated amyloid-beta (Aβ). Roche developed this compound for potential use as a disease-modifying medicine which aims to prevent dementia progression through reduction of amyloid plaque deposits and improvement of cognitive functions.

Clinical Trial Phase / FDA-Approval: Gantenerumab is currently in Phase III clinical trials (Graduate 1 and Graduate 2 studies) for early Alzheimer's disease. However, in November 2022, Roche announced that with no discernible slowing of cognitive deterioration and a lower-than-anticipated decrease in amyloid burden, gantenerumab fell short of the primary goal. Further analysis is ongoing to determine potential future applications.

Mechanism of Action: Gantenerumab is an anti-amyloid-beta monoclonal antibody that targets multiple regions of Aβ peptides, including:

1. **Selective Binding to Amyloid Plaques**
   - Unlike some antibodies that primarily bind to soluble Aβ protofibrils, Gantenerumab has a high affinity for insoluble amyloid plaques and fibrillar Aβ.
   - This allows it to reduce amyloid burden more effectively (theoretically).
2. **Microglia-Mediated Clearance**
   - The Fc region of Gantenerumab binds to Fcγ receptors on microglial cells, activating an immune response that leads to phagocytosis and degradation of amyloid plaques.
3. **Prevention of Further Aβ Aggregation**
   - Binding to Aβ fibrils - reduces the seeding effect - preventing further aggregation and plaque expansion.
4. **Impact on Tau Pathology**
   - While primarily targeting amyloid, reducing Aβ burden indirectly affects tau hyperphosphorylation, which is a key contributor to neurodegeneration in AD.

Key Pharmacokinetic Parameters: Plasma half-life of the drug reaches 28 days. Administration of the drug takes place through subcutaneous (s.c.) injection. Proteolytic enzymes metabolize the drug which the reticuloendothelial system removes from the body.

Adverse Drug Reactions: Amyloid-related imaging abnormalities (ARIA), such as injection site reactions (pain, redness, swelling), headaches, cerebral oedema (ARIA-E), and microhaemorrhages (ARIA-H), dizziness, flu-like symptoms and rare cases of hypersensitivity reactions.

Uses: The pharmaceutical product is being studied for treating early and mild Alzheimer's disease. The medicine may be used as part of combination treatment approaches with other disease-modifying treatments in future applications.

Dose: 1,020 mg SC monthly (dose in GRADUATE trials).

7. Zagotenemab

Introduction: The Eli Lilly pharmaceutical company developed Zagotenemab (LY3303560) as a monoclonal antibody that binds to tau protein aggregates which leads to Alzheimer's disease pathogenesis. This drug exists as part of a tau-targeted therapeutic method to decrease tau propagation while inhibiting the development of neurofibrillary tangles.

Clinical Trial Phase / FDA-Approval: Zagotenemab is currently in Phase II clinical trials (Tau NextGen and TRAILBLAZER-ALZ studies).

Mechanism of Action: Zagotenemab operates as a therapeutic monoclonal antibody targeting tau aggregates thereby blocking their transmission through neuronal cells. The mechanism includes:

1. **Selective Binding to Misfolded Tau**
   - Zagotenemab detects mid-region tau epitopes which appears in abnormally folded tau aggregates but not in normal physiological tau.
2. **Prevention of Tau Propagation**
   - Pathogenic tau spreads between neurons, facilitating disease progression.
   - Zagotenemab blocks tau transmission, reducing tau seeding and neurofibrillary tangles (NFT) formation.
3. **Microglia-Mediated Clearance**
   - Similar to Gantenerumab, the Fc region of Zagotenemab interacts with microglial Fc receptors, promoting phagocytosis and degradation of extracellular tau aggregates.
4. **Reduction of Neurotoxicity**
   - By reducing tau burden, Zagotenemab lowers neuronal dysfunction and synaptic toxicity.

Key Pharmacokinetic Parameters: The size of Zagotenemab makes its penetration into the central nervous system slow because of its large size. Plasma half-life is 20-30 days. The substance gets eliminated through proteolytic degradation (non-hepatic clearance) and reticuloendothelial clearance.

Adverse Drug Reactions: Injection-site reactions, fatigue and headache, ARIA (though less common compared to anti-Aβ therapies) and mild cognitive worsening in some cases (unclear mechanism).

Uses: Potential future use in combination therapies for tau-targeted AD treatments. Investigational therapy for other tauopathies such as frontotemporal dementia (FTD).

Dose: 70–210 mg SC every 4 weeks (Clinical trial dosing).

Key Therapeutic Targets

1. **Amyloid-Beta Pathway:** Monoclonal antibodies such as aducanumab, Lecanemab, Donanemab, and gantenerumab are all designed to reduce amyloid-beta levels, albeit through different epitopes and binding mechanisms. Clinical data suggest that while these antibodies can successfully lower brain amyloid plaque burden, their clinical impact on cognition is sometimes modest, controversial, or dependent on early intervention. Yet, the FDA's conditional approvals of some of these agents underscore their potential as the first disease-modifying therapies for AD.

2. **Tau-Targeting Therapies:** In addition to beta-amyloid, there is increasing attention on therapies that targets tau pathology. Among them, Zagotenemab and other anti-tau antibodies aim to prevent the spread of tau aggregates across the brain. Although still in development, tau-targeting drugs could be beneficial either as standalone therapies or in combination with amyloid-targeting agents.

3. **Neuroinflammation:** Chronic inflammation is now considered a core feature of the disease. Agents like Anavex 2-73 and GV-971 are designed to mitigate inflammation either centrally or via the gut-brain axis. This marks a growing trend toward multifaceted approaches, recognizing that neurodegeneration involves complex interactions between immune cells, glial cells, and pathological proteins.

4. **Synaptic Health and Neuroprotection:** Multiple experimental treatments focus on preserving synaptic function and preventing excitotoxicity. While memantine already modulates glutamatergic pathways in conventional treatment, next-generation compounds may offer more nuanced or potent neuroprotective effects.

Other Emerging Approaches

- **Gene Therapy:** Although still in its infancy for neurodegenerative diseases, gene therapy aim to deliver neuroprotective genes or correct pathogenic mutations. These remain largely experimental but could eventually offer personalized treatments for EOAD with known genetic mutations.

- **Cell-Based Therapies:** Stem cell transplantation to replace damaged neurons or support neuroregeneration is a theoretical approach, but it faces numerous challenges in clinical translation, including graft viability, immune response, and integration into existing neural circuits.

- **Combination Therapies:** Because Alzheimer's disease is complex, a mix of medications that target tau, amyloid, and inflammation may yield synergistic effects. Ongoing trials are examining whether combining monoclonal antibodies with neuroprotective agents can provide superior clinical benefits compared to monotherapy.

Conclusion

The treatment of Alzheimer's disease has significantly improved over the last ten years, shifting from traditional medication-based symptom management to biologic therapies that target underlying mechanisms such as tau pathology, amyloid-beta build-up, neuroinflammation, and synaptic loss. Even though new antibodies like aducanumab and lecanemab show promise, there are still issues, such as side effects, high costs, and limited efficacy, and results vary. New approaches, such as investigations into the gut-brain axis and gene and cell-based treatments, give hope. The goal of ongoing research is to improve these methods, find appropriate patient populations, and create combination therapies that can postpone or stop cognitive decline and, in the end, enhance quality of life.

References

1. Al-Kuraishy HM, Sulaiman GM, Mohammed HA, Mohammed SG, Al-Gareeb AI, Albuhadily AK, Dawood RA, Al Ali A, Abu-Alghayth MH. Amyloid-β and heart failure in Alzheimer's disease: the new vistas. Frontiers in Medicine. 2025 Feb 4;12:1494101.

2. Bovis K, Davies-Branch M, Day PJ. Dysregulated Neurotransmission and the Role of Viruses in Alzheimer's Disease. ACS Chemical Neuroscience. 2025 Mar 6.
3. Van Olst L, Simonton B, Edwards AJ, Forsyth AV, Boles J, Jamshidi P, Watson T, Shepard N, Krainc T, Argue BM, Zhang Z. Microglial mechanisms drive amyloid-β clearance in immunized patients with Alzheimer's disease. Nature medicine. 2025 Mar 6:1-3.
4. Chen C, Zhang Z, Liu Y, Hong W, Karahan H, Wang J, Li W, Diao L, Yu M, Saykin AJ, Nho K. Comprehensive characterization of the transcriptional landscape in Alzheimer's disease (AD) brains. Science Advances. 2025 Jan 3;11(1):eadn1927.
5. Bondi MW, Edmonds EC, Salmon DP. Alzheimer's disease: past, present, and future. Journal of the International Neuropsychological Society. 2017 Oct;23(9-10):818-31.
6. Cummings J, Aisen PS, DuBois B, Frölich L, Jack CR, Jones RW, Morris JC, Raskin J, Dowsett SA, Scheltens P. Drug development in Alzheimer's disease: the path to 2025. Alzheimer's research & therapy. 2016 Dec;8:1-2.
7. Anand R, Gill KD, Mahdi AA. Therapeutics of Alzheimer's disease: Past, present and future. Neuropharmacology. 2014 Jan 1;76:27-50.
8. Liu PP, Xie Y, Meng XY, Kang JS. History and progress of hypotheses and clinical trials for Alzheimer's disease. Signal transduction and targeted therapy. 2019 Aug 23;4(1):29.
9. Jack CR Jr. Advances in Alzheimer's disease research over the past two decades. Lancet Neurol. 2022;21(6):450–52.
10. Giacobini E, Becker RE. One hundred years after the discovery of Alzheimer's disease. A turning point for therapy?. Journal of Alzheimer's disease. 2007 Aug 24;12(1):37-52.
11. Chowdhury S, Chowdhury NS. Novel anti-amyloid-beta (Aβ) monoclonal antibody lecanemab for Alzheimer's disease: a systematic review. Int J ImmunopatholPharmacol. 2023;37:1–9.
12. Kwon HS, Koh SH. Monoclonal Antibodies–A New Horizon in Alzheimer's Treatment. Journal of Clinical Neurology. 2025 Jan 1;21(1):1-2.
13. Macfarlane S, Grimmer T, Teo K, O'Brien TJ, Woodward M, Grunfeld J, Mander A, Brodtmann A, Brew BJ, Morris P, Short C. Blarcamesine for the treatment of Early Alzheimer's Disease: Results from the ANAVEX2-73-AD-004 Phase IIB/III trial. The Journal of Prevention of Alzheimer's Disease. 2025 Jan 1;12(1):100016.
14. Rani A, Khan J, Choudhary L, Kumar M, Jha A, Pandey G, Nand B. Unraveling the Therapeutic Potential of Alzheimer's Drugs: A Comprehensive Review. Tetrahedron. 2025 Feb 1:134517.
15. Neațu M, Covaliu A, Ioniță I, Jugurt A, Davidescu EI, Popescu BO. Monoclonal antibody therapy in Alzheimer's disease. Pharmaceutics. 2023 Dec 29;16(1):60.
16. Esquer A, Blanc F, Collongues N. immunotherapies targeting amyloid and tau protein in Alzheimer's disease: Should we move away from diseases and focus on biological targets? A systematic review and expert opinion. Neurology and Therapy. 2023 Dec;12(6):1883-907.
17. Vaz M, Silvestre S. Alzheimer's disease: Recent treatment strategies. European journal of pharmacology. 2020 Nov 15;887:173554.
18. Aljassabi A, Zieneldien T, Kim J, Regmi D, Cao C. Alzheimer's disease immunotherapy: current strategies and future prospects. Journal of Alzheimer's Disease. 2024 Apr 2;98(3):755-72.
19. Triumbari EK, Chiaravalloti A, Schillaci O, Mercuri NB, Liguori C. Positron emission tomography/computed tomography imaging in therapeutic clinical trials in Alzheimer's disease: an overview of the current state of the art of research. Journal of Alzheimer's Disease. 2024 Oct 18;101(s1):S603-28.
20. Gu X, Qi L, Qi Q, Zhou J, Chen S, Wang L. Monoclonal antibody therapy for Alzheimer's disease focusing on intracerebral targets. BioScience Trends. 2024 Feb 29;18(1):49-65.
21. Winblad B, Amouyel P, Andrieu S, et al. Defeating Alzheimer's disease and other dementias: A priority for European science and society. Lancet Neurol. 2016;15(5):455–532.
22. Weller J, Budson A. Current understanding of Alzheimer's disease diagnosis and treatment. *F1000Res*.2018;7:1161.Lane CA, Hardy J, Schott JM. Alzheimer's disease. *Eur J Neurol*. 2018;25(1):59–70.
23. Scheltens P, De Strooper B, Kivipelto M, Holstege H, Chételat G, Teunissen CE, Cummings J, van der Flier WM. Alzheimer's disease. The Lancet. 2021 Apr 24;397(10284):1577-90.
24. Bateman RJ, Xiong C, Benzinger TL, Fagan AM, Goate A, Fox NC, Marcus DS, Cairns NJ, Xie X, Blazey TM, Holtzman DM. Clinical and biomarker changes in dominantly inherited Alzheimer's disease. New England Journal of Medicine. 2012 Aug 30;367(9):795-804.
25. Birks JS, Harvey RJ. Donepezil for dementia due to Alzheimer's disease. *Cochrane Database Syst Rev*. 2018(6):CD001190.
26. Karran E, De Strooper B. The amyloid cascade hypothesis: are we poised for success or failure?. Journal of neurochemistry. 2016 Oct;139:237-52.
27. Selkoe DJ, Hardy J. The amyloid hypothesis of Alzheimer's disease at 25 years. EMBO molecular medicine. 2016 Jun;8(6):595-608.
28. Wang X, Sun G, Feng T, Zhang J, Huang X, Wang T, Xie Z, Chu X, Yang J, Wang H, Chang S. Sodium oligomannate therapeutically remodels gut microbiota and suppresses gut bacterial amino acids-shaped neuroinflammation to inhibit Alzheimer's disease progression. Cell research. 2019 Oct;29(10):787-803.

29. Arroyo-Pacheco N, Sarmiento-Blanco S, Vergara-Cadavid G, Castro-Leones M, Contreras-Puentes N. Monoclonal therapy with lecanemab in the treatment of mild Alzheimer's disease: A systematic review and meta-analysis. Ageing Research Reviews. 2025 Feb 1;104:102620.
30. Cai W, Zhang H, Wu Y, Yao Y, Zhang J. Comparative the efficacy and safety of Gosuranemab, Semorinemab, Tilavonemab, and Zagotenemab in patients with Alzheimer's disease: a systematic review and network meta-analysis of randomized controlled trials. Frontiers in Aging Neuroscience. 2025 Jan 29;16:1465871.
31. Bateman RJ, Li Y, McDade EM, Llibre-Guerra JJ, Clifford DB, Atri A, Mills SL, Santacruz AM, Wang G, Supnet C, Benzinger TL. Safety and efficacy of long-term gantenerumab treatment in dominantly inherited Alzheimer's disease: an open-label extension of the phase 2/3 multicentre, randomised, double-blind, placebo-controlled platform DIAN-TU trial. The Lancet Neurology. 2025 Apr 1;24(4):316-30.
32. Fluegge K, Fluegge K. Comment on Wang et al. Simufilam Reverses Aberrant Receptor Interactions of Filamin A in Alzheimer's Disease. Int. J. Mol. Sci. 2023, 24, 13927. International Journal of Molecular Sciences. 2025 Mar 11;26(6):2480.

Chapter 13

Recent Advances in the Management of Bipolar Mood Disorder

Author: Dr. Pranab Das

Introduction

Bipolar mood disorder, previously referred to as manic-depressive disease, is a persistent mental condition characterised by alternating episodes of mania or hypomania and depression, interspersed by intervals of normal mood (euthymia). Impacting 1–3% of the global populace, it is a primary contributor to disability and elevated mortality, frequently coexisting with other medical disorders that exacerbate suicide risk. The intricate clinical manifestation and recurrent characteristics create considerable difficulties for precise diagnosis and sustained therapy. Primary symptoms include heightened activity, diminished sleep, and hazardous behaviour during manic episodes, contrasted by profound melancholy, anhedonia, and suicide thoughts during depression periods. Diagnosis is based on standardised criteria from the DSM-5 and ICD-11, which highlight symptom duration, intensity, and functional impact.

Treatment predominantly consists of lithium, anticonvulsants, and antipsychotics, which might diminish the frequency of episodes when administered consistently. Nonetheless, adverse effects, treatment resistance in certain subgroups, and the many manifestations of bipolar disorder necessitate ongoing research. Progress in comprehending the pathophysiology of the disorder; encompassing monoaminergic dysregulation, circadian rhythm disturbance, neuroinflammation, and compromised neuroplasticity, has facilitated the development of targeted therapeutics. Current advancements encompass innovative pharmaceuticals, enhanced formulations, and supplementary therapies focused on neuroprotection and mood stabilisation. This chapter examines the clinical characteristics and classifications of bipolar disorder, delineates conventional treatments, and presents innovative therapeutic approaches that show potential for enhanced outcomes.

Historical Perspective

Over the past century, there has been a significant evolution in our understanding and treatment of bipolar mood disorder (BPD). The foundation for modern diagnostic classifications was laid by Emil Kraepelin in the late 19th century, who formally classified "manic-depressive insanity" as a separate nosological entity. Hippocrates and Aretaeus of Cappadocia both described varying mood states that resemble modern-day manic-depressive illness.

John Cade's 1949 discovery of lithium marked a significant advancement in pharmacological management. Lithium is still essential for mood stabilisation, particularly for preventing suicide and manic episodes. Anticonvulsants like valproate, carbamazepine, and lamotrigine were developed in the ensuing decades, expanding the range of available treatments, especially for patients with mixed or rapid cycling states.

Second-generation antipsychotics (SGAs), like olanzapine, risperidone, and quetiapine, were used as mood stabilisers in the 1980s and 1990s, especially for bipolar mania. Later, these medications were included as adjuncts or monotherapy in official treatment guidelines. They were extremely valuable because of their capacity to control both mood symptoms and psychotic traits.

More recently, the focus of treatment has shifted from symptom suppression to neuroprotection and functional recovery. The approval of lumateperone, cariprazine, and lurasidone for bipolar depression fills a crucial therapeutic gap. The management paradigm has been further enhanced by adjunctive psychosocial therapies, such as interpersonal social rhythm therapy, family-focused therapy, and cognitive-behavioural therapy (CBT).

In order to predict relapse and customise treatments, current research focusses on digital monitoring, genetics, and biomarkers. Furthermore, there is hope for quicker and more customised interventions thanks to the active research of novel agents like ketamine, neurosteroids, and targeted anti-inflammatory therapies.

Types of Bipolar Disorder

Bipolar disorder is a heterogeneous disorder, encompassing various subtypes and clinical presentations. The common diagnostic subtypes include:

1. **Bipolar I Disorder:** Characterised by the presence of at least one complete manic episode, which could be followed or preceded by significant depressed or hypomanic episodes. Bipolar I Mania can be severe enough to necessitate hospitalization or be accompanied by psychotic features.
2. **Bipolar II Disorder:** Characterised by at least one episode of profound depression and one episode of hypomania. Patients with Bipolar II do not experience full-blown mania; however, they often have recurrent, significant depressive episodes that impair daily functioning.
3. **Cyclothymic Disorder:** A persistent mood disorder that lasts for at least two years (one year for kids and teenagers), with multiple episodes of hypomanic symptoms and depressive episodes that don't quite fit the definition of a major depressive episode.
4. **Other Specified / Unspecified Bipolar Disorder:** These classifications include people who have bipolar-like mood symptoms but do not entirely fit the criteria for cyclothymia, bipolar I, or bipolar II, reflecting the broad spectrum of bipolar-related conditions.

Distinguishing between these subtypes is essential for formulating treatment plans and prognostic expectations, as treatment response can vary significantly among subgroups.

Brief Note on Conventional Medicines

The core purpose of standard treatment for bipolar disorder focuses on achieving mental balance and preventing recurrent episodes of mood fluctuations while decreasing their intensity and frequency. Patients with bipolar disorder receive standard treatments through combining mood stabilizers with antipsychotic medications along with adjunctive agents which help treat acute mania and depression together with serving as maintenance therapy. This table below provides an abridged breakdown of the traditional treatment approaches that doctors commonly apply currently:

Table 1: Concise Overview of Conventional Medications Utilised in the Management of Bipolar Mood Disorder.

Drug/ Drug Class	Mechanism of Action	Common Dosage Forms	Usual Side Effects
Lithium	Modulates neurotransmission via multiple pathways, including second messengers (e.g. IP3) by inhibiting ionositolmonophosphatase enzyme, thereby reducing intracellular recycling of ionositol and neurotrophic factors - stabilizes mood.	Oral tablets, capsules, syrups.	Tremor, weight gain, polyuria, hypothyroidism, renal impairment.
Valproate (Valproic Acid)	Increases GABA (inhibitory neurotransmitter) levels - stabilizes neuronal membranes and modulates ion channels.	Oral tablets, capsules, i.v. formulation.	GI disturbances, weight gain, tremors, hepatotoxicity, teratogenicity.
Carbamazepine	Blocks voltage-gated sodium channels - stabilizing overexcited neurons.	Oral tablets, suspension.	Dizziness, sedation, ataxia, hyponatremia.
Lamotrigine	Decreases glutamate release and blocks voltage-sensitive sodium channels; it is very useful in preventing bipolar depression.	Oral tablet (chewable/ dispersible tablets).	Skin rash, headache, blurred vision, potential for Stevens-Johnson syndrome.
Atypical Antipsychotics (e.g. Olanzapine, Quetiapine, Risperidone)	Blocks D2 receptors and modulate serotonin receptors; some have mood-stabilizing properties.	Long-acting injectables, oral pills, and tablets that dissolve in the mouth.	Sedation, weight gain, metabolic syndrome, extrapyramidal symptoms, hyperprolactinemia.

Although these medications effectively reduce manic symptoms and stabilize mood, therapeutic outcomes may be tampered by medication side effects, partial response, or relapse over time. Psychoeducation, psychotherapy, and lifestyle modifications are typically recommended alongside medications to optimize patient adherence and long-term stabilization.

Newer Drugs / Recent Advances

Researchers aim to develop better bipolar disorder treatments through enhanced efficacy alongside wider therapeutic windows as well as decreased toxicity and pathologicalfactor based treatment of the disorder (e.g. neuroinflammation, circadian rhythm dysregulation, neurotrophic factors). A summary has been provided showing promising newer therapeutic agents as well as investigational approaches under clinical trialor under investigation. The development of drugs for bipolar disorder remains difficult because this condition presents extensive variability and requires data collection about long-term outcomes as well as managing comorbidities.

1. Cariprazine

Introduction: The atypical antipsychotic drug cariprazine, a derivative of piperazine, was initially created in Hungary. It functions as an antagonist at serotonin 5-HT2A receptors and as a partial agonist at central dopamine D2, dopamine D3, and serotonin 5-HT1A receptors. Numerous mental illnesses, such as major depressive disorder, bipolar disorder, and schizophrenia, have been studied in relation to cariprazine.

Clinical Trial Phase / FDA-Approved: Health Canada authorised the medication in April 2022 after it was initially approved in the US by FDA under the brand name Vraylar.

Mechanism of Action:

1. 5-HT2A antagonism:

Serotonin (5-HT) stimulates 5-HT2A receptors present in the glutamatergic neurones in pre-frontal cortex (PFC) - increase glutamate release - released glutamate stimulates dopaminergic neurones in emotional striatum - increase dopamine (DA) release in emotional striatum. In mania, this pathway becomes hyperactive, resulting in increase in DA release in emotional striatum. Hence, by 5-HT2A antagonism - decrease in DA release in emotional striatum - relieves manic symptoms.

5-HT - Stimulates 5-HT2A receptors in pituitary lactotrophs - stimulates prolactin release. Hence, 5-HT2A antagonist decreases prolactin release and does not cause hyperprolactinaemia.

2. D2 partial agonism:

D2 partial agonism produces submaximal D2 response without producing side-effects of D2 antagonists - antipsychotic and antimanic effect is perceived without any hyperprolactinaemia.

3. 5-HT1A partial agonism:

5-HT - stimulates 5-HT1A receptors present in glutamatergic neurones in substantia nigra (SN) - increase glutamate release - glutamate stimulates GABA interneurons - increase GABA release - GABA inhibits DA neurones in motor striatum - decrease DA release in motor striatum - DIP. Hence, 5-HT1A partial agonist increases DA release in motor striatum - reduces DIP.

5-HT stimulates 5-HT1A receptors in glutamatergic neurones of Ventral Tegmental Area (VTA) - increase glutamate release - glutamate stimulates GABA interneurons - increase GABA release - GABA inhibits DA neurones in PFC - decrease DA release in PFC - negative and depressive symptoms. 5-HT1A partial agonist - Stimulates glutamatergic neuronessubmaximally thereby reducing glutamate release - Reducing the activation of GABA interneurones - improvement of negative and depressive symptoms.

Key Pharmacokinetic Parameters: Cariprazine shows 91-97% plasma protein binding. CYP3A4 and, to a lesser extent, CYP2D6 extensively metabolise cariprazine to produce two main metabolites: didesmethylcariprazine (DDCAR) and desmethylcariprazine (DCAR). The metabolites DCAR and DDCAR have pharmacological activity. It is mainly excreted by faeces (63%) and partly by urine (21%).

Adverse Drug Reactions: Akathisia, nausea, insomnia and sedation. It has a favourable side-effect profile with minimal sedation and a lower risk of weight gain compared to other SGAs.

Uses: It is now used to treat bipolar disorder's depressive episodes, manic or mixed episodes, and schizophrenia.

Dose: 1.5–6 mg once daily orally.

2. Lumateperone

Introduction: The glutamate, dopamine, and serotonin systems are all impacted by lumeteperone, a novel antipsychotic. It has a unique mode of action because it acts as a postsynaptic D2 antagonist, a partial agonist at presynaptic dopamine D2 receptors, and an antagonist at serotonin 5-HT2A receptors. Lumateperone is approved to treat schizophrenia and is being studied for bipolar depression. With minimal risk of weight gain and metabolic side effects, its safety profile is favourable.

Clinical Trial Phase / FDA-Approval: FDA-approved (2021) for Bipolar Depression (I & II) as monotherapy and adjunctive therapy.

Mechanism of Action:

1. **D2 Receptor Modulation**
   - Partial agonist at presynaptic D2 receptors - reducing dopamine overactivity.
   - Antagonist at postsynaptic D2 receptors - stabilizing dopamine transmission.
2. **5-HT2A Antagonism**
   - Enhances glutamatergic transmission - improving mood stabilization.
3. **Glutamate NMDA Modulation**
   - Enhances AMPA receptor activity, increasing synaptic plasticity and mood regulation.
4. **GABAergic Enhancement**
   - Indirectly enhances GABA-A transmission, promoting calming effects in bipolar disorder.

Key Pharmacokinetic Parameters: Lumateperoneis able to permeate multidrug resistance protein 1 (MDR 1) and is very lipophilic at a pH of 7.4, which are characteristics that allow the antipsychotic to be absorbed in the small intestine and the blood brain barrier. Lumateperone is approximately 97% plasma protein bound. Lumateperone is extensively metabolized. The carbonyl side chain is reduced by ketone reductase to produce the primary active metabolite. It is mainly excreted by stools and partly by urine.

Adverse Drug Reactions: Drowsiness, dizziness, nausea, seizures and hypotension.

Uses: Used to manage both positive and negative symptoms of schizophrenia.

Dose: 42 mg once daily orally.

3. KarXT (Xanomeline-Trospium)

Introduction: A muscarinic receptor agonist/antagonist combination called KarXT has been developed to treat schizophrenia and bipolar disorder. With few side effects related to dopamine, it lessens psychotic symptoms.

Clinical Trial Phase / FDA-Approval: Currently in Phase III trials for bipolar psychosis.

Mechanism of Action:

1. **Xanomeline (M1/M4 Muscarinic Agonist)**
   - Enhances cholinergic signalling in cortical and limbic areas.
   - Reduces mania symptoms and stabilizes mood.
2. **Trospium (Peripheral Anticholinergic Agent)**
   - Blocks peripheral muscarinic receptors, reducing gastrointestinal and cardiovascular side effects.

Key Pharmacokinetic Parameters: Xanomeline is efficiently absorbed via oral administration, achieving therapeutic plasma concentrations within two to three hours. Trospium is a quaternary ammonium compound that inhibits central nervous system penetration, thereby restricting its action to peripheral muscarinic receptors. The plasma half-life ranges from 12 to 14 hours. It undergoes metabolism in the liver through CYP450 enzymes and is primarily excreted in urine.

Adverse Drug Reactions: Dry mouth, nausea, minimal weight gain and no extrapyramidal side effects.

Uses: Bipolar mania and Schizophrenia (under development).

Dose: 125–150 mg xanomeline / 30–40 mg trospium BID (clinical trial dose).

4. Seltorexant

Introduction: Seltorexant is currently being investigated for the treatment-resistant insomnia and bipolar depression.

Clinical Trial Phase / FDA-Approval: Phase III clinical trials for bipolar depression.

Mechanism of Action:

1. **Selective Orexin-2 Receptor Antagonism**
    - Orexins are secreted from lateral hypothalamus.
    - Orexins stimulates OXR1 and OXR2 receptors in histaminergic neurones - increase histamine release in brain - wakefulness.
    - Orexin receptor antagonist thereby decreases tendency of wakefulness and induces sleep.
    - Hence it promotes sleep and emotional stability by reducing hyperarousal in bipolar disorder.
2. **Cortisol Reduction**
    - Lowers stress-related cortisol levels, improving mood stability.

Key Pharmacokinetic Parameters: Elevated oral bioavailability (80%), guaranteeing efficient systemic absorption. The plasma half-life is 10 to 12 hours. It is broken down in the liver by CYP3A4 enzymes. It has significant plasma protein binding (80%) and is predominantly excreted through stool.

Adverse Drug Reactions: Mild daytime sedation, headache, dizziness, nausea, constipation, suicidal ideation, cognitive impairment, and hypotension.

Uses: Adjunctive therapy for bipolar depression and sleep disturbances.

Dose: 20 mg orally at bedtime (in clinical trials).

5. Esketamine

Intoduction: Esketamine, a ketamine derivative, is a fast-acting antidepressant sanctioned for treatment-resistant depression (TRD). Administered as a nasal spray, esketamine preferentially targets the glutamatergic system by functioning as an NMDA receptor antagonist, resulting in a quick antidepressant effect—typically within hours. Esketamine signifies a transformative advancement in the management of bipolar mood disorder characterised by recurrent depressive episodes, particularly for those unresponsive to traditional treatments.

Clinical Trial Phase / FDA-Approval: Ongoing Phase III clinical trials for bipolar depression.

Mechanism of Action: Esketamine, the S-enantiomer of racemic ketamine, is a non-competitive antagonist of the N-methyl-D-aspartate (NMDA) receptor, an ionotropic glutamate receptor. It binds to the allosteric site (not the glutamate binding site) and blocks the receptor. Receptor blockade leads to decrease calcium influx in the GABAergic interneurons in the pre-frontal cortex (PFC) - reduced GABA release - removal of inhibitor response of GABA on glutamatergicor excitatory neurones - increased glutamate release. Since NMDA receptors are blocked, hence the released glutamate now binds to the available AMPA receptors - AMPA receptor stimulation - promotes BDNF - promotes synaptic growth - ultimately contributing to mood stabilisation and rapid antidepressant effects.

Key Pharmacokinetic Parameters: This drug's nasal spray administration facilitates fast absorption. The average absolute bioavailability is roughly 48% following the administration of esketamine nasal spray. Peak esketamine plasma concentration is attained 20 to 40 minutes following the final nasal spray of esketamine. It is mostly metabolised to the noresketamine metabolite by cytochrome P450 enzymes CYP2B6 and CYP3A4, with minimal involvement from CYP2C9 and CYP2C19. It is predominantly eliminated by urine.

Adverse Drug Reactions: Sleepiness, dizziness, dissociation, perceptual disturbances, hypertension, and nausea.

Uses: Esketamine is indicated in combination with an oral antidepressant for the treatment of treatment-resistant depression in adults. It is also undergoing clinical trials for the treatment of bipolar illness.

Dose: 56 or 84 mg intranasally twice weekly for 4 weeks.

6. Other recent advances in bipolar disorder treatment:

Table 1: Recent advancements in the medical management of bipolar disorder.

Drug Name / Approach	Mechanism of Action	Clinical Trial Phase	Adverse Reactions	Distinctive/Salient Features
Anti-Inflammatory Agents (e.g. Minocycline, Celecoxib, N-acetylcysteine)	Target neuroinflammation and oxidative stress, which may be elevated in certain bipolar phenotypes.	Phase II/III for adjunctive therapy in bipolar disorder.	GI discomfort, rash, headache.	Early data suggests adjunctive benefits in improving mood stability and depressive symptoms.
Agomelatine (Melatonin Receptor Agonist / 5-HT2C Antagonist)	Resynchronizes circadian rhythms; has antidepressant effects and minimal sexual side effects.	Approved in some regions for Major depressive disorder (MDD); under evaluation as add-on in bipolar depression.	Headache, dizziness, nausea, liver enzyme elevation.	Circadian rhythm regulation and potential to stabilize mood cycles.
Targeted Gene Therapy / CRISPR-Based Approaches	Potential future direction: modifies specific genetic risk factors (e.g. CACNA1C) implicated in bipolar disorder.	Preclinical and early-phase research.	Unknown (long-term data needed); safety and ethical concerns.	Personalized medicine approach for individuals with well-characterized genetic mutations.

Key Therapeutic Targets

1. **D2/D3 Partial Agonists (Atypical Antipsychotics):** Cariprazine, lurasidone, and Lumateperone exemplify the next generation of atypical antipsychotics with more selective receptor profiles, potentially offering efficacy in both manic and depressive phases. These agents aim to reduce extrapyramidal side effects and metabolic risks while delivering robust mood stabilization.
2. **Modulating Glutamate Transmission:** Novel approaches, such as low-dose ketamine or esketamine, may rapidly relieve depressive symptoms by modulating the NMDA receptor and promoting synaptic plasticity. Although used clinically in treatment-resistant unipolar depression, their role in bipolar disorder is under active investigation, balancing rapid efficacy against the risk of mania induction and potential misuse.

3. **Anti-Inflammatory Approaches:** Growing evidence suggests that inflammatory and oxidative stress markers may be elevated in bipolar disorder, correlating with symptom severity. Agents like minocycline, celecoxib, and N-acetylcysteine have shown preliminary benefit as adjunctive therapies, highlighting the potential for targeting neuroinflammation to enhance mood stabilization.
4. **Circadian Rhythm Regulation:** Dysregulated sleep-wake cycles and disturbed circadian rhythms are closely intertwined with bipolar disorder pathophysiology. Therapies such as agomelatine aim to restore circadian homeostasis, thereby improving mood regulation. This approach can be particularly relevant for individuals experiencing seasonal or rapid-cycling patterns.
5. **Gene Therapy and Personalized Medicine:** Although still in the realm of experimental research, identifying genetic polymorphisms linked to bipolar disorder may pave the way for gene-editing therapies or highly individualized treatment plans. CRISPR-based editing to correct or modify at-risk alleles holds promise but also poses significant scientific, ethical, and safety challenges.

Conclusion

Effective care of bipolar mood disorder necessitates a comprehensive strategy that include pharmacotherapy, psychotherapy, lifestyle adjustments, and patient education. Although traditional mood stabilisers such as lithium, anticonvulsants, and second-generation antipsychotics are advantageous for numerous individuals, persistent issues like symptom unpredictability, adverse effects, and treatment resistance necessitate the pursuit of new medicines. Novel pharmaceutical techniques focus on neuroinflammation, oxidative stress, and circadian rhythm disturbances, whereas rapid-acting interventions such as NMDA receptor antagonists and prospective genetic-based methodologies offer the potential for more individualised treatment. As our comprehension of the neurobiology of bipolar disease advances, personalised treatment strategies provide optimism for enduring recovery and enhanced results, albeit existing constraints.

References

1. Oliva V, Fico G, De Prisco M, Gonda X, Rosa AR, Vieta E. Bipolar disorders: an update on critical aspects. The Lancet Regional Health–Europe. 2025 Jan 1;48.
2. Poletti S, Mazza MG, Benedetti F. Inflammatory mediators in major depression and bipolar disorder. Translational Psychiatry. 2024 Jun 8;14(1):247.
3. Chancel R, Lopez-Castroman J, Baca-García E, Mateos Alvarez R, Courtet P, Conejero I. Biomarkers of bipolar disorder in late life: an evidence-based systematic review. Current Psychiatry Reports. 2024 Mar;26(3):78-103.
4. López-Muñoz F, Shen WW, D'ocon P, Romero A, Álamo C. A history of the pharmacological treatment of bipolar disorder. International journal of molecular sciences. 2018 Jul 23;19(7):2143.
5. Geddes JR, Miklowitz DJ. Treatment of bipolar disorder. The lancet. 2013 May 11;381(9878):1672-82.
6. Healy D. Mania: A short history of bipolar disorder. JHU Press; 2008 Jun 23.
7. McIntyre RS, Berk M, Brietzke E, Goldstein BI, López-Jaramillo C, Kessing LV, Malhi GS, Nierenberg AA, Rosenblat JD, Majeed A, Vieta E. Bipolar disorders. The Lancet. 2020 Dec 5;396(10265):1841-56.
8. Miklowitz DJ, Johnson SL. Bipolar disorder. Psychopathology: History, Diagnosis, and Empirical Foundations, Third Edition. 2017 Jan 30:317-63.
9. Grande I, Berk M, Birmaher B, Vieta E. Bipolar disorder. The Lancet. 2016 Apr 9;387(10027):1561-72.
10. Malhi GS, Gessler D, Outhred T. The use of lithium for the treatment of bipolar disorder: recommendations from clinical practice guidelines. Journal of affective disorders. 2017 Aug 1;217:266-80.
11. National Institute of Mental Health. *Bipolar Disorder*. NIMH. 2020. Available at: https://www.nimh.nih.gov/health/topics/bipolar-disorder (Accessed on 02 Apr 2025).
12. Kapczinski F, Magalhães PV, Balanzá-Martinez V, Dias VV, Frangou S, Gama CS, Gonzalez-Pinto A, Grande I, Ha K, Kauer-Sant'Anna M, Kunz M. Staging systems in bipolar disorder: an I nternational S ociety for B ipolar D isorders T ask F orce R eport. Acta psychiatricascandinavica. 2014 Nov;130(5):354-63.
13. Gitlin M. Lithium side effects and toxicity: prevalence and management strategies. International journal of bipolar disorders. 2016 Dec;4:1-0.
14. Miklowitz DJ, Chung B. Family-focused therapy for bipolar disorder: Reflections on 30 years of research. Family process. 2016 Sep;55(3):483-99.

15. Durgam S, Starace A, Li D, Migliore R, Ruth A, Németh G, Laszlovszky I. The efficacy and tolerability of cariprazine in acute mania associated with bipolar I disorder: a phase II trial. Bipolar disorders. 2015 Feb;17(1):63-75.
16. McIntyre RS, Rosenblat JD, Nemeroff CB, Sanacora G, Murrough JW, Berk M, Brietzke E, Dodd S, Gorwood P, Ho R, Iosifescu DV. Synthesizing the evidence for ketamine and esketamine in treatment-resistant depression: an international expert opinion on the available evidence and implementation. American Journal of Psychiatry. 2021 May 1;178(5):383-99.
17. Harrison PJ. Using our brains: the findings, flaws, and future of postmortem studies of psychiatric disorders. Biological psychiatry. 2011 Jan 15;69(2):102-3.
18. Koziej S, Kowalczyk E, Soroka E. Cariprazine in Psychiatry: A Comprehensive Review of Efficacy, Safety, and Therapeutic Potential. Medical Science Monitor: International Medical Journal of Experimental and Clinical Research. 2024 Sep 20;30:e945411-1.
19. Tarchi L, Bugini S, Dani C, Cassioli E, Rossi E, Lucarelli S, Ricca V, Caini S, Castellini G. Efficacy of Cariprazine in the Psychosis Spectrum: A Systematic Review and Network Meta-Analysis of Randomised Controlled Trials in Schizophrenia and Bipolar Disorder. CNS drugs. 2024 Dec;38(12):961-71.
20. Li S, Xu C, Hu S, Lai J. Efficacy and tolerability of FDA-approved atypical antipsychotics for the treatment of bipolar depression: a systematic review and network meta-analysis. European Psychiatry. 2024 Mar 15:1-26.
21. Zhang Y, Zhou C, Liu Y, Hao Y, Wang J, Song B, Yu J. Adverse event signal mining and severe adverse event influencing factor analysis of Lumateperone based on FAERS database. Frontiers in Pharmacology. 2024 Sep 23;15:1472648.
22. Sparacino G, Verdolini N, Vieta E, Pacchiarotti I. Existing and emerging pharmacological approaches to the treatment of mania: A critical overview. Translational Psychiatry. 2022 Apr 23;12(1):169.
23. Xiao W, Moncy JC, Ghazi-Noori AR, Woodham RD, Rezaei H, Bramon E, Ritter P, Bauer M, Young AH, Fu CH. Enhanced network synchronization connectivity following transcranial direct current stimulation (tDCS) in bipolar depression: effects on EEG oscillations and deep learning-based predictors of clinical remission. Journal of Affective Disorders. 2025 Jan 15;369:576-87.
24. Santucci MC, Ansari M, Nikayin S, Radhakrishnan R, Rhee TG, Wilkinson ST. Efficacy and Safety of Ketamine/Esketamine in Bipolar Depression in a Clinical Setting. The Journal of Clinical Psychiatry. 2024 Oct 2;85(4):57118.
25. Li J, Ma L, Sun H, Li M, Cao Y, Peng Y, Xu J. Efficacy of racemic ketamine or esketamine monotherapy for reducing suicidal ideation in uni-or bipolar depression: a systematic review and meta-analysis. European Archives of Psychiatry and Clinical Neuroscience. 2024 Oct 9:1-3.

Chapter 14

Recent Advances in the Management of Migraine

Author: Dr. Pranab Das

Introduction

Migraine is a prevalent, debilitating primary headache illness marked by recurrent bouts of moderate to severe pain, frequently associated with nausea, photophobia, and phonophobia. Global epidemiology data indicates that migraine impacts over 1 billion people globally and is a predominant source of impairment across all age demographics. In recent decades, substantial advancements have been achieved in elucidating the pathophysiological processes of migraine, including the involvement of calcitonin gene-related peptide (CGRP), neuroinflammation, and cortical spreading depression.

These advancements have resulted in innovative therapeutic targets and more customised treatments. Despite the existence of several pharmaceutical and non-pharmacological interventions, a significant number of patients with migraines fail to attain adequate headache management. The challenge is exacerbated by insufficient compliance with therapy, adverse pharmaceutical effects, and comorbidities that complicate treatment. The revelation of new molecular pathways and the creation of targeted medicines, such CGRP antagonists and monoclonal antibodies, have significantly transformed migraine care in the past decade. This chapter explores traditional and novel migraine therapeutics, highlighting recent advancements that aim to enhance patient outcomes and alleviate the global disease burden.

Historical Perspective

Over the past century, pharmacologic treatment for migraine has changed dramatically due to a growing understanding of its neurovascular pathophysiology. Ergot alkaloids like ergotamine, which Arthur Stoll first synthesised at Sandoz in 1918, were part of early treatment strategies in the middle of the 20th century. More specific serotonin receptor agonists eventually replaced these. A significant advancement occurred in the 1990s when Glaxo scientists created sumatriptan, the first 5-HT1B/1D receptor agonist that provided quick and efficient relief from acute migraine attacks. As a result, a class of medications called triptans was created, and these drugs became the mainstay of treatment for acute migraines.

The use of triptans in patients with cardiovascular disorders was restricted due to their vasoconstrictive effects, which prompted a search for safer substitutes. Developments in migraine pathophysiology in the 2010s brought attention to the function of calcitonin gene-related peptide (CGRP), a neuropeptide implicated in vasodilation and pain transmission. CGRP receptor antagonists, or gepants, were created as a result, and ubrogepant and rimegepant became non-vasoconstrictive acute treatment options. In parallel, research was conducted on monoclonal antibodies that target CGRP or its receptor, like eptinezumab, which offer long-term preventive benefits with infrequent dosing. Another category of innovations included 5-HT1F receptor agonists, such as lasmiditan, which were created to completely avoid vasoconstriction.

Zavegepant, the first intranasal CGRP receptor antagonist, was approved more recently, offering a quick-acting, non-invasive solution for acute migraine relief. These advancements mark a change from symptomatic care to precision therapies based on mechanisms. Millions of people worldwide now enjoy better quality of life thanks to modern migraine treatment that is more individualised, safer, and effective thanks to an expanding arsenal of targeted agents.

Definition

Migraine is defined as a primary headache disorder characterized by recurrent headaches that typically last 4 to 72 hours, manifesting with unilateral, pulsating pain of moderate to severe intensity. Attacks can be aggravated by routine physical activities and are commonly accompanied by nausea and/or sensitivity to light (photophobia) or sound (phonophobia). The International Classification of Headache Disorders (ICHD) outlines several migraine subtypes, such as migraine with aura, migraine without aura, chronic migraine, and others. Each subtype has its own distinct clinical features but shares overlapping pathophysiological mechanisms involving trigeminal nerve activation and neuropeptide release.

Types of Migraine

1. **Migraine Without Aura:** The most prevalent form of migraine, characterized by pulsatile, throbbing headache typically on one side of the head. Headache may be accompanied by photophobia, phonophobia, and nausea but without preceding sensory disturbances (aura).
2. **Migraine With Aura:** Preceded by transient visual or sensory phenomena (e.g. zigzag lines, flashing lights, tingling sensations), which usually evolve gradually over several minutes and resolve within an hour. Aura symptoms are often followed by the onset of headache.
3. **Chronic Migraine:** Defined as headache on 15 or more days per month for at least three months, with features of migraine on at least eight of those days. Chronic migraine imposes significant disability and may be associated with medication overuse and comorbid conditions such as anxiety or depression.
4. **Other Subtypes:** Includes conditions like hemiplegic migraine, retinal migraine, and vestibular migraine. Although less common, these subtypes can present with atypical features like motor weakness or vertigo and often require specialized diagnostic considerations.

Brief Note on Conventional Medicines

Traditional migraine therapies are broadly classified into acute (abortive) treatments and preventive (prophylactic) treatments. Acute treatments aim to alleviate symptoms during an attack, while preventive treatments reduce the frequency and severity of attacks over the long term. Below is a concise summary of conventional drugs widely used for migraine:

Table 1: Concise overview of traditional pharmaceuticals employed in the management of Migraine.

Drug Name / Drug Class	Mechanism of Action	Adverse Drug Reactions	Uses
Sumatriptan (Triptan, 5-HT1B/1D Agonist)	Sumatriptan selectively activates 5-HT1B and 5-HT1D serotonin receptors in cranial blood vessels, leading to vasoconstriction and reduced neurogenic inflammation. It also inhibits trigeminal nerve activation, preventing further pain transmission.	Chest tightness, dizziness, hypertension, ischemic events.	Acute migraine attacks (moderate to severe) &cluster headaches.
Ergotamine (Ergot Alkaloid, 5-HT1 Agonist)	Ergotamine acts as a partial agonist at 5-HT1 receptors, causing vasoconstriction of cranial blood vessels. It also binds to dopamine and adrenergic receptors, further reducing neurogenic inflammation.	Nausea, vomiting, vasospasm, ischemia (risk of gangrene), rebound headaches.	Acute migraine attacks (less preferred due to side effects).
Propranolol (Beta-Blocker, Non-Selective)	Propranolol blocks beta-adrenergic receptors, reducing sympathetic nervous system activity. This decreases vascular reactivity, stabilizing blood vessels and preventing migraine triggers. It also modulates cortical excitability, reducing migraine frequency.	Fatigue, dizziness, bradycardia, hypotension, worsening of asthma.	Migraine prophylaxis.
Valproate (Antiepileptic, GABA Enhancer & Na+ Channel Blocker)	Valproate enhances GABAergic inhibition, reducing neuronal hyperexcitability. It also inhibits voltage-gated Na+ and T-type Ca2+ channels, preventing migraine aura and cortical spreading depression (CSD).	Hepatotoxicity, pancreatitis, weight gain, sedation, teratogenicity (contraindicated in pregnancy).	Migraine prophylaxis.

NSAIDs (Ibuprofen, Naproxen, Aspirin)	NSAIDs inhibit cyclooxygenase (COX-1 & COX-2), reducing prostaglandin (PGE2) synthesis. This lowers inflammation and pain transmission in the trigeminal pathway.	Gastritis, GI ulcers, increased bleeding risk, renal toxicity (long-term use).	Mild to moderate migraine attacks.
Metoclopramide (Dopamine D2 Antagonist, Anti-emetic)	Metoclopramide blocks D2 dopamine receptors in the chemoreceptor trigger zone (CTZ), preventing migraine-associated nausea and vomiting. It also enhances gastric emptying, improving oral drug absorption.	Extrapyramidal symptoms (EPS), sedation, hyperprolactinemia (galactorrhoea).	Migraine-associated nausea and vomiting.

Conventional preventive therapies, such as beta-blockers and anticonvulsants, can reduce migraine frequency by up to 50% in some patients. However, side effects, drug interactions, and partial response rates often necessitate ongoing refinement or adjunctive measures.

Newer Drugs / Recent Advances

The burgeoning understanding of migraine pathophysiology, particularly the central role of CGRP and related pathways, has led to the development of novel and highly targeted therapies. Several new classes of medications and therapeutic approaches are poised to reshape migraine management. Below is a summary of some of the most promising recent advances:

1. Ubrogepant (CGRP Receptor Antagonist)

Introduction: Ubrogepant is an oral calcitonin gene-related peptide (CGRP) receptor antagonist (gepant class) developed for the acute treatment of migraine attacks in adults. It is the first-in-class oral CGRP receptor antagonist approved by the U.S. Food and Drug Administration (FDA) for this indication. CGRP is a neuropeptide that plays a crucial role in migraine pathophysiology by causing vasodilation, neurogenic inflammation, and pain transmission. Ubrogepant blocks CGRP receptors, preventing these migraine-inducing processes. Unlike triptans, which act as serotonin (5-HT1B/1D) receptor agonists and cause vasoconstriction, ubrogepant offers a non-vasoconstrictive alternative, making it safer for patients with cardiovascular disease.

Clinical Trial Status / FDA-Approval: FDA-approved for the acute treatment of migraine. Ongoing trials evaluating efficacy in migraine prophylaxis.

Mechanism of Action: Ubrogepant exerts its therapeutic effects by selectively blocking CGRP receptors in the trigeminal system, which is involved in migraine pathogenesis.

1. **CGRP and Migraine Pathophysiology:** During a migraine attack, CGRP levels increase in the trigeminal ganglion and blood vessels, leading to:
   - Neurogenic vasodilation (widening of blood vessels).
   - Neurogenic inflammation (activation of pain-sensitive pathways).
   - Sensitization of trigeminal nociceptors, amplifying pain perception.

2. **Ubrogepant Binding to CGRP Receptors:**
   - Ubrogepant is a high-affinity, selective CGRP receptor antagonist.
   - It binds to CGRP receptors in the trigeminal ganglion, brainstem, and meningeal blood vessels, preventing CGRP from exerting its above-mentionedeffects.
3. **Inhibition of CGRP-Mediated Effects:**
   - By blocking CGRP receptors, ubrogepant reduces vasodilation, inhibits inflammatory signalling, and prevents activation of central pain pathways.
   - This results in relief from headache, light sensitivity (photophobia), sound sensitivity (phonophobia), and nausea during a migraine attack.

Key Pharmacokinetic Parameters: It is rapidly absorbed after oral administration, with peak plasma concentration (Tmax) reached within 1.5 hours. Food delays it's absorption but does not significantly reduce efficacy. High concentration is attained in the trigeminal ganglion and meningeal blood vessels, the primary sites of migraine pathophysiology.

Adverse Drug Reactions: Nausea, dizziness, dry mouth, hepatotoxicity, and hypersensitivity reactions.

Uses: Acute migraine treatment in patients.

Dose: 50 mg or 100 mg orally, as needed. Second dose may be taken at least 2 hours after the first, if needed.

2. Rimegepant (CGRP Receptor Antagonist)

Introduction: Rimegepant is a small-molecule calcitonin gene-related peptide (CGRP) receptor antagonist approved for the acute and preventive treatment of migraine in adults. Unlike triptans, which cause vasoconstriction by acting on serotonin (5-HT1B/1D) receptors, rimegepant directly blocks CGRP receptors, thereby inhibiting the vasodilation, neurogenic inflammation, and pain transmission associated with migraine attacks. It is the first orally disintegrating tablet (ODT) gepant that can be used both for acute relief and preventive therapy, offering a significant advantage for migraine management.

Clinical Trial Status / FDA-Approval: FDA-approved for acute and preventive migraine treatment.

Mechanism of Action: Rimegepant functions as a selective CGRP receptor antagonist, preventing the activity of CGRP, a key neuropeptide involved in migraine pathophysiology.

1. **CGRP and Migraine Pathogenesis:** During a migraine attack, CGRP is released from trigeminal sensory neurons, leading to:
   - Dilation of meningeal blood vessels (vasodilation).
   - Neurogenic inflammation via mast cell degranulation.
   - Pain signal transmission via trigeminal nerve activation.
2. **Binding to CGRP Receptors:**
   - Rimegepant acts as a high-affinity competitive antagonist of CGRP receptors.
   - It binds to CGRP receptors in the trigeminal ganglion, dura mater, and brainstem, blocking CGRP from exerting its effects.
3. **Inhibition of Vasodilation and Pain Transmission:**
   - By preventing CGRP receptor activation, rimegepant inhibits meningeal vasodilation and neurogenic inflammation, thereby reducing headache severity and associated symptoms.

- Unlike triptans, rimegepant does not cause vasoconstriction, making it a safer option for patients with cardiovascular disease.

Key Pharmacokinetics Parameters: It is well absorbed after oral administration, with peak plasma concentration (Tmax) reached within 1.5–2 hours. Orally disintegrating tablet (ODT) formulation enables faster onset than standard oral tablets. Food delays absorption but does not impact efficacy. It is primarily metabolized by CYP3A4 and CYP2C9 enzymes in the liver and is excreted mostly in faeces.

Adverse Drug Reactions: Nausea, somnolence, hepatic enzyme elevations and anaphylaxis.

Uses: Rimegepant is FDA-approved for both acute migraine treatment and migraine prevention.

Dose: 75 mg orally as needed for acute migraine (maximum 1 dose per 24 hours).

3. Eptinezumab (CGRP Monoclonal Antibody)

Introduction: Eptinezumab is a humanized monoclonal antibody (IgG1 subtype) specifically designed for the prevention of episodic and chronic migraine in adults. It is the first and only intravenous (i.v.) calcitonin gene-related peptide (CGRP) antagonist approved for migraine prophylaxis. Unlike other CGRP-targeting drugs (such as erenumab, fremanezumab, and galcanezumab), which are administered subcutaneously, eptinezumab is delivered intravenously, allowing for rapid onset of action and sustained migraine prevention.

Clinical Trial Phase / FDA-Approval: FDA-approved (2020) for migraine prevention.

Mechanism of Action: Eptinezumab works by selectively binding to CGRP, a neuropeptide that plays a central role in migraine pathophysiology.

1. **CGRP and Migraine Pathophysiology:**
   - CGRP is released from trigeminal sensory neurons during a migraine attack.
   - It induces vasodilation, neurogenic inflammation, and pain transmission via the trigeminovascular system.
   - Elevated CGRP levels correlate with migraine frequency and severity.
2. **Eptinezumab Binds to Free CGRP:**
   - Unlike erenumab (which blocks CGRP receptors), eptinezumab directly binds to soluble CGRP peptides in circulation.
   - This prevents CGRP from activating its receptor (CGRP-R), thereby inhibiting its migraine-inducing effects.
3. **Inhibition of CGRP-Mediated Vasodilation and Pain Transmission:**
   - Eptinezumab blocks CGRP-induced dilation of meningeal blood vessels, reducing neurogenic inflammation.
   - It prevents the activation of nociceptive (pain-sensitive) neurons in the trigeminal system.
4. **Rapid and Sustained CGRP Suppression:**
   - Due to i.v. administration, eptinezumab achieves peak plasma levels immediately, leading to rapid migraine relief.
   - It's long half-life ensures continuous migraine prevention for up to 12 weeks after a single infusion.

Key Pharmacokinetic Parameters: It has a wide tissue distribution, particularly in the trigeminal vascular system. It undergoes slow proteolytic degradation in the reticuloendothelial system (RES). It is not metabolized via cytochrome P450 (CYP450) enzymes, minimizing drug interactions. It is primarily cleared via hepatic and reticuloendothelial pathways and exhibits minimal renal clearance.

Adverse Drug Reactions: Hypersensitivity reactions, nasopharyngitis, fatigue, dizziness, and elevated liver enzymes.

Uses: Migraine prevention in patients with frequent attacks (>4/month).

Dose: 100 mg IV infusion over 30 minutes every 3 months.

4. Lasmiditan (Selective 5-HT1F Agonist)

Introduction: Lasmiditan is a first-in-class, selective serotonin (5-HT1F) receptor agonist approved for the acute treatment of migraine with or without aura in adults. Unlike triptans, which act on 5-HT1B/1D receptors and cause vasoconstriction, lasmiditan provides effective migraine relief without affecting vascular tone, making it a safer alternative for patients with cardiovascular risk factors. Lasmiditan was developed by Eli Lilly and Company and was approved by the U.S. Food and Drug Administration (FDA) as the first and only ditan-class drug for migraine treatment.

Clinical Trial Status / FDA-Approval: FDA-approved for acute migraine treatment.

Mechanism of Action: Lasmiditan is a highly selective 5-HT1F receptor agonist that exerts its anti-migraine effects by acting on the trigeminal system and central pain pathways, reducing neurogenic inflammation and pain transmission.

1. **Activation of 5-HT1F Receptors:**
   - Lasmiditan binds selectively to 5-HT1F receptors, which are expressed in trigeminal neurons and the central nervous system (CNS).
   - Unlike triptans, it does not activate 5-HT1B/1D receptors, thus avoiding vasoconstriction.
2. **Inhibition of CGRP and Glutamate Release:**
   - 5-HT1F receptor activation by Lasmiditanleads to inhibition of adenylate cyclase via Gi-protein signalling.
   - This results in reduced release of calcitonin gene-related peptide (CGRP) and glutamate, both of which are key mediators of migraine pathophysiology.
3. **Reduction of Trigeminal Nerve Activity and Central Pain Modulation:**
   - By inhibiting trigeminal afferent activation, lasmiditan reduces pain signal transmission from the trigemino-vascular system to the brainstem.
   - Its high penetration into the CNS allows it to modulate central pain processing, further enhancing its anti-migraine effects.
4. **No Vasoconstrictive Effects:**
   - Unlike triptans, which cause vasoconstriction of cerebral and coronary arteries, lasmiditan's action is entirely neuronal, making it safer for patients with cardiovascular disease.

Key Pharmacokinetic Parameters: It has high oral bioavailability. Shows high CNS penetration, enabling central modulation of migraine pain. Not significantly metabolised by CYP3A4, making it safe with many concurrent medications. It is primarily excreted in urine.

Adverse Drug Reactions: Dizziness, drowsiness. riving paraesthesia, nausea, and serotonin syndrome.

Uses: Acute migraine attacks, especially in patients with cardiovascular risks.

Dose: 50 mg, 100 mg, or 200 mg orally, as needed (maximum dose is 200 mg per 24 hours).

5. Zavegepant (Intranasal CGRP Antagonist)

Introduction: Zavegepant is a third-generation calcitonin gene-related peptide (CGRP) receptor antagonist (gepant class) developed for the acute treatment of migraine. It is the first and only CGRP antagonist available as a nasal spray, providing rapid relief for migraine attacks. Unlike oral CGRP antagonists (e.g. rimegepant, ubrogepant), Zavegepant bypasses the gastrointestinal (GI) tract, making it faster-acting and suitable for patients with nausea and vomiting during migraines. The U.S. Food and Drug Administration (FDA) approved Zavegepant in 2023 for adults experiencing migraine with or without aura.

Clinical Trial Status / FDA Approved: FDA approved (2023).

Mechanism of Action: Zavegepant selectively blocks CGRP receptors in the trigeminal system, inhibiting vasodilation, neurogenic inflammation, and pain signalling.

Stepwise Mechanism of Action:

1. **Role of CGRP in Migraine Pathophysiology:** During a migraine attack, CGRP is released from trigeminal neurons, leading to:
   - Vasodilation (widening of meningeal blood vessels).
   - Neurogenic inflammation via mast cell activation.
   - Activation of trigeminal pain pathways.
2. **Binding to CGRP Receptors:**
   - Zavegepant is a high-affinity CGRP receptor antagonist.
   - It binds to CGRP receptors in the trigeminal ganglion and dura mater, preventing CGRP from triggering migraine-inducing pathways.
3. **Inhibition of Vasodilation and Pain Transmission:**
   - Zavegepant blocks CGRP-mediated dilation of blood vessels, reducing headache severity.
   - It inhibits neurogenic inflammation, preventing further sensitization of pain pathways.
4. **Rapid Onset Due to Nasal Administration:**
   - As a nasal spray, Zavegepant bypasses the GI tract, allowing faster absorption into the bloodstream and quicker migraine relief.

Key Pharmacokinetic Parameters: It is rapidly absorbed after intranasal administration. Peak plasma concentration (Tmax) reached within 30 minutes. It has a high penetration in trigeminal ganglia and meningeal blood vessels. It is primarily excreted via faeces.

Adverse Drug Reactions: Nasal irritation and congestion, nausea, altered state and hypersensitivity reactions.

Uses: Fast relief of acute migraine attacks.

Dose: 10 mg intranasally as a single dose.

6. Other recent advances in the treatment of migraine

Table 2: Other latest developments in migraine treatment.

Drug Name / Approach	Mechanism of Action	Clinical Trial Phase	Adverse Drug Reactions	Distinctive / Salient Features
Neuromodulation Devices (e.g. Transcranial Magnetic Stimulation, Non-invasive Vagus Nerve Stimulation, Remote Electrical Neuromodulation).	Modulate neuronal excitability and pain pathways via external or implantable devices.	Cleared / Approved in some regions; further research continuing.	Local site discomfort, rare nerve irritation, mild dizziness.	Non-pharmacological approach for acute and prophylactic therapy, beneficial for patients intolerant to medications or who prefer device use.
Anti-CGRP Vaccines (Emerging research)	Aim to induce long-term antibody production against CGRP or its receptor, providing sustained migraine prophylaxis.	Phase I/II trials.	Potential immunological responses, injection-site issues.	Could offer extended protection without frequent dosing; however, still highly experimental.
Combination Therapies (e.g. CGRP mAb + Traditional Preventive Agent)	Simultaneous targeting of multiple pathways (e.g. CGRP blockade plus beta-blocker or anticonvulsant).	Phase I/II trials.	Potential additive side effects depending on agents used.	May enhance efficacy in patients with partial response to a single agent, personalizing regimens for refractory cases.

Key Therapeutic Targets

1. **CGRP Pathway:** The most notable recent breakthrough in migraine treatment has been the successful targeting of CGRP—either by antagonizing its receptor (erenumab) or by neutralizing the peptide itself (fremanezumab, galcanezumab, eptinezumab). CGRP plays a central role in mediating neurogenic inflammation and vasodilation during migraine attacks, and interrupting this pathway can dramatically reduce attack frequency and severity.

2. **Serotonin Subtypes Beyond 5-HT1B/1D:** While triptans act on 5-HT1B/1D, ditans selectively agonize 5-HT1F receptors, avoiding vasoconstrictive effects but retaining analgesic properties. This makes ditans suitable for patients with cardiovascular contraindications to triptans.

3. **Neuromodulation:** Innovations in neuromodulatory devices, including single-pulse transcranial magnetic stimulation (sTMS) and non-invasive vagus nerve stimulation (nVNS), reflect an increasing interest in non-pharmacological methods. These devices attempt to modulate cortical excitability or trigeminal pain pathways. They can be particularly beneficial in patients who experience frequent side effects or have multiple comorbidities that limit medication use.

4. **Long-acting Prophylaxis (Vaccine-like Approaches):** Researchers are exploring the possibility of vaccine-like therapies to induce a patient's immune system to generate antibodies against CGRP. This would theoretically offer a longer duration of prophylaxis without monthly or quarterly injections, although this strategy remains in the early stages of research.

5. **Combination and Personalized Therapies:** Given the multifactorial nature of migraine, a combination of treatments—whether it is adding a CGRP monoclonal antibody to a beta-blocker or pairing a neuromodulation device with existing preventive medications—may provide more robust symptomatic relief and prophylaxis. Personalized medicine approaches, including genetic markers or biomarker analysis, are on the horizon to tailor treatments to individual patient profiles.

Conclusion

A complex neurological condition, migraines have a major impact on healthcare systems, productivity, and quality of life. Even though traditional treatments like beta-blockers, NSAIDs, and triptans have been helpful, their drawbacks have prompted the creation of more specialised therapies. Recent developments include intranasal medications like zavegepant, monoclonal antibodies like eptinezumab, 5-HT1F receptor agonists like lasmiditan, and CGRP receptor antagonists like ubrogepant and rimegepant. Better safety, efficacy, and a lower chance of medication overuse headaches are provided by these more recent options. Research is still being done to improve these treatments and make more individualised, potentially disease-modifying strategies possible, despite obstacles like expense and restricted access. The treatment of migraines has the potential to improve patient safety, efficacy, and quality of life for people all over the world.

References

1. GBD 2019 Diseases and Injuries Collaborators. Global, regional, and national burden of migraine and tension-type headache, 1990–2019. *Lancet Neurol*. 2022;21(12):954–976.
2. Lipton RB. Preventive treatment of migraine. CONTINUUM: Lifelong Learning in Neurology. 2024 Apr 1;30(2):364-78.
3. Bentivegna E, Galastri S, Onan D, Martelletti P. Unmet needs in the acute treatment of migraine. Advances in Therapy. 2024 Jan;41(1):1-3.
4. Lipton RB, Bigal ME, Diamond M, Freitag F, Reed ML, Stewart WF. Migraine prevalence, disease burden, and the need for preventive therapy. Neurology. 2011 Nov 22;77(21):1905.
5. Humphrey PP, Feniuk W, Perren MJ, Beresford IJ, Skingle M, Whalley ET. Serotonin and migraine. Annals of the new York Academy of Sciences. 1990 Jan 1;600:587-98.
6. Ashina M, Katsarava Z, Do TP, Buse DC, Pozo-Rosich P, Özge A, Krymchantowski AV, Lebedeva ER, Ravishankar K, Yu S, Sacco S. Migraine: epidemiology and systems of care. The Lancet. 2021 Apr 17;397(10283):1485-95.
7. Parisi P, Belcastro V, Verrotti A, Striano P, Trenitè DK. "Ictal epileptic headache" and the revised International Headache Classification (ICHD-3) published in Cephalalgia 2018, vol. 38 (1) 1–211: Not just a matter of definition!. Epilepsy &Behavior. 2018 Oct 1;87:243-5.
8. Natoli JL, Manack A, Dean B, Butler Q, Turkel CC, Stovner L, Lipton RB. Global prevalence of chronic migraine: a systematic review. Cephalalgia. 2010 May;30(5):599-609.
9. Edvinsson L. Rimegepant for the acute and preventive treatment of migraine: a narrative review of the evidence. Expert Rev Neurother. 2024;24(12):1141–55.
10. Jones A, O'Gorman C, Tabuteau H. Treatment of Migraine Pain and Associated Symptoms with AXS-07: Results from MOVEMENT, a Long-term Efficacy and Safety Study. InAmerican Headache Society Virtual Annual Scientific Meeting Jun 2021 Jun 3 (pp. 3-6).
11. Ogunlaja OI, Goadsby PJ. Headache: treatment update. Eneurologicalsci. 2022 Dec 1;29:100420.
12. Antonaci F, Ghiotto N, Wu S, Pucci E, Costa A. Recent advances in migraine therapy. Springerplus. 2016 May 17;5(1):637.
13. Szkutnik-Fiedler D. Pharmacokinetics, pharmacodynamics and drug–drug interactions of new anti-migraine drugs—Lasmiditan, gepants, and calcitonin-gene-related peptide (CGRP) receptor monoclonal antibodies. Pharmaceutics. 2020 Dec 3;12(12):1180.
14. Olesen J, Ashina M. Emerging migraine treatments and drug targets. Trends in pharmacological sciences. 2011 Jun 1;32(6):352-9.
15. Tfelt-Hansen P, De Vries P, Saxena PR. Triptans in migraine: a comparative review of pharmacology, pharmacokinetics and efficacy. Drugs. 2000 Dec;60:1259-87.
16. Diener HC, Limmroth V. Advances in pharmacological treatment of migraine. Expert opinion on investigational drugs. 2001 Oct 1;10(10):1831-45.
17. González-Hernández A, Marichal-Cancino BA, MaassenVanDenBrink A, Villalón CM. Side effects associated with current and prospective antimigraine pharmacotherapies. Expert opinion on drug metabolism & toxicology. 2018 Jan 2;14(1):25-41.

18. Edvinsson L, Linde M. New drugs in migraine treatment and prophylaxis: telcagepant and topiramate. The Lancet. 2010 Aug 21;376(9741):645-55.
19. Macone AE, Perloff MD. Triptans and migraine: advances in use, administration, formulation, and development. Expert opinion on pharmacotherapy. 2017 Mar 4;18(4):387-97.
20. Negro A, Martelletti P. Gepants for the treatment of migraine. Expert opinion on investigational drugs. 2019 Jun 3;28(6):555-67.
21. Haanes KA, Edvinsson L. Pathophysiological mechanisms in migraine and the identification of new therapeutic targets. CNS drugs. 2019 Jun 5;33(6):525-37.
22. Al-Hassany L, Goadsby PJ, Danser AJ, MaassenVanDenBrink A. Calcitonin gene-related peptide-targeting drugs for migraine: how pharmacology might inform treatment decisions. The Lancet Neurology. 2022 Mar 1;21(3):284-94.
23. Edvinsson L, Haanes KA, Warfvinge K, Krause DN. CGRP as the target of new migraine therapies—successful translation from bench to clinic. Nature Reviews Neurology. 2018 Jun;14(6):338-50.
24. Diener HC, Charles A, Goadsby PJ, Holle D. New therapeutic approaches for the prevention and treatment of migraine. The Lancet Neurology. 2015 Oct 1;14(10):1010-22.
25. Shewale AR, Poh W, Reed ML, Liu J, Cadiou F, Ezzati A, Burslem K, Manthena S, Lipton RB. Ubrogepant users' real-world experience: Patients on ubrogepant, characteristics and outcomes (UNIVERSE) study. Headache: The Journal of Head and Face Pain. 2024 Nov;64(10):1244-52.
26. Tassorelli C, Jensen RH, Goadsby PJ, Charles AC, Tepper SJ, Snoer AH, Josiassen MK, Linander CB, Ettrup A, Sperling B, Boneva N. Long-term safety, tolerability, and efficacy of eptinezumab in chronic cluster headache (CHRONICLE): an open-label safety trial. The Lancet Neurology. 2025 May 1;24(5):429-40.
27. Croop R, Berman G, Kudrow D, Mullin K, Thiry A, Lovegren M, L'Italien G, Lipton RB. A multicenter, open-label long-term safety study of rimegepant for the acute treatment of migraine. Cephalalgia. 2024 Apr;44(4):03331024241232944.
28. Vila-Pueyo M, Page K, Murdock PR, Loraine HJ, Woodrooffe AJ, Johnson KW, Goadsby PJ, Holland PR. The selective 5-HT1F receptor agonist lasmiditan inhibits trigeminal nociceptive processing: Implications for migraine and cluster headache. British journal of pharmacology. 2022 Feb;179(3):358-70.
29. Suresh V, Bardhan M, Dave T, Shamim MA, Suresh D, Satish P, Dhakal B, Bhonsale A, Roy P, Padhi BK, Monteith T. Zavegepant for acute treatment of migraine: a systematic review and meta-analysis of randomized controlled trials. Clinical Neuropharmacology. 2024 May 1;47(3):72-81.

Section 4

Cardiovascular System

Chapter 15

Recent Advances in the Management of Shock

Author: Dr. Pranab Das

Introduction

The principal characteristics of shock involve insufficient tissue blood flow coupled with inadequate oxygen delivery for cellular function because of this life-threatening state. The medical developments of present times have failed to diminish shock as an ongoing life-threatening issue that afflicts critically ill patients. Multiple causes including haemorrhage and sepsis begin shock events and immediate recognition combined with medical treatment must occur to stop end-organ failure and death.

The primary approach of standard shock treatments aims to both maintain blood pressure and achieve sufficient blood volume and keep cardiac output stable. A customized treatment strategy should be employed because shock syndromes display diverse characteristics. New studies aim to enhance fluid treatment protocols while selecting better vasopressors in addition to creating new pharmacological solutions to enhance patient results. Hemodynamic tracking systems combined with molecular diagnostic methods allow medical staff to provide individualized shock therapy by rapidly treating its fundamental causes. This section examines shock definitions and classes and then details traditional treatment methods followed by new therapeutic strategies which can boost care quality.

Historical Perspective

Since its initial conception, the treatment of shock—a potentially fatal illness marked by insufficient tissue perfusion—has undergone substantial change. Shock was first defined as the "collapse of the vital powers" in the 18th century, but as physiology and treatment progressed, the concept has evolved from a haemodynamic one to a cellular and molecular one.

Early in the 20th century, shock was mostly linked to trauma and bleeding, as was frequently seen in World War I and II battlefield medicine. The foundation of early management was laid by the introduction of whole blood transfusions, intravenous fluid therapy, and basic monitoring (blood pressure and pulse). The Korean and Vietnam Wars also fuelled advancements in resuscitation, which resulted in the identification of hypovolemic and cardiogenic shock subtypes as well as the widespread use of colloids and crystalloids.

Intensive care units (ICUs) and sophisticated monitoring devices, like pulmonary artery catheters, became more common between the 1970s and 1990s, enabling accurate haemodynamic profiling. Vasoactive substances, such as dopamine, norepinephrine, and dobutamine, were also developed during this time and were specifically designed to treat shock subtypes such as anaphylactic, cardiogenic, and septic shock.

Since the historic Rivers trial in 2001, research has focused on early goal-directed therapy (EGDT) in the twenty-first century, especially in sepsis. This changed the emphasis to aggressive fluid resuscitation, early detection, and the use of vasopressors. Global care was further standardised by the Surviving Sepsis Campaign guidelines. Furthermore, recent advancements in shock diagnosis and treatment include biomarker-guided therapy, point-of-care ultrasound, and customised resuscitation techniques.

Novel vasopressors (like angiotensin II), extracorporeal life support (ECLS) for cardiogenic shock, and immunomodulators for septic shock are examples of recent advancements. Furthermore, there is potential for revolutionising shock classification and treatment through precision medicine techniques utilising genomics, metabolomics, and AI-guided monitoring.

Definition

Shock is an acute state of circulatory failure resulting in inadequate cellular oxygen supply and utilization due to hypoperfusion of organs. While hypotension (mean arterial pressure <65 mmHg or systolic blood pressure <100 mmHg) often accompanies shock, it is not universally present in its early stages. The essential feature is the cardiovascular system's incapacity to supply enough oxygen-rich blood to fulfil tissue metabolic needs. If uncorrected, prolonged tissue hypoxia leads to cellular dysfunction, organ failure, and eventually death.

Types of Shock

A thorough comprehension of the various types of shock is necessary for suitable, focused management. Although shock can be classified in various ways, four main categories are widely recognized:

1. **Hypovolemic Shock:** Characterized by reduced intravascular volume, commonly stemming from haemorrhage (trauma, severe dehydration, burns) or gastrointestinal bleeding (ruptured aneurysm). In hypovolemic shock, reduced preload leads to decreased cardiac output and insufficient end-organ perfusion.
2. **Cardiogenic Shock:** Arises from heart pump malfunction, usually brought on by anabrupt myocardial infarction, arrhythmias, or end-stage cardiomyopathy. Low cardiac output and elevated filling pressures mark this subtype, necessitating inotropic support and careful fluid administration.
3. **Distributive (Vasodilatory) Shock:** Caused by profound vasodilation and altered vascular permeability, typically observed in septic shock (the most common), anaphylactic shock or neurogenic shock. Although cardiac output may be high or normal initially, the profound drop in systemic vascular resistance (SVR) impairs effective tissue perfusion.
4. **Obstructive Shock:** Results from obstruction to blood flow, as seen in major pulmonary embolism, cardiac tamponade, or tension pneumothorax. Similar to cardiogenic shock, it is associated with decreased cardiac output, but the primary issue lies external to the myocardium itself (e.g. mechanical obstruction).

Although shock can present in overlapping and mixed forms, such as a trauma patient experiencing both haemorrhagic and septic shock, classifying the type of shock is essential for guiding initial resuscitation strategies, which may include fluid administration, vasopressor use, or surgical and procedural interventions.

Brief Note on Conventional Therapies

Management of shock has historically centered on stabilizing the hemodynamics through fluid resuscitation, vasopressor and/or inotrope support, and addressing the underlying aetiology. Below is a concise summary of the conventional pharmacological and supportive therapies often employed in shock management.

Table 1: Concise overview of traditional therapies utilised in shock management.

Therapeutic Modality	Mechanism of Action	Common Dosage Forms	Usual Side Effects & Salient Features
Crystalloids (e.g. Normal Saline, Ringer's lactate)	Expand intravascular volume, increase preload and cardiac output.	IV infusion	Fluid overload, electrolyte imbalance, oedema.
Colloids (e.g. Albumin, Dextrans)	Retain fluid in intravascular space through high osmotic pressure.	IV infusion	Risk of anaphylaxis (synthetic colloids), costs higher than crystalloids.
Vasopressors (e.g. Norepinephrine, Dopamine)	Increase vascular tone and raises mean arterial pressure (MAP).	IV infusion (titrated)	Tachyarrhythmias, peripheral ischemia, hyperglycaemia.
Inotropes (e.g. Dobutamine, Milrinone)	Enhances myocardial contractility and thereby improve cardiac output.	IV infusion (titrated)	Tachyarrhythmias, hypotension (especially milrinone).
Vasodilators (e.g. Nitroglycerine, Nitroprusside)	Reduces preload (nitrates) afterload (nitroprusside); used selectively in cardiogenic shock to improve forward flow (cardiac output).	IV infusion (titrated)	Hypotension, reflex tachycardia, headache, potential cyanide toxicity (nitroprusside).
Corticosteroids (e.g. Hydrocortisone)	Anti-inflammatory effect - reduces vasopressor requirements (particularly in septic shock).	IV, oral	Hyperglycaemia, immunosuppression, adrenal suppression over long-term use.

Conventional therapies primarily aim to restore perfusion and mitigate end-organ damage. However, optimal fluid type, volume, and vasopressor selection remain debated topics in critical care. Furthermore, in sepsis-induced distributive shock, early appropriate antibiotic therapy is equally pivotal. In cardiogenic shock, timely percutaneous interventions or mechanical circulatory support devices can be life-saving. As research elucidates the complexities of shock pathophysiology, new agents are continually being explored to complement or enhance these traditional measures.

Newer Drugs / Recent Advances in Shock Management

Recent advances in shock management underscore the importance of precision medicine—delivering medications in their appropriate dosage, frequency, and timing, depending on the patient's physiological status and underlying pathology. Below is a summary of notable newer pharmacological agents or strategies under investigation or use in the critical care setting.

1. Angiotensin II

Introduction: Laboratory-made vasoactive peptide Angiotensin II serves as an approved medication to treat distributive and septic shock cases. The synthetic substance replicates RAAS natural processes to increase blood pressure.

Clinical Trial Phase / FDA-Approval: FDA gave its approval to use Angiotensin II for the treatment of septic shock and distributive shock. Public evaluations for long-term safety and effectiveness of this drug are ongoing through Phase IV of post-marketing research.

Mechanism of Action:

1. **Direct Vasoconstriction via AT1 Receptor Activation**

   The main blood-pressure increasing effect occurs when Angiotensin II binds with the angiotensin type 1 receptor (AT1R) present on vascular smooth muscle cells.

   - AT1R is a G-protein coupled receptor (GPCR), which upon activation, triggers Gq protein signalling.
   - Phospholipase C (PLC), which is activated by this, catalyses the conversion of phosphatidylinositol 4,5-bisphosphate (PIP2) into:
     i. Inositol triphosphate (IP3): Mobilizes intracellular calcium (Ca^{2+}) from the sarcoplasmic reticulum, causing smooth muscle contraction.
     ii. Diacylglycerol (DAG): Activates protein kinase C (PKC), further enhancing vasoconstriction.

2. **Increased Aldosterone Release from the Adrenal Cortex**

   Angiotensin II causes the adrenal cortex's zona glomerulosa to secrete more aldosterone, which results in:

   - Sodium and water retention in the kidneys via upregulation of epithelial sodium channels (ENaCs) in the distal tubules.
   - Expansion of intravascular volume, thereby improving cardiac output and systemic perfusion.

3. **Modulation of Sympathetic Nervous System Activity**

   Angiotensin II enhances norepinephrine (NE) release from sympathetic nerve terminals, leading to:

   - Augmented vasoconstriction through α_1-adrenergic receptor activation.
   - Increased heart rate and myocardial contractility, contributing to improved cardiac output in shock states.

4. **Regulation of Renal Hemodynamics and Filtration**

   Angiotensin II plays a critical role in kidney function during shock, acting on renal arterioles to maintain the glomerular filtration rate (GFR):

   - Efferent arteriole constriction (blood leaving the glomerulus) - Preserves filtration pressure - preventing acute kidney injury (AKI) in shock.
   - Sodium retention via direct stimulation of sodium-hydrogen exchanger 3 (NHE3) in proximal tubules - Helps to sustain intravascular volume.

5. **Endothelial Effects and Inflammatory Modulation**

   - Angiotensin II influences endothelial function by increasing endothelin-1 levels, further potentiating vasoconstriction.
   - Anti-inflammatory effects: Angiotensin II reduces pro-inflammatory cytokines (TNF-α, IL-6) and modulates immune response in septic shock.

Key Pharmacokinetic Parameters: The plasma half-life duration of this biologically active substance amounts to 30 seconds. It is eliminated from body via renal and hepatic pathways. It is metabolized by aminopeptidases in the blood and tissues and is broken down into inactive metabolites (angiotensin III and IV).

Adverse Drug Reactions: Hypertension, thrombosis risk, hypertension, tachyarrhythmias and renal impairment.

Uses: Septic shock refractory to catecholamines and distributive shock (due to systemic vasodilation).

Dose: Initial dose - 20 ng/kg/min IV infusion; titrate up to 80 ng/kg/min.

2. Selepressin

Introduction: Selepressin is a selective vasopressin V1A receptor agonist, developed to treat septic shock without causing fluid overload or excessive vasoconstriction.

Clinical Trial Phase / FDA-Approval: In Phase III clinical trials at the current moment for septic shock.

Mechanism of Action:

1. **Selective Activation of V1A Receptors on Vascular Smooth Muscle**

   Selpressin primarily binds to vasopressin 1A (V1A) receptors, which are vascular smooth muscle's G-protein-coupled receptors (GPCRs).

   Gq Protein Activation:

   a. V1A receptor activation leads to Gq protein stimulation, triggering phospholipase C (PLC) activation.
   b. PLC catalyzes Phosphatidylinositol 4,5-bisphosphate (PIP2) which is transformed into:
      i. Inositol triphosphate (IP3) - Stimulates intracellular calcium (Ca^{2+}) release from the sarcoplasmic reticulum.
      ii. Diacylglycerol (DAG) - Activates protein kinase C (PKC), which further promotes vasoconstriction.

2. **Smooth Muscle Contraction and Vasoconstriction**
   - Vascular smooth muscle contraction results from myosin light-chain kinase (MLCK) activation caused by elevated intracellular calcium.
   - The outcome is higher mean arterial pressure (MAP) and the resistance of the systemic arteries (SVR).

3. **No V2 Receptor Activation - Prevention of Fluid Overload**

   Unlike vasopressin, Selepressin does not bind to V2 receptors in the kidneys, which:

   - Prevents water retention and hyponatremia (common adverse effects of vasopressin).
   - Reduces capillary leakage, limiting pulmonary and peripheral oedema.

   This makes Selepressin particularly useful in septic shock, where excessive fluid accumulation worsens respiratory distress and multi-organ failure.

4. **Reduction of Inflammatory Cytokine Release**
   - Selepressin inhibits cytokines that promote inflammation (TNF-α, IL-6, IL-1β), reducing the excessive immune response in septic shock.
   - Decreases nitric oxide (NO) production, limiting excessive vasodilation and endothelial damage.
   - Improves microvascular perfusion, preventing tissue hypoxia and organ dysfunction.

5. **Restoration of Endothelial Integrity**
   - Reduces vascular permeability by stabilizing endothelial gap junctions, thereby limiting fluid leakage.

- Prevents capillary hyperpermeability, which is a major cause of hypotension and organ failure in septic shock.

Key Pharmacokinetic Parameters: Plasma t1/2 is about 4 hours. It is metabolised in liver and excreted in urine. Route of administration is intravenous.

Adverse Drug Reactions: Hypertension, headache, fatigue, myalgia, and peripheral ischemia.

Uses: Septic shock with refractory hypotension (undergoing phase III trials).

Dose: 2.5 ng/kg/min continuous IV (dose in SOFA, SEPSIS-ACT trials).

3. Methylene Blue

Introduction: Methylene blue functions as an oxidative enzyme inhibitor as well as an agent that scavenges nitric oxide (NO). Scientists investigate whether methylene blue can reverse the condition of vasoplegic shock.

Clinical Trial Phase / FDA-Approval: Phase III trials for vasoplegic and septic shock.

Mechanism of Action:

1. **Inhibition of Soluble Guanylate Cyclase (sGC) and NO Pathway**

   A major cause of refractory vasodilatory shock (e.g. septic shock, vasoplegic syndrome) is the overproduction of NO (nitric oxide). Endothelial cells' inducible nitric oxide synthase (iNOS) produces NO, which attaches to soluble guanylate cyclase (sGC) to cause:

   - Increased cGMP production, which activates protein kinase G (PKG).
   - PKG-mediated vascular smooth muscle relaxation, causing hypotension and reduced systemic vascular resistance (SVR).

   Methylene Blue Counteracts This Process:

   1. Direct inhibition of sGC - Blocks NO-induced cGMP production, preventing excessive vasodilation.
   2. Competitive inhibition of NO - Reduces NO availability by acting as a scavenger.
   3. Restoration of vascular tone - Improves perfusion, raises blood pressure (BP), and increases systemic vascular resistance (SVR).

2. **Vasopressor Effect via Catecholamine-Sparing Mechanism**

   Unlike norepinephrine or vasopressin, methylene blue does not rely on adrenergic receptor stimulation to increase blood pressure. This makes it useful in patients with catecholamine-refractory shock where adrenergic receptors are desensitized.

3. **Mitochondrial Protection and ATP Generation**

   - In septic shock, mitochondrial dysfunction leads to impaired ATP production and cellular energy failure.
   - Methylene blue enhances mitochondrial electron transport by:
     i. Acting as an alternative electron acceptor in the electron transport chain (ETC).
     ii. Reducing reactive oxygen species (ROS) generation and oxidative stress.

   This effect improves cellular oxygen utilization, reducing the likelihood of multi-organ failure in prolonged shock states.

4. **Reduction of Endothelial Permeability and Capillary Leakage**
   - Methylene blue stabilizes endothelial function by reducing NO-mediated hyperpermeability.
   - This limits capillary leak syndrome, a key contributor to fluid loss and oedema in septic shock.

Key Pharmacokinetic Parameters: It is administered intravenously (i.v.) as a continuous infusion. It is highly hydrophilic, limiting tissue penetration. Metabolised in liver (CYP450 enzyme) and excreted by urine.

Adverse Drug Reactions: Methemoglobinemia, serotonin syndrome (with SSRIs), hypotension, thrombosis, and cardiac arrhythmias.

Uses: Refractory vasoplegic shock (e.g. post-cardiac surgery, sepsis).

Dose: 1–2 mg/kg IV over 20–30 min; may repeat or follow with infusion (0.25–2 mg/kg/hr).

4. Ularitide

Introduction: Ularitide is a synthetic natriuretic peptide developed for cardiogenic shock and acute heart failure.

Clinical Trial Phase / FDA-Approval: Currently in Phase III trials.

Mechanism of Action:

1. **Activation of Natriuretic Peptide Receptor-A (NPR-A) Leading to cGMP-Mediated Vasodilation**

   Ularitide mimics endogenous ANP by binding to endothelial cells and vascular smooth muscle natriuretic peptide receptor-A (NPR-A). NPR-A activation stimulates intracellular guanylate cyclase (GC) which leads to increased cGMP levels. cGMP activates protein kinase G (PKG), leading to:

   - Smooth muscle relaxation and vasodilation.
   - Arteriolar dilation - reduced systemic vascular resistance (SVR) - Decreased afterload.
   - Venous dilation - increased venous capacitance - Decreased preload and improved cardiac filling.

   This results in improved left ventricular function and reduced pulmonary congestion, which provides key benefits in cardiogenic shock.

2. **Enhancement of Renal Function via Natriuresis and Diuresis**

   Ularitide prevents fluid overload by increasing renal salt and water excretion, thereby reducing pulmonary and peripheral oedema.

   1. Direct Natriuretic Action: Inhibits resorption of sodium in the renal tubules.
   2. It enhances afferent arteriole dilatation and efferent arteriole constriction, hence increasing the glomerular filtration rate (GFR) - diuretic effect.
   3. Reduces renal medullary interstitial pressure, leading to increased urine output.

3. **Reduction of Myocardial Wall Stress and Oxygen Demand**
   - By lowering afterload and preload, Ularitide reduces ventricular wall tension, lowering myocardial oxygen consumption.
   - This protects the ischemic myocardium in cardiogenic shock and cardiac failure, preventing further damage.

4. **Suppression of RAAS (Renin-Angiotensin-Aldosterone System)**
   - Ularitide inhibits renin release, reducing angiotensin II and aldosterone levels.
   - This avoids salt retention and vasoconstriction, supporting its vasodilatory and natriuretic effects.

Key Pharmacokinetic Parameters: Plasma half-life is 10 minutes. It is metabolized by neutral endopeptidases (NEP) in the kidney and other tissues and is excreted by renal route.

Adverse Drug Reactions: Hypotension, nausea, vomiting and electrolyte imbalance.

Uses: Cardiogenic shock and acute decompensated heart failure.

Dose: 15–30 ng/kg/min continuous IV infusion.

5. Landiolol

Introduction: An extremely short-acting beta-1 adrenergic antagonist is landiolol, useful in managing cardiogenic shock and tachyarrhythmias.

Clinical Trial Phase / FDA-Approval: Phase III trials for cardiogenic shock. Approved in Japan and Europe.

Mechanism of Action:

1. **Selective β1-Adrenergic Receptor Blockade**

   Landiolol competitively inhibits cardiac β1-adrenergic receptors, which lessen catecholamines' (epinephrine and norepinephrine) impact on cardiac function and thereby it:

   I. **Reduces Heart Rate (Negative Chronotropic Effect)**
      - By blocking β1 receptors in the sinoatrial (SA) node, Landiolol decreases the rate of spontaneous depolarization, reducing sinus tachycardia and preventing arrhythmias.
      - This helps maintain stable cardiac output without excessive myocardial demand.

   II. **Slows Atrioventricular (AV) Conduction (Negative Dromotropic Effect)**
      - Landiolol prolongs AV nodal conduction, preventing rapid ventricular responses in atrial fibrillation (AF) and supraventricular tachycardia (SVT).

   III. **Minimal Negative Inotropic Effect**
      - Unlike non-selective beta-blockers, Landiolol does not significantly impair myocardial contractility, making it safe for use in shock states.

2. **Modulation of Sympathetic Overactivity in Shock**

   In septic shock, cardiogenic shock, and vasoplegic syndromes, excessive sympathetic activation leads to:

   - Tachycardia, which worsens cardiac efficiency.
   - Increased myocardial oxygen consumption, leading to ischemia.
   - Endothelial dysfunction, exacerbating vasodilation and hemodynamic instability.

   Landiolol counteracts these effects by:

   - Blocking cardiac β1-adrenergic receptors, which lessen catecholamines' (epinephrine and norepinephrine) impact on cardiac function.
   - Reducing myocardial workload, preventing ischemic injury.

- Restoring autonomic balance, decreasing production of inflammatory cytokines (TNF-α, IL-6) in septic shock.

Key Pharmacokinetic Parameters: It is administered intravenously (i.v.) only because of its short duration of action. The plasma half-life is about four minutes. It shows little blood-brain barrier penetration, minimising central nervous system effects. It exhibits moderate plasma protein binding (50-60%), primarily to albumin. It is metabolized by hepatic esterases and is excreted via renal route.

Adverse Drug Reactions: Bradycardia and hypotension.

Uses: Cardiogenic shock with tachyarrhythmias.

Dose: Starting: 1–10 μg/kg/min IV infusion, titrate as needed.

6. Other recent advances in the treatment of shock:

Table 2: Other latest developments in therapy for shock.

Drug/Strategy	Mechanism of Action	Clinical Trial Phase / Status	Adverse Reactions	Distinctive / Salient Features
Levosimendan	K+-ATP channel opener and calcium sensitiser that increases cardiac contractility without substantially raising myocardial oxygen demand.	Used in some countries for cardiogenic shock; ongoing trials for broader applications.	Hypotension, headache, potential arrhythmias.	May improve outcomes in low-output states, has anti-inflammatory and vasodilatory effects.
Beta-blockers in Septic Shock (e.g. Esmolol)	Reduces heart rate and myocardial oxygen demand; can improve stroke volume in hyperdynamic septic shock.	Phase II/III studies assessing morbidity and mortality outcomes.	Bradycardia, hypotension, AV block.	Emerging concept: controlling excessive sympathetic drive to optimize cardiac performance and end-organ perfusion.
Tocilizumab / Other IL-6 Inhibitors	Blockade of IL-6 to reduce hyperinflammatory state in septic shock or cytokine storm.	Under investigation for severe infections and cytokine-release syndromes which leads to septic shock.	Elevated liver enzymes, risk of infection, infusion reactions.	Targeting inflammatory mediators may attenuate organ dysfunction in septic shock or cytokine storm scenarios.
Cell-Based Therapies (e.g. Mesenchymal Stem Cells)	Potential to modulate immune response, improve microvascular blood flow, and enhance tissue repair.	Early-phase clinical trials (Phase I/II).	Unknown long-term immune responses, risk of infection transmission.	Novel immunomodulatory approach to reverse organ dysfunction; still experimental.

Key Emerging Concepts in Shock Management

1. **Precision Fluid Therapy:** The use of dynamic fluid responsiveness assessments (e.g. pulse pressure variation, stroke volume variation, passive leg raise test) has refined fluid therapy, minimizing fluid overload and optimizing end-organ perfusion. Research on balanced crystalloids vs. normal saline suggests potential benefits in renal outcomes and mortality for the former, although debate persists.

2. **Personalized Vasopressor Selection:** Current clinical trials evaluate the safety and effectiveness of catecholamines (norepinephrine, epinephrine, dopamine), vasopressin analogues (selepressin), and synthetic agents (angiotensin II) in specific subsets of shock. Tailoring vasopressor choice to individual hemodynamic profiles may enhance survival by avoiding excessive vasoconstriction or tachyarrhythmias.

3. **Immunomodulatory Therapies:** Sepsis-induced shock is characterized by a dysregulated immune response, prompting investigation into immune-targeted therapies. Tocilizumab and other biologics that inhibit specific cytokines have shown promise in reducing systemic inflammation and organ dysfunction under certain conditions, although large-scale validation is pending.

4. **Mechanical Circulatory Support:** Advanced mechanical devices—extracorporeal membrane oxygenation (ECMO), Impella pumps, intra-aortic balloon pumps—are increasingly used in refractory cardiogenic shock or acute decompensated heart failure. While not "pharmacological," these interventions represent critical advances when drugs alone are insufficient.

5. **Rapid Diagnostics and Biomarkers:** Emerging molecular diagnostics (e.g. pathogen detection with PCR-based assays) and biomarkers (procalcitonin, presepsin) enhance early identification of sepsis, allowing targeted antibiotic therapy and timely intervention. Such precision diagnostics guide the judicious use of novel immunomodulatory treatments.

Conclusion

Shock continues to be a predominant concern in critical care owing to its intricate mechanisms and elevated death rates. Efficient care necessitates the swift identification of shock types—distributive, obstructive, cardiogenic, or hypovolemic—subsequently followed by prompt fluid resuscitation, vasopressor administration, and focused treatment of underlying aetiologies. Standard therapy encompasses crystalloids, norepinephrine, and inotropes, however novel techniques increasingly focus on specific pathophysiological pathways utilising drugs such as angiotensin II, selepressin, levosimendan, and immunomodulators. Advancements in precision medicine—such as biomarker-directed medicines and individualised haemodynamic monitoring—present encouraging opportunities for boosting outcomes, minimising organ failure, and improving survival rates in critically sick patients.

References

1. Kessing LV. Why is lithium [not] the drug of choice for bipolar disorder? a controversy between science and clinical practice. International journal of bipolar disorders. 2024 Jan 16;12(1):3.
2. Poletti S, Mazza MG, Benedetti F. Inflammatory mediators in major depression and bipolar disorder. Translational Psychiatry. 2024 Jun 8;14(1):247.
3. Vieta E. Neuroprogression in bipolar disorder: Why right is wrong. Psychological Medicine. 2024 Jul;54(10):2344-6.
4. GrepMed. Shock classification types - pathophysiology comparison [Internet]. GrepMed; 2023 [cited 2025 May 16]. Available from: https://www.grepmed.com/images/15918/types-classification-shock-comparison-criticalcare.
5. Cecconi M, Evans L, Levy M, Rhodes A. Sepsis and septic shock. The Lancet. 2018 Jul 7;392(10141):75-87.
6. Van Diepen S, Katz JN, Albert NM, Henry TD, Jacobs AK, Kapur NK, Kilic A, Menon V, Ohman EM, Sweitzer NK, Thiele H. Contemporary management of cardiogenic shock: a scientific statement from the American Heart Association. Circulation. 2017 Oct 17;136(16):e232-68.
7. Bonanno FG. Management of hemorrhagic shock: physiology approach, timing and strategies. Journal of clinical medicine. 2022 Dec 29;12(1):260.
8. Cecconi M, De Backer D, Antonelli M, et al. Consensus on circulatory shock and hemodynamic monitoring. *Task force of the European Society of Intensive Care Medicine. Intensive Care Med.* 2014;40(12):1795–815.
9. Vincent JL, De Backer D. Circulatory shock. *N Engl J Med.* 2013;369(18):1726–34.
10. Singer M, Deutschman CS, Seymour CW, Shankar-Hari M, Annane D, Bauer M, Bellomo R, Bernard GR, Chiche JD, Coopersmith CM, Hotchkiss RS. The third international consensus definitions for sepsis and septic shock (Sepsis-3). Jama. 2016 Feb 23;315(8):801-10.

11. Cannon CM, Braxton CC, Kling-Smith M, Mahnken JD, Carlton E, Moncure M. Utility of the shock index in predicting mortality in traumatically injured patients. Journal of Trauma and Acute Care Surgery. 2009 Dec 1;67(6):1426-30.
12. Rhodes A, Evans LE, Alhazzani W, Levy MM, Antonelli M, Ferrer R, Kumar A, Sevransky JE, Sprung CL, Nunnally ME, Rochwerg B. Surviving sepsis campaign: international guidelines for management of sepsis and septic shock: 2016. Intensive care medicine. 2017 Mar;43:304-77.
13. Muir WW, Hughes D, Silverstein DC. Fluid therapy in animals: physiologic principles and contemporary fluid resuscitation considerations. Frontiers in Veterinary Science. 2021 Oct 20;8:744080.
14. Khanna A, English SW, Wang XS, Ham K, Tumlin J, Szerlip H, Busse LW, Altaweel L, Albertson TE, Mackey C, McCurdy MT. Angiotensin II for the treatment of vasodilatory shock. New England Journal of Medicine. 2017 Aug 3;377(5):419-30.
15. Shankar-Hari M, Spencer J, Sewell WA, Rowan KM, Singer M. Bench-to-bedside review: Immunoglobulin therapy for sepsis-biological plausibility from a critical care perspective. Critical care. 2012 Apr;16:1-4.
16. Westphal GA, Koenig Á, Caldeira Filho M, Feijó J, de Oliveira LT, Nunes F, Fujiwara K, Martins SF, Gonçalves AR. Reduced mortality after the implementation of a protocol for the early detection of severe sepsis. Journal of critical care. 2011 Feb 1;26(1):76-81.
17. Chaba A, Zarbock A, Forni LG, Hästbacka J, Korneva E, Landoni G, Pickkers P, Bellomo R. Angiotensin II for Catecholamine Resistant Vasodilatory Shock in Patients with Acute Kidney Injury: A Post-Hoc Analysis of the ATHOS-3 Trial. Shock. 2023 Jan 23:10-97.
18. Vincent JL, Annoni F. Vasopressor Therapy. Journal of Clinical Medicine. 2024 Dec 3;13(23):7372.
19. Alkazemi A, Almoosawy SA, Murad A, Alfares A. Methylene Blue for Septic Shock: A Systematic Review and Meta-analysis of Randomized and Prospective Observational Studies. Journal of Intensive Care Medicine. 2024 Nov 22:08850666241300312.
20. Rehberg S, Frank S, Černý V, Cihlář R, Borgstedt R, Biancofiore G, Guarracino F, Schober A, Trimmel H, Pernerstorfer T, Siebers C. Landiolol for heart rate control in patients with septic shock and persistent tachycardia. A multicenter randomized clinical trial (Landi-SEP). Intensive Care Medicine. 2024 Oct;50(10):1622-34.
21. Whitehouse T, Hossain A, Perkins GD, Gordon AC, Bion J, Young D, McAuley D, Singer M, Lord J, Gates S, Veenith T. Landiolol and organ failure in patients with septic shock: the STRESS-L randomized clinical trial. Jama. 2023 Nov 7;330(17):1641-52.
22. Manzi L, Buongiorno F, Narciso V, Florimonte D, Forzano I, Castiello DS, Sperandeo L, Paolillo R, Verde N, Spinelli A, Cristiano S. Acute Heart Failure and Non-Ischemic Cardiomyopathies: A Comprehensive Review and Critical Appraisal. Diagnostics. 2025 Feb 23;15(5):540.
23. Sharifan A. Global analysis of vasoactive agents in septic shock management: Exploring trends and bridging knowledge gaps. Journal of Translational Critical Care Medicine. 2024 Dec 1;6(4):e24-00032.
24. Li S, Jiang J, Pi D, Li J, Bai X, Lu Y, Xu F, Li X, Li J. Clinical efficacy and safety of vasopressin and its analogues in patients with septic shock: a meta-analysis and trial sequential analysis.
25. Leisman DE, Wieruszewski PM, Busse LW, Chawla LS, Hibbert KA, Handisides DR, Khanna AK, Ostermann M, McCurdy MT, Adams CD, Hodges TN. An index of the initial blood pressure response to angiotensin II treatment and its association with clinical outcomes in vasodilatory shock. Critical Care. 2025 Feb 19;29(1):81.

Chapter 16

Recent Advances in the Management of Myocardial Infarction

Author: Dr. Pranab Das

Introduction

The typical causes of myocardial infarction (MI) are rupture of the atherosclerotic plaque and subsequent thrombus formation in a coronary artery. MI remains one of the leading causes of morbidity and mortality worldwide, despite tremendous progress in prevention, early detection, and treatment. The death rate from MI has significantly decreased over the last 20 years, in part because of better emergency care, which includes PCI, better medication, and following evidence-based recommendations.

Traditional treatments have demonstrated effectiveness in lowering mortality and preventing recurrent MI events. These include dual antiplatelet therapy, ACE inhibitors, beta-blockers, and statins. However, a sizable fraction of patients continues to suffer from complications like heart failure, recurrent ischaemia, or fatal arrhythmias in spite of these achievements. Current developments seek to improve acute and long-term care even more. These include more recent lipid-lowering treatments that go beyond the reach of conventional statins, biologics that target inflammatory pathways, mechanical circulatory support devices, and novel antithrombotic agents. The advent of innovative treatments, such as gene and stem cell therapies and high-sensitivity cardiac troponin assays, has given clinicians more complete tools to customise treatment for each patient, improving outcomes and quality of life. The main terms and categories of myocardial infarction are described in this section, along with a brief overview of traditional treatment methods and an exploration of the newest and most promising medications influencing the state of modern medicine.

Historical Perspective

Over the past century, there has been a significant shift in our understanding and treatment of myocardial infarction (MI), also known as a heart attack. The first accounts of MI date from the 19th century, when pathologists connected myocardial necrosis and coronary artery blockage during autopsies. But MI wasn't clinically recognised until the early 1900s, thanks to the development of electrocardiography (ECG) in the 1910s, which transformed diagnosis.

Because there were no proven treatments for coronary thrombosis, the management of MI in the middle of the 20th century was primarily conservative and concentrated on bed rest and morphine administration. A significant turning point was the establishment of coronary care units (CCUs) in the 1960s, which decreased mortality by closely monitoring patients and intervening early in arrhythmias.

When the role of thrombus formation in acute MI was discovered in the 1970s and 1980s, reperfusion therapy became the new standard of care. A period of pharmacological reperfusion began with the introduction of intravenous thrombolytics like streptokinase and later tissue plasminogen activator (tPA). The 1990s saw the introduction of primary percutaneous coronary intervention (PCI), which swiftly rose to prominence as the gold standard because it produced better results than thrombolysis.

Results have significantly improved over the past 20 years due to advancements in pharmacotherapy, including dual antiplatelet therapy (DAPT), statins, beta-blockers, and ACE inhibitors. More recently, drug-eluting stents (DES), high-sensitivity troponins, and more recent P2Y12 inhibitors (such as ticagrelor and prasugrel) have improved long-term prognosis and diagnosis.

Individualised risk assessment, microvascular protection, early invasive techniques, and secondary prevention—including lifestyle modifications and AI-powered risk modelling—have become the main areas of focus in the modern era. Further advancements in the treatment of MI include biological therapies that target inflammation and cardiac regeneration as well as mechanical circulatory support.

Definition

Myocardial cell death (necrosis) brought on by protracted cardiac myocytes ischaemia is known as myocardial infarction. The Fourth Universal Definition of Myocardial Infarction states that the diagnosis is dependent on the presence of myocardial ischaemia symptoms, as well as an increase in cardiac biomarkers (ideally troponin) with at least one value above the 99th percentile of upper reference limit:

1. Ischemic symptoms,
2. New significant ECG modification or addition of a new left bundle branch block (LBBB),
3. Imaging evidence of a regional irregularity in wall motion or a recent loss of viable myocardium, or
4. Identification of a coronary thrombus by angiography or autopsy.

Types (STEMI vs. NSTEMI)

In clinical settings, MI can also be classified by the underlying pathological mechanism (type 1, brought on by the rupture of plaque; type 2, brought on by an imbalance between the supply and demand of oxygen; type 3, sudden cardiac death with suggestive findings of ischemia; etc.). However, the most pragmatic approach for acute management remains distinguishing STEMI from NSTEMI due to different immediate reperfusion strategies.

1. **ST-Segment Elevation Myocardial Infarction (STEMI)**
   - Characterized either a fresh left bundle branch block (LBBB) or persistent ST-segment elevations in ≥2 contiguous leads on the ECG.
   - Usually signifies that an epicardial coronary artery is completely blocked.
   - Urgent reperfusion therapy (primary PCI if available within recommended timelines, or fibrinolysis if PCI is not feasible) is the standard of care to minimize myocardial damage.
2. **Non-ST-Segment Elevation Myocardial Infarction (NSTEMI)**
   - Presents with ischemic symptoms and elevated cardiac biomarkers but without persistent ST-segment elevation.
   - Commonly connected to intermittent or partial coronary artery blockage.
   - Management involves early invasive angiography (within 24–72 hours, depending on risk stratification) followed by percutaneous or surgical revascularization if indicated, in addition to medical therapy.

Brief Note on Conventional Medicines

Standard therapy for acute myocardial infarction focuses on re-establishing blood flow to the ischemic myocardium (via PCI or fibrinolysis in eligible STEMI patients), inhibiting further thrombosis, controlling ischemic pain, and preventing adverse left ventricular (LV) remodelling. Below is a concise summary of conventional agents.

Table 1: Concise overview of conventional medications utilised in myocardial infarction treatment.

Drug Class / Drug Names	Mechanism of Action	Common Dosage Forms	Usual Side Effects
Antiplatelets (e.g. Aspirin, Clopidogrel, Prasugrel, Ticagrelor)	Inhibits platelet activation, adhesion and aggregation, reduce thrombus formation.	Oral tablets	Bleeding (gastrointestinal, intracranial), dyspnoea (ticagrelor).
Anticoagulants (e.g. Unfractionated Heparin, LMWH, Fondaparinux)	Inhibit clotting factors (thrombin, factor Xa), preventing thrombus formation and propagation.	i.v. infusion (UFH), s.c. injection (LMWH & Fondaparinux)	Bleeding, thrombocytopenia (particularly with heparin).
Beta-Blockers (e.g. Metoprolol, Esmolol, Labetalol, Carvedilol)	Reduce myocardial oxygen demand, contractility, and heart rate.	Oral tablets, i.v. injection	Bradycardia, hypotension, fatigue, bronchospasm in susceptible individuals.
ACE Inhibitors / ARBs (e.g. Enalapril, Lisinopril, Valsartan)	Prevents left ventricular remodelling and afterload by blocking the renin-angiotensin-aldosterone pathway.	Oral tablets	Cough (ACE inhibitors), hyperkalaemia, renal impairment, angioedema.
Statins (e.g. Atorvastatin, Rosuvastatin)	Lower LDL cholesterol, stabilize plaques, and exert pleiotropic anti-inflammatory effects.	Oral tablets	Myalgias, elevated liver enzymes, rare rhabdomyolysis.
Nitrates (e.g. Nitro-glycerine)	Vasodilation (venous>arterial), reduces preload, helps to relieve angina.	Sublingual tablets, oro-mucosal spray, i.v. infusion, oral tablets, transdermal patches.	Headache, hypotension, reflex tachycardia, tolerance (when used continuously).

These therapies collectively reduce mortality, limit infarct size, and prevent recurrent cardiac events. Notably, immediate revascularization by PCI or fibrinolysis (STEMI) or early invasive strategy (NSTEMI) is central to favourable outcomes. Nevertheless, ongoing research seeks to refine and expand upon this established therapeutic foundation.

Newer Drugs / Recent Advances

Despite extensive progress, there remains a subset of patients with ongoing ischemia, increased bleeding risk, or incomplete myocardial recovery following conventional therapy. Consequently, the focus of research has shifted toward innovative pharmacologic agents, next-generation devices, and precision interventions that tackle residual risk factors (e.g. inflammation, hyperlipidaemia, microvascular obstruction). Below is a summary of selected novel agents and strategies.

1. Zalunfiban

Introduction: Zalunfiban is a new antagonist of the integrin αIIbβ3 receptor that was created to treat ST-elevation myocardial infarction (STEMI). It serves as a substitute for conventional glycoprotein IIb/IIIa inhibitors such as abciximab by preventing platelet aggregation and thrombus formation.

Clinical Trial Phase / FDA-Approval: STEMI patients having percutaneous coronary intervention (PCI) are presently enrolled in Phase III clinical trials.

Mechanism of Action: Zalunfiban selectively binds to the integrin αIIbβ3, thereby blocking the binding of von Willebrand factor (vWF) and fibrinogen to platelets via this receptor. This action inhibits platelet aggregation, reducing thrombus formation in coronary arteries. Unlike traditional IIb/IIIa inhibitors, Zalunfiban exhibits a shorter half-life and rapid reversibility, making it ideal for emergency MI management.

Key Pharmacokinetic Parameters: Rapid onset of action. Shows high plasma protein binding. Unlike oral P2Y12 inhibitors, Zalunfiban does not require hepatic metabolism, making it independent of liver function variability and is excreted out in urine. Plasma half-life is short, allowing quick reversal of effects.

Adverse Drug Reactions: Increased risk of bleeding, thrombocytopenia, hypotension, nausea, and vomiting.

Uses: Acute STEMI and NSTEMI management and adjunct therapy during PCI.

Dose: 3–6 μg/kg IV bolus, followed by infusion (in clinical trials).

2. Finerenone

Introduction: Patients with type 2 diabetes and chronic kidney disease (CKD) can lower their cardiovascular risk by using finerenone, a nonsteroidal, selective mineralocorticoid receptor antagonist (MRA). It helps avoid post-MI unfavourable ventricular remodelling and cardiac fibrosis.

Clinical Trial Phase / FDA-Approval: FDA-approved for CKD-related cardiovascular risk but under investigation (Phase II trial) for MI prevention.

Mechanism of Action:

1. **Inhibition of Mineralocorticoid Receptor (MR) -Induced Fibrosis**
   - Post-MI, there is excessive collagen deposition in the myocardium due to Mineralocorticoid Receptor (MR) activation.
   - Finerenone blocks MR in cardiac fibroblasts, preventing:
     i. Activation of transforming growth factor-beta (TGF-β), which reduces myofibroblast differentiation.
     ii. Excessive collagen synthesis (COL1A1, COL3A1 genes) and thereby prevents myocardial stiffening.
     iii. Fibrotic scar expansion which ultimately leads to preservation of left ventricular (LV) function.
2. **Reduction of Inflammation Post-MI**
   - MI triggers a pro-inflammatory response, leading to immune cell infiltration and cytokine release.
   - MR activation increases pro-inflammatory cytokines (IL-6, TNF-α) and promotes M1 macrophage (proinflammatory macrophage) recruitment, exacerbating cardiac injury.
   - Finerenone prevents MI-driven inflammation by:
     i. Inhibiting NF-κB activation, reducing inflammatory gene expression.
     ii. Blocking macrophage infiltration - limiting cardiac damage.
     iii. Inhibits the shift towards M1 macrophages (proinflammatory) and promotes polarization toward the M2 phenotype (anti-inflammatory macrophage).

3. **Improvement of Endothelial Function & Microvascular Integrity**
   - MR activation damages endothelial cells, reducing nitric oxide (NO) availability which leads to vascular dysfunction and microvascular occlusion.
   - Finerenone preserves endothelial function by:
     i. Increasing eNOS (endothelial nitric oxide synthase) - restores NO production.
     ii. Reducing oxidative stress (inhibits NADPH oxidase, ROS formation).
     iii. Preventing endothelial apoptosis - improves coronary microcirculation.
4. **Prevention of Adverse Cardiac Remodelling & Heart Failure**
   - MR activation in cardiomyocytes causes hypertrophy and LV dysfunction, increasing the risk of heart failure post-MI.
   - Finerenone protects against adverse remodelling by:
     i. Blocking hypertrophic signalling pathways (MAPK, ERK1/2).
     ii. Reducing cardiomyocyte apoptosis.
     iii. Preventing left ventricular dilation and dysfunction.

Key Pharmacokinetic Parameters: Oral bioavailability is 43%. It is metabolised in liver (CYP3A4 enzyme) and undergoes renal (major) and faecal (minor) excretion. It is highly plasma protein-bound. Plasma half-life is around 2–3 hours.

Adverse Drug Reactions: Hyperkalaemia, hypotension, dizziness and fatigue.

Uses: Prevention of heart failure in post-MI patients and reducing cardiovascular risk in diabetic CKD patients.

Dose: 10–20 mg orally once daily.

3. Semaglutide

Introduction: Semaglutide is a GLP-1 receptor agonist marketed under the brand name Wegovy. It was originally developed for diabetes and weight loss, but recent studies show its potential in reducing MI risk in obese and diabetic patients.

Clinical Trial Phase / FDA-Approval: Currently in Phase III trials.

Mechanism of Action: Semaglutide is a glucagon-like peptide-1 receptor agonist (GLP-1RA) primarily used for type 2 diabetes (T2D) and obesity. However, recent clinical trials (SELECT, SOUL, EVOKE, EVOKE+) have demonstrated cardioprotective effects.

1. **Direct Cardioprotective Effects of GLP-1 Receptor Activation**

   Semaglutide activates GLP-1 receptors (GLP-1R) in cardiomyocytes, vascular smooth muscle cells and endothelial cells, leading to:
   - Increased cAMP which leads to activation of PKA & PI3K/Akt Pathway.
   - Enhanced nitric oxide (NO) production leading to vasodilation.
   - Mitochondrial protection ultimately resulting in reduced oxidative stress.

2. **Anti-Inflammatory Effects in Post-MI Setting**

   After an MI, a pro-inflammatory cascade is triggered, leading to cardiac damage and remodelling. Semaglutide suppresses inflammation by:

   - Reducing cytokines (IL-6, TNF-α, MCP-1, CRP) and thereby lowers systemic and local inflammation.
   - Inhibiting NF-κB pathway - Prevents endothelial dysfunction.
   - Reducing macrophage infiltration - Limits post-MI immune overactivation.

3. **Endothelial Protection & Anti-Atherosclerotic Effects**

   MI often occurs due to atherosclerosis and plaque rupture. Semaglutide improves endothelial function and stabilizes plaques. Mechanism:

   Enhances nitric oxide (NO) production - Improves vasodilation & reduces arterial stiffness and also reduces endothelial oxidative stress, ultimately leading to protection against plaque formation. It also decreases vascular smooth muscle proliferation and thereby limits atherosclerosis progression. It also lowers LDL-C & triglycerides, ultimately reducing plaque burden.

4. **Cardiac Remodelling & Heart Failure Prevention Post-MI**

   Post-MI, heart failure results from inappropriate remodelling of the heart. Semaglutide protects against adverse remodelling by:

   - Reducing fibrosis by inhibiting TGF-β and collagen deposition.
   - Enhancing cardiomyocyte survival, thereby decreasing apoptosis via PI3K/Akt pathway.
   - Preserving left ventricular function (LVEF) which improves myocardial contractility.
   - Reducing hypertrophy by inhibiting ERK1/2 signalling.

5. **Metabolic & Energy Benefits for Myocardium**

   Post-MI, cardiac metabolism shifts from fatty acid oxidation to glucose metabolism to preserve energy. Semaglutide enhances myocardial energy efficiency by:

   - Increasing glucose uptake via AMPK activation.
   - Reducing myocardial oxygen demand.
   - Enhancing mitochondrial function thereby reducing oxidative stress.

Key Pharmacokinetic Parameters: It is available in subcutaneous (s.c.) and oral dosage forms. S.C. bioavailability is around 89% with once-weekly injection, whereas oral bioavailability is around 0.8%, requiring a high-dose formulation. Time to peak concentration (Tmax) for s.c. injection is around 1–3 days after injection whereas for oral formulation it is around 1–4 hours post-administration. It is highly plasma protein-bound (99%), leading to prolonged action. It is degraded slowly by enzymatic cleavage (similar to endogenous GLP-1). No CYP450 involvement, reducing drug interaction risks. Primarily excreted via hepatic metabolism, with minimal renal clearance.

Adverse Drug Reactions: Nausea, vomiting, constipation, pancreatitis, cholelithiasis, cholecystitis and hypoglycaemia.

Uses: Cardiovascular risk reduction in diabetic and obese patients. Weight loss in high-risk cardiovascular patients.

Dose: 0.25 mg weekly, titrate to 1–2 mg weekly SC.

4. Selatogrel

Introduction: Selatogrel is a reversible P2Y12 receptor antagonist developed as a subcutaneous emergency therapy for acute MI.

Clinical Trial Phase / FDA-Approval: Currently in Phase III trials for acute MI.

Mechanism of Action: Platelets play a central role in thrombosis during MI. Upon vascular injury or plaque rupture:

1. Adenosine diphosphate (ADP) is released from platelets and endothelial cells.
2. ADP binds to $P2Y_{12}$ receptors on platelets, activating them.
3. Glycoprotein IIb/IIIa (GP IIb/IIIa), which binds fibrinogen to activated platelets, is expressed by platelet aggregates (thrombus).
4. This leads to coronary artery occlusion, worsening MI.

Selatogrel inhibits the receptor for P2Y12, preventing ADP-induced platelet aggregation. In contrast to clopidogrel, it has a rapid onset and shorter half-life, allowing a more feasible MI treatment.

Key Pharmacokinetic Parameters: Rapid (subcutaneous) absorption and high bioavailability (85%) guarantee efficient systemic distribution. Liver enzymes mainly break it down through phase II conjugation and hydrolysis. Its short half-life (8–12 hours) allows for quick action offset. Mostly it is eliminated by hepatic metabolism, with little excretion in the kidneys.

Adverse Drug Reactions: Bleeding risk, dyspnoea, bradycardia, hypotension,as well as injection site reactions (pain, redness, swelling), which include discomfort, oedema and redness at the injection site.

Uses: Emergency self-administered MI therapy. Alternative to oral P2Y12 inhibitors.

Dose: 16 mg SC single dose (in development).

5. Inclisiran

Introduction: Inclisiran is a PCSK9 inhibitor that lowers LDL cholesterol and lowers the risk of recurrent MI.

Clinical Trial Phase / FDA-Approval: FDA-approved for hypercholesterolemia and atherosclerosis management and is in currently undergoing Phase II trial for MI treatment.

Mechanism of Action:

1. **Role of PCSK9 in Myocardial Infarction (MI) Pathophysiology**

   PCSK9 is a liver-secreted protein that regulates LDL receptor (LDLR) degradation. High PCSK9 levels leads to:

   a. Reduced LDL receptor availability - Less LDL-C clearance.

   b. Increased LDL-C in blood - Promotes atherosclerosis.

   c. Plaque instability - Higher risk of MI due to rupture.

2. **Pharmacodynamic Mechanism of Inclisiran**

   PCSK9 is silenced by the small interfering RNA (siRNA) in hepatocytes.

   A. RNA Interference (RNAi) Mechanism in the Liver:

   i. Inclisiran enters hepatocytes via GalNAc-mediated delivery.
   ii. It attaches itself to the RISC (RNA-induced silencing complex).

iii. RISC cleaves PCSK9 mRNA - Prevents PCSK9 protein synthesis.
iv. Lower PCSK9 levels lead to increased LDL receptor expression on hepatocytes.
v. More LDL-C is removed from the bloodstream, reducing plaque burden and MI risk.

B. Anti-Atherosclerotic & Plaque-Stabilizing Effects

- Inclisiran prevents MI by reducing atherosclerosis progression: Lowers LDL-C levels (by 50-60%), thereby slows down plaque build-up.
- Reduces macrophage-driven inflammation - Prevents plaque rupture.
- Stabilizes high-risk "vulnerable plaques" - Reduces risk of sudden coronary artery occlusion.

C. Improves Endothelial Function & Prevents Thrombosis

- LDL-C reduction improves nitric oxide (NO) availability in the endothelium - enhances vasodilation.
- Helps in repairing defective endothelium by reducing oxidative stress - Prevents microvascular damage.
- Lowers thrombogenic factors (e.g. fibrinogen, PAI-1) - Reduces clot formation post-MI.

Key Pharmacokinetic Parameters: It is administered subcutaneously (s.c.) every 6 months after two initial doses at 0 and 3 months. Peak plasma concentration (Tmax) is achieved within 4–6 hours post-injection. It shows extensive hepatic uptake, where it silences PCSK9 mRNA, reducing circulating PCSK9 levels. It is metabolized intracellularly via endonucleases, leading to the development of small inactive metabolites. Its effective half-life is around 16–21 days, supporting long dosing intervals. Plasma clearance is primarily via renal (major) and hepatic (minor) pathways.

Adverse Drug Reactions: Injection site reactions (pain, redness, swelling), hepatic dysfunction, myalgia, nasopharyngitis and elevated liver enzymes.

Uses: LDL cholesterol reduction and prevention of recurrent MI.

Dose: 284 mg SC on Day 1, Day 90, then Q6M (The expanded meaning of Q6M is "quaque 6 mensis" which refers to once every 6 months).

6. Other recent advances in treatment of MI:

Table 2: Other recent developments in myocardial infarction intervention.

Drug / Strategy	Mechanism of Action	Clinical Trial Phase / Status	Adverse Reactions	Distinctive / Salient Features
Cangrelor (i.v. P2Y12 inhibitor)	Direct, rapid, reversible inhibition of platelet ADP receptor (P2Y12).	FDA-Approved for use in MI patients undergoing percutaneous coronary intervention (PCI).	Bleeding, rare allergic reactions.	Ultra-short-acting i.v. antiplatelet, useful in emergent PCI.
Bivalirudin (Direct Thrombin Inhibitor)	Binds to thrombin (both free and clot-bound), preventing fibrin formation.	FDA-approved for use in MI patients undergoing percutaneous coronary intervention (PCI).	Bleeding (less as compared to heparin + GP IIb/IIIa inhibitor combinations).	Lower bleeding risk in PCI, especially in high-risk or older patients.
PCSK9 Inhibitors (e.g. Alirocumab, Evolocumab)	Monoclonal antibodies that block PCSK9 from degrading LDL receptors, substantially reducing LDL levels.	FDA-approved for high-risk atherosclerosis. Ongoing trials for treatment in MI.	Injection site reactions (pain, redness, swelling), potential neurocognitive effects.	Effective in secondary prevention, drastically reduce LDL-C; beneficial post-MI for high-risk individuals.
Colchicine (Anti-inflammatory)	Inhibits microtubule polymerization, reducing neutrophil activation and inflammation.	Approved for gout; repurposed for cardiovascular disease; first anti-inflammatory drug which is FDA-approved for secondary prevention of cardiovascular events, including: Myocardial infarction (MI), stroke and coronary revascularization.	GI upset, diarrhoea, rare cytopenia with long-term use.	Recent trials (COLCOT, LoDoCo2) suggest reduced ischemic events in post-MI patients via anti-inflammatory effects.
SGLT2 Inhibitors (e.g. Dapagliflozin, Empagliflozin)	Lower glucose reabsorption in the proximal tubule, also exerting cardiovascular and reno-protective effects.	Approved for HF, T2DM; under investigation for acute MI.	Genitourinary infections, euglycemic ketoacidosis.	Demonstrated reductions in HF hospitalization; ongoing trials evaluating post-MI remodelling and outcomes.
Cell-based Therapies (e.g. Stem Cell Transplant)	Potential regeneration of damaged myocardium, improved angiogenesis, and contractility.	Early-phase clinical trials ongoing.	Unknown long-term safety; arrhythmogenic risks, immune response may occur.	Aimed at restoring myocardial tissue post-infarction; ongoing research is promising.

Novel Anti-Inflammatory Agents (e.g. Canakinumab, IL-6 inhibitors)	Target pro-inflammatory cytokines to reduce vascular inflammation and plaque progression.	Phase II/III trials for secondary prevention; some evidence from CANTOS.	Increased risk of infection, potential immune-related side-effects.	Identifies a subgroup of post-MI patients with elevated inflammatory markers (e.g. CRP) who may benefit from therapy.

Key Emerging Concepts

1. **Advanced Antiplatelet and Anticoagulant Strategies:** Intravenous P2Y12 inhibitors like cangrelor or more selective thrombin inhibitors like bivalirudin provide tailored solutions for patients at high bleeding risk or needing urgent PCI. Balancing efficacy and safety remain paramount, prompting ongoing trials examining de-escalation or duration-titration of antithrombotic therapy.
2. **Aggressive Lipid-Lowering Strategies:** High-intensity statin therapy remains foundational post-MI, but a significant portion of patients have persistent, elevated LDL or remain at risk for recurrent events. PCSK9 inhibitors and inclisiran offer profound LDL-lowering effects, reducing atheroma progression and recurrent ischemic events. They also demonstrate that more aggressive, personalized lipid management can significantly impact long-term outcomes.
3. **Inflammation as a Therapeutic Target:** Landmark trials, such as CANTOS, suggest that reducing inflammation (independent of lipid levels) confers cardiovascular benefits by lowering rates of recurrent MI and other major adverse cardiac events. Colchicine and canakinumab highlight this new dimension in post-MI care, although cost, side effects, and patient selection criteria are areas requiring further clarity.
4. **Metabolic Modulation / Cardiorenal Protection:** Inhibitors of the sodium-glucose cotransporter-2 (SGLT2) were first created to treat type 2 diabetes mellitus, now shows broad cardiovascular and renal protective effects, including in heart failure. Current research evaluates whether these benefits extend specifically to post-MI remodelling, potentially preventing the transition to ischemic cardiomyopathy.
5. **Cell-Based and Gene Therapies:** The potential for stem cells or genes to regenerate editing technologies has garnered attention for myocardial repair, yet robust clinical data remains limited. Challenges include cell survival, targeted delivery, and immunogenicity, given the intricate interactions between many cell types in the infarcted myocardium. Nevertheless, these remain exciting avenues for future therapeutic breakthroughs.

Conclusion

Recent advancements in medical guidelines and revascularisation techniques have markedly decreased mortality rates associated with myocardial infarction (MI). Standard treatments for STEMI and NSTEMI include aspirin, P2Y12 inhibitors, beta-blockers, ACE inhibitors or ARBs, statins, and rapid reperfusion, all of which are well-established. Residual risks continue to stimulate innovation in the development of next-generation antiplatelets, anticoagulants, PCSK9 inhibitors, SGLT2 inhibitors, and anti-inflammatory medications. Personalised treatment informed by high-sensitivity troponin testing, advanced imaging, and genetic profiling is increasingly central to patient care. Regenerative therapies exhibit potential; however, obstacles persist in improving their safety and efficacy. Future improvements will rely on the integration of pharmacological advancements with individualised patient strategies to further decrease morbidity and mortality associated with myocardial infarction.

References

1. Matter MA, Paneni F, Libby P, Frantz S, Stähli BE, Templin C, Mengozzi A, Wang YJ, Kündig TM, Räber L, Ruschitzka F. Inflammation in acute myocardial infarction: the good, the bad and the ugly. European heart journal. 2024 Jan 7;45(2):89-103.
2. Liu J, Liu F, Liang T, Zhou Y, Su X, Li X, Zeng J, Qu P, Wang Y, Chen F, Lei Q. The roles of Th cells in myocardial infarction. Cell Death Discovery. 2024 Jun 15;10(1):287.
3. Jolly SS, d'Entremont MA, Pitt B, Lee SF, Mian R, Tyrwhitt J, Kedev S, Montalescot G, Cornel JH, Stanković G, Moreno R. Routine spironolactone in acute myocardial infarction. New England Journal of Medicine. 2025 Feb 13;392(7):643-52.
4. Yndigegn T, Lindahl B, Mars K, Alfredsson J, Benatar J, Brandin L, Erlinge D, Hallen O, Held C, Hjalmarsson P, Johansson P. Beta-blockers after myocardial infarction and preserved ejection fraction. New England Journal of Medicine. 2024 Apr 18;390(15):1372-81.
5. Hajar R. Evolution of myocardial infarction and its biomarkers: A historical perspective. Heart views. 2016 Oct 1;17(4):167-72.
6. Anderson JL, Morrow DA. Acute myocardial infarction. New England Journal of Medicine. 2017 May 25;376(21):2053-64.
7. Reed GW, Rossi JE, Cannon CP. Acute myocardial infarction. *Lancet*. 2017;389(10065):197–210.
8. Ibanez B, James S, Agewall S, Antunes MJ, Bucciarelli-Ducci C, Bueno H, Caforio AL, Crea F, Goudevenos JA, Halvorsen S, Hindricks G. 2017 ESC Guidelines for the management of acute myocardial infarction in patients presenting with ST-segment elevation: The Task Force for the management of acute myocardial infarction in patients presenting with ST-segment elevation of the European Society of Cardiology (ESC). European heart journal. 2018 Jan 7;39(2):119-77.
9. Thygesen K, Alpert JS, Jaffe AS, Chaitman BR, Bax JJ, Morrow DA, White HD, Executive Group on behalf of the Joint European Society of Cardiology (ESC)/American College of Cardiology (ACC)/American Heart Association (AHA)/World Heart Federation (WHF) Task Force for the Universal Definition of Myocardial Infarction. Fourth universal definition of myocardial infarction (2018). Circulation. 2018 Nov 13;138(20):e618-51.
10. Collet JP, Thiele H, Barbato E, Barthélémy O, Bauersachs J, Bhatt DL, Dendale P, Dorobantu M, Edvardsen T, Folliguet T, Gale CP. 2020 ESC Guidelines for the management of acute coronary syndromes in patients presenting without persistent ST-segment elevation: The Task Force for the management of acute coronary syndromes in patients presenting without persistent ST-segment elevation of the European Society of Cardiology (ESC). European heart journal. 2021 Apr 7;42(14):1289-367.
11. Sun B, Liang C, Sun P, Li L, Zhao L, Li P, Li Y, Foo RS, Chan MY, Yang Q, Zhou X. Mortality Risk and Treatment Disparities in the Chinese SMuRF-less STEMI Patients: A Nationwide Cohort Study. medRxiv. 2025:2025-04.
12. Bhatt DL, Stone GW, Mahaffey KW, Gibson CM, Steg PG, Hamm CW, Price MJ, Leonardi S, Gallup D, Bramucci E, Radke PW. Effect of platelet inhibition with cangrelor during PCI on ischemic events. New England Journal of Medicine. 2013 Apr 4;368(14):1303-13.
13. Ray KK, Landmesser U, Leiter LA, Kallend D, Dufour R, Karakas M, Hall T, Troquay RP, Turner T, Visseren FL, Wijngaard P. Inclisiran in patients at high cardiovascular risk with elevated LDL cholesterol. New England Journal of Medicine. 2017 Apr 13;376(15):1430-40.
14. Tardif JC, Kouz S, Waters DD, Bertrand OF, Diaz R, Maggioni AP, Pinto FJ, Ibrahim R, Gamra H, Kiwan GS, Berry C. Efficacy and safety of low-dose colchicine after myocardial infarction. New England journal of medicine. 2019 Dec 26;381(26):2497-505.
15. Ridker PM, Everett BM, Thuren T, MacFadyen JG, Chang WH, Ballantyne C, Fonseca F, Nicolau J, Koenig W, Anker SD, Kastelein JJ. Antiinflammatory therapy with canakinumab for atherosclerotic disease. New England journal of medicine. 2017 Sep 21;377(12):1119-31.
16. Madonna R, Van Laake LW, Davidson SM, Engel FB, Hausenloy DJ, Lecour S, Leor J, Perrino C, Schulz R, Ytrehus K, Landmesser U. Position Paper of the European Society of Cardiology Working Group Cellular Biology of the Heart: cell-based therapies for myocardial repair and regeneration in ischemic heart disease and heart failure. European heart journal. 2016 Jun 14;37(23):1789-98.
17. Milluzzo RP, Franchina GA, Capodanno D, Angiolillo DJ. Selatogrel, a novel P2Y12 inhibitor: a review of the pharmacology and clinical development. Expert Opinion on Investigational Drugs. 2020 Jun 2;29(6):537-46.
18. Grundy SM, Hansen B, Smith Jr SC, Cleeman JI, Kahn RA, Conference Participants. Clinical management of metabolic syndrome: report of the American Heart Association/National Heart, Lung, and Blood Institute/American Diabetes Association conference on scientific issues related to management. Circulation. 2004 Feb 3;109(4):551-6.
19. Kuzmich N, Andresyuk E, Porozov Y, Tarasov V, Samsonov M, Preferanskaya N, Veselov V, Alyautdin R. PCSK9 as a Target for Development of a New Generation of Hypolipidemic Drugs. Molecules. 2022 Jan 10;27(2):434.
20. Koren MJ, Rodriguez F, East C, Toth PP, Watwe V, Abbas CA, Sarwat S, Kleeman K, Kumar B, Ali Y, Jaffrani N. An "inclisiran first" strategy vs usual care in patients with atherosclerotic cardiovascular disease. Journal of the American College of Cardiology. 2024 May 21;83(20):1939-52.
21. Barkas F, Ray K. An update on inclisiran for the treatment of elevated LDL cholesterol. Expert Opinion on Pharmacotherapy. 2024 Mar 3;25(4):349-58.
22. Millhuff AC, Blankenship JC. Strategies to optimize initial P2Y12 inhibitor therapy in STEMI patients. Cardiovascular Revascularization Medicine. 2024 Sep 25.

23. De Luca G, Verburg A, Hof AV, Ten Berg J, Kereiakes DJ, Coller BS, Gibson CM. Current and Future Roles of Glycoprotein IIb–IIIa Inhibitors in Primary Angioplasty for ST-Segment Elevation Myocardial Infarction. Biomedicines. 2024 Sep 4;12(9):2023.
24. Parker WA, Storey RF. The role of platelet P2Y12 receptors in inflammation. British journal of pharmacology. 2024 Feb;181(4):515-31.
25. Hansen MK, Olesen KK, Gyldenkerne C, Thrane PG, Stødkilde-Jørgensen N, Mortensen MB, Maeng M. Eligibility for and preventive potential of semaglutide in overweight and obese patients with myocardial infarction. Journal of the American College of Cardiology. 2024 Mar 5;83(9):956-8.
26. Ahmed M, Ahsan A, Shafiq A, Maniya MT, Jain H, Iqbal J, Naveed MA, Ahmed R, Rana JS, Fudim M, Fonarow GC. Cardiovascular Efficacy and Safety of Finerenone: A Meta-Analysis of Randomized Controlled Trials. Clinical Cardiology. 2025 Feb;48(2):e70065.

Chapter 17

Recent Advances in the Management of Hypertension

Author: Dr. Pranab Das

Introduction

Hypertension, characterised by consistently elevated arterial blood pressure, is a significant global health issue and a primary contributor to cardiovascular disease, stroke, and renal failure. With over a billion individuals impacted globally, it remains a significant challenge despite public health initiatives and clinical guidelines advocating for lifestyle modifications and pharmacological interventions. A considerable proportion of individuals are either undiagnosed or inadequately managed, underscoring the disparity between treatment guidelines and actual clinical results.

Despite the availability of various antihypertensive medications, including ACE inhibitors, ARBs, calcium channel blockers, beta-blockers, and diuretics, numerous patients continue to face challenges in achieving target blood pressure levels. Resistant hypertension, along with comorbidities such as diabetes and chronic kidney disease, complicates patient management. Recent research has concentrated on innovative therapies such as renal denervation, biologics, and personalised medicine. This chapter delineates the clinical profile of hypertension, standard treatment modalities, and innovative strategies designed to enhance management and mitigate cardiovascular risk.

Historical Perspective

The comprehension and management of hypertension have shown significant evolution throughout the last century. Historically referred to as the "silent killer," hypertension remained inadequately comprehended until the mid-20th century, when research began to reveal a definitive correlation between increased blood pressure and cardiovascular disease and mortality. Initial therapeutic options were constrained and predominantly ineffectual, frequently comprising bed rest, low-sodium diets, or, in severe instances, surgical sympathectomy.

The 1950s heralded the advent of pharmacological intervention with the introduction of ganglionic blockers and reserpine, both of which exhibited significant adverse effects. The identification of thiazide diuretics in the late 1950s transformed hypertension treatment by offering efficient blood pressure lowering with improved tolerance. The 1970s and 1980s witnessed the emergence of beta-blockers, angiotensin-converting enzyme (ACE) inhibitors, and calcium channel blockers, which established themselves as fundamental classes in hypertension treatment.

Over time, pivotal clinical trials, including the Veterans Administration Cooperative Study (1967), the SHEP trial (1991), and the ALLHAT study (2002), demonstrated the effectiveness of these treatments in decreasing stroke, heart failure, and mortality, thereby reinforcing hypertension management as a fundamental aspect of cardiovascular disease prevention.

Over the past twenty years, efforts have concentrated on optimising therapy with angiotensin receptor blockers (ARBs), employing fixed-dose combination pills to enhance adherence, and the introduction of device-based interventions like renal denervation for resistant hypertension. The recent incorporation of personalised medicine, genetics, and digital health tools has advanced hypertension management, providing prospects for tailored treatment options based on individual risk profiles.

Definition

According to the 2017 American College of Cardiology/American Heart Association (ACC/AHA) recommendations, hypertension (HTN) is defined as a systolic blood pressure (SBP) of 130 mmHg or higher and/or a diastolic blood pressure (DBP) of 80 mmHg or higher. The European Society of Cardiology (ESC) and the European Society of Hypertension (ESH) are two examples of other international guidelines that may include slightly different cut-offs (e.g. ≥140/90 mmHg). The MOHFW (Ministry of Health and Family Welfare) India guidelines of hypertension outlines hypertension as BP ≥140/90 mmHg. The fundamental idea is still that persistently high blood pressure puts excessive strain on arterial systems, speeds up atherosclerosis, and greatly raises the chance of end-organ damage (heart, kidneys, brain, etc.).

Types

Hypertension can be broadly classified into two major categories:

1. **Primary (Essential) Hypertension**
   - Represents around 90–95% of all hypertensive cases.
   - No distinct cause, but rather it is multifactorial—encompassing genetic predisposition, lifestyle factors (dietary sodium, obesity, physical inactivity), and neurohormonal dysregulation.
2. **Secondary Hypertension**
   - Comprises of approximately 5–10% of hypertensive instances.
   - Caused by recognisable diseases, including hyperaldosteronism, pheochromocytoma, Cushing's syndrome, thyroid disorders (hyperthyroidism), renal artery stenosis, or obstructive sleep apnoea.
   - In addition to controlling blood pressure, treatment aims to treat the underlying cause.

Recognition of these subtypes is crucial because correcting reversible aetiologies (e.g. surgically removing a pheochromocytoma) can yield dramatic improvements in secondary hypertension. Meanwhile, essential hypertension often requires a more prolonged pharmacological approach coupled with comprehensive lifestyle modifications.

Brief Note on Conventional Medicines

Clinical practice guidelines recommend initiating antihypertensive therapy with one or more agents from the following classes, based on patient comorbidities, side-effect profiles, and the severity of hypertension. Below is a concise summary of these conventional options:

Table 1: Concise Overview of Conventional Medications Utilized in the Management of Hypertension.

Drug Class / Drug Names	Mechanism of Action	Common Dosage Forms	Usual Side Effects
Diuretics (such as potassium-sparing diuretics, loop diuretics, and thiazides)	Reduces preload or end-diastolic volume and blood volume and increase excretion of water and sodium.	Oral tablets, i.v. injection.	Electrolyte disturbances (hyponatremia, hypokalaemia), hyperuricemia, dehydration.
Beta-Blockers, such as bisoprolol and metoprolol.	Blocks beta-1 receptors of heart, thereby reducing heart rate and cardiac output and subsequent fall in BP.	Oral tablets, i.v. injection.	Bradycardia, fatigue, bronchospasm in susceptible individuals, masking of hypoglycaemia.
ACE Inhibitors, such as Ramipril and Enalapril	Reduce aldosterone secretion, lower angiotensin II formation by inhibiting the angiotensin-converting enzyme (ACE).	Oral tablets	Cough, hyperkalaemia, renal impairment, angioedema.
ARBs (e.g. Losartan, Valsartan)	Block angiotensin II type 1 receptor (AT1 receptor) and reduces effects of angiotensin II.	Oral tablets	Hyperkalaemia, renal impairment, less cough than ACE inhibitors.
Calcium Channel Blockers (e.g. Amlodipine, Diltiazem)	Inhibit L-type calcium channels in vascular smooth muscle or cardiac tissue, causing vasodilation and/ or decreased heart rate.	Oral tablets	Peripheral oedema, flushing, headache, bradycardia (non-dihydropyridines).
Alpha-1 Blockers (e.g. Prazosin)	Relax vascular smooth muscle by blocking alpha-1 adrenergic receptors.	Oral tablets	Orthostatic hypotension, dizziness, reflex tachycardia.

Lifestyle interventions including limiting salt intake, losing weight, getting more exercise, and reduced alcohol intakeremain essential adjuncts to pharmacotherapy. While many patients achieve target BP with these medications, a significant percentage either discontinue treatment due to side effects or exhibit resistant hypertension. Such challenges necessitate new approaches to optimize efficacy and tolerability.

Newer Drugs / Recent Advances

The pursuit of more effective and better-tolerated antihypertensive therapies, alongside adjunctive interventions, has led to several notable developments. These advances include novel molecules acting on previously underexplored pathways, combination therapies, and even device-based solutions. Below is a summary of promising new drugs and strategies under investigation or recently introduced in the medical management.

1. Aprocitentan

Introduction: Aprocitentan was created as a dual endothelin receptor antagonist (ETRA) to treat resistant hypertension.

Clinical Trial Phase / FDA-Approval: FDA approved in March 2024 for patients with uncontrolled hypertension.

Mechanism of Action:

1. **Endothelin Pathway Blockade:**

   Vasoconstriction and elevated blood pressure result from endothelin-1 (ET-1) binding to ETA and ETB receptors on vascular smooth muscle cells. ET-1 interacts with and stimulates ETA and ETB receptors (GPCRs) on vascular smooth muscle cells. This stimulates Gq protein of GPCR, resulting in the activation of phospholipase C (PLC). Phospholipase C hydrolyses phosphatidylinositol 4,5-bisphosphate (PIP2) to produce inositol trisphosphate (IP3) and diacylglycerol (DAG). IP3 induces the release of Ca^{2+} from the sarcoplasmic reticulum. Elevated intracellular Ca^{2+} associates with calmodulin. This initiates myosin light chain kinase (MLCK) activation. MLCK phosphorylates myosin light chains, facilitating cross-bridge formation with actin, which results in vascular smooth muscle contraction and ultimately induces vasoconstriction. DAG also activates Protein Kinase C (PKC) which sensitizes contractile proteins to calcium. Aprocitentan selectively inhibits both ETA and ETB receptors, hence obstructing endothelin-induced vasoconstriction.

2. **Vasodilation & Blood Pressure Reduction:**

   By inhibiting the endothelin receptors, blood vessels relax (vasodilation), reducing peripheral resistance. This results in a drop in blood pressure, especially in individuals with resistant hypertension.

3. **Long Half-Life for Sustained Effect:**

   Aprocitentan has a long half-life (40-45 hours), allowing once-daily dosing and sustained antihypertensive effects.

Key Pharmacokinetic Parameters: Peak plasma concentration in attained in 6–8 hours. It is well absorbed orally and exhibits high degree of binding to plasma proteins (99%), mostly to albumin. It is converted into active and inactive metabolites by CYP3A4. The plasma half-life is about 40-45 hours and is primarily excreted by faeces.

Adverse Drug Reactions: Peripheral oedema, headache, anaemia, fatigue, nasal congestion, and hepatic dysfunction.

Uses: Resistant hypertension (approved use) and pulmonary arterial hypertension (PAH) (off-label use).

Dose: 12.5 mg to 25 mg once daily (oral).

2. Baxdrostat

Introduction: Baxdrostat is a selective aldosterone synthase inhibitor designed for patients with treatment-resistant hypertension.

Clinical Trial Phase/FDA-Approval: Currently undergoing Phase III clinical trials for resistant hypertension.

Mechanism of Action:

1. **Inhibition of Aldosterone Synthase (CYP11B2)**
   - Baxdrostat specifically inhibits aldosterone synthase (CYP11B2), an enzyme responsible for converting deoxycorticosterone to aldosterone in the adrenal cortex.
   - This prevents aldosterone synthesis, reducing its effects on sodium and water retention, which are key factors in hypertension.
2. **Selective Targeting of CYP11B2 (Minimal Effect on Cortisol)**
   - Aldosterone synthase (CYP11B2) is structurally similar to 11β-hydroxylase (CYP11B1), the enzyme that produces cortisol.

- Unlike older inhibitors, Baxdrostat selectively inhibits CYP11B2 while sparing CYP11B1, thereby avoiding cortisol deficiency and associated risks (e.g. adrenal insufficiency).

3. **Reduction in Sodium Retention and Vascular Resistance**
   - Lower aldosterone levels diminish the kidneys' reabsorption of salt, which lowers blood pressure and fluid retention.
   - Additionally, aldosterone promotes vascular inflammation and fibrosis, which contributes to arterial stiffness and hypertension. By blocking aldosterone synthesis, Baxdrostat lowers blood pressure and enhances vascular function.

Key Pharmacokinetic Parameters: High oral bioavailability. Almost 94% drug is primarily bound to albumin. It is metabolised by the CYP3A4 enzyme in the liver. It's major metabolite is an inactive hydroxylated derivative. Faecal elimination (85%), with minor renal excretion (15%).

Adverse Drug Reactions: Headache, nausea, fatigue, hyperkalaemia, hypotension and mild adrenal insufficiency.

Uses: Resistant hypertension and primary aldosteronism (both under investigation).

Dose: 2 mg to 5 mg once daily (oral) (clinical trial dose).

3. ARNI (Sacubitril/Valsartan)

Introduction: ARNI (Angiotensin Receptor-Neprilysin Inhibitor) is a combination drug of sacubitril and valsartan that lowers blood pressure and cardiovascular risk.

Clinical Trial Phase / FDA-Approval: FDA approved for hypertension and heart failure.

Mechanism of Action:

1. **Neprilysin Inhibition**
   - Neprilysin is an endopeptidase that degrades vasoactive peptides, including:
     1. Atrial Natriuretic Peptide (ANP).
     2. B-type Natriuretic Peptide (BNP).
     3. C-type Natriuretic Peptide (CNP).
     4. Bradykinin, Adrenomedullin, and Substance P.
   - Sacubitril blocks neprilysin, increasing the certain natriuretic peptides' amount, which promotes:
     - i. Vasodilation.
     - ii. Diuresis and natriuresis (increased urine and sodium excretion).
     - iii. Reduced cardiac preload and afterload.
2. **Increased Natriuretic Peptide Activity**
   - Higher ANP, BNP, and CNP levels enhance vasodilation and lower blood pressure.
   - Bradykinin levels also increase, which contributes to vasodilation and reduced inflammation.
3. **Reduces Cardiac Remodelling and Fibrosis**
   - Elevated BNP and ANP decrease fibrosis and hypertrophy, improving heart function.
   - Adrenomedullin helps to reduce vascular resistance and protects endothelial function.
4. **Complementary Role of Valsartan (ARNI Combination)**
   - Valsartan blocks angiotensin II type-1 receptors (AT1R), reducing vasoconstriction and sodium retention.

- This prevents angiotensin II-mediated activation of neprilysin, vasoconstriction and elevation of BP, enhancing sacubitril's effects.

5. **Results in Net Hemodynamic Benefits**
   - Reduced preload and afterload - Lower cardiac workload.
   - Decreased systemic vascular resistance (SVR) - Lower BP.
   - Increased diuresis & natriuresis - Reduced congestion in heart failure patients.

Key Pharmacokinetic Parameters: Well absorbed orally. Oral bioavailability is around 70-80%. It is almost 94% primarily bound to albumin. It is metabolised by the CYP3A4 enzyme within the liver. The plasma half-life is 8–12 hours.

Adverse Drug Reactions: Headache, nausea, hypokalaemia, hypotension, and fatigue.

Uses: Resistant heart failure with reduced ejection fraction (HFrEF) and hypertension – currently under Phase III trial.

Dose: 100 mg twice daily (sacubitril 49 mg/valsartan 51 mg).

4. Zilebesiran

Introduction: Zilebesiran is an RNA interference (RNAi) therapy targeting angiotensinogen, reducing blood pressure for up to six months per injection.

Clinical Trial Phase / FDA-Approval: Phase II trials ongoing for hypertension.

Mechanism of Action:

1. **RNA Interference (RNAi) on AGT mRNA**
   - Zilebisiran selectively binds to AGT mRNA in the liver.
   - This triggers RNA-induced silencing complex (RISC), leading to AGT mRNA degradation.
2. **Reduction in Angiotensinogen Levels**
   - Lower AGT levels leads to decreased angiotensin I (Ang I) and angiotensin II (Ang II) production.
   - Ang II is a potent vasoconstrictor, so reducing it leads to vasodilation and lowers blood pressure.
3. **Long-Lasting Antihypertensive Effect**
   - A single dose can suppress AGT for months, offering an advantage over daily antihypertensive pills.

Key Pharmacokinetic Parameters: Administration occurs through subcutaneous (s.c.) injection. The Tmax duration ranges from 4 to 8 hours. Zilebisiran exhibits high bioavailability through selective hepatic uptake facilitated by GalNAc-mediated liver targeting, resulting in its primary accumulation in hepatocytes. It undergoes intracellular metabolism in hepatocytes via the RNA-induced silencing complex (RISC). Drug-drug interactions are minimised due to the absence of involvement of cytochrome P450 (CYP) enzymes. The plasma half-life ranges from 4 to 8 weeks, with metabolites being excreted via urine and bile.

Adverse Drug Reactions: Injection site reactions (pain, redness, swelling), fatigue, hypotension, hyperkalaemia, hypotension, and potential hepatotoxicity.

Uses: Hypertension (long-term control) (under investigation).

Dose: 300 mg to 600 mg subcutaneously every 6 months (investigational dose).

5. Firibastat

Introduction: Firibastat is a brain-penetrant aminopeptidase A inhibitor (BAPAI), reducing neurogenic hypertension.

Clinical Trial Phase / FDA-Approval: Currently in Phase II trials for hypertension.

Mechanism of Action:

A. **Prodrug Activation & Blood-Brain Barrier (BBB) Penetration**
   - Firibastat is a prodrug that crosses the blood-brain barrier (BBB).
   - Once inside the brain, it is metabolized by central enzymes into EC33, its active form.

B. **Inhibition of Brain Aminopeptidase A (APA)**
   - In the brain, an enzyme called aminopeptidase A (APA) changes angiotensin II (Ang II) into Ang III.
   - Ang III has a strong vasopressor action by stimulating sympathetic activation, vasoconstriction, and sodium retention.
   - Firibastat blocks APA, reducing Ang III formation, which results in:
     I. Reduced sympathetic tone - Decreased vasoconstriction.
     II. Lowered aldosterone levels - Increased sodium excretion (natriuresis).

C. **Effects on Blood Pressure & Cardiovascular Function**
   - Decreasing Ang III leads to:
     I. Vasodilation - Lower systemic vascular resistance (SVR).
     II. Increased diuresis - Decreased blood volume & preload.
     III. Reduced cardiac workload - Protection against heart failure progression.

Key Pharmacokinetic Parameters: It has high oral bioavailability. Tmax is around 1-2 hours post administration. 90% bound to plasma protein albumin. Firibastat is converted to EC33 by plasma and brain esterases. Not significantly affected by cytochrome P450 (CYP) enzymes, reducing drug-drug interactions and is excreted mainly in urine.

Adverse Drug Reactions: Headache, fatigue, nausea, hypotension, and mild alteration of cognitive function.

Uses: Resistant hypertension (under investigation).

Dose: 250 mg twice daily (oral) (clinical trial dosing).

6. Esaxerenone

Introduction: Esaxerenone is a nonsteroidal mineralocorticoid receptor antagonist (MRA) used for hypertension.

Clinical Trial Phase / FDA-Approval: Approved in Japan for hypertension and diabetic kidney disease and also currently in Phase III trials in other countries.

Mechanism of Action:

A. **Selective Mineralocorticoid Receptor Antagonism (MRA)**
   - Aldosterone, a key component of BP regulation, binds to MRs in the kidney, heart, and arteries as a component of the renin-angiotensin-aldosterone system (RAAS).

- Excess aldosterone leads to:
  I. Hypertension (via sodium retention and volume expansion).
  II. Kidney damage (via fibrosis and inflammation).
  III. Cardiac remodelling (by causing fibroblast proliferation, neutrophil & macrophage infiltration leading to hypertrophy and fibrosis).
- Esaxerenone competes with aldosterone at the MR binding site and thereby blocking this receptor, preventing these harmful effects.

B. Cardiovascular & Renal Protection

1. Reduces Sodium Retention & Lowers Blood Pressure

- Blocks MR activation in kidney tubules - Increases sodium excretion (natriuresis) - Lowers blood pressure.

2. Prevents Fibrosis & Inflammation

- Inhibits aldosterone-driven pro-inflammatory & pro-fibrotic gene expression.
- Reduces TGF-β (fibrosis mediator) & NF-κB (inflammation mediator).

3. Protects Heart & Blood Vessels

- Prevents cardiac hypertrophy & vascular stiffness caused by aldosterone excess.
- Improves endothelial function & reduces oxidative stress.

Key Pharmacokinetic Parameters: It shows high (90%) oral bioavailability. Tmax is 1-3 hours. Food barely affects its absorption. 90% of the drug are bonded to plasma proteins. It is primarily metabolised by CYP3A4 enzyme and with little effect on CYP2C19 and CYP2D6 and mainly excreted by faeces.

Adverse Drug Reactions: Hyperkalaemia, hypotension, and renal impairment.

Uses: Primary hypertension and diabetic nephropathy (under investigation).

Dose: 1.25 mg to 2.5 mg once daily (oral).

7. Cicletanine

Introduction: Cicletanine is a vasodilatory and natriuretic drug under investigation for resistant hypertension.

Clinical Trial Phase / FDA-Approval: Undergoing Phase II trial for hypertension.

Mechanism of Action:

A. Phosphodiesterase-9 (PDE9) Inhibition

- Cicletanine selectively inhibits PDE9, an enzyme that degrades cyclic guanosine monophosphate (cGMP).
- Increased cGMP levels lead to:
  i. Smooth muscle relaxation - Vasodilation - Blood pressure reduction.
  ii. Reduced vascular stiffness and cardiac workload.
  iii. Enhanced nitric oxide (NO)-mediated enhancement of vascular function.

B. Natriuretic and Diuretic Effects

- Cicletanine enhances renal sodium excretion (natriuresis), contributing to blood pressure reduction.
- This occurs via renal tubular effects that differ from conventional diuretics.

C. **Endothelial & Anti-Inflammatory Effects**
   - Reduces oxidative stress and inflammation, improving endothelial function.
   - Protects against vascular remodelling and fibrosis.

D. **Pulmonary Vasodilation (Potential Use in Pulmonary Hypertension)**
   - PDE9 inhibition reduces pulmonary artery pressure, making it a potential treatment for pulmonary hypertension (PH).

Key Pharmacokinetic Parameters: It shows high oral bioavailability. It is 90% bound to plasma protein albumin. Hepatic metabolism occurs via cytochrome P450 (CYP3A4, CYP2C9) enzymes. Active and inactive metabolites contribute to its sustained effects and is primarily excreted in urine.

Adverse Drug Reactions: Headache, dizziness, nausea, hypotension, and QT prolongation.

Uses: Resistant hypertension (under investigation).

Dose: 50 mg to 100 mg once daily (oral) (trial dosing).

8. Other major developments in the treatment of hypertension:

Table 2: Additional significant advancements in hypertension management.

Drug / Strategy	Mechanism of Action	Clinical Trial Phase / Status	Adverse Reactions	Distinctive / Salient Features
Selective Natriuretic Peptide Receptor Agonists (e.g. Ularitide)	Induces natriuresis, diuresis, and vasodilation via natriuretic peptide pathways.	Phase II/III in acute heart failure and hypertension.	Hypotension, possible renal function fluctuations.	Potential to reduce volume overload quickly; further data needed for long-term BP control.
Mineralocorticoid Receptor Antagonist-Like Drugs (Next-gen eplerenone analogues)	More selective blockade of the mineralocorticoid receptor to prevent sodium retention and cardiovascular fibrosis.	Early-stage clinical trials.	Hyperkalaemia, some sexual hormone-related side effects.	Improved receptor selectivity promises fewer off-target effects compared to spironolactone.
Renal Denervation	Ablation of sympathetic nerves in the renal artery to reduce sympathetic overdrive contributing to hypertension.	Trials ongoing in the US.	Procedure-related vascular complications, limited success in some trials.	Minimally invasive; potential for durable BP reduction without daily medications in select populations.
Baroreflex Activation Therapy	Implantable gadget that activates carotid baroreceptors sinus, reducing sympathetic tone and BP.	Approved in some regions for resistant hypertension; more trials ongoing.	Device-related complications, infection risk, possible nerve damage.	Adjunct for severely resistant patients; can be combined with pharmacotherapy to enhance BP control.
Combination Pills / Polypills (e.g. triple combination including ARB + CCB + diuretic)	Improves patient adherence, provides multi-modal BP control in a single pill.	Widely implemented; continuous outcome data.	Similar to constituent drugs (e.g. hypotension, electrolyte issues).	Simplifies dosing schedules, enhances compliance, and optimizes BP-lowering effect.

Key Emerging Concepts

1. **Aldosterone and Beyond:** Traditionally, mineralocorticoid receptor antagonists (e.g. spironolactone) have been used in resistant hypertension, but side effects, such as hyperkalaemia and gynecomastia, limit their use. Emerging agents like Baxdrostat (an aldosterone synthase inhibitor) aim to achieve more precise blockade of aldosterone production, potentially reducing volume overload and improving BP control without causing significant off-target effects.

2. **Endothelin Pathway:** Endothelin-1 is a potent vasoconstrictor implicated in certain forms of resistant and salt-sensitive hypertension. Aprocitentan, an endothelin receptor antagonist, has shown promise in lowering BP in individuals inadequately controlled on standard therapies. Though side effects such as oedema and headache may limit its widespread adoption, it represents a new avenue for those with difficult-to-treat hypertension.

3. **Renal Denervation and Device-Based Therapies:** The overactivation of the sympathetic nerve system substantially contributes to hypertension pathogenesis. Renal denervation, once met with skepticism after initial trials failed to demonstrate robust efficacy, is experiencing renewed interest with improved procedural techniques and patient selection criteria. Baroreflex activation therapy is another device-based option, particularly for those with resistant hypertension, though it requires surgical implantation and long-term follow-up for device maintenance.

4. **Combination Strategies:** Recognizing that many patients need more than one antihypertensive agent to achieve target BP, combination pills simplify treatment regimens, thereby enhancing adherence. Recent guidelines endorse using dual or even triple fixed-dose combinations early in treatment, especially among those suffering from stage 2 hypertension or significantly elevated baseline BP. The emergence of polypills that incorporate antihypertensive, antiplatelet, and lipid-lowering agents seeks to address not only hypertension but broader cardiovascular risk in one regimen.

5. **Personalized and Precision Medicine:** Advances in genomics, proteomics, and digital health have begun to inform personalized approaches to hypertension management. Ongoing research investigates genetic polymorphisms (e.g. in renin-angiotensin system genes), biomarkers (e.g. plasma renin activity), and wearable sensors (e.g. continuous BP monitors) to tailor therapy selection, dosage, and monitoring. Though widespread implementation remains in early stages, the aim is to optimize therapeutic outcomes and minimize side effects by choosing the appropriate medication for the patient at the appropriate time.

Conclusion

Management of hypertension has advanced considerably, with established therapies such as ACE inhibitors, ARBs, beta-blockers, diuretics, and calcium channel blockers demonstrating efficacy in reducing cardiovascular risk. Nonetheless, numerous patients continue to struggle with achieving optimal control, highlighting the necessity for innovative strategies. Novel pharmacologic targets, including neprilysin and aldosterone synthase inhibitors, alongside device-based interventions such as renal denervation, present promising alternatives for the management of resistant hypertension. Innovations such as fixed-dose combination pills and personalised medicine, informed by genetic insights and advanced monitoring, seek to improve adherence and treatment accuracy. As care transitions to patient-centered approaches, these developments may significantly enhance blood pressure management and alleviate the global impact of hypertension-related conditions.

References

1. Arvanitis LV, Mewaldt C, Krawisz A, Secemsky EA. Approach to Resistant Hypertension: A Review of Recent Pharmacological Advances. Current Treatment Options in Cardiovascular Medicine. 2025 Dec;27(1):1-0.

2. Lim H, Agustian H, Febriana V, Supit AI. Sacubitril/Valsartan Role in Patients with Resistant Hypertension: A Systematic Review. Hellenic Journal of Cardiology. 2025 Jan 27.
3. Guthi VR, Kumar DS, Kumar S, Kondagunta N, Raj S, Goel S, Ojah P. Hypertension treatment cascade among men and women of reproductive age group in India: analysis of National Family Health Survey-5 (2019–2021). The Lancet Regional Health-Southeast Asia. 2024 Apr 1;23.
4. McLaughlin V, Farber HW, Highland KB, Hemnes AR, Chakinala MM, Chin KM, Han M, Cho M, Tobore T, Rahman M, Kim NH. Disease characteristics, treatments, and outcomes of patients with pulmonary arterial hypertension treated with selexipag in real-world settings from the SPHERE registry (SelexiPag: tHeusErsdRugrEgistry). The Journal of Heart and Lung Transplantation. 2024 Feb 1;43(2):272-83.
5. Williams B, Mancia G, Spiering W, AgabitiRosei E, Azizi M, Burnier M, Clement DL, Coca A, De Simone G, Dominiczak A, Kahan T. 2018 ESC/ESH Guidelines for the management of arterial hypertension: The Task Force for the management of arterial hypertension of the European Society of Cardiology (ESC) and the European Society of Hypertension (ESH). European heart journal. 2018 Sep 1;39(33):3021-104.
6. Calhoun DA, Jones D, Textor S, Goff DC, Murphy TP, Toto RD, White A, Cushman WC, White W, Sica D, Ferdinand K. Resistant hypertension: diagnosis, evaluation, and treatment: a scientific statement from the American Heart Association Professional Education Committee of the Council for High Blood Pressure Research. Hypertension. 2008 Jun 1;51(6):1403-19.
7. Whelton PK, Carey RM, Aronow WS, Casey DE, Collins KJ, Dennison Himmelfarb C. Guideline for high blood pressure in adults-American College of Cardiology. J Am Coll Cardiol. 2018;71:e127-248.
8. Padmanabhan S, Joe B. Towards precision medicine for hypertension: a review of genomic, epigenomic, and microbiomic effects on blood pressure in experimental rat models and humans. Physiological reviews. 2017 Oct 1;97(4):1469-528.
9. Appel LJ, Brands MW, Daniels SR, Karanja N, Elmer PJ, Sacks FM. Dietary approaches to prevent and treat hypertension: a scientific statement from the American Heart Association. Hypertension. 2006 Feb 1;47(2):296-308.
10. Preeti, Sambhakar S, Malik R, Bhatia S, Al-Harrasi A, Saharan R, et al. Lipid horizons: recent advances and future prospects in LBDDS for oral administration of antihypertensive agents. Int J Hypertens. 2024;2024:2430147.
11. Azizi M, Sapoval M, Gosse P, Monge M, Bobrie G, Delsart P, Midulla M, Mounier-Véhier C, Courand PY, Lantelme P, Denolle T. Optimum and stepped care standardised antihypertensive treatment with or without renal denervation for resistant hypertension (DENERHTN): a multicentre, open-label, randomised controlled trial. The Lancet. 2015 May 16;385(9981):1957-65.
12. Seravalle G, Dell'Oro R, Grassi G. Baroreflex activation therapy systems: current status and future prospects. Expert Review of Medical Devices. 2019 Dec 2;16(12):1025-33.
13. Milluzzo RP, Franchina GA, Capodanno D, Angiolillo DJ. Selatogrel, a novel P2Y12 inhibitor: a review of the pharmacology and clinical development. Expert Opinion on Investigational Drugs. 2020 Jun 2;29(6):537-46.
14. Kuzmich N, Andresyuk E, Porozov Y, Tarasov V, Samsonov M, Preferanskaya N, Veselov V, Alyautdin R. PCSK9 as a Target for Development of a New Generation of Hypolipidemic Drugs. Molecules. 2022 Jan 10;27(2):434.
15. Dey S, Frishman WH, Aronow WS. Baxdrostat: an aldosterone synthase inhibitor for the treatment of systemic hypertension. Cardiology in Review. 2025 May 1;33(3):243-5.
16. Lin L, Bian W, Luo Q, Wang L, Liu N, Yang M, Cen J, Cai K, Hua J, Gu H, Qi H. Sacubitril-Valsartan Lowers Blood Pressure in Patients on Dialysis-A Randomized Controlled Multicenter Study. Kidney Diseases. 2025.
17. Evbayekha E, Idowu AB, LaRue S. Sacubitril/Valsartan vs ACE Inhibitors or ARBs: A Systematic Review and Meta-Analysis of Randomized Trials. JACC: Advances. 2025 Mar 1;4(3):101598.
18. Chopra VK, Chopra VK. Newer Antihypertensive Drugs. MEDICAL JOURNAL March 2025.:40.
19. Thomas S. Aprocitentan (TRYVIO). Amrita Journal of Medicine. 2024 Apr 1;20(2):83-5.
20. Muras MS, Lorenc T, Marcinkowski K, Michalik M, Mikszta N, Mikszta J, Marcinkowska J. The New Drugs in the Treatment of Hypertension and Resistant Hypertension: A Review of Therapies. Quality in Sport. 2025 Apr 5;40:59480.
21. NA N. Angiotensin Receptor-Neprilysin Inhibitor (ARNI). MEDICAL JOURNAL March 2025.:41.
22. Schinzari F, Montenero R, Cardillo C, Tesauro M. Emerging Pharmacological Approaches for the Treatment of Arterial Hypertension. Biomedicines. 2025 Mar 25;13(4):790.
23. Yamamoto E, Usuku H, Sueta D, Suzuki S, Nakamura T, Matsui K, Matsushita K, Iwasaki T, Sakaino N, Sakanashi T, Hirayama K. Efficacy and safety of esaxerenone in hypertensive patients with left ventricular hypertrophy (ESES-LVH) study: a multicenter, open-label, prospective, interventional study. Advances in Therapy. 2024 Mar;41(3):1284-303.
24. Butler HM, McCrorey MK, Palygina L, Lacey R, Van Beusecum JP. Salt-sensitive hypertension: role of endothelial and vascular dysfunction and sex. Frontiers in Pharmacology. 2025 Mar 12;16:1565962.
25. Ilatovskaya DV, Behr A, Staruschenko A, Hall G, Palygin O. Mechanistic insights into redox damage of the podocyte in hypertension. Hypertension. 2025 Jan;82(1):14-25.

Chapter 18

Recent Advances in the Management of Heart Failure

Author: Dr. Pranab Das

Introduction

Heart failure (HF) is a complex clinical condition that arises when the heart's ability to pump an adequate volume of blood to satisfy the body's metabolic requirements is impaired. Despite ongoing advancements in pharmacological and device-based therapies, heart failure remains a major contributor to morbidity, mortality, and healthcare costs globally. Current estimates indicate that more than 64 million individuals are impacted worldwide, with projections anticipating an increase corresponding to ageing demographics and the growing prevalence of risk factors such as diabetes, hypertension, and ischaemic heart disease.

Recent advancements in specific pharmacological agents, such as sodium-glucose cotransporter-2 (SGLT2) inhibitors and angiotensin receptor-neprilysin inhibitors (ARNIs), have redefined the standard-of-care treatment for several patients. Furthermore, innovative device therapeutics and regenerative medicine strategies have potential for individuals with refractory or terminal conditions. This chapter offers a comprehensive overview of heart failure definitions and classifications, evaluates traditional therapy, and examines recent advancements that are set to revolutionise heart failure management.

Historical Perspective

The management of heart failure (HF) has significantly evolved over the past century, transitioning from basic supportive care to well-defined, evidence-based treatment approaches. During the early 20th century, management of heart failure predominantly involved bed rest, fluid restriction, and the administration of digitalis and diuretics, which offered limited symptomatic relief without impacting disease progression. The introduction of loop diuretics in the 1960s markedly enhanced fluid management; however, the underlying pathophysiology of heart failure was not well comprehended.

The contemporary phase of heart failure therapy commenced in the 1980s, marked by the introduction of neurohormonal modulation as a therapeutic focus. Significant clinical trials, including CONSENSUS (1987) and SOLVD (1991), established that angiotensin-converting enzyme (ACE) inhibitors enhanced symptoms and decreased mortality in patients with reduced ejection fraction (HFrEF). The introduction of beta-blockers, supported by trials such as MERIT-HF and COPERNICUS, solidified neurohormonal blockade as a fundamental component of therapy.

During the late 1990s and early 2000s, mineralocorticoid receptor antagonists (MRAs) such as spironolactone and eplerenone were introduced, demonstrating a reduction in mortality in trials such as RALES and EMPHASIS-HF. These advancements established the basis for guideline-directed medical therapy (GDMT). The recent approval of angiotensin receptor–neprilysin inhibitors (ARNIs), specifically sacubitril/valsartan, marked a significant advancement, showing superiority over enalapril in the PARADIGM-HF trial.

Recent advancements encompass sodium-glucose co-transporter 2 (SGLT2) inhibitors, originally designed for diabetes, which have demonstrated significant advantages in both HFrEF and HFpEF populations, as evidenced by trials such as DAPA-HF and EMPEROR-Preserved. Innovations in device therapy, including implantable cardioverter defibrillators (ICDs), cardiac resynchronisation therapy (CRT), and advanced left ventricular assist devices (LVADs), have transformed the management of advanced heart failure. The historical development of heart failure treatment demonstrates a progression from symptom management to disease modification, and currently, to personalised, mechanism-based strategies.

Definition

A structural or functional cardiac abnormality that affects the ventricle's filling or ejection capability is described as heart failure (HF), a clinical syndrome characterised by typical symptoms (e.g. fatigue, dyspnoea) and signs (e.g. elevated jugular venous pressure, oedema, pulmonary crackles. A complicated interaction between neurohormonal stimulation, maladaptive remodelling, and increasing haemodynamic deterioration is frequently present in the pathogenesis of HF. A detailed history, physical examination, echocardiogram, and evaluation of biomarkers—most notably B-type natriuretic peptide, or BNP, or its precursor NT-proBNP—are typically used in the diagnosis process.

Types of Heart Failure

Ejection fraction (EF), a crucial indicator that shows the proportion of blood expelled from the ventricle during systole, can be used to categorize heart failure. Although EF is an imperfect measure, it is widely used to classify HF and guide therapeutic decisions.

1. **Heart Failure with Reduced Ejection Fraction (HFrEF)**
   - Another name for it is systolic HF, typically defined by an EF ≤40%.
   - Characterized by diminished contractility, significant left ventricular (LV) dilation, and neurohormonal dysregulation.
   - Many clinical trials have focused on HFrEF, leading to evidence-based therapies that confer mortality benefits.
2. **HFpEF, or Heart Failure with Preserved Ejection Fraction**
   - Defined by an EF ≥50%.
   - Often presents having diastolic dysfunction, in which despite having nearly normal systolic function, increased filling pressures are caused by poor ventricular relaxation or filling.
   - Common in older persons, frequently accompanied by concomitant conditions, including hypertension, obesity, and diabetes. Effective treatment options have been more elusive, although recent trials offer some optimism.
3. **Mildly Reduced Ejection Fraction Heart Failure (HFmrEF)**
   - Typically defined by an EF between 41% and 49%.
   - Represents an intermediate phenotype that may share characteristics with both HFrEF and HFpEF.
   - Growing recognition of HFmrEF has led to targeted research to clarify optimal management strategies.

While these EF-based categories guide therapy, understanding that HF is clinically diverse is crucial, because varying aetiologies (ischemic, non-ischaemic), comorbidity profiles, and disease trajectories requires individualized management.

Brief Note on Conventional Medicines

For decades, the cornerstone of HF treatment (particularly HFrEF) has consisted of therapies aimed at antagonizing maladaptive neurohormonal pathways and preventing adverse cardiac remodelling. Below is a concise summary of widely used conventional agents:

Table 1: Concise overview of conventional medications in the management of Heart Failure.

Drug Class & Drug Name	Mechanism of Action	Common Dosage Forms	Usual Side Effects
ACE (Angiotensin Converting Enzyme) Inhibitors (e.g. Enalapril, Lisinopril)	Block conversion of angiotensin I to angiotensin II, thus reducing vasoconstriction, increase in peripheral resistance, afterload, aldosterone release, and adverse cardiac remodelling.	Oral tablets	Cough, hyperkalaemia, renal impairment, angioedema.
Angiotensin Receptor Blockers (ARBs) (e.g. Losartan, Valsartan)	Block angiotensin II type 1 receptor (AT1R), mitigating vasoconstriction and aldosterone release.	Oral tablets	Hyperkalaemia, renal impairment, less cough than ACE inhibitors.
Beta-Blockers (e.g. Carvedilol, Bisoprolol, Metoprolol succinate)	Inhibits β-adrenergic receptors, reducing sympathetic overdrive, heart rate, and myocardial oxygen demand.	Oral tablets, i.v. injection	Bradycardia, hypotension, fatigue, bronchospasm in susceptible individuals.
Mineralocorticoid Receptor Antagonists (e.g. Spironolactone, Eplerenone)	Block aldosterone's effects on sodium retention and cardiac/vascular fibrosis.	Oral tablets	Hyperkalaemia, gynecomastia (spironolactone).
Diuretics (e.g. Loop diuretics like Furosemide, Bumetanide)	Reduce fluid overload and preload by increasing sodium/water excretion.	Oral tablets, i.v. injection	Electrolyte imbalances, hypotension, dehydration, ototoxicity (especially high-dose Furosemide).
Vasodilators (Hydralazine + Isosorbide Dinitrate)	Vasodilators that reduce afterload (hydralazine) and preload (nitrates). Often used in patients with HFrEF or those intolerant to ACEI/ARB.	Oral tablets	Headache, hypotension, reflex tachycardia, drug-induced lupus (hydralazine).

These therapies have collectively improved survival rates and quality of life. Nonetheless, many patients remain at risk for disease progression, recurrent hospitalizations, and end-organ complications, indicating a need for newer therapies addressing additional pathophysiological mechanisms.

Newer Drugs / Recent Advances

Recent years have seen a surge of novel therapeutic agents and strategies that build upon and expand beyond standard neurohormonal blockade. The information laid below provides an overview of several notable treatments that have reshaped or may reshape the HF management landscape.

1. Empaglifozin

Introduction: Empagliflozin, initially developed for the treatment of type 2 diabetes mellitus (T2DM), has demonstrated potential in recent studies for reducing hospitalisations due to heart failure and cardiovascular events as a sodium-glucose cotransporter-2 (SGLT2) inhibitor.

Clinical Trial Phase / FDA-Approval: FDA approved (2021) for HFrEF and HFpEF based on the EMPEROR-Reduced and EMPEROR-Preserved trials.

Mechanism of Action:

1. **Primary Mechanism: SGLT2 Inhibition**

   Empagliflozin exerts its primary action in the kidneys by specifically blocking the proximal renal tubules' SGLT2 protein. Approximately 90% of the filtered glucose is reabsorbed by SGLT2 under normal physiological circumstances. By inhibiting this transporter, empagliflozin promotes glucosuria, leading to a reduction in blood glucose levels without relying on insulin secretion. This insulin-independent system, which makes it especially advantageous for patients with insulin resistance or β-cell dysfunction. By inhibiting the same transported it also reduces sodium reabsorption leading to natriuresis - decrease sodium and water in plasma - decrease blood volume and blood pressure - decrease end-diastolic volume - decrease in preload.

2. **Secondary Mechanisms**

   Besides glucose-lowering effects, empagliflozin has several pleiotropic benefits:

   a. **Cardiovascular Protection**

   Empagliflozin has been demonstrated to lower heart failure hospitalisation rates and cardiovascular death. This occurs via:

   - Diuresis and natriuresis: By inhibiting sodium and glucose reabsorption, empagliflozin increases urinary sodium excretion, leading to a mild diuretic effect that reduces blood volume and preload on the heart.
   - Prevention of cardiac fibrosis and remodelling: It inhibits the NF-κB and HIF-1α pathways, reducing oxidative stress and inflammation, which aid in preventing atrial fibrillation and myocardial fibrosis.

   b. **Renal Protection**

   Empagliflozin reduces chronic kidney disease (CKD) development by lowering glomerular hyperfiltration. It decreases intraglomerular pressure, thereby slowing down nephron loss also by downregulating pro-inflammatory cytokines, empagliflozin helps to protect renal function.

   c. **Metabolic Benefits**

   - Weight loss: Due to glucosuria and calorie excretion, patients on empagliflozin experience mild weight reduction.
   - Improved lipid profile: It indirectly reduces triglycerides and increases HDL cholesterol, contributing to better cardiovascular health.

Key Pharmacokinetic Parameters: High oral bioavailability (75%), food intake does not significantly affects absorption, plasma protein binding is almost 86%, mainly bound to albumin, hepatic metabolism is via glucuronidation (UGT1A9 and UGT2B7) and is excreted via urine. Plasma half-life is 12 hours.

Adverse Drug Reactions: Urinary tract infections, polyuria, dehydration, mild hypoglycaemia, hypotension, acute kidney injury, fracture risk and diabetic ketoacidosis (rare).

Uses: Heart failure (HFrEF and HFpEF) and type 2 diabetes mellitus.

Dose: 10 mg once daily (oral).

2. Vericiguat

Introduction: Vericiguat is a stimulant of soluble guanylate cyclase (sGC), improving vascular function and reducing heart failure progression.

Clinical Trial Phase / FDA-Approval: FDA approved for HFrEF based on the VICTORIA trial.

Mechanism of Action: Vericiguat directly stimulates soluble guanylate cyclase (sGC), both independently and in synergy with nitric oxide (NO). The key steps in its mechanism are:

1. **sGC Activation:**
   - Vericiguat binds directly to sGC, leading to its activation even in the presence of reduced NO levels.
   - This compensates for endothelial dysfunction, which is common in heart failure and cardiovascular diseases.
2. **cGMP Production:**
   - Once activated, sGCcatalyzes the conversion of GTP to cGMP, a second messenger involved in vasodilation and myocardial relaxation.
   - Increased intracellular cGMP levels activated protein kinase G (PKG).
3. **Downstream Effects:**

   Activation of protein kinase G (PKG) causes reduction in intracellular calcium and activates myosin light chain phosphatase (MLCP), which causes:
   - Vascular smooth muscle relaxation - reduces vascular resistance (vasodilation) - Improves blood flow and reduces afterload.
   - Inhibits cardiac fibrosis - Prevents heart failure progression.
   - Improves endothelial function - Enhances nitric oxide availability.

Additional Effects of Vericiguat

Beyond its primary role in enhancing cGMP signalling, vericiguat exerts pleiotropic cardiovascular benefits:

a. Myocardial Function Improvement

- By reducing left ventricular hypertrophy and fibrosis, vericiguat improves cardiac contractility and prevents worsening of heart failure.

b. Vasodilation and Blood Pressure Regulation

- Vericiguat enhances vasodilation, thereby reducing systemic vascular resistance leading to a mild reduction in BP.
- Unlike nitrates, it does not lead to tachyphylaxis (loss of effectiveness over time).

c. Reno-protective Effects

- Studies indicate that vericiguat may reduce renal arterial resistance and enhance kidney perfusion, providing additional benefits in individuals suffering from chronic renal disease and heart failure.

Key Pharmacokinetic Parameters: It is orally administered with a peak plasma concentration (Tmax) of 4 hours. Bioavailability is enhanced with food intake. Exhibits 98% plasma protein binding. It is metabolised in liver by UGT1A9 and UGT1A1-mediated glucuronidation. Plasma half-life is 20 hours, mainly excreted by faeces.

Adverse Drug Reactions: Hypotension, syncope, anaemia, headache, dizziness, fatigue, and teratogenicity.

Uses: HFrEF with high risk of hospitalization.

Dose: 2.5 - 5 mg once daily.

3. Omecamtiv Mecarbil

Introduction: Omecamtiv Mecarbil, a specific cardiac myosin activator, is currently undergoing trail evaluation for treatment of heart failure with systolic dysfunction.

Clinical Trial Phase/FDA-Approval: Phase III clinical trials (GALACTIC-HF study completed, METEORIC-HF ongoing).

Mechanism of Action: Omecamtiv mecarbil (OM) attaches itself specifically to the cardiac β-myosin catalytic domain and improves cardiac function, leading to:

1. **Increased Actin-Myosin Cross-Bridge Formation**
   - Omecamtiv mecarbil (OM) stabilizes myosin in a strong actin-bound state, increasing the proportion of myosin heads engaged in excitation-contraction coupling.
2. **Prolonged Systolic Ejection Time (SET)**
   - Omecamtiv mecarbil (OM) delays myosin detachment from actin, which prolongs the force-generating phase of the cardiac cycle, leading to stronger and more efficient contractions.
3. **Increased Stroke Volume Without Increasing Oxygen Demand**
   - Unlike β-adrenergic agonists (e.g. dobutamine), Omecamtiv mecarbil does not increase intracellular calcium or cyclic AMP (cAMP), thus avoiding increased oxygen consumption and arrhythmogenic effects.
4. **Additional Effects of Omecamtiv Mecarbil**
   a. **Improvement in Cardiac Output**
      - Omecamtiv mecarbil (OM) enhances left ventricular systolic function by raising cardiac output and stroke volume in heart failure patients.
      - Unlike other inotropes, OM doesn't raise blood pressure or heart rate, making it a safer option for long-term heart failure treatment.

Key Pharmacokinetic Parameters: Oral bioavailability increases with food. Plasma protein binding is 93%. It is metabolized in liver by CYP3A4 and CYP2D6 enzymes. Major metabolic pathways include oxidation and glucuronidation. It is mainly eliminated via hepatic process and renal clearance is minimal.

Adverse Drug Reactions: Arrhythmias (atrial fibrillation and ventricular tachycardia), myocardial ischaemia, headache, dizziness, and fatigue.

Uses: Systolic heart failure (HFrEF).

Dose: 25 mg or 50 mg twice daily (oral).

4. Tirzepatide

Introduction: Tirzepatide is a dual GLP-1 and GIP receptor agonist initially developed for diabetes but recently studies showing cardioprotective effects.

Clinical Trial Phase / FDA-Approval: Currently undergoing Phase III trials (SUMMIT and SURPASS-HF ongoing).

Mechanism of Action: Tirzepatide is a dual agonist of the glucagon-like peptide-1 (GLP-1) receptor and glucose-dependent insulinotropic polypeptide (GIP), created initially to treat type 2 diabetes mellitus (T2DM) and obesity, it has shown potential cardiovascular benefits, particularly in heart failure (HF). Its mechanism of action in HF involves metabolic, anti-inflammatory, and direct myocardial effects.

1. **Primary Mechanism: GIP and GLP-1 Receptor Activation**

   Tirzepatide exerts its effects by simultaneously stimulating GIP and GLP-1 receptors, leading to improvements in the control of metabolism, inflammation, and cardiac function.

   a. **GLP-1 Receptor Activation**
      - Increases cAMP levels in cardiomyocytes, improving calcium handling and contractility.
      - Enhances natriuresis and diuresis by inhibition of Na^+/H^+ exchanger 3 (NHE3) in proximal tubules, reducing preload and afterload.
      - Reduces inflammation and fibrosis, limiting cardiac remodelling.

   b. **GIP Receptor Activation**
      - Enhances lipid metabolism, reducing myocardial fat accumulation.
      - Increases nitric oxide (NO) availability, leading to improved endothelial function and vasodilation.
      - Reducing oxidative stress, limiting cardiomyocyte apoptosis.

   c. **Combined Effects on Cardiac Function**
      - Improves left ventricular ejection fraction (LVEF) by enhancing contractility.
      - Reduces left ventricular hypertrophy (LVH) by modulating cardiac fibrosis and hypertrophy pathways.

2. **Additional Effects in Heart Failure**

   a. **Effects on Inflammation Reduction**
      - Tirzepatide decreases systemic inflammation in heart failure with preserved ejection fraction (HFpEF) by lowering pro-inflammatory cytokines (TNF-α, IL-6).
      - Inhibits NLRP3 inflammasome activation, reducing myocardial injury.

   b. **Anti-Fibrotic Effects**
      - Suppresses TGF-β signalling, reducing collagen deposition and fibrosis.
      - Protects against myocardial stiffness and diastolic dysfunction.

   c. **Weight Loss and Insulin Sensitivity**
      - Improves metabolic efficiency, leading to reduced cardiac workload.
      - Decreases visceral fat and ectopic fat deposition, limiting lipotoxicity-induced myocardial dysfunction.

Key Pharmacokinetic Parameters: Tirzepatideis given once weekly via subcutaneous injection and has a long half-life. Bioavailability is around 80% after subcutaneous administration. Peak plasma concentration

(Tmax) is around 24 hours post-injection. It is primarily metabolized via proteolytic degradation, similar to endogenous GLP-1 and is not significantly affected by cytochrome P450 (CYP) enzymes, thereby limiting drug-drug interactions. Plasma half-life is about 5 days, allowing weekly administration. Elimination is primarily via urinary excretion of metabolites, with minor faecal elimination.

Adverse Drug Reactions: Nausea, vomiting, diarrhoea, hypoglycaemia, and pancreatitis.

Uses: FDA-approved for Type 2 DM and obesity and under investigation for heart failure with metabolic syndrome.

Dose: 2.5 mg once weekly.

5. Dapagliflozin

Introduction: Dapagliflozin is an SGLT2 inhibitor, improving cardiac and renal outcomes in heart failure.

Clinical Trial Phase / FDA-Approval: FDA approved for HFrEF and HFpEF.

Mechanism of Action:

1. **Primary Mechanism: SGLT2 Inhibition and Natriuresis**

   Dapagliflozin blocks SGLT2 in the proximal renal tubules, resulting in natriuresis and diuresis along with excretion of glucose in urine. This results in:

   a. **Reduced preload and afterload**

      - Increased natriuresis (sodium excretion) and diuresis lowers intravascular volume and ventricular wall stress, leading to improved hemodynamic consequence.

   b. **Lowers blood pressure without increasing heart rate**

      - Unlike traditional diuretics, SGLT2 inhibitors maintain electrolyte balance, preventing excessive sympathetic activation.

2. **Additional Mechanisms in Heart Failure**

   a. **Myocardial Energy Efficiency and Mitochondrial Function**

      - Dapagliflozin enhances myocardial ATP production, shifting cardiac metabolism from glucose to ketones and fatty acids, which are more oxygen-efficient energy sources for failing hearts.

   b. **Anti-Inflammatory and Anti-Fibrotic Effects**

      - Reducing cytokines that promote inflammation (TNF-α, IL-6, IL-1β), limiting chronic inflammation in heart failure.
      - Inhibits cardiac fibrosis by reducing TGF-β signalling, preventing ventricular remodelling.

Key Pharmacokinetic Parameters: Oral bioavailability is almost 78%. It is metabolized mainly by the liver via UDP-glucuronosyltransferase (UGT1A9). No significant CYP450 metabolism, reducing drug interaction risk. The primary metabolite is inactive 3-O-glucuronide which is mainly excreted by urine.

Adverse Drug Reactions: Dehydration, urinary tract infections, polyuria, mild hypoglycaemia, diabetic ketoacidosis, and Fournier's gangrene (rare).

Uses: FDA-approved for Diabetes mellitus type 2, HFrEF, and HFpEF.

Dose: 10 mg once daily (oral).

6. Other recent advances in the treatment of heart failure:

Table 2: Other recent innovations in heart failure management.

Drug / Strategy	Mechanism of Action	Clinical Trial Phase / Status	Adverse Reactions	Distinctive/Salient Features
Endocubitril/ Valsartan is an example of an angiotensin receptor-neprilysin inhibitor (ARNI).	Combines ARB with neprilysin inhibition to enhance natriuretic peptides, reducing afterload and remodelling.	Approved for HFrEF, studied in HFpEF.	Hypotension, hyperkalaemia, renal impairment, angioedema.	Shown to reduce mortality more than ACE inhibitors in HFrEF (PARADIGM-HF trial); ongoing evaluation for HFpEF.
Semaglutide & Other GLP-1 Receptor Agonists	Enhance insulin secretion, reduces appetite, promote weight loss, may have cardioprotective anti-inflammatory effects.	Approved for T2DM; HF trials ongoing.	GI intolerance, potential pancreatitis risk.	Emerging data suggest beneficial effects on cardiac structure and function; ongoing studies in HF with obesity or diabetic HF.
Iron Supplementation (i.v. Iron Carboxymaltose)	Addresses iron insufficiency, increasing energy, exercise capacity metabolism, and quality of life in HF.	Approved for iron-deficient HF patients.	Hypersensitivity reactions (rare), headache.	Ferric carboxymaltose significantly reduces hospitalizations, improves functional status in iron-deficient HFrEF.
Gene / Cell-Based Therapies	Aim to regenerate damaged myocardium or restore defective molecular pathways.	Preclinical and early-phase clinical trials.	Potential immune reactions, arrhythmias, limited long-term data.	Remains exploratory; includes stem cell injections or gene editing targeting sarcomeric proteins and advanced molecular signals.

Key Therapeutic Areas

1. **ARNIs and Expanded Indications:** Sacubitril/Valsartan has supplanted ACE inhibitors in many patients with HFrEF due to its superior mortality and hospitalization benefits. Ongoing research investigates its role in HFpEF, where initial trials (e.g. PARAGON-HF) have shown trends but not definitive results. Subgroup analyses, however, hint at benefit in certain HFpEF phenotypes, suggesting that patient selection might be critical.

2. **SGLT2 Inhibitors Across the HF Spectrum:** SGLT2 inhibitors, initially developed for glucose control in type 2 diabetes, have demonstrated robust benefits in HFrEF—even among patients without diabetes—by reducing hospitalization rates and improving survival. Recent data also confirm their utility in HFpEF, making them among the first pharmacologic agents to show a meaningful outcome advantage in that population.

3. **Myosin Modulators and Other Novel Pathways:** Omecamtiv Mecarbil exemplifies a new class of "myotropes" or direct myosin activators aimed at enhancing systolic performance without exacerbating intracellular calcium overload (a problem with older inotropes). While trial results have been mixed, certain subgroups—particularly those with low ejection fraction and high natriuretic peptides—may derive notable benefit. Similarly, vericiguat's success underscores the importance of novel vasodilatory pathways in advanced HF.
4. **Iron Repletion:** Iron deficiency is highly prevalent among HF patients and correlates with worse exercise tolerance and increased hospitalizations. Intravenous iron formulations (e.g. ferric carboxymaltose) have been validated in multiple trials for symptomatic improvement and reduced hospitalizations in iron-deficient HFrEF, illustrating the multifactorial nature of HF therapy.
5. **Gene and Regenerative Therapies:** Despite substantial research in cell-based approaches—such as stem cell transplantation—to repair or replace damaged myocardium, definitive clinical success has been elusive. Variability in cell types, methods of delivery, and outcome measures complicates interpretation. Advances in genetic editing tools (e.g. CRISPR/Cas9) and engineered tissues remain in the early stages but could eventually offer curative modalities for specific HF aetiologies (e.g. inherited cardiomyopathies).

Device-Based and Advanced Therapies

Even with optimal medical therapy, many patients with refractory or severe HF can need device-based or surgical interventions. These include:

1. **Implantable Cardioverter-Defibrillators (ICDs):** Indicated in order to lower the risk of sudden cardiac death in those with significantly reduced EF.
2. **Cardiac Resynchronization Therapy (CRT):** Biventricular pacing is used to rectify dyssynchronous contraction in selected patients with wide QRS durations, improving cardiac efficiency and outcomes.
3. **Mechanical Circulatory Support (MCS):** Includes left ventricular assist devices (LVADs), which are frequently used as destination therapy for patients who are not eligible for transplantation or as a bridge to transplantation. Recent LVAD models feature improved design for reduced thrombosis and device-related complications.
4. **Heart Transplantation:** It is still the only treatment that works for some individuals with end-stage heart failure and in those who are suitable surgical candidates. Advances in immunosuppression and donor allocation have improved survival, though donor availability remains limited.
5. **Baroreflex Activation Therapy:** Investigated in resistant hypertension (see previous chapter), but also shows potential in HF by modulating sympathetic overdrive. More robust evidence is still needed.

These interventions can be life-extending and life-improving for patients with severe or refractory HF, but they require thorough patient selection, specialized centres, and consideration of cost and long-term complications.

Conclusion

Management of heart failure has evolved from merely alleviating symptoms to a comprehensive, targeted strategy that enhances survival rates and quality of life. Standard therapies, including beta-blockers, ACE inhibitors/ARBs, and MRAs, have been augmented by the introduction of ARNIs and SGLT2 inhibitors, alongside the development of novel agents and device-based treatments that broaden therapeutic options. Despite advancements, disparities persist, particularly in HFpEF. Future advancements in personalised medicine, gene therapy, and regenerative strategies show significant potential. An integrated, patient-focused strategy is crucial for enhancing outcomes in the complex context of heart failure.

References

1. Anker SD, Butler J, Filippatos G, Ferreira JP, Bocchi E, Böhm M, Brunner–La Rocca HP, Choi DJ, Chopra V, Chuquiure-Valenzuela E, Giannetti N. Empagliflozin in heart failure with a preserved ejection fraction. New England Journal of Medicine. 2021 Oct 14;385(16):1451-61.
2. Bozkurt B. Contemporary pharmacological treatment and management of heart failure. Nature Reviews Cardiology. 2024 Aug;21(8):545-55.
3. Maddox TM, Januzzi Jr JL, Allen LA, Breathett K, Brouse S, Butler J, Davis LL, Fonarow GC, Ibrahim NE, Lindenfeld J, Masoudi FA. 2024 ACC expert consensus decision pathway for treatment of heart failure with reduced ejection fraction: a report of the American College of Cardiology Solution Set Oversight Committee. Journal of the American College of Cardiology. 2024 Apr 16;83(15):1444-88.
4. Burnier M. Hypertension in chronic kidney disease and future heart failure. Current opinion in cardiology. 2025 May 1;40(3):158-63.
5. McMurray JJ, Solomon SD, Inzucchi SE, Køber L, Kosiborod MN, Martinez FA, Ponikowski P, Sabatine MS, Anand IS, Bělohlávek J, Böhm M. Dapagliflozin in patients with heart failure and reduced ejection fraction. New England Journal of Medicine. 2019 Nov 21;381(21):1995-2008.
6. Rist A, Sevre K, Wachtell K, Devereux RB, Aurigemma GP, Smiseth OA, Kjeldsen SE, Julius S, Pitt B, Burnier M, Kreutz R. The current best drug treatment for hypertensive heart failure with preserved ejection fraction. European journal of internal medicine. 2024 Feb 1;120:3-10.
7. Yang J, Ye W, Wang K, Wang A, Deng J, Chen G, Cai Y, Li Z, Chen Y, Lin D. Empagliflozin promotes skin flap survival by activating AMPK signaling pathway. European Journal of Pharmacology. 2025 Jan 15;987:177207.
8. Puymirat E. Should SGLT2 inhibitors be prescribed after myocardial infarction with left ventricular dysfunction?. Archives of Cardiovascular Diseases. 2024 Nov 1;117(11):613-5.
9. Christ T, Schwedhelm E, Eschenhagen T. Dapagliflozin and atrial fibrillation: elevated dosing to achieve class I antiarrhythmic effects?. Basic Research in Cardiology. 2024 Jun;119(3):505-7.
10. Badreldin H, Elshal M, El-Karef A, Ibrahim T. Empagliflozin protects the heart from atrial fibrillation in rats through inhibiting the NF-κB/HIF-1α regulatory axis and atrial remodeling. International Immunopharmacology. 2024 Dec 25;143:113403.
11. Polhemus D, Almodiel D, Harb T, Ziogos E, Amat-Codina N, Ranek M, Santhanam L, Gerstenblith G, Leucker TM. Vericiguat prevents high glucose-mediated impaired vascular smooth muscle cGMP production and vasorelaxation. Scientific Reports. 2025 Feb 10;15(1):4939.
12. Aimo A, Castiglione V, Vergaro G, et al. The place of vericiguat in the landscape of treatment for heart failure with reduced ejection fraction. Heart Fail Rev. 2022;27:1165–71.
13. Fritsch A, Meyer M, Blaustein RO, Trujillo ME, Kauh E, Roessig L, Boettcher M, Becker C. Clinical pharmacokinetic and pharmacodynamic profile of vericiguat. Clinical Pharmacokinetics. 2024 Jun;63(6):751-71.
14. Natale F, Fusco C, Stigliani R, Golino P, Cimmino G. Renal arterial resistance index before and after vericiguat administration: Should it be considered the fantastic five?. International Journal of Cardiology. 2024 Nov 15;415:132467.
15. Cacciapuoti F, Mauro C, Capone V, Chianese S, Tarquinio LG, Gottilla R, Marsico F, Crispo S, Cacciapuoti F. The Role of Vericiguat in Early Phases of Anterior Myocardial Infarction: A Potential Game-Changer?. Medicina. 2024 Sep 28;60(10):1595.
16. Boettcher M, Thomas D, Mueck W, Loewen S, Arens E, Yoshikawa K, Becker C. Safety, pharmacodynamic, and pharmacokinetic characterization of vericiguat: results from six phase I studies in healthy subjects. European journal of clinical pharmacology. 2021 Apr;77:527-37.
17. Ding C, Guo C, Fang L, Li Y, Wang Z, Dong Z. Determination of vericiguat in rat plasma by UPLC-MS/MS and its application to drug interaction. Journal of Chromatography A. 2023 Oct 25;1709:464401.
18. Ruehs H, Klein D, Frei M, Grevel J, Austin R, Becker C, Roessig L, Pieske B, Garmann D, Meyer M. Population pharmacokinetics and pharmacodynamics of vericiguat in patients with heart failure and reduced ejection fraction. Clinical pharmacokinetics. 2021 Nov;60(11):1407-21.
19. Rao VN, Diez J, Gustafsson F, Mentz RJ, Senni M, Jankowska EA, Bauersachs J. Practical patient care considerations with use of vericiguat after worsening heart failure events. Journal of Cardiac Failure. 2023 Mar 1;29(3):389-402.
20. Vohra M, Amir M, Osoro I, Sharma A, Kumar R. Impact of vericiguat on heart failure with reduced ejection fraction: a review. Global Health Journal. 2023 Sep 1;7(3):123-9.
21. Boettcher M, Nowotny B, Krausche R, Becker C. Evaluation of the influence of sildenafil on the safety, tolerability, pharmacokinetics, and pharmacodynamics of vericiguat in healthy adults. Clinical Pharmacokinetics. 2023 Feb;62(2):321-33.
22. Hammer A, Niessner A, Sulzgruber P. Vericiguat: a fifth cornerstone in the treatment of heart failure with reduced ejection fraction?. ESC Heart Failure. 2023 Oct 8;10(6):3735.
23. Planelles-Herrero VJ, Hartman JJ, Robert-Paganin J, Malik FI, Houdusse A. Mechanistic and structural basis for activation of cardiac myosin force production by omecamtivmecarbil. Nature communications. 2017 Aug 4;8(1):190.
24. Woody MS, Greenberg MJ, Barua B, Winkelmann DA, Goldman YE, Ostap EM. Positive cardiac inotrope omecamtivmecarbil activates muscle despite suppressing the myosin working stroke. Nature communications. 2018 Sep 21;9(1):3838.

25. Governali S, Caremani M, Gallart C, Pertici I, Stienen G, Piazzesi G, Ottenheijm C, Lombardi V, Linari M. Orthophosphate increases the efficiency of slow muscle-myosin isoform in the presence of omecamtivmecarbil. Nature communications. 2020 Jul 7;11(1):3405.
26. Felker GM, Solomon SD, Metra M, Mcmurray JJ, Diaz R, Claggett B, Lanfear DE, Vandekerckhove H, Biering-Sørensen T, Lopes RD, Arias-Mendoza A. Cardiac Troponin and Treatment Effects of OmecamtivMecarbil: Results From the GALACTIC-HF Study. Journal of cardiac failure. 2024 Jun 1;30(6):755-63.
27. Psotka MA, Teerlink JR. Direct myosin activation by omecamtivmecarbil for heart failure with reduced ejection fraction. Heart Failure. 2017:465-90.
28. Shoji S, Mentz RJ. Beyond quadruple therapy: the potential roles for ivabradine, vericiguat, and omecamtivmecarbil in the therapeutic armamentarium. Heart Failure Reviews. 2024 Sep;29(5):949-55.
29. Palaparthy R, Banfield C, Alvarez P, Yan L, Smith B, Johnson J, Monsalvo ML, Malik F. Relative bioavailability, food effect, and safety of the single-dose pharmacokinetics of omecamtivmecarbil following administration of different modified-release formulations in healthy subjects. International Journal of Clinical Pharmacology and Therapeutics. 2015 Dec 28;54(3):217.
30. Trivedi A, Oberoi RK, Jafarinasabian P, Zhang H, Flach S, Abbasi S, Dutta S, Lee E. Effect of varying degrees of renal impairment on the pharmacokinetics of omecamtivmecarbil. Clinical Pharmacokinetics. 2021 Aug;60:1041-8.
31. Teerlink JR, Diaz R, Felker GM, McMurray JJ, Metra M, Solomon SD, Adams KF, Anand I, Arias-Mendoza A, Biering-Sørensen T, Böhm M. Cardiac myosin activation with omecamtivmecarbil in systolic heart failure. New England Journal of Medicine. 2021 Jan 14;384(2):105-16.
32. Docherty KF, McMurray JJ, Diaz R, Felker GM, Metra M, Solomon SD, Adams KF, Böhm M, Brinkley DM, Echeverria LE, Goudev AR. The effect of omecamtivmecarbil in hospitalized patients as compared with outpatients with HFrEF: an analysis of GALACTIC-HF. Journal of Cardiac Failure. 2024 Jan 1;30(1):26-35.

Chapter 19

Newer Anti-Arrhythmic Drugs

Author: Dr. Pranab Das

Introduction

Cardiac arrhythmias are disturbances in the heart's rhythm that can range from asymptomatic premature beats to life-threatening ventricular tachyarrhythmias or complete heart block. Arrhythmias impose a significant global burden, contributing to increased morbidity, mortality, and healthcare costs. Therapeutic approaches historically focus on restoring or maintaining normal sinus rhythm or controlling ventricular rate while preventing disease progression and reducing sudden cardiac death. The development of antiarrhythmic drugs spans many decades, guided by the classical Vaughan Williams classification (Class I to IV) or the more contemporary Sicilian Gambit approach. Despite the availability of numerous agents—such as blockers of sodium channels, beta-blockers, potassium channel blockers, and calcium channels blockers, the management of arrhythmias remains challenging. Adverse effects, proarrhythmia (i.e., the potential for these drugs to induce new or more dangerous arrhythmias), and incomplete efficacy continue to limit the success of conventional therapies.

Recent developments in electrophysiology, pharmacogenomics, and molecular cardiology have sparked the creation of new and safer antiarrhythmic agents. These include drugs targeting specific molecular pathways (e.g. atrial-selective mechanisms, late sodium current) or novel sites of action (e.g. gap junctions). Non-pharmacological therapies—such as radiofrequency ablation, cardiac resynchronization therapy (CRT), implanted cardioverter-defibrillators (ICDs)—also play significant roles, but there remains a pressing need for antiarrhythmic agents with better safety and efficacy profiles. An overview of recent advances is given in this chapter, which briefly reviews conventional antiarrhythmics, and highlights newer developments poised to improve the pharmacological management of these conditions.

Historical Perspective

The progression of arrhythmia management demonstrates a significant transition from basic symptom control to advanced, mechanism-specific therapies. During the early 20th century, arrhythmias were primarily diagnosed via clinical observation and auscultation, while treatment options were restricted to digitalis and quinidine. The introduction of electrocardiography in the 1900s facilitated enhanced diagnostic accuracy, establishing the groundwork for contemporary electrophysiology. In the 1960s and 1970s, the Vaughan Williams classification established a systematic pharmacological framework that categorised antiarrhythmic drugs according to their primary electrophysiological effects on cardiac ion channels.

Traditional agents such as amiodarone, lidocaine, and procainamide are useful; however, their common side effects and proarrhythmic risks have led to a gradual transition to non-pharmacological methods. The 1980s and 1990s saw notable advancements in catheter-based techniques, particularly radiofrequency ablation, which provided curative options for various supraventricular and ventricular arrhythmias. During this period, the advent of implantable cardioverter-defibrillators (ICDs) and cardiac resynchronisation therapy (CRT) significantly transformed the prevention of sudden cardiac death and the management of arrhythmias in patients with heart failure.

The field has increasingly focused on atrial-selective drug development to reduce the risk of ventricular proarrhythmia, with novel agents such as vernakalant, ranolazine, and dronedarone demonstrating potential efficacy. Recent developments in mapping systems, high-density electrode catheters, and contact force sensing have improved ablation outcomes. Additionally, emerging targets like gap junction modulation and gene-based therapies suggest potential future therapeutic options. The increasing focus on personalised and precision medicine, which includes genetics, wearable monitoring, and AI-driven diagnostics, indicates an ongoing evolution in the identification and treatment of arrhythmias, promising safer, more effective, and individualised patient care.

Definition

According to ACC/AHA, arrhythmia is characterised as any alteration from the normal cardiac rhythm, arising from irregularities in impulse generation or conduction, which may be regular or irregular, and can occur at a slow or rapid rate. The term arrhythmia encompasses bradyarrhythmias (slower-than-normal rhythms) and tachyarrhythmias (faster-than-normal rhythms). Common examples include:

- **Atrial arrhythmias:** Atrial fibrillation (AF), atrial flutter, and supraventricular tachycardias (SVT).
- **Ventricular arrhythmias:** Ventricular tachycardia (VT), ventricular fibrillation (VF), premature ventricular complexes (PVCs).
- **Conduction disturbances:** Heart block (AV nodal block), bundle branch blocks.

Clinically, arrhythmias are assessed based on their hemodynamic stability, symptomatic burden (e.g. palpitations, syncope), and potential for progression to lethal arrhythmias.

Types

The Vaughan Williams classification of anti-arrhythmic drugs is traditionally used to categorize different types of antiarrhythmics:

1. **Class I:** Sodium-channel blockers (e.g. Ia: Quinidine, Procainamide; Ib: Lidocaine; Ic: Flecainide).
2. **Class II:** Beta-blockers (e.g. Metoprolol, Propranolol).
3. **Class III:** Potassium-channel blockers (e.g. Amiodarone, Sotalol, Dofetilide).
4. **Class IV:** Calcium-channel blockers (e.g. Verapamil, Diltiazem).

While useful, the Vaughan Williams system does not fully capture the complexities of newer agents, many of which have overlapping mechanisms or novel targets. Moreover, arrhythmia management often focuses on rhythm control versus rate control tactics, particularly in atrial fibrillation.

Brief Note on Conventional Antiarrhythmics

Conventional antiarrhythmic therapies have been a mainstay in managing both supraventricular and ventricular arrhythmias, though their usage can be limited by side effects and proarrhythmic risk. Below is a concise summary of these mainstream agents:

Table 1: Concise Overview of Traditional Antiarrhythmics.

Drug Class	Mechanism of Action	Common Dosage Forms	Usual Side Effects
Class I [Sodium Channel Blockers like Quinidine (Ia)]	Slow or block conduction (Phase 0), reduce excitability.	Oral tablets, i.v. injection.	Proarrhythmia (especially in structural heart disease), dizziness, blurred vision.
Class II (Beta-Blockers like Propanolol)	Inhibit β-adrenergic receptors, lower automaticity and conduction velocity in nodal tissue.	Oral tablets, i.v. injection.	Bradycardia, hypotension, fatigue, potential bronchospasm in susceptible individuals.
Class III (Potassium Channel Blockers like Amiodarone, Sotalol)	Prolonged repolarization (Phase 3) and refractoriness.	Oral tablets, i.v. injection.	QT prolongation, danger of thyroid dysfunction & goitre (Amiodarone), and torsades de pointes (particularly with Sotalol and Dofetilide).
Class IV (Calcium Channel Blockers like Verapamil, Diltiazem)	Slows AV nodal conduction, reduce automaticity in SA node.	Oral tablets, i.v. injection.	Hypotension, bradycardia, oedema, constipation (especially Verapamil).
Digoxin	Increases vagal tone, decreases AV nodal conduction, mild positive inotrope.	Oral tablets, i.v. formulation.	Narrow therapeutic index, GI disturbances, arrhythmias (toxicity).
Adenosine	Transient block of AV node conduction (via A1 receptor stimulation), terminating re-entrant SVTs (PSVTs).	Rapid IV bolus injection.	Flushing, chest discomfort, dyspnoea.

Although efficacious in specific arrhythmic contexts, these therapies often have narrow therapeutic windows and non-negligible side effects, driving continuous efforts to develop safer, more targeted agents.

Newer Drugs / Recent Advances

Rationale for Novel Agents

Many conventional antiarrhythmic drugs either lack selectivity (potentially affecting both atrial and ventricular tissue) or exhibit significant extracardiac toxicities (e.g. amiodarone's lung, liver, and thyroid concerns). Hence, the drive toward developing atrial-selective agents, late sodium current inhibitors, and gap-junction modulators aims to enhance efficacy while minimizing systemic or ventricular proarrhythmic effects. Below is a summary of notable newer antiarrhythmic agents or strategies under investigation or recently introduced into clinical practice:

1. Flecainide

Introduction: Flecainide is a medication classified as a Class Ic antiarrhythmic that is used to treat atrial fibrillation and other supraventricular arrhythmias. It stabilizes cardiac electrical activity and reduces the likelihood of AF recurrence.

Clinical Trial Phase / FDA-Approval: FDA-approved for paroxysmal AF, ventricular tachycardia,and supraventricular tachycardia (SVT).

Mechanism of Action:

1. **Primary Mechanism: Sodium Channel Blockade (NaV1.5 Inhibition)**

Flecainide blocks fast voltage-gated sodium channels (NaV1.5) in cardiac myocytes, leading to:

i. **Reduced Phase 0 Depolarization**
   b. Slows the rapid influx of sodium (Na^+) during the cardiac action potential's phase 0.
   c. This decreases conduction speed and stops the quick spread of electrical impulses, stabilizing ectopic pacemaker activity.

ii. **Prolonged PR and QRS Intervals on ECG**
   a. Due to the slowed conduction across atria, ventricles, and Purkinje fibres, the QRS complex is widened.
   b. The PR interval may also be prolonged due to AV nodal delay.

2. **Secondary Mechanisms of Action**

a. **Use-Dependent Blockade**
   - Flecainide exhibits stronger sodium channel blockade at higher heart rates (use-dependent effect).
   - This makes it effective in tachyarrhythmias, as it preferentially suppresses rapidly firing ectopic foci.

b. **Potassium Channel Effects (Minor Role in Prolonging Repolarization)**
   - Flecainide weakly inhibits potassium channels (K^+ currents), leading to a slight increase in action potential duration (APD).
   - This contributes to its pro-arrhythmic risk in structural heart disease.

c. **Calcium Handling and Antiarrhythmic Effects in Catecholaminergic Polymorphic Ventricular Tachycardia (CPVT)**
   - Flecainide blocks ryanodine receptor 2 (RyR2)-mediated calcium release, preventing calcium-triggered arrhythmias in CPVT.
   - This unique mechanism makes it a first-line therapy in CPVT.

Key Pharmacokinetic Parameters: Oral bioavailability is 90%. Oral absorption is unaffected by food. It is mostly broken down by CYP2D6 enzymes in the liver. Due to slowed and delayed elimination, dose modifications are required in cases of renal and hepatic impairment. It has a 12-27-hour plasma half-life.

Adverse Drug Reactions: Dizziness, blurred vision, and increasing heart failure in individuals with structural heart disease, as well as proarrhythmia (ventricular tachycardia, torsades de pointes in some people).

Uses: Supraventricular tachycardia (SVT), ventricular tachycardia (VT), and atrial fibrillation and flutter for rhythm control, particularly in catecholaminergic polymorphic VT (CPVT).

Dose: 50–100 mg twice daily.

2. Vernakalant

Introduction: Vernakalant is a potassium and sodium channel blocker. It has atrial-selective effects, making it safer than other Class I antiarrhythmic agents.

Clinical Trial Phase / FDA-Approval: Approved in Europe and Canada for acute AF conversion but not FDA-approved in the U.S.

Mechanism of Action:

1. **Primary Mechanism: Multi-Channel Blockade**

Vernakalant acts via selective blockade of atrial ion channels, distinguishing it from conventional antiarrhythmic drugs.

a. Potassium (K^+) Channel Blockade

1. **Inhibition of ultra-rapid delayed rectifier K+ current (IKur)**
    - Because ventricular cells lack IKur, it is selective for atrial myocytes.
    - Increases the length of the atrial action potential (APD) without appreciably altering the ventricular repolarization.

b. Sodium (Na^+) Channel Blockade

- Blocks peak and late-phase sodium currents (INa).
- Slows atrial conduction velocity, terminating re-entrant circuits responsible for AF.

c. Atrial Selectivity: Minimal Ventricular Effects

- Vernakalant prolongs atrial refractoriness without significantly affecting the ventricles.
- Reduces atrial re-entry circuits, facilitating AF's transition to sinus rhythm.

2. **Additional Mechanisms in Atrial Fibrillation (AF) Treatment**

a. Rate-Dependent Blockade

- More effective at high atrial rates, which occur during AF episodes.
- This property makes it ideal for rapid cardioversion of AF.

Key Pharmacokinetic Parameters: Administration is via i.v. route leading to a rapid onset of action. It is metabolized primarily by cytochrome P450 (CYP2D6). It is mostly removed via renal excretion (80%) and plasma half-life is approximately three to five hours.

Adverse Drug Reactions: Dysgeusia, hypotension, nausea, dizziness, and bradycardia.

Uses: Rapid cardioversion of recent-onset atrial fibrillation.

Dose: 3 mg/kg IV over 10 minutes.

3. Ranolazine

Introduction: The anti-ischemic drug ranolazine also has anti-arrhythmic effects, making it useful in treating atrial fibrillation (AF) and ventricular arrhythmias.

Clinical Trial Phase / FDA-Approval: Approved for chronic angina. Currently undergoing Phase II/III trials for atrial fibrillation (AF) and ventricular tachycardia (VT).

Mechanism of Action:

1. **Primary Mechanism: Late Sodium Current (INa+-Late) Inhibition**

    Ranolazine selectively blocks late-phase sodium influx (INa+-Late) in ventricular and atrial myocytes, leading to:

    i. **Reduced Intracellular Sodium Accumulation**

        a. Late sodium current is prolonged in ischemic or failing hearts, causing excess intracellular Na^+ accumulation.

b. By blocking INa+-Late, ranolazine limits Na^+ overload, preventing downstream arrhythmic effects.

ii. Reduced Calcium Overload via Na^+/Ca^{2+} Exchange

a. Excess intracellular Na^+ inhibits Na^+/Ca^{2+} exchanger (NCX), leading to Ca^{2+} overload.

b. Ranolazine reduces intracellular Ca^{2+}, preventing early afterdepolarizations (EADs) and delayed afterdepolarizations (DADs), which are the key triggers of arrhythmias.

iii. Stabilization of Action Potential Duration (APD)

a. Ranolazine shortens prolonged APD in atrial fibrillation, restoring normal conduction.

b. It reduces repolarization dispersion, lowering the risk of re-entrant arrhythmias.

2. Additional Mechanisms in Arrhythmia Treatment

a. Effects on Potassium (K^+) Currents

- Weak IKr inhibition (delayed rectifier potassium current).
- Minimal QT prolongation compared to other Class III antiarrhythmics, reducing torsades de pointes risk.

b. Atrial Selectivity

- More effective in atrial than ventricular arrhythmias due to higher atrial dependence on INa+-Late.

c. Anti-Fibrillatory Effects

- Suppresses atrial fibrillation triggers by reducing atrial ectopy and re-entry circuits.
- Enhances atrial electrical stability, particularly in heart failure or ischemic cardiomyopathy patients.

Ranolazine inhibits late sodium currents, prevents calcium overload, and stabilizes cardiac repolarization, making it an effective antiarrhythmic agent. It can be useful especially for atrial fibrillation and ventricular arrhythmias in ischemic heart disease.

Key Pharmacokinetic Parameters: Oral bioavailability is 35-50%, as its first-pass metabolism is substantial. It is metabolized in liver (CYP3A4, CYP2D6). Plasma half-life is around 7 hours and is excreted mainly in urine.

Adverse Drug Reactions: Dizziness, nausea, constipation, QT prolongation, bradycardia, hypotension, and renal impairment.

Uses: FDA-approved for chronic stable angina and under investigation for AF suppression and VT reduction.

Dose: 500 mg to 1000 mg twice daily (trial dosing).

4. AZD7009

Introduction: AZD7009 is a novel antiarrhythmic agent targeting AF suppression through selective INa+ and IKr blockade.

Clinical Trial Phase / FDA-Approval: Currently in Phase II clinical trial.

Mechanism of Action:

1. **Primary Mechanism: Multi-Channel Blockade**
   a. Sodium Channel (INa+) Blockade
      - Inhibits peak and late sodium currents (INa+ and INa+-Late).
      - Slows atrial conduction velocity, preventing re-entrant circuits that sustain atrial fibrillation.
      - Use-dependent blockade: The effect increases at higher atrial rates, making it ideal for AF termination.

   b. Potassium Channel (IKr / IKur) Blockade
      - Inhibits IKr (hERG potassium current), which leads to mild QT prolongation without excessive torsades de pointes risk.
      - Blocks ultra-rapid delayed rectifier current, or IKur (atrial-specific), thereby prolongs atrial action potential duration.
      - Minimal effects on ventricular repolarization, unlike conventional Class III drugs.

   c. Calcium Channel (ICa-L) Blockade
      - Mild inhibition of L-type calcium channels, reducing atrial excitability and triggered activity.
      - Helps to suppress ectopic pacemaker activity.

2. **Additional Mechanisms in Arrhythmia Treatment**
   a. Rate-Dependent Effects
      - Stronger blockade occurs at higher atrial rates, selectively targeting rapid atrial rhythms in AF.
      - Unlike Class I antiarrhythmics, it does not excessively slow conduction at normal heart rates, reducing bradycardia risk.

   b. Anti-Fibrillatory Effects
      - Prolongs atrial effective refractory period (ERP) without significant ventricular ERP changes.
      - Suppresses re-entry circuits, preventing AF recurrence.

   c. Atrial Selectivity and Reduced Ventricular Proarrhythmic Risk
      - Unlike traditional Class III antiarrhythmics, AZD7009 selectively targets atrial tissue.
      - Minimal impact on ventricular conduction, reducing the risk of ventricular arrhythmias.

Key Pharmacokinetic Parameters: Phase II trials are being conducted to produce an oral formulation for long-term therapy of AF and an intravenous formulation for acute conversion. It is metabolized primarily by cytochrome P450 (CYP3A4 and CYP2D6) enzymes. No active metabolites with significant pharmacological effects are generated. Plasma half-life is 4–6 hours and is excreted mainly by urine.

Adverse Drug Reactions: Mild QT prolongation, gastrointestinal upset, bradycardia, and AV block.

Uses: Under investigation for atrial fibrillation and atrial flutter.

Dose: 0.5 to 2.5 mg/kg over 10–20 minutes (investigational dose).

5. Mexiletine

Introduction: Mexiletine is a Class Ib sodium channel blocker used for ventricular arrhythmias, particularly in Long QT Syndrome (LQT3).

Clinical Trial Phase / FDA-Approval: FDA-approved for ventricular arrhythmias.

Mechanism of Action:

1. **Primary Mechanism: Sodium Channel Blockade (INa+ Inhibition)**

Mexiletine primarily blocks voltage-gated sodium channels (NaV1.5) in cardiac myocytes, leading to:

1. **Inhibition of Phase 0 Depolarization**
   - Mexiletine reduces the sodium (Na^+) influx during the action potential's first phase (Phase 0).
   - This slows conduction velocity, particularly in ventricular tissue, preventing re-entrantarrhythmias.
2. **Use-Dependent Blockade**
   - Mexiletine preferentially blocks sodium channels during high-frequency depolarizations, making it most effective in tachyarrhythmias.
   - This selective effect on depolarized tissues reduces the risk of excessive conduction slowing.
3. **Shortens the Refractory Period and Action Potential Duration (APD)**
   - Unlike Class Ia (quinidine, procainamide) or Class III agents (amiodarone, sotalol), mexiletine does not significantly prolong APD.
   - This prevents excessive repolarization delay and reduces the risk of TdP, or torsades de pointes.

2. **Additional Mechanisms in Arrhythmia Treatment**

   a. **Anti-Fibrillatory Effects**
   - Mexiletine suppresses ventricular ectopy and re-entry circuits, making it effective for ventricular fibrillation (VF) and ventricular tachycardia (VT) prevention.
   - Reduces the incidence of ischemia-induced ventricular arrhythmias, often seen in post-myocardial infarction (MI) patients.

   b. **Potassium and Calcium Current Modulation**
   - Mild suppression of late sodium currents (Na-Late) - Reduces calcium overload and afterdepolarizations, which helps suppress arrhythmic triggers.
   - No significant inhibition of potassium (K^+) currents, making it safer than Class III drugs in terms of QT prolongation risk.

Key Pharmacokinetic Parameters: Oral bioavailability is 90%. Consuming food slows down absorption but has no effect on total bioavailability. Hepatic metabolism is via cytochrome P450 (CYP2D6, CYP1A2, CYP3A4 enzymes). Plasma half-life is 10 hours and it is mainly excreted via urine.

Adverse Drug Reactions: CNS effects (dizziness, tremors), nausea, QT prolongation, hepatotoxicity, and vomiting.

Uses: Ventricular arrhythmia, off-label use in myotonic disorders and neuropathic pain and is under investigation for Long QT Syndrome Type 3 (LQT3).

Dose: 200–300 mg every 8 hours (TID dosing).

6. Other recent advances in the course of treatment of arrhythmia:

Table 2: Additional latest developments in medical management of arrhythmia.

Drug Name / Strategy	Mechanism of Action	Clinical Trial Phase / Status	Adverse Reactions	Distinctive / Salient Features
Dronedarone	Multichannel blockade (sodium, potassium, calcium) but categorised as Class III anti-arrhythmic, structurally related to amiodarone but less lipophilic.	FDA-Approved for AF, ongoing post-marketing data.	GI upset, possible worsening of HF, liver injury in some cases.	Developed to reduce amiodarone's organ toxicities; recommended primarily in less severe structural heart disease.
Eleclazine (GS-6615)	Selective inhibitor of late sodium current, reducing intracellular sodium/calcium overload.	Phase II/III for various arrhythmias like LQTS3, AF, VT and ischaemia-induced arrythmia.	Headache, dizziness, limited long-term data.	Potential to reduce torsades de pointes in congenital long QT syndrome; also being explored for AF and VT.
XEN-D0103	Selective Kv1.5 (IKur) channel blockade, designed for atrial fibrillation termination.	Phase II trials completed.	Potential local irritation, mild GI disturbances.	Highly atrial-selective approach aims to avoid proarrhythmia in ventricles.
GAP-134 (Rotigaptide)	Increases gap junction conductance (connexin 43), potentially improving conduction and reducing AF.	Phase II trials in atrial fibrillation.	Minimal so far in small studies; potential to cause hypotension.	Focuses on modifying conduction rather than purely ion channel blockade.
Gene Therapy	Experimental: modifies ion-channel expression or conduction pathways (e.g. reprogramming nodal tissue).	Preclinical and early-phase trial.	Unknown long-term effects, potential immunogenicity.	Could provide personalized, disease-specific solutions in inherited arrhythmias or refractory AF.

Key Emerging Concepts

1. **Atrial-Selective Blockade:** Drugs like vernakalant and XEN-D0103 target channels predominantly expressed in atrial tissue (e.g. IKur). This specificity aims to prevent atrial fibrillation without prolonging ventricular repolarization, thereby lowering the risk of proarrhythmia such as torsades de pointes.

2. **Late Sodium Current Inhibition:** Cardiac action potential's plateau phase is prolonged by late sodium current (INa), which exacerbates intracellular calcium overload, and predisposes to arrhythmogenic activity. Agents like ranolazine and eleclazine shows promise in various atrial and ventricular arrhythmias by dampening these late currents without significantly affecting early sodium influx vital for normal conduction.

3. **Multichannel Modulators with Reduced Toxicity:** Dronedarone was introduced to retain amiodarone's multichannel blockade profile but with fewer thyroid, hepatic, or pulmonary side effects. Although it is linked to decreased long-term toxicity, patients with permanent atrial fibrillation or severe heart failure should still exercise caution because of the higher risk of negative outcomes in these subgroups.

4. **Gap-Junction Modulation:** Gap junctions facilitate electrical coupling between myocardial cells. Agents that enhance gap-junction conductance, like GAP-134 (rotigaptide), might stabilize conduction, reducing the propensity for re-entrant arrhythmias. Although early-phase results are promising, more data is needed before routine clinical application.
5. **Personalized / Precision Approaches:** Ongoing advances in genomics and molecular cardiology raise the possibility of gene therapy to correct inherited arrhythmogenic syndromes (e.g. catecholaminergic polymorphic VT, long QT syndromes). In the future, expression-modulating viral vectors or CRISPR-based techniques could tailor antiarrhythmic strategies to each patient's genetic makeup.

Conclusion

Arrhythmias, particularly atrial fibrillation and ventricular tachyarrhythmias, continue to provide a significant clinical problem. Although conventional antiarrhythmics offer essential therapy, their limitations in efficacy and safety necessitate the development of more selective, safer, and personalised medicines. Recent medications like as vernakalant, dronedarone, and late sodium current inhibitors signify advancements in targeted atrial therapy with reduced adverse effects. Innovative techniques, such as conduction modulators, gene therapy, and personalised therapies, present intriguing future avenues. Ultimately, effective arrhythmia management depends on a customised amalgamation of pharmacotherapy, interventions such as ablation and implantable cardioverter-defibrillators (ICDs), and rigorous risk-factor mitigation, informed by continuous research and advancing clinical knowledge.

References

1. Nagpal AK, Pundkar A, Singh A, Gadkari C. Cardiac arrhythmias and their management: An in-depth review of current practices and emerging therapies. Cureus. 2024 Aug 9;16(8).
2. Taylor DA, Watts SW. Antiarrhythmic drugs. Brody's Human Pharmacology-E-Book: Brody's Human Pharmacology-E-Book. 2024 Feb 2;392.
3. Fye WB. A history of the origin, evolution, and impact of electrocardiography. Am J Cardiol. 1994;73(13):937–949.
4. Roden DM. Antiarrhythmic drugs: Historical insights into mechanisms, clinical applications, and unresolved questions. Heart Rhythm. 2004;1(1):11–19.
5. January CT, Wann LS, Calkins H, Chen LY, Cigarroa JE, Cleveland Jr JC, Ellinor PT, Ezekowitz MD, Field ME, Furie KL, Heidenreich PA. 2019 AHA/ACC/HRS focused update of the 2014 AHA/ACC/HRS guideline for the management of patients with atrial fibrillation: a report of the American College of Cardiology/American Heart Association Task Force on Clinical Practice Guidelines and the Heart Rhythm Society in collaboration with the Society of Thoracic Surgeons. Circulation. 2019 Jul 9;140(2):e125-51.
6. Lecturio. Class I antiarrhythmic drugs [Internet]. Lecturio; [cited 2025 May 16]. Available from: https://www.lecturio.com/concepts/class-1-antiarrhythmic-drugs/.
7. Vaughan Williams EM. A classification of antiarrhythmic actions reassessed after a decade of new drugs. *J Clin Pharmacol.* 1984;24(3):129–47.
8. Roy D, Pratt CM, Torp-Pedersen C, Wyse DG, Toft E, Juul-Moller S, Nielsen T, Rasmussen SL, Stiell IG, Coutu B, Ip JH. Vernakalant hydrochloride for rapid conversion of atrial fibrillation: a phase 3, randomized, placebo-controlled trial. Circulation. 2008 Mar 25;117(12):1518-25.
9. Murdock DK, Overton N, Kersten M, Kaliebe J, Devecchi F. The effect of ranolazine on maintaining sinus rhythm in patients with resistant atrial fibrillation. Indian Pacing and Electrophysiology Journal. 2008 Aug 1;8(3):175.
10. Dobrev D, Nattel S. New antiarrhythmic drugs for treatment of atrial fibrillation. The Lancet. 2010 Apr 3;375(9721):1212-23.
11. Lubitz SA, Yin X, Fontes JD, Magnani JW, Rienstra M, Pai M, Villalon ML, Vasan RS, Pencina MJ, Levy D, Larson MG. Association between familial atrial fibrillation and risk of new-onset atrial fibrillation. Jama. 2010 Nov 24;304(20):2263-9.
12. Burashnikov A, Di Diego JM, Zygmunt AC, Belardinelli L, Antzelevitch C. Atrial-selective sodium channel block as a strategy for suppression of atrial fibrillation. Annals of the New York Academy of Sciences. 2008 Mar;1123(1):105-12.
13. Bogert NV, Therre M, Din S, Furkel J, Zhou X, El-Battrawy I, Heineke J, Schweizer PA, Akin I, Katus HA, Frey N. Macrophages enhance sodium channel expression in cardiomyocytes. Basic Research in Cardiology. 2024 Dec;119(6):1063-73.
14. Cupelli M, Ginjupalli VK, Reisqs JB, Sleiman Y, El-Sherif N, Gourdon G, Puymirat J, Chahine M, Boutjdir M. Calcium handling abnormalities increase arrhythmia susceptibility in DMSXL myotonic dystrophy type 1 mice. Biomedicine & Pharmacotherapy. 2024 Nov 1;180:117562.

15. Van Ham WB, Meijboom EE, Ligtermoet ML, Monshouwer-Kloots J, Riele AS, Asselbergs FW, van Rooij E, Bourfiss M, van Veen TA. An hiPSC-CM approach for electrophysiological phenotyping of a patient-specific case of short-coupled TdP. Stem cell research & therapy. 2024 Dec 18;15(1):470.
16. Mao Z, Wheeler JJ, Townsend R, Gao Y, Kshirsagar S, Keirns JJ. Population pharmacokinetic–pharmacodynamic analysis of vernakalant hydrochloride injection (RSD1235) in atrial fibrillation or atrial flutter. Journal of pharmacokinetics and pharmacodynamics. 2011 Oct;38:541-62.
17. Duggan ST, Scott LJ. Spotlight on intravenous vernakalant in recent-onset atrial fibrillation. Drugs & aging. 2011 Jun;28:501-4.
18. Hall AJ, Mitchell AR. Introducing vernakalant into clinical practice. Arrhythmia & electrophysiology review. 2019 Mar;8(1):70.
19. Tamargo J. Other antiarrhythmic drugs. Antiarrhythmic Drugs. 2020:265-306.
20. Glover BM, Dorian P. Anti-arrhythmic Drugs. Clinical Handbook of Cardiac Electrophysiology. 2016:249-64.
21. Jost N, Christ T, Magyar J. New strategies for the treatment of atrial fibrillation. Pharmaceuticals. 2021 Sep;14(9):926.
22. Hauguel-Moreau M, Guedeney P, Dauphin C, Auffret V, Clerc JM, Marijon E, Elbaz M, Aldebert P, Beygui F, Abi Khalil W, Da Costa A. Flecainide to Prevent Atrial Arrhythmia After Patent Foramen Ovale Closure: AFLOAT Study, A Randomized Clinical Trial. Circulation. 2024 Nov 19;150(21):1659-68.
23. Hoteit A, Moumneh MB, Nahlawi A, Hebbo E, Abdulhai F, Abi-Saleh B, Khoury M, Refaat M, Moumneh MB, Khoury Sr M. Efficacy and Safety of Intravenous Vernakalant in Rapid Cardioversion of Recent Onset Atrial Fibrillation: A Retrospective Single-Centre Study. Cureus. 2024 Apr 19;16(4).
24. Murai K, Vasigh A, Alexy T, Tóth K, Czopf L. The Role of Ranolazine in the Treatment of Ventricular Tachycardia and Atrial Fibrillation: A Narrative Review of the Clinical Evidence. Biomedicines. 2024 Jul 26;12(8):1669.
25. Alhourani N, Wolfes J, Könemann H, Ellermann C, Frommeyer G, Güner F, Lange PS, Reinke F, Köbe J, Eckardt L. Relevance of mexiletine in the era of evolving antiarrhythmic therapy of ventricular arrhythmias. Clinical Research in Cardiology. 2024 Jun;113(6):791-800.

Chapter 20

Newer Anti-Thrombotic Agents

Author: Dr. Pranab Das

Introduction

Many cardiovascular and cerebrovascular disorders are caused by thrombosis, which is the development of blood clots inside blood vessels. One of the main causes of morbidity and death globally is venous thromboembolism (VTE), which comprises pulmonary embolism (PE) and deep vein thrombosis (DVT). Similarly, ischemic strokes and acute coronary syndromes (myocardial infarction) are caused by arterial thrombosis. In the last few decades, an increasing amount of evidence has underscored the need for effective antithrombotic therapies to mitigate these risks.

Traditionally, vitamin K antagonists (VKAs), low-molecular-weight heparin (LMWH), and unfractionated heparin (UFH)—along with antiplatelet agents like aspirin—have formed the cornerstone of thromboprophylaxis and treatment. However, the limitations of these conventional agents, including the need for regular monitoring (VKAs), parenteral administration (UFH, LMWH), and bleeding complications, have fuelled the development of newer oral anticoagulants, platelet inhibitors, and novel combination regimens. Advances in molecular biology and translational research have provided insight into specific coagulation factors and platelet signalling pathways, enabling the design of targeted therapies with more favourable safety profiles, simplified administration, and potentially superior efficacy. This chapter reviews the essentials of thrombosis and conventional antithrombotic approaches and highlights the latest therapies—focusing on new anticoagulant mechanisms, next-generation antiplatelet drugs, and emerging adjunctive strategies.

Historical Perspective

The initiation of antithrombotic therapy commenced with the identification of heparin in the early 20th century, representing a significant advancement in the prevention and management of thromboembolic disorders. Subsequently, warfarin, a vitamin K antagonist, was introduced and served as the foundation of oral anticoagulation for many years. Warfarin, while effective, necessitated regular monitoring, exhibited multiple drug and food interactions, and possessed a narrow therapeutic index, presenting challenges in clinical practice.

The development of antiplatelet agents concurrently broadened therapeutic options. Acetylsalicylic acid (aspirin) became the first widely used antiplatelet drug, later followed by agents like dipyridamole and ticlopidine. The introduction of clopidogrel in the 1990s markedly enhanced secondary prevention strategies for cardiovascular disease, particularly in acute coronary syndromes and following stent implantation.

The constraints of conventional agents prompted a paradigm shift in the early 21st century, resulting in the emergence of direct oral anticoagulants (DOACs), which encompass direct thrombin inhibitors and factor Xa inhibitors. The agents provided predictable pharmacokinetics, reduced interactions, and eliminated the necessity for routine monitoring, thereby significantly simplifying anticoagulation management. During this period, novel P2Y12 inhibitors like prasugrel and ticagrelor demonstrated superior potency and consistency in platelet inhibition relative to clopidogrel, thereby enhancing antiplatelet therapy.

Recent efforts have concentrated on the development of antithrombotic drugs that exhibit enhanced safety profiles, specifically with a focus on minimising bleeding risk. Inhibitors of factors XI and XII, PAR-1 antagonists such as vorapaxar, and strategies for dual-pathway inhibition are designed to maintain antithrombotic effectiveness while reducing the risk of haemorrhagic complications. These developments indicate a trend towards precision medicine, wherein therapies are customised based on individual thrombotic risk and bleeding susceptibility. The evolution of antithrombotic therapy is transforming cardiovascular and cerebrovascular care, striving to achieve an optimal balance between clot prevention and bleeding management.

Definition

Thrombosis refers to the pathological process wherein a clot (thrombus) forms inappropriately within a blood vessel, impeding or obstructing blood flow. Two primary manifestations include:

- **Arterial Thrombosis:** Often superimposed on atherosclerotic plaques, leading to myocardial infarction, ischemic stroke, or limb ischemia. Platelet-rich ("white") clots typically predominate in arterial circulation due to high shear stress.
- **Venous Thrombosis:** Frequently occurring in areas of stasis or hypercoagulability (e.g. deep leg veins), leading to DVT and potentially fatal pulmonary embolism if dislodged. Fibrin-rich ("red") clots are more common in venous circulation, although platelets also contribute.

  These processes are often explained by endothelial damage, stasis or turbulent blood flow, and hypercoagulability which are the three components of Virchow's triad and these factors acts as predisposing factors. Modern antithrombotic therapy aims to inhibit key pathways involved in clot initiation, amplification, and propagation, while minimizing the inherent risk of bleeding.

Types

From a pharmacological standpoint, two primary categories can be used to broadly classify anti-thrombotic agents:

1. **Antiplatelet Agents**
   - Interfere with platelet activation or aggregation.
   - Commonly used in arterial thrombosis prevention and treatment (e.g. aspirin, P2Y12 inhibitors like clopidogrel, prasugrel, ticagrelor).
2. **Anticoagulants**
   - Inhibit factors in the coagulation cascade, reducing fibrin formation.
   - Essential for treating or preventing venous thromboembolism and in conditions like atrial fibrillation to prevent cardioembolic stroke. Examples include heparins, direct oral anticoagulants (DOACs) and vitamin K antagonists (warfarin).

   While some therapies blend characteristics of both pathways (e.g. dual pathway inhibition, factor XI inhibitors with partial effects on platelet function), the traditional division helps guide clinical decisions regarding the most appropriate regimen for arterial vs. venous thrombosis.

Brief Note on Conventional Medicines

The following table provides a concise summary of the well-established or "conventional" antithrombotic agents that have long been cornerstones of treatment.

Table 1: Concise overview of current antithrombotic medications.

Drug Class / Drug Names	Mechanism of Action	Common Dosage Forms	Usual Side Effects
Unfractionated Heparin (UFH)	Increases the potency of antithrombin III's inactivation of thrombin (Factor IIa) and Factor Xa by binding to it.	Intravenous, subcutaneous.	Bleeding, osteoporosis (long-term), and heparin-induced thrombocytopenia (HIT).
Heparins with low molecular weights, such as enoxaparin	Preferentially inactivate Factor Xa via antithrombin III, with less effect on thrombin (Factor IIa).	Subcutaneous injection.	Bleeding, osteoporosis (long-term), and heparin-induced thrombocytopenia (HIT). Compared to UFH, bleeding is less likely to occur, although it is still possible.
Vitamin K Antagonists (e.g. Warfarin)	Inhibits vitamin K-dependent gamma-carboxylation of clotting factors (II, VII, IX, X) and proteins C/SX-1, reducing thromboxane A2 production, and thus preventing platelet aggregation.	Oral tablets	Bleeding, narrow therapeutic index, requires INR monitoring, numerous drug/food interactions.
Aspirin (ASA)	Cyclooxygenase-1 (COX-1) is irreversibly inhibited, which lowers the formation of thromboxane A2 and, consequently, platelet aggregation is inhibited.	Oral tablet	Gastrointestinal irritation, bleeding risk, hypersensitivity.
P2Y12 Inhibitors (e.g. Clopidogrel)	Platelet activation and aggregation can be avoided by blocking the ADP receptor (P2Y12) on the platelet surface.	Oral tablet	Bleeding, variable response due to genetic polymorphisms (especially with clopidogrel).
Glycoprotein IIb/IIIa Inhibitors (e.g. Abciximab)	Prevent fibrinogen from binding to platelets, inhibiting platelet aggregation.	i.v. infusion	Bleeding (risk of thrombocytopenia), typically used in percutaneous coronary intervention (PCI).

Figure 1 illustrates how anticoagulant drugs exert their effects at crucial points in the clotting process.

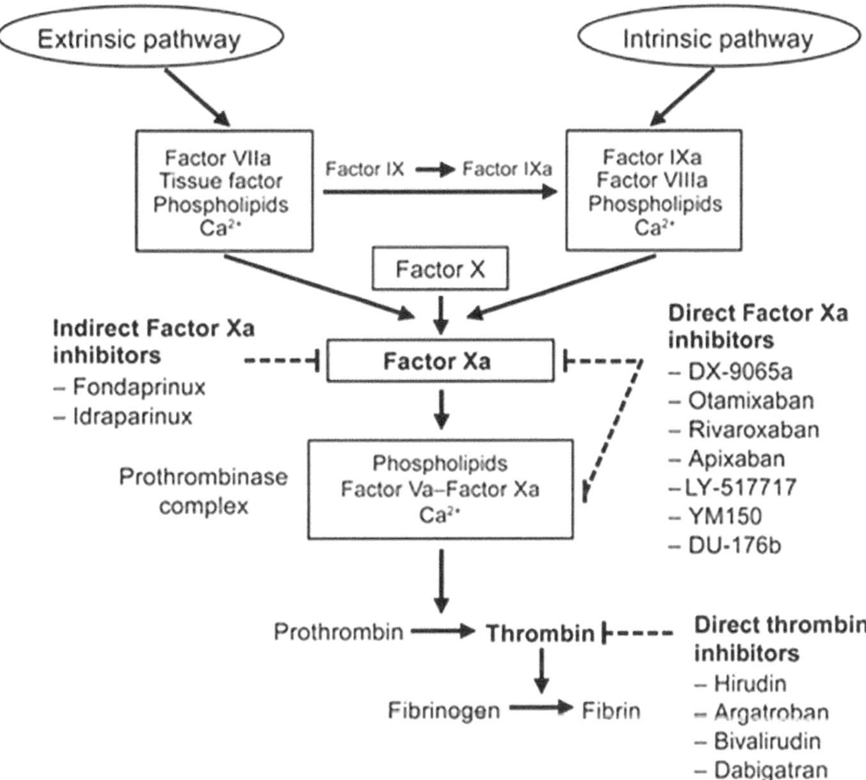

Figure 1: Key points in the clotting process where anticoagulant medications act (Source: Burghaus R et al.).

Although these agents have substantially reduced morbidity and mortality from thrombotic events, their use can be complicated by significant bleeding risks, inter-patient variability in response, and logistical challenges (e.g. frequent monitoring). Thus, a major objective in developing newer agents is improving ease of use and safety—ideally maintaining or enhancing efficacy while minimizing bleeding and monitoring requirements.

Newer Drugs / Recent Advances

Breakthroughs in the knowledge of the biology of coagulation have cleared the path for a variety of newer antithrombotic agents. These include direct oral anticoagulants (DOACs), next-generation factor XI/XIa inhibitors, novel antiplatelets [including protease-activated receptor (PAR) inhibitors], and dual-pathway strategies. Below is an overview, followed by a more detailed discussion of each category.

1. Rivaroxaban

Introduction: Rivaroxaban, a direct oral Factor Xa inhibitor, provides a substitute for warfarin in the treatment of venous thromboembolism (VTE) and stroke management. It provides predictable anticoagulation without the need for routine monitoring.

Clinical Trial Phase / FDA-Approval: FDA-approved for stroke prevention in AF, VTE prophylaxis, and acute coronary syndrome.

Mechanism of Action:

1. **Primary Mechanism: Factor Xa Inhibition**
   a. **Direct Inhibition of Factor Xa**
      - Rivaroxaban binds directly to both clot-bound and free Factor Xa, which stops prothrombin from becoming thrombin (IIa).

- Unlike warfarin, it does not require antithrombin III for its action.

b. Suppression of Thrombin Formation
   - Thrombin (IIa) is a key enzyme responsible for fibrin clot formation.
   - By inhibiting Factor Xa, rivaroxaban reduces thrombin production, limiting clot development.

c. Prevention of Platelet Activation
   - Thrombin also promotes platelet aggregation.
   - Rivaroxaban indirectly reduces platelet activation, decreasing thrombotic risk in cardiovascular conditions.

Key Pharmacokinetic Parameters: It shows high oral bioavailability (around 80–100%). Binding to plasma proteins is around 92-95% (mainly albumin). It undergoes CYP3A4-mediated hepatic metabolism. It is excreted mainly via urine and plasma half-life is 5–9 hours.

Adverse Drug Reactions: Bleeding complications (intracranial, gastrointestinal), nausea, dyspepsia, anaemia, and liver enzyme elevation.

Uses: Thromboprophylaxis following orthopaedic surgery, treatment and prevention of VTE (DVT and PE), and stroke prevention in non-valvular atrial fibrillation.

Dose: 15 mg twice daily for the first 21 days, followed by 20 mg once daily thereafter.

2. Dabigatran

Introduction: Dabigatran, a direct oral thrombin inhibitor (DOTI), offers a fixed-dose option to warfarin without necessitating regular coagulation monitoring.

Clinical Trial Phase / FDA-Approval: FDA-approved for stroke prevention in AF, VTE treatment, and thromboprophylaxis.

Mechanism of Action:

1. **Inhibition of Thrombin (Factor IIa):**
   - Dabigatran stops thrombin from cleaving fibrinogen into fibrin by binding to its active site in a reversible way. This prevents clot formation and thrombus propagation.
   - It also inhibits thrombin-induced platelet aggregation, further reducing thrombus formation.
2. **Independent of Antithrombin III:**
   - Unlike heparin Dabigatran and low molecular weight heparins (LMWHs) does not require antithrombin III as a cofactor. This direct inhibition leads to predictable pharmacokinetics, eliminating the need for routine monitoring.
3. **Rapid Onset of Action:**
   - Esterases in the liver and plasma quickly transform the pro-drug dabigatran etexilate into its active form, dabigatran.
   - This rapid conversion contributes to its fast beginning of action (within 30 minutes to 2 hours after administration).
4. **Presence of an Reversal Agent:**
   - Idarucizumab, a monoclonal antibody that binds to dabigatran with high affinity and neutralises its anticoagulant effects in circumstances of life-threatening bleeding or urgent surgery, can be used to reverse the effects of dabigatran.

5. **Clinical Superiority Over Warfarin:**
   - Clinical trials such as RE-LY (Randomized Evaluation of Long-term Anticoagulation Therapy) demonstrated that dabigatran is as effective in preventing stroke and systemic embolism, with lower rates of intracranial haemorrhage as compared to warfarin.

Key Pharmacokinetic Parameters: Hepatic and plasma esterases transform the prodrug dabigatran etexilate into active dabigatran. 6-7% is the oral bioavailability (poor because of P-glycoprotein efflux). Tmax, or peak plasma concentration, is achieved within one to three hours after the injection. A plasma half-life of 12 to 17 hours is seen with dabigatran. Because CYP450 enzymes cannot metabolise dabigatran, there are fewer drug-drug interactions. It is excreted mainly in urine.

Adverse Drug Reactions: Major bleeding risk (especially gastrointestinal bleeding), dyspepsia, nausea, headache, fatigue and hepatotoxicity (rare).

Uses: Stroke prevention in AF, treatment and prevention of DVT (deep vein thrombosis) and PE (pulmonary embolism).

Dose: 150 mg twice daily.

3. Milvexian

Introduction: Milvexian is a Factor XIa inhibitor, representing a new class of anticoagulants that provide effective clot prevention with a lower bleeding risk.

Clinical Trial Phase / FDA-Approval: Undergoing Phase III clinical trials for post-operative thromboprophylaxis and stroke prevention in AF.

Mechanism of Action:

a. **Selective and Reversible Factor XIa Inhibition**
   - Milvexian directly binds to Factor XIa, inhibiting its activity.
   - In contrast to the thrombin inhibitors (like dabigatran) or Factor Xa inhibitors (like rivaroxaban), milvexian targets an upstream step in the coagulation cascade, preventing thrombin generation while maintaining haemostasis.

b. **The Intrinsic Coagulation Pathway is Inhibited**
   - A crucial part of the clot formation propagation phase is played by Factor XIa.
   - By inhibiting Factor XIa, milvexian prevents thrombus formation while preserving normal haemostasis, reducing the risk of spontaneous bleeding.
   - Unlike heparins, it does not require antithrombin III for its activity.

c. **Minimal Impact on Primary Haemostasis**
   - Unlike vitamin K antagonists (VKAs) and direct orally acting anticoagulants (DOACs), milvexian does not inhibit thrombin or platelet function, reducing the risk of spontaneous and life-threatening bleeding.
   - Milvexian may be safer in high-risk bleeding populations (e.g. elderly, patients with gastrointestinal bleeding history).

Key Pharmacokinetic Parameters: Oral bioavailability is 25-30%. Food intake has no significant effect on absorption. Plasma protein binding is 85-90%. It is primarily metabolized via CYP3A4 enzymes in the liver. Plasma half-life is 12-16 hours. It is mainly excreted by faeces.

Adverse Drug Reactions: Gastrointestinal disturbances, headache, dizziness, elevated liver enzymes and minimal bleeding risk compared to traditional anticoagulants.

Uses: Stroke prevention in AF, postoperative VTE prevention, secondary prevention of acute Coronary Syndrome (ACS) and myocardial infarction (MI) (under investigation).

Dose: 25 mg to 200 mg once or twice daily (oral) (trial dosing).

4. Vorapaxar

Introduction: Vorapaxar is an antagonist of the thrombin receptor (PAR-1) used to prevent recurrent cardiovascular events in individuals with atherothrombosis.

Clinical Trial Phase / FDA-Approval: FDA-approved for secondary prevention of peripheral artery disease and myocardial infarction.

Mechanism of Action:

a. **Inhibition of PAR-1 Receptor on Platelets**
   - Thrombin activates platelets through attaching to the receptor-1 (PAR-1).
   - Vorapaxar competitively inhibits PAR-1, preventing thrombin from triggering platelet activation and aggregation.
   - Unlike P2Y12 inhibitors that prevent platelet activation mediated by ADP, vorapaxar specifically targets thrombin-induced platelet aggregation, a key driver of thrombosis.

b. **Prevention of Thrombus Formation Without Disrupting Haemostasis**
   - Since platelet aggregation is a central process in clot formation, vorapaxar reduces the risk of arterial thrombosis.
   - However, it does not significantly affect primary haemostasis, preserving normal bleeding functions compared to anticoagulants like warfarin or direct oral anticoagulants (DOACs).

c. **Long Half-Life and Sustained PAR-1 Inhibition**
   - Vorapaxar has a long half-life (8 days), resulting in sustained platelet inhibition for up to 4 weeks after discontinuation.
   - Due to this prolonged effect, no particular reversal agent exists, and bleeding complications may require platelet transfusion.

Key Pharmacokinetic Parameters: Oral bioavailability is 100%. CYP3A4-mediated hepatic metabolism is observed with this drug. Plasma protein binding is 99%, primarily to albumin. Undergoes faecal excretion. Plasma half-life is 8 days.

Adverse Drug Reactions: Intracranial haemorrhage in high-risk patients, headache, fatigue, and hypotension.

Uses: Secondary prevention of stroke and myocardial infarction.

Dose: 2.08 mg once daily (equivalent to 2.5 mg vorapaxar sulfate).

5. Bentracimab

Introduction: Bentracimab is a monoclonal antibody designed as a reversal agent for ticagrelor-induced bleeding.

Clinical Trial Phase / FDA-Approval: Currently under FDA priority review for ticagrelor reversal.

Mechanism of Action:

a. **High-Affinity Binding to Ticagrelor and Its Metabolites**
   - Ticagrelor works by binding reversibly to the P2Y12 receptor, preventing ADP-induced platelet aggregation.
   - Bentracimab binds directly to ticagrelor and its highly affinitized active metabolite (AR-C124910XX), neutralizing their inhibitory effects on platelet function.
   - This restores normal platelet aggregation and clot formation within 5-10 minutes of administration.

b. **Immediate and Sustained Reversal of Ticagrelor's Effects**
   - Unlike traditional platelet transfusions, bentracimab immediately restores platelet function, making it particularly useful in life-threatening bleeding events or emergency surgery.
   - Its effects are sustained for 12-24 hours, depending on the dose.

c. **No Effect on Normal Haemostasis**
   - Since bentracimab only binds to ticagrelor and its metabolites, it does not affect baseline platelet function or other coagulation pathways.
   - This minimizes the risk of prothrombotic complications compared to non-specific reversal strategies.

Key Pharmacokinetic Parameters: It is given over ten to fifteen minutes as an intravenous (i.v.) infusion. Onset of action occurs within 5 minutes and achieving near-complete reversal of ticagrelor's effects. Sustained and prolonged duration of action for 12-24 hours, depending on dose and infusion regimen. It is not metabolized by liver enzymes (CYP450-independent), reducing drug-drug interactions and is cleared via renal clearance and proteolytic degradation.

Adverse Drug Reactions: Injection-site reactions, headache, dizziness, and allergic reactions.

Uses: Reversal of ticagrelor-induced bleeding.

Dose: Initial IV bolus of 6 g followed by a continuous infusion of 6 g over 4 hours.

Conclusion

The field of antithrombotic therapy has undergone significant advancements, with newer agents offering improved efficacy, safety, and reversibility. Rivaroxaban and dabigatran have replaced warfarin as first-line anticoagulants, while milvexian represents a promising next-generation option. Vorapaxar provides additional platelet inhibition for secondary prevention, and bentracimab offers a critical reversal option in life-threatening bleeding situations. These advances have transformed thromboprophylaxis and continue to shape the future of cardiovascular medicine.

References

1. Doshi G, Nailwal N. A review on molecular mechanisms and patents of marine-derived anti-thrombotic agents. Current Drug Targets. 2021 Feb 1;22(3):318-35.
2. Raimova GM, Khoshimov NN, Nasirov KE, Turaev AS, Savutova ME. Anti-thrombotic action of sulfated polysaccharides on thrombosis caused by thromboplastin. Research Journal of Pharmacy and Technology. 2021;14(11):6085-8.
3. Schaefer A, Flierl U, Bauersachs J. Anti-thrombotic strategies in patients with atrial fibrillation undergoing PCI. Clinical research in cardiology. 2021 Jun;110(6):759-74.
4. Wendelboe AM, Raskob GE. Global burden of thrombosis: epidemiologic aspects. Circulation research. 2016 Apr 29;118(9):1340-7.
5. Weitz JI, Eikelboom JW, Samama MM. New antithrombotic drugs: antithrombotic therapy and prevention of thrombosis: American college of chest physicians evidence-based clinical practice guidelines. Chest. 2012 Feb 1;141(2):e120S-51S.

6. Esmon CT. Basic mechanisms and pathogenesis of venous thrombosis. Blood reviews. 2009 Sep 1;23(5):225-9.
7. Burghaus R, Coboeken K, Gaub T, Kuepfer L, Sensse A, Siegmund HU, et al. Evaluation of the efficacy and safety of rivaroxaban using a computer model for blood coagulation. PLoS One. 2011;6(4):e17626.
8. Mega JL, Simon T. Pharmacology of antithrombotic drugs: an assessment of oral antiplatelet and anticoagulant treatments. The Lancet. 2015 Jul 18;386(9990):281-91.
9. Ruff CT, Giugliano RP, Braunwald E, Hoffman EB, Deenadayalu N, Ezekowitz MD, Camm AJ, Weitz JI, Lewis BS, Parkhomenko A, Yamashita T. Comparison of the efficacy and safety of new oral anticoagulants with warfarin in patients with atrial fibrillation: a meta-analysis of randomised trials. The Lancet. 2014 Mar 15;383(9921):955-62.
10. Weitz JI, Fredenburgh JC. Factors XI and XII as targets for new anticoagulants. Frontiers in medicine. 2017 Feb 24;4:19.
11. Morrow DA, Braunwald E, Bonaca MP, Ameriso SF, Dalby AJ, Fish MP, Fox KA, Lipka LJ, Liu X, Nicolau JC, Ophuis AO. Vorapaxar in the secondary prevention of atherothrombotic events. New England Journal of Medicine. 2012 Apr 12;366(15):1404-13.
12. Eikelboom JW, Connolly SJ, Bosch J, Dagenais GR, Hart RG, Shestakovska O, Diaz R, Alings M, Lonn EM, Anand SS, Widimsky P. Rivaroxaban with or without aspirin in stable cardiovascular disease. New England Journal of Medicine. 2017 Oct 5;377(14):1319-30.
13. Connolly SJ, Ezekowitz MD, Yusuf S, Eikelboom J, Oldgren J, Parekh A, Pogue J, Reilly PA, Themeles E, Varrone J, Wang S. Dabigatran versus warfarin in patients with atrial fibrillation. New England journal of medicine. 2009 Sep 17;361(12):1139-51.
14. Rodrigues A, Gonçalves LR, Gregório T, Baldaia C, Santo GC, Gouveia J. Urgent Reversal of Direct Oral Anticoagulants in Critical and Life-Threatening Bleeding: A Multidisciplinary Expert Consensus. Journal of Clinical Medicine. 2024 Jan;13(22):6842.
15. Levy JH, Shaw JR, Castellucci LA, Connors JM, Douketis J, Lindhoff-Last E, Rocca B, Samama CM, Siegal D, Weitz JI. Reversal of direct oral anticoagulants: Guidance from the SSC of the ISTH: R1. Journal of Thrombosis and Haemostasis. 2024 Jul 17.
16. Laudani C, Capodanno D, Angiolillo DJ. The pharmacology of antiplatelet agents for primary, secondary, and tertiary prevention of ischemic stroke. Expert Opinion on Pharmacotherapy. 2024 Jul 2;25(10):1373-90.
17. Gelbenegger G, Jilma B. Clinical pharmacology of antiplatelet drugs. Expert Review of Clinical Pharmacology. 2022 Oct 3;15(10):1177-97.
18. Bontinis A, Bontinis V, Giannopoulos A, Kontes I, Manaki V, Pitoulias AG, Chorti A, Ktenidis K. The routine use of Rivaroxaban as thromboprophylaxis following endovenous thermal ablation. Vasa. 2025 Jan 31.
19. Birchansky J, Frishman WH. Milvexian: A Focus on a New Oral Anticoagulant that Targets Factor XIa for Thromboembolism Prophylaxis. Cardiology in Review. 2025 Jan 1;33(1):93-7.
20. Gupta R, Lin M, Mehta A, Aedma SK, Shah R, Ranchal P, Vyas AV, Singh S, Kluck B, Combs WG, Patel NC. Protease-activated receptor antagonist for reducing cardiovascular events–A review on Vorapaxar. Current Problems in Cardiology. 2023 Mar 1;48(3):101035.
21. Rim MH, Dean C, Aliaj E, Dandino M, Tanriverdi T, Levitsky AM. Recent and anticipated novel drug approvals (4Q 2024 through 3Q 2025). American Journal of Health-System Pharmacy. 2025 Mar 15;82(6):291-6.

Chapter 21

Newer Hypolipidemic Drugs

Author: Dr. Pranab Das

Introduction

A major modifiable risk factor for atherosclerotic cardiovascular disease (ASCVD) is dyslipidaemia, which is characterised by abnormal levels of triglycerides or cholesterol. Global morbidity and mortality from coronary artery disease and stroke remain high despite improvements in cardiovascular care. Statins and other lipid-lowering medications have long been the cornerstone of ASCVD prevention. Many patients, however, either do not achieve their desired lipid levels or are statin intolerant, which calls for alternative or combination treatment approaches, especially in situations like severe hypertriglyceridemia or familial hypercholesterolaemia.

Numerous innovative treatments have surfaced as a result of increased understanding of lipid metabolism. These include new oral medications like bempedoic acid, siRNA-based medications, PCSK9 inhibitors, and ANGPTL3 inhibitors. After a brief review of dyslipidaemia and its traditional treatments, this chapter focusses on new and developing treatments, their mechanisms, clinical effectiveness, and possible effects on lowering cardiovascular risk.

Historical Perspective

Over the past century, there has been a significant evolution in the management of dyslipidaemia due to the evident correlation between elevated low-density lipoprotein cholesterol (LDL-C) and atherosclerotic cardiovascular disease (ASCVD). The journey started in the 1950s when bile acid sequestrants were found to have a cholesterol-lowering effect. In the 1970s, Akira Endo's ground-breaking work began when he isolated compactin from Penicillium citrinum, which paved the way for the development of statins. Because statins are so effective at blocking HMG-CoA reductase, their approval in 1987 was a significant milestone that solidified statins as the mainstay of lipid-lowering treatment.

Even with their broad success, statins were insufficient for some patients, especially those who had statin intolerance or familial hypercholesterolaemia. The result of this was the 2002 release of ezetimibe, which blocks the absorption of intestinal cholesterol through the NPC1L1 transporter. When Nabil Seidah and associates discovered proprotein convertase subtilisin/kexin type 9 (PCSK9) and explained its function in the breakdown of LDL receptors in 2003, a significant paradigm shift took place. This finding paved the way for the creation of the 2015-approved monoclonal antibodies evolocumab and alirocumab, which improved LDL receptor recycling and dramatically reduced LDL-C.

In the field of lipid management, RNA-based treatments have become increasingly effective in recent times. A small interfering RNA (siRNA) that targets PCSK9 mRNA, inclisiran was approved in 2020 and provides long-lasting LDL-C reduction with biannual dosing. An additional non-statin alternative was made available with the development of bempedoic acid, an oral ATP citrate lyase inhibitor that was authorised in 2020. Other substances being studied include ANGPTL3 inhibitors, like evinacumab, which reduce LDL-C and triglycerides, especially in homozygous familial hypercholesterolaemia. For patients with complex lipid disorders and statin intolerance, these developments represent a step towards precision lipid management.

Definition

Dyslipidaemia broadly refers to abnormal levels of lipids in the blood that predispose individuals to atherosclerosis. The key lipid components implicated in cardiovascular risk include:

- **Low-Density Lipoprotein Cholesterol (LDL-C):** "Bad" cholesterol, whose elevation drives plaque formation in arterial walls.
- **High-Density Lipoprotein Cholesterol (HDL-C):** "Good" cholesterol, which aids in reverse cholesterol transport.
- **Triglycerides (TG):** Elevated triglycerides can contribute to pancreatitis and, when combined with other risk factors, heighten cardiovascular risk.

Although LDL-C reduction has taken centre stage in cardiovascular prevention, emerging data underscore the importance of addressing hypertriglyceridemia and low HDL-C in specific patient populations as well. Dyslipidaemia is often secondary to diet, obesity, metabolic syndrome, and genetic predispositions, but it can also be exacerbated by comorbidities (e.g. diabetes, hypothyroidism) or medications (e.g. steroids, antipsychotics). Proper management requires a comprehensive evaluation of lipid profiles, patient risk stratification, and individualized therapy.

It is through chylomicrons that dietary fats are transported; using VLDL for the transportation of triacyl glycerol resulting from de novo synthesis; a representation of the regulation of cholesterol synthesis and the uptake of LDL may be found in Figures 1, 2, and 3, respectively.

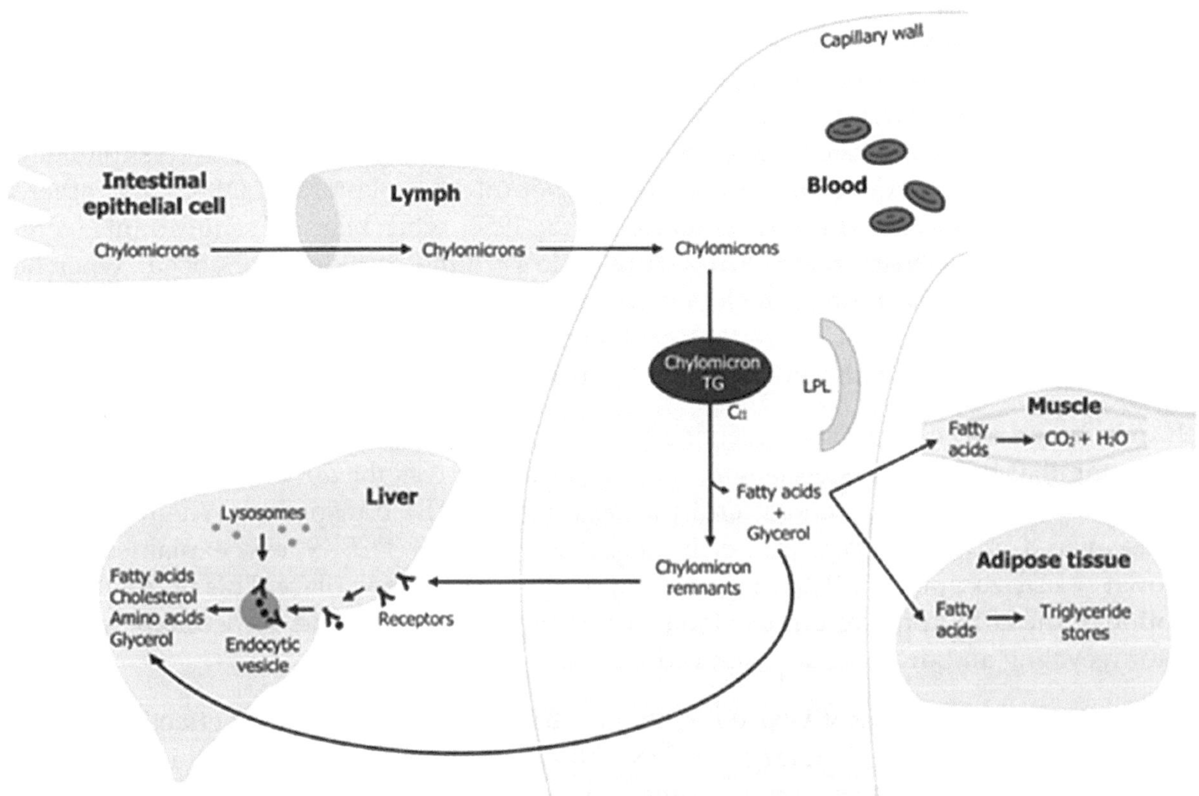

Figure 1: Transport of dietary lipids via chylomicrons (Source: Grey K. Lipoprotein metabolism and cholesterol synthesis).

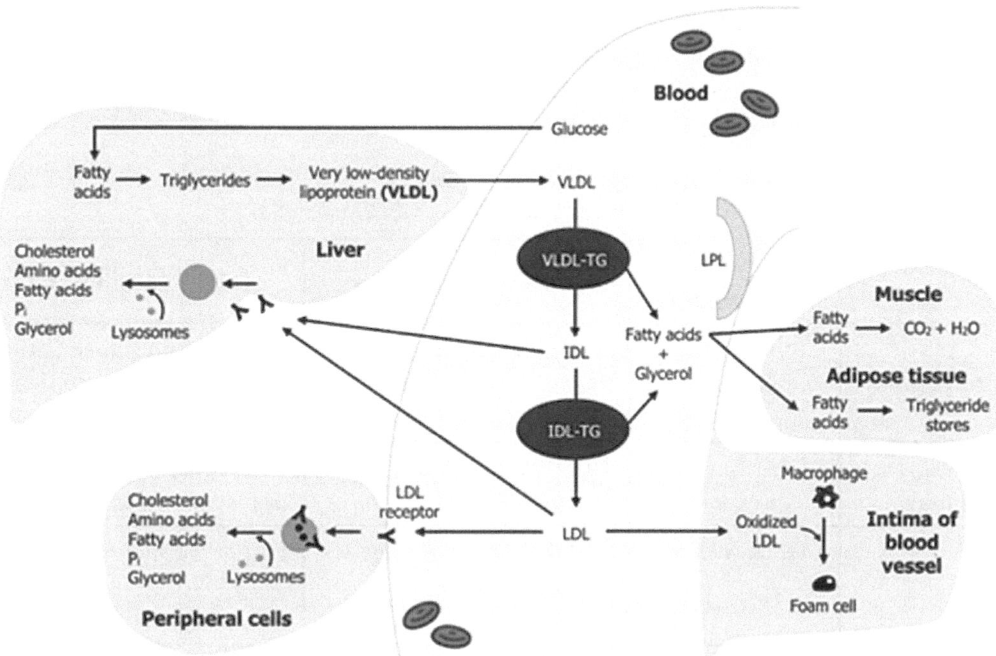

Figure 2: Transport of triacyl glycerol from de novo synthesis using VLDL (Source: Grey K. Lipoprotein metabolism and cholesterol synthesis).

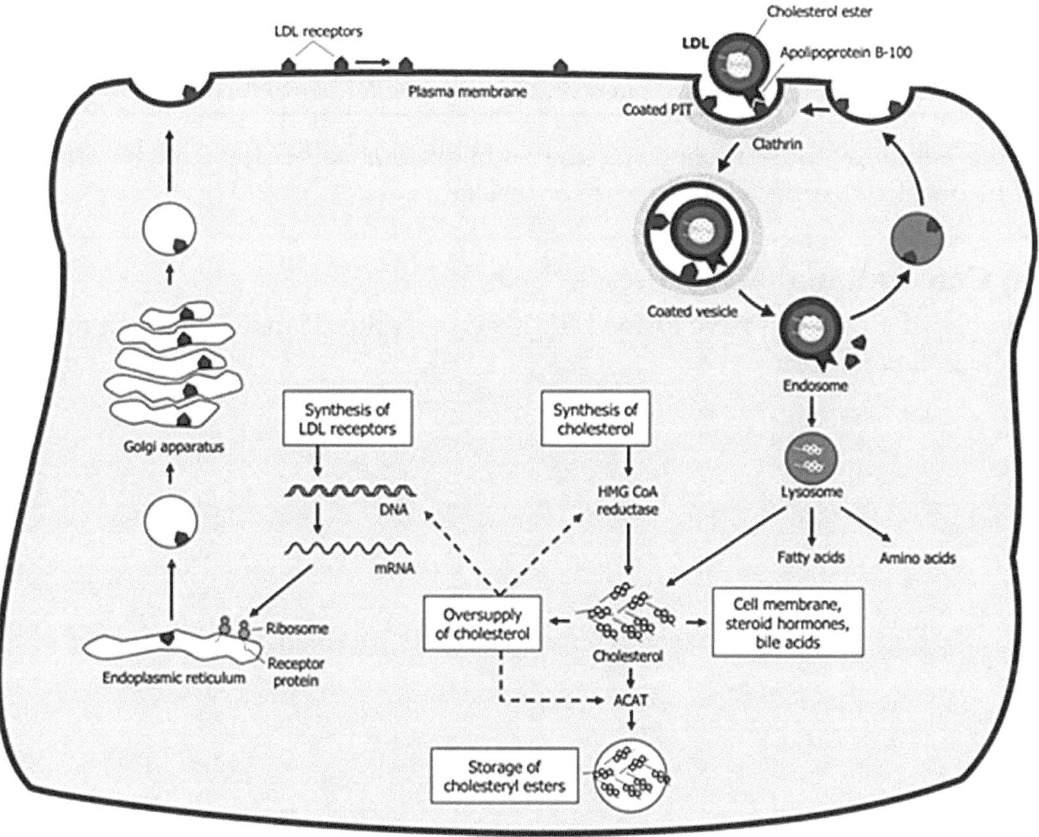

Figure 3: Uptake of LDL and regulation of cholesterol synthesis (Source: Grey K. Lipoprotein metabolism and cholesterol synthesis).

Types

Several classification systems categorize dyslipidaemias based on lipid patterns or aetiology. One frequently used approach is the Fredrickson classification, which divides dyslipidaemias into Types I–V based on the predominant lipoprotein abnormality:

Table 1: Different categories of dyslipidaemia.

Types	Elevated Lipoproteins	Lipid Abnormality	Common Causes
Type I (Hyperchylomicronaemia)	Chylomicrons	↑ Triglycerides (>1000 mg/dL)	Lipoprotein lipase (LPL) deficiency, ApoC-II deficiency (Rare, autosomal recessive)
Type IIa (Familial Hypercholesterolemia)	LDL	↑ LDL-C (>190 mg/dL), Normal TG	LDL receptor mutation, ApoB-100 defect (Familial hypercholesterolemia)
Type IIb (Familial Combined Hyperlipidaemia)	LDL & VLDL	↑ LDL-C, ↑ Triglycerides	Hepatic overproduction of VLDL
Type III (Dysbetalipoproteinemia)	IDL (Remnant Lipoproteins)	↑ Total cholesterol, ↑ Triglycerides	ApoE2 homozygosity (defective remnant clearance)
Type IV (Hypertriglyceridemia)	VLDL	↑ Triglycerides (200-500 mg/dL), Normal LDL	Increased hepatic VLDL production (common in metabolic syndrome, insulin resistance)
Type V (Mixed Hyperlipidaemia)	Chylomicrons & VLDL	↑ Triglycerides (>1000 mg/dL), Normal/↑ LDL	LPL deficiency + increased VLDL production (rare)

Recognition of the aetiology aids in choosing the right pharmacotherapy and identifying when newer treatments may be beneficial, especially in severe or resistant cases.

Brief Note on Conventional Medicines

Conventional hypolipidemic drugs have formed the basis of dyslipidaemia treatment for decades. Below is a concise overview in tabular form:

Table 2: Concise overview of classical hypolipidemic agents.

Drug Class / Drug Name	Mechanism of Action	Adverse Drug Reactions	Uses
Statins (e.g. Atorvastatin, Rosuvastatin)	Inhibit HMG-CoA reductase, the enzyme responsible for cholesterol synthesis in the liver. This leads to upregulation of LDL receptors in liver, increasing hepatic LDL clearance and reducing plasma LDL levels. Statins also decrease triglycerides and have anti-inflammatory, endothelial-protective, and plaque-stabilizing effects.	Common ADRs: Muscle pain, myopathy, fatigue, nausea, liver enzyme elevation. Serious ADRs: Rhabdomyolysis (rare), hepatotoxicity.	Primary hyperlipidaemia, prevention of cardiovascular disease (CVD), secondary prevention post-MI/stroke, familial hyperchole-sterolemia.
Bile Acid Sequestrants (e.g. Cholestyramine, Colestipol)	Bind bile acids in the intestine, preventing their reabsorption. This leads to upregulation of hepatic LDL receptors to synthesize more bile acids, thereby reducing plasma LDL levels.	Common ADRs: Constipation, bloating, nausea. Serious ADRs: Vitamin A, D, E, K deficiencies (due to fat malabsorption), increased triglycerides in some patients.	Primary hyperchole-sterolemia, adjunct therapy with statins, bile acid diarrhoea, pruritus in liver disease.
Fibrates (e.g. Fenofibrate, Gemfibrozil)	Activate peroxisome proliferator-activated receptor-alpha (PPAR-α), leading to increased lipoprotein lipase (LPL) activity, enhancing triglyceride breakdown and increasing HDL levels. They also reduce hepatic VLDL production.	Common ADRs: GI discomfort, headache. Serious ADRs: Myopathy (increased risk when combined with statins), gallstones, hepatotoxicity.	Hypertrigly-ceridemia, mixed dyslipidaemia, Type III hyperlipopro-teinemia, prevention of pancreatitis in severe hypertrigl-yceridemia
Niacin (Vitamin B3)	Inhibits hepatic triglyceride synthesis, reducing VLDL production, thereby lowering LDL and increasing HDL levels. Also reduces lipolysis in adipose tissue, decreasing free fatty acid flux to the liver.	Common ADRs: Flushing, itching, GI upset. Serious ADRs: Hepatotoxicity, hyperuricemia (may precipitate gout), insulin resistance.	Hyperchole-sterolemia, hypertriglyceridemia, used with statins in mixed dyslipidaemia.
Ezetimibe	Inhibits NPC1L1 transporter in the small intestine, reducing cholesterol absorption, leading to lower LDL and total cholesterol levels. Unlike statins, it does not affect triglycerides significantly.	Common ADRs: Fatigue, diarrhoea, headache. Serious ADRs: Rare hepatotoxicity, myopathy (when used with statins).	Primary hyperchole-sterolemia (especially in statin-intolerant patients), combination therapy with statins for additional LDL reduction.

While statins remain the foundational therapy for LDL-C reduction, many patients require additional lipid-lowering strategies. Combination therapies (e.g. statin + ezetimibe) are increasingly common for those failing to achieve LDL-C targets. Still, a notable proportion of patients experience statin intolerance or exhibit a suboptimal response, prompting interest in novel treatments.

Newer Drugs / Recent Advances

Recent years have seen a proliferation of innovative therapies that specifically target components of lipid metabolism. These agents often build on or bypass mechanisms conventional drugs do not fully address. Below is a summary of key novel therapies:

1. Evolocumab (PCSK9 Inhibitor)

Introduction: Evolocumab is a fully humanised monoclonal antibody (IgG2) that selectively inhibits proprotein convertase subtilisin/kexin type 9 (PCSK9). It is used primarily in patients with familial hypercholesterolemia (FH), statin-resistant hyperlipidaemia, and high cardiovascular risk.

Clinical Trial Phase / FDA-Approval: FDA-approved for familial hypercholesterolemia (FH) and atherosclerotic cardiovascular disease (ASCVD). Major trials: FOURIER, DESCARTES, OSLER-1, GLAGOV (demonstrated 50-60% LDL reduction).

Mechanism of Action: Evolocumab is a fully humanised monoclonal antibody (IgG2) that specifically inhibits proprotein convertase subtilisin/kexin type 9 (PCSK9). PCSK9 is a key regulator of LDL receptor (LDLR) degradation, making it an important target for lowering low-density lipoprotein cholesterol (LDL-C).

1. **LDL Receptor (LDLR) Recycling and PCSK9 Interaction**
   - Normally, LDLR binds to LDL-C on hepatocytes and facilitates its uptake and clearance from circulation.
   - PCSK9 binds to LDLR on the hepatocyte surface, promoting internalization and lysosomal degradation of LDL receptors, reducing LDL-C clearance.
   - This results in higher LDL-C levels in circulation, increasing the risk of atherosclerosis and cardiovascular disease (CVD).
2. **Inhibition of PCSK9 by Evolocumab**
   - Evolocumab binds to circulating PCSK9, preventing its interaction with LDL receptors.
   - Without PCSK9-mediated degradation, LDL receptors recycle back to the hepatocyte membrane, increasing the number of functional receptors.
   - This leads to enhanced LDL-C clearance, reducing plasma LDL-C by approximately 50-60%.
3. **Synergistic Effect with Statins**
   - Statins upregulate LDL receptor expression, increasing LDL clearance.
   - However, statins also increase PCSK9 levels, which can limit LDL receptor availability.
   - Evolocumab counteracts this effect by inhibiting PCSK9, leading to greater LDL reduction when used with statins (approximately 75% reduction).

Key Pharmacokinetic Parameters: It is administered by subcutaneous injection, reaching peak plasma concentration (Tmax) in 3-4 days. Evolocumab exhibits extensive plasma protein binding, with a volume of distribution of about 3.3 L. It does not cross the blood-brain barrier. It is degraded by reticuloendothelial and proteolytic pathways. It is cleared primarily via monoclonal antibody degradation pathways (not renally excreted).

Adverse Drug Reactions: Injection-site reactions, flu-like symptoms, cognitive impairment, myalgias and increased risk of diabetes.

Uses: Primary hypercholesterolemia, familial hypercholesterolemia (FH) and cardiovascular disease prevention (ASCVD, post-MI, stroke prevention).

Dose: 40 mg subcutaneously every 2 weeks or, 420 mg subcutaneously once monthly. Both regimens are considered therapeutically equivalent.

2. Inclisiran (siRNA Therapy for LDL Reduction)

Introduction: Inclisiran is an RNA-based therapy that reduces PCSK9 production at the genetic level. Unlike monoclonal antibodies (Evolocumab), Inclisiran offers longer-lasting LDL reduction with twice-yearly dosing.

Clinical Trial Phase / FDA-Approval: FDA-approved for hypercholesterolemia and ASCVD prevention. ORION Trials (ORION-9, ORION-10, ORION-11) confirm 50% LDL reduction.

Mechanism of Action: Inclisiran is a novel small interfering RNA (siRNA) therapy that reduces low-density lipoprotein cholesterol (LDL-C) by inhibiting proprotein convertase subtilisin/kexin type 9 (PCSK9) synthesis at the genetic level. Unlike PCSK9 monoclonal antibodies (e.g. Evolocumab), which neutralize circulating PCSK9, Inclisiran silences the PCSK9 gene in hepatocytes, offering a longer duration of action.

1. **Hepatic Uptake via GalNAc Conjugation**
   - Inclisiran is conjugated with N-acetylgalactosamine (GalNAc), allowing specific hepatocyte uptake via the asialoglycoprotein receptor (ASGPR).
   - This ensures liver-targeted delivery, minimizing systemic exposure and side effects.
2. **RNA Interference and PCSK9 mRNA Degradation**
   - Once inside hepatocytes, Inclisiran binds to the RNA-induced silencing complex (RISC), a key enzyme in RNA interference (RNAi).
   - The RISC complex guides Inclisiran to PCSK9 messenger RNA (mRNA), leading to mRNA degradation and inhibition of PCSK9 protein synthesis.
3. **Increased LDL Receptor Recycling and LDL Clearance**
   - Without PCSK9, LDL receptors (LDLR) are not degraded and continue to recycle back to the cell surface.
   - This results in enhanced LDL clearance from circulation, leading to 50-60% LDL reduction.
4. **Prolonged LDL-Lowering Effect**
   - Since Inclisiran acts at the mRNA level, it has a sustained duration of action, requiring only two doses per year.

Key Pharmacokinetic Parameters: It is administered as a subcutaneous (s.c.) injection, reaching peak plasma levels within 4-8 hours. It shows high hepatic uptake (90%), minimizing systemic side effects. Inclisiran is highly specific to the liver, with minimal plasma protein binding. It is metabolized by endogenous RNA degradation pathways. It is primarily excreted via hepatic pathways, with minimal renal excretion.

Adverse Drug Reactions: Mild injection-site reactions, mild flu-like symptoms, mild liver enzyme elevations but shows no significant muscle toxicity or neurocognitive issues.

Uses: Primary Hypercholesterolemia, Familial Hypercholesterolemia and Atherosclerotic Cardiovascular Disease (ASCVD) Prevention.

Dose: 284 mg administered subcutaneously; the dosage pattern is as follows: Administer the initial dose on Day 0; the subsequent dose at 3 months, followed by doses every 6 months afterward.

3. Bempedoic Acid (ATP-Citrate Lyase Inhibitor)

Introduction: Bempedoic acid is an oral lipid-lowering agent that reduces hepatic cholesterol synthesis, upstream of HMG-CoA reductase. It is particularly beneficial for statin-intolerant patients and those requiring additional LDL reduction.

Clinical Trial Phase / FDA-Approval: FDA-approved for hypercholesterolemia and ASCVD prevention. CLEAR trials (CLEAR Wisdom, CLEAR Harmony) confirm 17-25% LDL reduction.

Mechanism of Action: Bempedoic acid is a first-in-class ATP-citrate lyase (ACL) inhibitor that reduces low-density lipoprotein cholesterol (LDL-C) levels by inhibiting hepatic cholesterol biosynthesis upstream of HMG-CoA reductase (the target of statins).

1. **Hepatic Activation of Bempedoic Acid**
   - Bempedoic acid is a prodrug, meaning it must be converted into its active form to exert its effect.
   - It is activated by very-long-chain acyl-CoA synthetase 1 (ACSVL1), an enzyme expressed only in hepatocytes.
   - This liver-specific activation ensures that bempedoic acid does not accumulate in muscle tissue, reducing myopathy risk (a major issue with statins).
2. **Inhibition of ATP-Citrate Lyase (ACL)**
   - Once activated, bempedoic acid inhibits ATP-citrate lyase (ACL), a key enzyme in the cholesterol biosynthesis pathway.
   - ACL converts citrate into acetyl-CoA, the precursor for cholesterol synthesis.
   - By blocking ACL, bempedoic acid reduces cholesterol synthesis upstream of HMG-CoA reductase, leading to a decrease in intracellular cholesterol levels.
3. **Upregulation of LDL Receptors (LDLR)**
   - Reduced cholesterol synthesis triggers LDL receptor (LDLR) upregulation, similar to statins.
   - Increased LDL receptor expression enhances LDL clearance from the bloodstream, lowering plasma LDL-C levels (17-25%).
4. **Additional Anti-Inflammatory and Metabolic Effects**
   - Bempedoic acid activates AMP-activated protein kinase (AMPK) in immune cells, reducing C-reactive protein (CRP) and systemic inflammation.
   - It may also enhance insulin sensitivity and glucose metabolism, offering potential metabolic benefits.

Key Pharmacokinetic Parameters: It is rapidly absorbed after oral administration, reaching peak plasma concentration (Tmax) within 3-4 hours. It is highly plasma protein-bound (99%), leading to a low volume of distribution. It does not cross the blood-brain barrier, reducing the risk of neurocognitive side effects. Prodrug is being converted to its active CoA derivative in hepatocytes via ACSVL1-mediated activation. It is not metabolized by CYP450 enzymes, minimizing drug-drug interactions and is mainly excreted via urine.

Adverse Drug Reactions: Hyperuricemia, mild myalgias, liver enzyme elevation, tendon rupture but shows no significant neurocognitive effects.

Uses: Primary Hypercholesterolemia, Atherosclerotic Cardiovascular Disease (ASCVD) Prevention and statin-intolerant patients requiring LDL reduction.

Dose: 180 mg orally once daily.

4. Evinacumab (ANGPTL3 Inhibitor)

Introduction: Evinacumab is a fully humanised monoclonal antibody targeting angiopoietin-like protein 3 (ANGPTL3). It is used in homozygous familial hypercholesterolemia (HoFH) and severe hypertriglyceridemia.

Clinical Trial Phase / FDA-Approval: FDA-approved for HoFH and severe hypercholesterolemia. ELIPSE-HoFH trial confirmed 50% LDL-C reduction in HoFH patients.

Mechanism of Action: Evinacumab is a fully humanised monoclonal antibody (IgG4) that targets angiopoietin-like protein 3 (ANGPTL3), a key regulator of lipid metabolism. Unlike statins and PCSK9 inhibitors, which depend on low-density lipoprotein receptor (LDLR)-mediated clearance, evinacumab lowers LDL cholesterol (LDL-C) independently of LDLR, making it effective even in homozygous familial hypercholesterolemia (HoFH) patients who have defective LDL receptors.

1. **Inhibition of ANGPTL3**
   - ANGPTL3 is a key inhibitor of lipoprotein lipase (LPL) and endothelial lipase (EL).
   - In normal physiology, ANGPTL3 suppresses LPL and EL, reducing triglyceride and LDL clearance.
   - Evinacumab binds to ANGPTL3, preventing it from inhibiting LPL and EL, leading to increased enzyme activity and enhanced lipid breakdown.
2. **Increased Lipoprotein Clearance: By blocking ANGPTL3, evinacumab facilitates:**
   - Increased lipolysis of triglyceride-rich lipoproteins (VLDL, chylomicrons).
   - Enhanced clearance of LDL-C and non-HDL cholesterol (non-HDL-C).
3. **LDL-C Reduction Independent of LDL Receptors**
   - Unlike statins or PCSK9 inhibitors, evinacumab lowers LDL-C via a receptor-independent pathway.
   - This makes it effective in HoFH patients, where LDLR function is impaired.
4. **Additional Effects on Triglycerides and HDL Metabolism**
   - Reduces circulating triglycerides (50-70%), making it effective in severe hypertriglyceridemia.
   - May increase HDL clearance, but the clinical significance remains under investigation.

Key Pharmacokinetic Parameters: It is administered via intravenous infusion over 60 minutes, reaching peak plasma concentration in 6-8 hours. It is highly plasma protein-bound with a large volume of distribution (3.5 L), suggesting widespread extracellular penetration. It does not cross the blood-brain barrier. It is cleared via monoclonal antibody degradation pathways, mainly through reticuloendothelial phagocytosis and lysosomal degradation. It does not undergoes hepatic CYP450 metabolism, minimizing drug-drug interactions. Elimination is via biphasic clearance:

- **At low concentrations:** Rapid clearance due to target-mediated elimination (binding to ANGPTL3).
- **At high concentrations:** Slower clearance via nonspecific monoclonal antibody pathways.

Adverse Drug Reactions: Mild flu-like symptoms, nasopharyngitis, no significant neurocognitive effects or myopathy and rare hypersensitivity reactions (<1%).

Uses: Severe hypercholesterolemia, homozygous FH, hypertriglyceridemia, and resistant dyslipidaemia.

Dose: 15 mg/kg IV infusion administered over 1 hour, every 4 weeks.

5. Pemafibrate (Selective PPAR-α Modulator)

Introduction: Pemafibrate is a next-generation fibrate that selectively activates PPAR-α, improving triglyceride metabolism and HDL function.

Clinical Trial Phase / FDA-Approval: Currently in Phase 3 trials for hypertriglyceridemia and metabolic syndrome. PROMINENT trial (ongoing) evaluating its cardiovascular benefits. Approved in Japan.

Mechanism of Action: Pemafibrate is a novel selective peroxisome proliferator-activated receptor alpha (PPAR-α) modulator (SPPARM-α) designed to enhance lipid metabolism with greater efficacy and fewer side effects compared to conventional fibrates (e.g. fenofibrate, gemfibrozil).

1. **Selective PPAR-α Activation**
   - PPAR-α is a nuclear receptor that regulates genes involved in fatty acid oxidation, lipoprotein metabolism, and inflammation.
   - Unlike traditional fibrates, pemafibrate selectively binds to PPAR-α found primarily in liver and skeletal muscles with high affinity, enhancing its lipid-lowering effects while minimizing adverse events.
2. **Enhanced β-Oxidation of Fatty Acids in the Liver**
   - Pemafibrate upregulates key enzymes involved in fatty acid β-oxidation in hepatocytes.
   - This results in reduced hepatic triglyceride (TG) synthesis and secretion, lowering triglycerides (TG) and very-low-density lipoprotein (VLDL) production.
3. **Increased Lipoprotein Lipase (LPL) Activity**
   - Pemafibrate stimulates lipoprotein lipase (LPL), an enzyme that hydrolyzes triglycerides in VLDL and chylomicrons.
   - This promotes clearance of circulating triglycerides (TG), reducing plasma TG levels by 45-50%.
4. **Modulation of HDL and LDL Metabolism**
   - Increases apolipoprotein A-I (ApoA-I) and ApoA-II expression, leading to higher high-density lipoprotein cholesterol (HDL-C) levels.
   - Decreases small dense LDL (sdLDL), a highly atherogenic LDL subtype.
5. **Anti-Inflammatory and Vascular Protective Effects**
   - Reduces vascular inflammation by inhibiting NF-κB and pro-inflammatory cytokines (e.g. IL-6, TNF-α).
   - Decreases oxidative stress and endothelial dysfunction, potentially reducing atherosclerosis risk.

Key Pharmacokinetics Parameters: It is rapidly absorbed after oral administration, reaching peak plasma concentration (Tmax) within 6 hours. It is highly plasma protein-bound (99%). It is primarily metabolized via hepatic UGT1A3 and UGT2B7 pathways (glucuronidation) and is excreted primarily in faeces.

Adverse Drug Reactions: Mild GI symptoms, increased liver enzymes, no significant rhabdomyolysis risk (unlike gemfibrozil) and minimal renal toxicity compared to older fibrates.

Uses: Hypertriglyceridemia, non-alcoholic fatty liver disease (NAFLD), adjunct therapy in metabolic syndrome and diabetes-related dyslipidaemia.

Dose: 0.2 mg orally twice daily (PROMINENT trial dosing).

Key Therapeutic Targets & Strategies

1. **PCSK9 Pathway:** The discovery that PCSK9 promotes LDL receptor degradation revolutionized lipid pharmacology. Monoclonal antibodies (e.g. alirocumab, evolocumab) and siRNA-based therapies (e.g. inclisiran) offer powerful LDL-C reductions on top of statins. These agents are particularly valuable for patients with familial hypercholesterolemia or those who remain at high risk despite maximally tolerated statin therapy.

2. **Upstream Enzyme Blockade:** Bempedoic acid represents a novel approach by inhibiting ATP citrate lyase (ACL), an enzyme upstream of HMG-CoA reductase. This allows further reduction in cholesterol synthesis without directly targeting the same pathway as statins, thereby mitigating some statin-associated side effects. Bempedoic acid is particularly helpful in patients who cannot tolerate high-dose statins or who demonstrate partial statin intolerance.

3. **ANGPTL3 Inhibition:** ANGPTL3 is a regulator of lipoprotein metabolism, influencing the breakdown of triglycerides and lipoproteins. Its inhibition (e.g. evinacumab) has shown promise for severe familial hypercholesterolemia, achieving additional LDL-C and triglyceride reductions beyond what is typically possible with existing therapies. This strategy underscores the growing recognition that multi-target lipid management may yield superior outcomes, especially in genetic dyslipidaemias.

4. **Refined Fibrate Therapy:** While traditional fibrates can be effective in lowering triglycerides, concerns over drug interactions (particularly with statins), potential hepatotoxicity, and variable cardiovascular outcomes have tempered their widespread use. Next-generation fibrates like pemafibrate aim to achieve potent PPAR-α\alpha activation with fewer adverse effects, potentially making them safer and more effective in patients with mixed or hypertriglyceridemia dyslipidaemia.

5. **Combination Therapy and Personalized Approaches:** In practice, combination regimens are increasingly common as clinicians tailor lipid-lowering therapy to an individual's genetic background, comorbidities, and tolerance profile. A patient with severe hypercholesterolemia might require a statin, ezetimibe, and a PCSK9 inhibitor. Another patient with predominant hypertriglyceridemia may benefit from a refined fibrate or omega-3 fatty acids coupled with dietary adjustments. Emerging genetic tools and biomarkers may further enable personalized lipid management, matching specific drugs to the patient's lipid phenotype or genotype.

Conclusion

Treatment options for dyslipidaemia have increased due to the development of newer hypolipidemic medications, which fill the gaps left by fibrates, ezetimibe, and statins. By blocking PCSK9, Evolocumab and Inclisiran have revolutionised LDL-C lowering techniques. Inclisiran offers the benefit of twice-yearly dosing. For patients intolerant to statins, bempedoic acid offers an oral substitute, and for severe lipid disorders, evinacumab targets ANGPTL3. The next-generation fibrate pemafibrate improves triglyceride metabolism while causing fewer adverse effects on the muscles. These medications are anticipated to play a major role in precision lipid management in high-risk and statin-intolerant populations as ongoing clinical trials improve dosage schedules, long-term safety, and cardiovascular outcome data.

References

1. Espinós C, Turró R, Abad R, et al. Bariatric endoscopy: an innovative approach to obesity management. *World J Gastrointest Endosc*. 2022;14(1):11–25.
2. Benjamin EJ, Muntner P, Alonso A, et al. Heart disease and stroke statistics—2019 update: a report from the American Heart Association. *Circulation*. 2019;139:e56–e528.
3. Arnett DK, Blumenthal RS, Albert MA, et al. 2019 ACC/AHA guideline on the primary prevention of cardiovascular disease. *Circulation*. 2019;140(11):e596–e646.

4. Ference BA, Ginsberg HN, Graham I, et al. Low-density lipoproteins cause atherosclerotic cardiovascular disease. 1. Evidence from genetic, epidemiologic, and clinical studies. *Eur Heart* J. 2017;38(32):2459–2472.
5. Nordestgaard BG, Chapman MJ, Ray K, et al. Lipoprotein(a) as a cardiovascular risk factor: current status. *Eur Heart* J. 2010;31(23):2844–2853.
6. Brown MS, Goldstein JL. How LDL receptors influence cholesterol and atherosclerosis. *Sci Am*. 1984;251(5):58–66.
7. Sabatine MS, Giugliano RP, Keech AC, et al. Evolocumab and clinical outcomes in patients with cardiovascular disease. *N Engl J Med.* 2017;376(18):1713–1722.
8. Ray KK, Landmesser U, Leiter LA, et al. Inclisiran in patients at high cardiovascular risk with elevated LDL cholesterol. *N Engl J Med*. 2017;376(15):1430–1440.
9. Goldberg AC, Leiter LA, Stroes ESG, et al. Effect of bempedoic acid vs placebo added to maximally tolerated statins on low-density lipoprotein cholesterol in patients at high risk for ASCVD. *JAMA.* 2019;322(18):1780–1788.
10. Raal F, Rosenson RS, Reeskamp LF, et al. Evinacumab for homozygous familial hypercholesterolemia. N Engl J Med. 2020;383(8):711–720.
11. Grey K. Lipoprotein metabolism and cholesterol synthesis [Internet]. In: Jakubowski H, editor. *Cell Biology, Genetics, and Biochemistry for Pre-Clinical Students*. Blacksburg (VA): Virginia Tech Publishing; 2021 [cited 2025 Jun 7]. Available from: https://pressbooks.lib.vt.edu/cellbio/chapter/lipoprotein-metabolism-and-cholesterol-synthesis/.
12. Ishibashi S. Pemafibrate, a new selective PPAR-alpha modulator: lessons from basic research to clinical practice. *Expert Opin Pharmacother*. 2019;20(2):173–185.
13. Khera AV, Everett BM, Caulfield MP, et al. Lipid-lowering therapies: a new era. *N Engl J Med*. 2023;388(3):274–288.
14. Ballantyne CM, Laufs U. PCSK9 inhibitors and siRNA: advances in lipid management. *Eur Heart J*.2022;43(19):1941–1953.
15. Brunton LL, Hilal-Dandan R, Knollmann BC, editors. Goodman & Gilman's The Pharmacological Basis of Therapeutics. 14th ed. New York: McGraw-Hill Education; 2022.
16. NICE Lipid Modification Guidelines. Bempedoic acid adverse effects. *Available from*: www.nice.org.uk.
17. Bays HE, Taub PR, Epstein E, et al. Ten things to know about lipid management in 2022. *J Clin Lipidol*.2022;16(2):117–137.
18. Stein EA, Raal FJ. New and emerging strategies for reducing LDL cholesterol. *Nat Rev Endocrinol*.2022;18(7):395–410.
19. Ray KK, Wright RS, Kallend D, et al. Two phase 3 trials of Inclisiran in patients with elevated LDL cholesterol. *N Engl J Med*. 2020;382(16):1507–1519.
20. Toth PP, Hull M, Granowitz C, et al. Inclisiran: a review of LDL-C lowering and current clinical trial results. *J Clin Lipidol.* 2021;15(4):415–428.
21. Kosmas CE, DeJesus E, Morcelo R, et al. Bempedoic acid and its role in lipid-lowering therapy. *Curr Atheroscler Rep*. 2020;22(12):71.
22. Stein EA, Raal FJ. An update on PCSK9 inhibition and its future directions. *Curr OpinLipidol.* 2021;32(5):265–272.
23. Yamazaki T, Sasaki Y, Hattori Y, et al. Pharmacological properties of Pemafibrate, a novel selective PPAR-α modulator. *J Clin Med*. 2020;9(5):1600.

Section 5

Respiratory System

Chapter 22

Recent Advances in the Management of Bronchial Asthma

Author: Dr. Pranab Das

Introduction

Bronchial asthma is a common chronic inflammatory disease of the airways, characterized by episodes of wheezing, coughing, chest tightness, and shortness of breath. The underlying pathophysiology involves airway hyperresponsiveness (AHR) and reversible airflow obstruction, both of which are driven by complex immunologic and inflammatory processes. Asthma affects millions of people worldwide, posing a significant burden in terms of healthcare costs, reduced quality of life, and lost productivity. Over the last few decades, the management of bronchial asthma has undergone substantial evolution, driven primarily by improved understanding of immunopathologic mechanisms and the heterogeneous phenotypes of the disease. Historically, short-acting bronchodilators and inhaled corticosteroids (ICS) have been the mainstay of therapy. However, in patients with severe or difficult-to-treat asthma, these traditional approaches often prove insufficient. In response, the development of targeted biologic therapies, novel inhaler devices, and personalized management strategies has emerged, aiming to achieve more precise disease control and prevention of exacerbations.

This chapter reviews the definition and classification of asthma, briefly summarizes conventional medications, and highlights the latest therapeutic advances—including biologic agents targeting specific immunologic pathways, newly formulated inhaler devices, and digital health innovations.

Historical Perspective

Over the past century, the understanding and management of bronchial asthma has changed from symptomatic relief to targeted immunomodulatory strategies. Early 19th- and early 20th-century treatments, like the use of theophylline and epinephrine, produced short-term bronchodilation but lacked long-term control. The anti-inflammatory properties of cortisone, which Philip Hench pioneered, opened the door for systemic corticosteroids in the 1950s, revolutionising the treatment of both acute and chronic asthma. By providing local anti-inflammatory action with fewer systemic effects, inhaled corticosteroids (ICS), particularly beclomethasone, revolutionised the treatment of asthma in the 1970s. Salmeterol and other long-acting beta-agonists (LABAs) were developed in the 1980s and 1990s and, when combined with ICS, produced sustained bronchodilation.

With the introduction of omalizumab, the first monoclonal antibody that targets IgE, in 2003 for severe allergic asthma, the turn of the century signalled a move towards biologic therapies. The treatment options for eosinophilic and Type 2-high asthma phenotypes were then expanded by interleukin-targeted therapies such as mepolizumab, reslizumab, and benralizumab (anti-IL-5/IL-5R), and later dupilumab (anti-IL-4Rα). These developments, which allowed for more individualised and successful interventions, were supported by expanding knowledge of asthma endotypes and immunopathology. Today, a new era of precision medicine in asthma care has begun, with an emphasis on small-molecule therapies, biologics for non-Type 2 asthma, and digital health tools for adherence and monitoring.

Definition

Asthma is defined as a chronic inflammatory disorder of the airways that leads to episodes of airflow limitation. Characteristic features include variable expiratory airflow obstruction, airway hyperresponsiveness, and airway remodelling if not well controlled over time. The inflammation in asthma involves multiple cell types (e.g. eosinophils, mast cells, T lymphocytes) and cytokines. Although asthma can present at any age, childhood onset is common, and genetic predisposition (e.g. atopy) often plays an important role. Reversibility of airflow obstruction, typically demonstrated by a significant improvement in forced expiratory volume in 1 second (FEV1) after bronchodilator administration or with a course of corticosteroids, is a key functional hallmark of asthma. However, not all asthma patients display obvious reversibility, particularly those with more chronic, severe disease or airway remodelling.

Types of Asthma

Asthma is a highly heterogeneous disease, and classification can be approached from multiple perspectives (e.g. clinical severity, triggers, immunologic phenotypes). The Global Initiative for Asthma (GINA) guidelines focus on treatment steps rather than rigid subtypes; however, certain phenotypic or endotypic classifications can guide personalized therapy:

1. **Allergic (Atopic) Asthma**
   - Usually begins in childhood.
   - Associated with elevated immunoglobulin E (IgE) levels and eosinophilia.
   - Common triggers include allergens (e.g. dust mites, pollen, animal dander).
2. Non-Allergic (Non-Atopic) Asthma
   - Often adult-onset.
   - Not driven by classical IgE-mediated processes.
   - May be triggered by factors such as respiratory infections or irritants (e.g. pollutants, chemicals).
3. Eosinophilic Asthma (Type 2 High)
   - Marked by sputum or blood eosinophilia and often responds well to inhaled corticosteroids.
   - Biologic agents targeting IL-5 or IL-4/IL-13 pathways can be beneficial in severe cases.
4. Neutrophilic Asthma (Type 2 Low)
   - Associated with neutrophilic infiltration and often less responsive to corticosteroids.
   - May be observed in occupational exposures or in obese asthmatics.
5. Exercise-Induced Bronchoconstriction (EIB)
   - Manifests primarily with bronchospasm triggered by exercise or exertion.
   - Often coexists with other forms of asthma but can occur independently.

Classifying asthma by these phenotypes or endotypes (particularly Type 2 high v/s Type 2 low inflammation) helps to determine the most appropriate and effective therapies, especially when considering advanced biologics.

Brief Note on Conventional Medicines

For many years, asthma management has relied on a stepwise approach focused on controlling inflammation and bronchodilation. Below is a concise overview of standard or "conventional" therapies:

Table 1: Concise overview of conventional medications utilized in the management of bronchial asthma.

Drug Class / Drug Names	Mechanism of Action	Adverse Drug Reaction	Uses
Short-Acting Beta-2 Agonists (SABAs) (e.g. Albuterol/ Salbutamol)	Relax bronchial smooth muscle, providing rapid but short-lived bronchodilation.	Tachycardia, tremor, potential hypokalaemia.	Used for acute relief of bronchospasm (rescue inhaler).
Inhaled Corticosteroids (ICS) (e.g. Budesonide, Fluticasone)	Reduce airway inflammation by inhibiting inflammatory cytokine production and reducing eosinophil infiltration.	Oral thrush (candidiasis), hoarseness, possible systemic effects at high doses.	First-line controller therapy for persistent asthma; reduces airway inflammation.
Long-Acting Beta-2 Agonists (LABAs) (e.g. Salmeterol, Formoterol)	Provide prolonged bronchodilation (12–24 hours) by stimulating beta-2 receptors in airway smooth muscle.	Similar to SABAs (tachycardia, tremor), but less acute.	Used in combination with ICS for long-term asthma control.
Leukotriene Receptor Antagonists (LTRAs) (e.g. Montelukast)	Block leukotriene-mediated bronchoconstriction and inflammation.	Headache, GI upset, rare neuropsychiatric events (mood changes).	Used as an add-on therapy in asthma, especially in aspirin-sensitive or exercise-induced asthma.
Long-Acting Muscarinic Antagonists (LAMAs) (e.g. Tiotropium)	Block cholinergic (muscarinic) receptors, reducing bronchoconstriction and mucus production.	Dry mouth, blurred vision, possible urinary retention in predisposed individuals.	Used as an add-on therapy for severe asthma; improves bronchodilation.
Oral Corticosteroids (OCS) (e.g. Prednisone)	Systemic anti-inflammatory effects; used for exacerbations or severe, uncontrolled asthma.	Weight gain, osteoporosis, hyperglycaemia, adrenal suppression, mood changes.	Used for acute exacerbations and severe persistent asthma.

While these therapies are highly effective for most patients, some individuals experience persistent symptoms, recurrent exacerbations, or side effects that compromise adherence and disease control. Consequently, recent years have witnessed a surge in novel treatment strategies designed to meet the needs of patients with moderate-to-severe or refractory asthma.

Newer Drugs / Recent Advances

Rationale for Innovation

Asthma's complexity—especially in the severe or difficult-to-treat spectrum—has necessitated precision medicine approaches, targeting specific inflammatory pathways. The identification of Type 2-driven inflammation (via IL-4, IL-5, IL-13, and IgE) paved the way for biologic agents. Meanwhile, improved inhaler technologies, combination formulations, and digital health tools aim to boost medication adherence and optimize drug delivery. Below is a summarizing notable newer or emerging therapy, followed by a detailed exploration of each category:

1. Benralizumab

Introduction: Benralizumab is a monoclonal antibody that targets the IL-5 receptor alpha (IL-5Rα) on eosinophils and basophils, leading to their depletion. It is used for severe eosinophilic asthma.

Clinical Trial Phase/FDA-Approval: FDA-approved for severe eosinophilic asthma. Evaluated in SIROCCO and CALIMA trials, showing reduced asthma exacerbations.

Mechanism of Action:

1. **IL-5Rα Blockade and Eosinophil Depletion**
   - IL-5 is the primary cytokine responsible for eosinophil growth, survival, and activation.
   - Eosinophils contribute to airway inflammation in asthma by releasing toxic granules (major basic protein, eosinophil peroxidase), leading to epithelial damage, bronchial hyperresponsiveness, and airway remodelling.
   - Benralizumab binds to IL-5Rα on eosinophils, blocking IL-5 signalling and inducing rapid eosinophil apoptosis.
   - Unlike other IL-5 inhibitors (mepolizumab, reslizumab), benralizumab directly depletes eosinophils through ADCC, a process mediated by natural killer (NK) cells.
   - This elimination of eosinophils leads to sustained suppression of airway inflammation.
2. **Reduction of Airway Hyperresponsiveness and Mucus Production**
   - Eosinophils stimulate mucus-secreting goblet cells, leading to airway obstruction and exacerbations in asthma.
   - Benralizumab reduces eosinophil-induced mucus hypersecretion, improving airflow and reducing asthma symptoms.
3. **Long-Term Effects on Airway Remodelling**
   - Chronic eosinophilic inflammation contributes to fibrosis, subepithelial thickening, and airway narrowing, known as airway remodelling.
   - By depleting eosinophils, benralizumab reduces airway structural damage, leading to long-term lung function preservation.

Key Pharmacokinetic Parameters: Benralizumab is administered via subcutaneous injection, with a bioavailability of approximately 70%. It follows target-mediated drug disposition (TMDD), meaning its clearance depends on the availability of IL-5Rα-expressing eosinophils. After administration, peak plasma concentration (Tmax) is reached within 3–7 days. The volume of distribution (Vd) is approximately 5.2 L, indicating moderate tissue distribution. Benralizumab is metabolized via proteolytic degradation rather than hepatic enzymes, minimizing the risk of drug-drug interactions. Its half-life ($t\frac{1}{2}$) is approximately 15–20 days, allowing for monthly or bi-monthly dosing regimens. The drug is eliminated through the reticuloendothelial system, with no significant renal or hepatic clearance.

Adverse Drug Reactions: Headache, sore throat, hypersensitivity reactions and increased risk of infections (herpes zoster).

Uses: Approved for severe eosinophilic asthma in patients 12 years and older.

Dose: 30 mg subcutaneously every 4 weeks for the first 3 doses, then every 8 weeks thereafter.

2. Tezepelumab

Introduction: Tezepelumab is a monoclonal antibody targeting thymic stromal lymphopoietin (TSLP), a key cytokine in airway inflammation.

Clinical Trial Phase / FDA-Approval: FDA-approved for severe asthma. Evaluated in PATHWAY and NAVIGATOR trials, showing improved lung function and fewer exacerbations.

Mechanism of Action:

1. **TSLP Inhibition and Inflammatory Suppression**
    - TSLP is an epithelial cytokine released in response to allergens, pollutants, and infections.
    - It activates multiple immune cells [dendritic cells, mast cells, eosinophils, basophils, and type 2 helper (Th2) cells], driving inflammation.
    - Tezepelumab binds to TSLP, preventing its interaction with the TSLP receptor complex, leading to:
        a. Reduced dendritic cell activation, decreasing antigen presentation to Th2 cells.
        b. Suppression of IL-4, IL-5, IL-13, and IL-17 production, reducing eosinophilic and neutrophilic inflammation.
        c. Downregulation of IgE synthesis, decreasing allergic airway inflammation.
2. **Airway Hyperresponsiveness and Smooth Muscle Relaxation**
    - TSLP contributes to airway smooth muscle contraction, leading to bronchial hyperresponsiveness (BHR).
    - By blocking TSLP, tezepelumab reduces airway hyperreactivity, improving bronchodilation and airflow.
3. **Mucus Hypersecretion and Airway Remodelling Prevention**
    - TSLP promotes mucus-producing goblet cell hyperplasia, leading to airway obstruction.
    - Tezepelumab inhibits goblet cell activation, reducing mucus accumulation.
    - Long-term use prevents airway remodelling, preserving lung function.

Key Pharmacokinetic Parameters: Tezepelumab is administered subcutaneously at a recommended dose of 210 mg every 4 weeks. It has a high bioavailability (approximately 80%), with peak plasma concentrations (Tmax) reached in 3–7 days. Like other monoclonal antibodies, tezepelumab is degraded by proteolysis into small peptides and amino acids. It does not undergo hepatic metabolism, reducing the risk of drug-drug interactions. It is eliminated primarily via the reticuloendothelial system, without renal or hepatic clearance.

Adverse Drug Reactions: Nasopharyngitis, headache, arthralgia, fatigue, injection-site reactions (pain, redness, swelling) and hypersensitivity reactions.

Uses: Approved for severe asthma, including non-eosinophilic asthma.

Dose: 210 mg subcutaneously every 4 weeks.

3. Dupilumab

Introduction: Dupilumab is a monoclonal antibody targeting IL-4 and IL-13, both critical cytokines in asthma pathogenesis.

Clinical Trial Phase / FDA-Approval: FDA-approved for moderate-to-severe asthma. Evaluated in LIBERTY ASTHMA QUEST and VENTURE trials, showing significant reduction in oral corticosteroid use.

Mechanism of Action:

1. **IL-4Rα Blockade and Inhibition of Type 2 Inflammation**
   - IL-4 and IL-13 are central cytokines in type 2 inflammation, responsible for:
     1. Eosinophil recruitment.
     2. Airway hyperresponsiveness (AHR).
     3. Goblet cell hyperplasia and mucus overproduction.
   - Dupilumab binds to IL-4Rα, preventing IL-4 and IL-13 from activating downstream signalling pathways.
   - This leads to:
     1. Reduced eosinophilic airway inflammation.
     2. Decreased IL-5 production, lowering eosinophil survival and recruitment.
     3. Suppression of airway hyperreactivity, improving lung function.
2. **Inhibition of Mucus Hypersecretion**
   - IL-13 is a key regulator of mucus production by inducing goblet cell hyperplasia.
   - Dupilumab reduces IL-13-driven mucus overproduction, decreasing airway obstruction.
   - This effect reduces asthma exacerbations and improves airflow.
3. **Prevention of Airway Remodelling and Fibrosis**
   - Chronic type 2 inflammation leads to fibrosis, subepithelial thickening, and airway narrowing, known as airway remodelling.
   - IL-13 promotes collagen deposition and fibroblast activation, worsening lung function over time.
   - By blocking IL-13 signalling, dupilumab prevents airway remodelling, preserving long-term pulmonary function.

Key Pharmacokinetic Parameters: Dupilumab is administered subcutaneously (s.c.) at a loading dose of 600 mg, followed by 300 mg every 2 weeks. It has a bioavailability of approximately 64-80%, with peak plasma concentration (Tmax) occurring within 3–7 days after injection. Like other monoclonal antibodies, dupilumab is metabolized via proteolytic degradation into small peptides and amino acids. It does not undergo hepatic metabolism, minimizing the risk of drug-drug interactions. The plasma half-life is around 21–28 days, allowing for biweekly dosing.

Adverse Drug Reactions: Conjunctivitis, keratitis, hypersensitivity reactions, injection site reactions, and eosinophilic pneumonia.

Uses: Approved for moderate-to-severe asthma and corticosteroid-dependent asthma in patients ≥12 years.

Dose: 400 mg or 600 mg, followed by 200 mg or 300 mg subcutaneously every 2 weeks, depending on patient's weight and indication.

4. Rilzabrutinib

Introduction: Rilzabrutinib is a Bruton's Tyrosine Kinase (BTK) inhibitor, under investigation for severe allergic asthma.

Clinical Trial Phase / FDA-Approval: Phase III trials ongoing.

Mechanism of Action:

1. **Inhibition of Bruton's Tyrosine Kinase (BTK) and Mast Cell Activation**
   - BTK is a crucial enzyme in B cell receptor (BCR) and Fc receptor signalling pathways, which are involved in allergic and non-allergic asthma.
   - Activation of BTK in mast cells leads to degranulation and the release of histamine, leukotrienes, and prostaglandins, contributing to bronchoconstriction and airway hyperresponsiveness.
   - Rilzabrutinib binds to BTK in a reversible manner, preventing mast cell degranulation and reducing the release of pro-inflammatory mediators.
2. **Suppression of IgE-Mediated and Non-IgE Inflammatory Pathways**
   - BTK is involved in the cross-linking of IgE on mast cells, a key mechanism in allergic asthma.
   - By blocking BTK signalling, rilzabrutinib reduces IgE-mediated mast cell activation, preventing excessive immune responses to allergens.
   - In addition to allergic pathways, BTK also regulates neutrophilic inflammation, which plays a role in non-type 2 (T2-low) asthma.
3. **Modulation of B Cell Function and Cytokine Production**
   - BTK activation in B cells enhances antigen presentation and cytokine production, including IL-4, IL-5, and IL-13, which contribute to airway inflammation.
   - By inhibiting BTK, rilzabrutinib suppresses B cell activation, reducing excessive cytokine release and decreasing inflammation.
   - This mechanism suggests potential benefits for both eosinophilic and non-eosinophilic asthma subtypes.

Key Pharmacokinetic Parameters: Rilzabrutinib is orally administered, with rapid absorption and peak plasma concentration (Tmax) occurring within 1–3 hours post-dose. It has a high bioavailability, allowing for twice-daily dosing in clinical studies. Rilzabrutinib is primarily metabolized via hepatic cytochrome P450 enzymes (CYP3A4, CYP2C9, CYP1A2) and undergoes oxidation and conjugation reactions. It is converted into multiple inactive metabolites. The drug has a half-life ($t\frac{1}{2}$) of approximately 4–8 hours, supporting twice-daily dosing. It is excreted primarily in urine and partly in faeces, with minimal renal clearance of the parent drug.

Adverse Drug Reactions: Headache, nausea, dizziness, increased infection risk, neutropenia, and lymphopenia.

Uses: Under investigation for use in asthma and chronic urticaria.

Dose: 200 mg orally twice daily used in early asthma trials.

5. Fevipiprant

Introduction: Fevipiprant is a prostaglandin D2 receptor antagonist (CRTh2 inhibitor), reducing inflammatory cell recruitment.

Clinical Trial Phase / FDA-Approval: Phase III trials completed, but not FDA-approved due to efficacy concerns.

Mechanism of Action:

1. **Inhibition of DP2 (CRTh2) Receptor on Immune Cells:**
   - The DP2 (CRTh2) receptor is activated by prostaglandin D2 (PGD2), leading to:
     1. Eosinophil recruitment and survival, worsening airway inflammation.
     2. Th2 lymphocyte activation, increasing IL-4, IL-5, and IL-13 secretion.
     3. ILC2 activation, amplifying type 2 inflammation in the lungs.
   - Fevipiprant blocks the DP2 receptor, preventing PGD2-induced inflammation, resulting in:
     I. Reduced eosinophil chemotaxis and activation.
     II. Decreased Th2 cytokine production, lowering airway inflammation.
     III. Suppression of mucus hypersecretion and airway remodelling.
2. **Eosinophil Apoptosis and Airway Inflammation Reduction**
   - Eosinophils drive airway inflammation and tissue damage in asthma.
   - Fevipiprant promotes eosinophil apoptosis by blocking DP2 signalling, reducing airway eosinophilia and improving lung function.
3. **Prevention of Airway Remodelling**
   - PGD2 signalling via DP2 contributes to fibrosis, smooth muscle hypertrophy, and goblet cell hyperplasia.
   - Fevipiprant inhibits these pathways, potentially preventing long-term airway remodelling.

Key Pharmacokinetic Parameters: Fevipiprant is rapidly absorbed after oral administration, reaching peak plasma concentration (Tmax) within 1-3 hours. It has a high oral bioavailability (approximately 70–80%) and demonstrates linear pharmacokinetics over therapeutic doses. The drug is moderately protein-bound (approximately 60–80%) in plasma and distributes well into tissues, including the lungs. Fevipiprant undergoes hepatic metabolism, primarily via cytochrome P450 enzymes (CYP3A4 and CYP2C8), forming inactive metabolites. It has a half-life ($t\frac{1}{2}$) of approximately 18–20 hours, allowing for once-daily dosing. The drug is excreted mainly through faeces (approximately 80%) and urine (approximately 20%), with minimal renal clearance. Importantly, no significant drug-drug interactions (DDIs) were observed in trials, making it a low-risk candidate for polypharmacy regimens in asthma management.

Adverse Drug Reactions: Nausea, diarrhoea, dyspepsia, headache, elevated liver enzymes, QT prolongation and increased risk of opportunistic infections.

Uses: Under investigation for use in severe asthma.

Dose: 150 mg or 450 mg once daily (oral) in Phase II/III studies.

6. Other recent advances in the treatment of bronchial asthma:

1. **Smart Inhalers / Digital Health:** Poor medication adherence is a major contributor to suboptimal asthma control. Smart inhalers incorporate sensors that track usage frequency, technique, and peak

flow or symptom scores. These data are transmitted to mobile applications or cloud platforms, offering real-time feedback and reminders for patients as well as usage insights for clinicians. By improving adherence and allowing earlier detection of deteriorating control, smart inhaler technology can reduce exacerbations and healthcare utilization. Furthermore, digital health solutions facilitate telemedicine-based asthma reviews, beneficial in remote or underserved populations. While privacy and data security concerns exist, the potential to personalize and optimize therapy is substantial.

2. **Triple Combination Inhalers:** Traditionally, patients requiring multiple medications have used separate inhalers (e.g. ICS/LABA plus a separate LAMA inhaler). Triple combination inhalers (ICS + LABA + LAMA in one device) streamline regimens, thereby potentially enhancing adherence and simplifying the patient's regimen. Several large trials have shown that single-inhaler triple therapy can reduce exacerbations more effectively than dual therapy in patients with frequent exacerbations or suboptimal control, particularly those with features of both asthma and chronic obstructive pulmonary disease (COPD) overlap. Though not universally indicated for all asthmatics, they are a valuable option in moderate-to-severe disease.

3. **Novel Pathways Under Investigation (IL-17, IL-33, GM-CSF):** There is ongoing research into other inflammatory pathways implicated in the pathogenesis of asthma, particularly in non–Type 2 endotypes. Agents targeting IL-17 or IL-33, granulocyte-macrophage colony-stimulating factor (GM-CSF), and other novel cytokines or alarmins could further expand the armamentarium for patients who do not respond to current biologics. While some early clinical trials have shown promise (e.g. IL-33 inhibitors may reduce exacerbations), results are not yet sufficiently robust or consistent for regulatory approval. Personalized biomarker-based selection will likely be key to identifying the subset of patients who derive greatest benefit from these newer approaches.

Table 2: Additional latest developments in the control of bronchial asthma.

Drug / Strategy	Mechanism of Action	Clinical Trial Phase / Status	Adverse Drug Reactions	Distinctive / Salient Features
Anti-IgE Therapy (Omalizumab)	Binds free IgE, preventing interaction with mast cells and basophils, thus reducing the allergic response.	FDA-Approved for moderate-to-severe allergic asthma.	Injection site reactions, rare anaphylaxis.	First targeted biologic for allergic asthma; demonstrated reduction in exacerbations and steroid use in IgE-mediated disease.
Smart Inhalers / Digital Health	Inhaler devices with sensors transmitting usage data to apps, reminders, or healthcare providers to improve adherence.	Widely available or in advanced development.	Few direct adverse events; potential privacy concerns.	Offer real-time monitoring of inhaler use and technique, personalized feedback, improved adherence, potentially reducing exacerbations.
Triple Combination Inhalers	Combine ICS, LABA, and LAMA in a single inhaler for comprehensive airway targeting (inflammation, bronchoconstriction).	FDA-Approved for moderate-to-severe asthma.	Similar to ICS + LABA + LAMA (oropharyngeal candidiasis, tachycardia).	Improve adherence with single-inhaler therapy; shown to reduce exacerbations v/s. dual therapy in selected populations.

Biologics Targeting Novel Pathways (e.g. IL-17, IL-33, GM-CSF)	Target alternative inflammatory mediators, under investigation for steroid-refractory or non–Type 2 asthma phenotypes.	Phase II/III clinical trials, not yet widely approved.	Vary by agent; infection risk, injection site reactions.	Potential breakthrough for patients with non-eosinophilic, Type 2–low, or steroid-insensitive disease; still requiring robust clinical validation.

Conclusion

Over the past century, the understanding and management of bronchial asthma has changed from symptomatic relief to targeted immunomodulatory strategies. Early 19th- and early 20th-century treatments, like the use of theophylline and epinephrine, produced short-term bronchodilation but lacked long-term control. The anti-inflammatory properties of cortisone, which Philip Hench pioneered, opened the door for systemic corticosteroids in the 1950s, revolutionising the treatment of both acute and chronic asthma. By providing local anti-inflammatory action with fewer systemic effects, inhaled corticosteroids (ICS), particularly beclomethasone, revolutionised the treatment of asthma in the 1970s. Salmeterol and other long-acting beta-agonists (LABAs) were developed in the 1980s and 1990s and, when combined with ICS, produced sustained bronchodilation. With the introduction of omalizumab, the first monoclonal antibody that targets IgE, in 2003 for severe allergic asthma, the turn of the century signalled a move towards biologic therapies. The treatment options for eosinophilic and Type 2-high asthma phenotypes were then expanded by interleukin-targeted therapies such as mepolizumab, reslizumab, and benralizumab (anti-IL-5/IL-5R), and later dupilumab (anti-IL-4Rα). These developments, which allowed for more individualised and successful interventions, were supported by expanding knowledge of asthma endotypes and immunopathology. Today, a new era of precision medicine in asthma care has begun, with an emphasis on small-molecule therapies, biologics for non-Type 2 asthma, and digital health tools for adherence and monitoring.

References

1. Global Initiative for Asthma (GINA). Global strategy for asthma management and prevention. 2022 update [Internet]. Available from: https://ginasthma.org.
2. Umarova TA, Kudratova ZE, Maxmudova D. Pathogenesis of bronchial asthma development at the present stage. InInternational Conference on Modern Science and Scientific Studies 2024 Dec 11:21-24.
3. Ora J, De Marco P, Gabriele M, Cazzola M, Rogliani P. Exercise-Induced Asthma: Managing Respiratory Issues in Athletes. Journal of Functional Morphology and Kinesiology. 2024 Jan 3;9(1):15.
4. Lommatzsch M, Buhl R, Canonica GW, Ribas CD, Nagase H, Brusselle GG, Jackson DJ, Pavord ID, Korn S, Milger K, Taube C. Pioneering a paradigm shift in asthma management: remission as a treatment goal. The Lancet Respiratory Medicine. 2024 Feb 1;12(2):96-9.
5. Barnes PJ. The evolution of asthma treatment over the last 100 years. J Allergy Clin Immunol. 2011;128(1):3–8.
6. Fahy JV. Type 2 inflammation in asthma—present in most, absent in many. Nature Reviews Immunology. 2015 Jan;15(1):57-65.
7. Kostakou E, Kaniaris E, Filiou E, Vasileiadis I, Katsaounou P, Tzortzaki E, Koulouris N, Koutsoukou A, Rovina N. Acute severe asthma in adolescent and adult patients: current perspectives on assessment and management. Journal of clinical medicine. 2019 Aug 22;8(9):1283.
8. Busse W, Corren J, Lanier BQ, McAlary M, Fowler-Taylor A, Della Cioppa G, van As A, Gupta N. Omalizumab, anti-IgE recombinant humanized monoclonal antibody, for the treatment of severe allergic asthma. Journal of allergy and clinical immunology. 2001 Aug 1;108(2):184-90.
9. Busse WW, Kraft M, Rabe KF, Deniz Y, Rowe P, Ruddy M, et al. Reduction in asthma exacerbations with triple combination therapy of budesonide-glycopyrronium-formoterol: a randomized clinical trial. *Lancet.* 2018;392(10154):1199–209.
10. Elsevier. Benralizumab [Internet]. ScienceDirect Topics. Amsterdam: Elsevier; [cited 2025 Jun 7]. Available from: https://www.sciencedirect.com/topics/immunology-and-microbiology/benralizumab.
11. Castro M, Corren J, Pavord ID, Maspero J, Wenzel S, Rabe KF, Busse WW, Ford L, Sher L, FitzGerald JM, Katelaris C. Dupilumab efficacy and safety in moderate-to-severe uncontrolled asthma. New England journal of medicine. 2018 Jun 28;378(26):2486-96.
12. FitzGerald JM, Bleecker ER, Nair P, Korn S, Ohta K, Lommatzsch M, Ferguson GT, Busse WW, Barker P, Sproule S, Gilmartin G. Benralizumab, an anti-interleukin-5 receptor α monoclonal antibody, as add-on treatment for patients with severe,

uncontrolled, eosinophilic asthma (CALIMA): a randomised, double-blind, placebo-controlled phase 3 trial. The Lancet. 2016 Oct 29;388(10056):2128-41.

13. Nair P, Wenzel S, Rabe KF, Bourdin A, Lugogo NL, Kuna P, Barker P, Sproule S, Ponnarambil S, Goldman M. Oral glucocorticoid–sparing effect of benralizumab in severe asthma. New England journal of medicine. 2017 Jun 22;376(25):2448-58.
14. Menzies-Gow A, Corren J, Bourdin A, Chupp G, Israel E, Wechsler ME, Brightling CE, Griffiths JM, Hellqvist Å, Bowen K, Kaur P. Tezepelumab in adults and adolescents with severe, uncontrolled asthma. New England Journal of Medicine. 2021 May 13;384(19):1800-9.
15. Rabe KF, Nair P, Brusselle G, Maspero JF, Castro M, Sher L, Zhu H, Hamilton JD, Swanson BN, Khan A, Chao J. Efficacy and safety of dupilumab in glucocorticoid-dependent severe asthma. New England journal of medicine. 2018 Jun 28;378(26):2475-85.
16. Hussain M, Liu G. Eosinophilic asthma: pathophysiology and therapeutic horizons. Cells. 2024 Feb 23;13(5):384.
17. Brusselle GG, Koppelman GH. Biologic therapies for severe asthma. New England Journal of Medicine. 2022 Jan 13;386(2):157-71.
18. Porsbjerg CM, Sverrild A, Lloyd CM, Menzies-Gow AN, Bel EH. Anti-alarmins in asthma: targeting the airway epithelium with next-generation biologics. European Respiratory Journal. 2020 Nov 12;56(5).
19. Ramakrishnan S, Russell RE, Mahmood HR, Krassowska K, Melhorn J, Mwasuku C, Pavord ID, Bermejo-Sanchez L, Howell I, Mahdi M, Peterson S. Treating eosinophilic exacerbations of asthma and COPD with benralizumab (ABRA): a double-blind, double-dummy, active placebo-controlled randomised trial. The Lancet Respiratory Medicine. 2025 Jan 1;13(1):59-68.
20. Carpagnano GE, Dragonieri S, Resta E, Lulaj E, Montagnolo F, Portacci A, Magaletti P, Soccio P, Lacedonia D, Scioscia G. Short-term Tezepelumab effectiveness in patients with severe asthma: a multicenter study. Journal of Asthma. 2025 Mar 4;62(3):456-64.
21. Pavord ID, Rabe KF, Israel E, Szefler SJ, Brusselle G, Pandit-Abid N, Altincatal A, Chen Z, Amin N, Khan AH, Lederer DJ. Dupilumab induces long-term on-treatment clinical remission in patients with type 2 asthma. The Journal of Allergy and Clinical Immunology: In Practice. 2025 Jan 1;13(1):132-42.
22. Talia J, Sarbjit S, Lee CH, Sun I, Mikol V, Mannet L, Gereige J. Rilzabrutinib Improves Chronic Spontaneous Urticaria in Patients With and Without Allergic Comorbidities: A Subgroup Analysis From the RILECSU Study. Journal of Allergy and Clinical Immunology. 2025 Feb 1;155(2):AB227.
23. Jaiswal R, Ahmad S, Pandey S, Ali A, Jaiswal R, Yadav R, Yadav R, Ahsan R, Dwivedi T. Innovative Approaches to Eczema Treatment: A Review of Fevipiprant and Its Potential as a New Therapeutic Agent. Prostaglandins & Other Lipid Mediators. 2024 Dec 29:106946.

Chapter 23

Recent Advances in the Management of Pulmonary Hypertension

Author: Dr. Pranab Das

Introduction

Elevated pulmonary arterial pressure is the hallmark of pulmonary hypertension (PH), a pathological condition that leads to progressive right ventricular (RV) dysfunction and, if treatment is not received, it eventually progresses to right heart failure. Pulmonary hypertension markedly diminishes quality of life and is linked to considerable morbidity and mortality. As our comprehension of the molecular underpinnings of pulmonary hypertension has advanced, so have our treatment strategies. In the last ten years, various innovative medicines and interventional methods have been developed to target the multiple pathways involved in disease pathogenesis—vasoconstriction, vascular remodelling, inflammation, and thrombosis.

Historically, pulmonary hypertension was seen as an uncommon and invariably lethal condition. Nonetheless, progress in diagnoses, targeted medicines, and multidisciplinary care has extended survival and enhanced symptom management for numerous patients. Notwithstanding these favourable advancements, problems remain, such as the precise phenotyping of various kinds of pulmonary hypertension, addressing drug resistance or inadequate responses, and guaranteeing equitable access to sophisticated treatments. This chapter offers a comprehensive overview of pulmonary hypertension, delineates traditional therapy, and emphasises innovative medicines and strategies that demonstrate potential in enhancing outcomes.

Historical Perspective

The development of targeted therapies and a better understanding of the pathobiology of pulmonary hypertension (PH) have helped to turn the disease from one that is consistently fatal to one that is manageable. Nitric oxide deficiency, elevated endothelin, and dysregulation of the prostacyclin pathway were recognised as key factors in pulmonary arterial hypertension (PAH), a subtype of PH, in the 1980s, marking the beginning of the therapeutic evolution. The first significant innovation was the creation of epoprostenol, a synthetic prostacyclin analogue, by Dr. Lewis Rubin and associates. Approved in 1995, it ushered in the era of prostacyclin-based therapy and showed survival benefit in PAH patients.

Actelion Pharmaceuticals' bosentan, the first oral endothelin receptor antagonist (ERA), was introduced in the late 1990s, making the endothelin pathway a target. Dr. Gérald Simonneau conducted extensive research on the drug. With its 2001 approval, it signalled a move towards oral therapies. At about the same time, phosphodiesterase-5 (PDE-5) inhibitors, such as sildenafil, which were first created to treat erectile dysfunction, were repurposed for PAH because of their ability to dilate the pulmonary vasculature. Following pivotal trials showing improved exercise capacity and haemodynamics, sildenafil was approved for PAH in 2005.

Other advancements included ambrisentan, a selective ERA, and tadalafil, another PDE-5 inhibitor, which offered once-daily dosing and improved tolerability. For patients who did not respond to PDE-5 inhibitors, riociguat, a soluble guanylate cyclase (sGC) stimulator, was created in 2013. This medication was the first to be approved for both chronic thromboembolic pulmonary hypertension (CTEPH) and PAH.

The development of oral prostacyclin receptor agonists, like selexipag, in the 2010s also made it possible to target the prostacyclin pathway without constant infusion. Subcutaneous and inhaled formulations, such as treprostinil, have enhanced drug delivery and patient convenience in more recent years. In order to improve long-term results, current approaches frequently include initial combination therapy that targets multiple pathways at once.

These advances highlight the move from symptom management to mechanism-based, precision therapy and reflect a growing understanding of PH as a multifactorial vascular disease. Currently, ongoing research is investigating new targets that could define the next era of treatment, such as metabolic modulators, tyrosine kinase inhibitors, and gene therapy.

Definition

The World Health Organization (WHO) currently defines pulmonary hypertension as a mean pulmonary artery pressure (mPAP) ≥20 mmHg (revised from the previous threshold of 25 mmHg), measured via right heart catheterization, together with a pulmonary vascular resistance (PVR) ≥3 Wood units in the presence of a normal pulmonary capillary wedge pressure (PCWP) (≤15 mmHg). According to its aetiology, PH is divided into five groups:

1. Pulmonary Arterial Hypertension (PAH) is Group 1.
2. Group 2: Left Heart Disease-Related PH.
3. Group 3: PH brought on by hypoxia and/or lung diseases.
4. Chronic Thromboembolic Pulmonary Hypertension (CTEPH) is Group 4.
5. Group 5: Uncertain Multifactorial Mechanisms in PH.

The pathophysiology, prognosis, and management considerations vary amongst each category. Group 1 (PAH), where several signalling pathways have been found and targeted, has seen the biggest advancements in pharmaceutical innovation.

Pathophysiology

Because of its unique pathology, which includes dysfunctions in three important pathways, pulmonary arterial hypertension (Group 1) is frequently the focus of drug development within the larger classification:

1. **Prostacyclin Pathway:** Decreased prostacyclin (PGI2) production results in reduced vasodilatory and antiproliferative effects.
2. **Nitric Oxide (NO) Pathway:** Reduced cyclic guanosine monophosphate (cGMP)-mediated vasodilation results from impaired nitric oxide synthesis and elevated phosphodiesterase-5 (PDE-5) activity.
3. **Endothelin Pathway:** Excessive vasoconstriction and vascular remodelling are brought on by endothelin-1 overproduction.

Brief Note on Conventional Medicines

Traditional or "conventional" therapies for PH include general supportive measures and first-generation targeted treatments. Below is a concise summary of these approaches:

Table 1: Concise overview of conventional medications utilized in the management of pulmonary hypertension.

Drug Class / Drug Name	Mechanism of Action	Adverse Drug Reactions	Uses
Diuretics (e.g. Furosemide)	Reduce volume overload (preload) and right ventricular strain by promoting natriuresis and diuresis.	Hypokalaemia, hyperglycaemia, orthostatic hypotension, hyperuricemia.	Used for symptomatic relief of fluid overload in PAH.
Anticoagulants (e.g. Warfarin, Rivaroxaban)	Reduce thrombotic complications, especially in CTEPH or advanced PAH.	Bleeding, haemorrhage, INR fluctuations (Warfarin).	Considered in PAH patients at high risk of thrombosis, particularly those with idiopathic PAH.
Calcium Channel Blockers (e.g. Amlodipine, Diltiazem)	Reduce pulmonary vasoconstriction, lower pulmonary vascular resistance (PVR), and enhance right ventricular function by blocking L-type calcium channels. Only in patients with vasoreactive PAH, this drug is effective.	Hypotension, flushing, lower limb oedema, dizziness, bradycardia (Diltiazem)	Used only in vasoreactive PAH (patients who respond to vasodilator testing). Not effective for severe PAH.
Endothelin Receptor Antagonists (e.g. Bosentan, Ambrisentan)	Block endothelin-1 (ET-1) receptors, reducing vasoconstriction, smooth muscle proliferation and vascular remodelling in pulmonary arteries. Improves exercise capacity and delays disease progression.	Hepatotoxicity (Bosentan), peripheral oedema, nasopharyngitis, anaemia.	First-line therapy for PAH (WHO Group 1). Used in mild to moderate PAH to improve exercise tolerance and symptoms.
Phospho-diesterase-5 Inhibitors (e.g. Sildenafil, Tadalafil)	PDE-5 inhibition raises cGMP levels, which promotes better oxygenation and NO-mediated pulmonary vasodilation, lowers the afterload in the right ventricle.	Priapism, headache, flushing, hypotension, and visual abnormalities (blue-tinged vision with sildenafil).	Utilised as the primary treatment in PAH WHO Group 1 to enhance haemodynamics and exercise capacity.
Prostacyclin Analogues (e.g. Epoprostenol, Treprostinil)	Imitate prostacyclin (PGI2), which causes antiproliferative effects on vascular smooth muscle, inhibition of platelet aggregation, and vasodilation.	Diarrhoea, hypotension, nausea, jaw pain, flushing, and site pain (i.v. or s.c. delivery).	Moderate to severe PAH.

With the help of these traditional treatments, PAH has changed from a disease that always results in death to one that many patients can manage but not cure. Individual reactions, however, differ, highlighting the necessity for more focused and sophisticated approaches.

Newer Drugs / Recent Advances

Current developments include new devices or interventions to support right heart function, more stable formulations of existing agents, and continued research into new targets. Key emergent therapies and methods are outlined below:

1. Sotatercept

Introduction: Developed to treat PAH, sotatercept is a first-in-class activin signalling inhibitor. It focusses on vascular remodelling, which is a major factor in the development of PAH. In 2024, the FDA authorised it as a PAH (WHO Group 1) add-on therapy.

Clinical Trial Phase / FDA-Approval: FDA-approved for the treatment of PAHs in 2024. Significant improvements in exercise capacity and haemodynamics were demonstrated by the pivotal Phase 3 STELLAR trial.

Mechanism of Action:

1. **Inhibition of Activin A and Other TGF-β Ligands:** Activins and other TGF-β ligands encourage vascular remodelling, endothelial dysfunction, and smooth muscle proliferation in PAH. By binding to activins before they interact with their receptors, sotatercept functions as a ligand trap, decreasing the pro-proliferative effects of activins.
2. **Restoring BMPR2 Signalling:** PAH is linked to abnormalities in bone morphogenetic protein receptor type 2 (BMPR2), a crucial modulator of vascular homeostasis. Sotatercept works to restore BMPR2 signalling by blocking activins, and thereby itexerts anti-fibrotic and anti-proliferative effects on pulmonary arteries.
3. **Mitigation of Pulmonary Vascular Resistance (PVR):** Sotatercept improves pulmonary haemodynamics by reducing fibrosis and smooth muscle proliferation.
4. **Improvement in Right Ventricular Function:** Sotatercept lessens the strain on the right ventricle by lowering pulmonary artery pressure, which stops the progression of right heart failure.

Key Pharmacokinetic Parameters: It is given via subcutaneous injection, sotatercept shows a slow absorption profile, reaching peak levels within 2–5 days post-administration. It shows high plasma protein binding of around 95%. Degraded via proteolysis in the reticuloendothelial system. No metabolism via cytochrome P450 (CYP450) enzymes, minimizing drug interactions. Plasma half-life is around 25-30 days, allowing for monthly dosing.

Adverse Drug Reactions: Fatigue, headache, dizziness, increased haemoglobin and haematocrit levels and mild gastrointestinal disturbances (nausea, diarrhoea).

Uses: Approved for PAH (WHO Group 1) as an add-on therapy to improve exercise capacity and haemodynamics.

Dose: Subcutaneously, 0.3 mg/kg or 0.7 mg/kg every three weeks.

2. Selexipag

Introduction: Selexipag is a selective agonist of the prostacyclin IP receptor that has anti-proliferative and vasodilatory effects on PAH.

Clinical Trial Phase / FDA-Approval: FDA-approved for PAH. GRIPHON trial showed a 40% reduction in PAH-related events.

Mechanism of Action:

1. **Selective IP Receptor Activation:** Selectipag binds to and activates the IP receptor, causing an increase in cyclic adenosine monophosphate (cAMP) levels that promote vasodilation and inhibit smooth muscle proliferation, in contrast to prostacyclin analogues (e.g., epoprostenol, treprostinil), which activate multiple prostanoid receptors.

2. **Vasodilation and Pulmonary Pressure Reduction:** Higher cAMP levels relax the smooth muscle cells in the pulmonary arteries (PASMCs), which lowers the right ventricular afterload and pulmonary vascular resistance (PVR).
3. **Impact on Pulmonary Arteries that Prevents Proliferation:** Smooth muscle proliferation and vascular remodelling are linked to PAH. Selectipag reduces vascular remodelling by blocking growth factor-mediated proliferation through IP receptor activation.
4. **Inhibition of Platelet Aggregation:** By preventing platelet aggregation, IP receptor activation lowers the risk of intravascular thrombosis in patients with PAH.

Key Pharmacokinetic Parameters: It has a 70% bioavailability and is taken orally twice a day. Selexipag is a prodrug, rapidly converted into its active metabolite (ACT-333679) by carboxylesterases in the liver. The active metabolite has 130 times greater affinity for IP receptors than the parent drug. Plasma half-life of parent drug is between 1–3 hours and of active metabolite is between 6–13 hours. It is primarily excreted via hepatic metabolism, with minimal renal clearance.

Adverse Drug Reactions: Flushing, jaw pain, nausea, diarrhoea, headache, hypotension and hepatic dysfunction.

Uses: First-line oral therapy for PAH to delay disease progression and improve symptoms.

Dose: 200 mcg orally twice daily.

3. Riociguat

Introduction: Riociguat increases nitric oxide signalling for pulmonary vasodilation by acting as a soluble guanylate cyclase (sGC) stimulator.

Clinical Trial Phase / FDA-Approval: FDA-approved for chronic thromboembolic pulmonary hypertension (CTEPH) and PAH. Trials of PATENT-1 and CHEST-1 demonstrated better haemodynamics and exercise tolerance.

Mechanism of Action:

1. **NO-Independent Pathway Direct sGC Stimulation**
   - Riociguat activates soluble guanylate cyclase (sGC) without the aid of nitric oxide (NO) by binding to it directly.
   - Guanosine triphosphate (GTP) is converted to cyclic GMP (cGMP) by sGC.
   - Protein kinase G (PKG) is activated by elevated cGMP levels.
   - PKG causes smooth muscle relaxation by phosphorylating myosin light-chain phosphatase, which dilates pulmonary arteries and lowers vascular resistance.
2. **Enhanced sGC Activity Sensitive to NO**
   - Riociguat also increases the production of cGMP by stabilising the NO-sGC binding, which makes sGC more sensitive to endogenous nitric oxide (NO).
   - As a result, the smooth muscle cells (PASMCs) in the pulmonary arteries relax more.
3. **A decrease in the resistance and pressure of the pulmonary arteries**
   - The pulmonary vascular smooth muscle relaxes as a result of elevated cGMP levels, lowering PAP and PVR.

4. **Inhibition of Pulmonary Arterial Remodelling:**
    - cGMP inhibits the proliferation of vascular smooth muscle cells, which lessens the pulmonary arteries' pathological remodelling.

Key Pharmacokinetic Parameters: It is rapidly absorbed orally, reaching peak plasma concentration (Tmax) within 1-1.5 hours post-administration. It is highly plasma protein-bound (95%), predominantly to albumin. It is primarily metabolized by CYP1A1, CYP3A4, and CYP2C8 enzymes. It's major metabolite is known as M1 which is pharmacologically active but weaker than Riociguat itself. Plasma half-life is around 7 hours. It is mainly excreted via urine.

Adverse Drug Reactions: Hypotension, dizziness, nausea, peripheral oedema and bleeding risk due to platelet inhibition.

Uses: Used in PAH (WHO Group 1) and CTEPH (WHO Group 4) to improve functional capacity.

Dose: 1 mg orally three times daily.

4. Macitentan

Introduction: Macitentan is an orphan medication used for long-term PAH management. It is a dual endothelin receptor antagonist (ERA) with improved tissue penetration.

Clinical Trial Phase / FDA-Approval: FDA-approved for PAH, the SERAPHIN trial demonstrated a 50% decrease in the rate of disease progression.

Mechanism of Action:

1. **Endothelin-1 (ET-1) inhibition Signalling**
    A. The strong vasoconstrictor and mitogen endothelin-1 (ET-1) is overexpressed in response to PAH.
    B. Two receptors allow ET-1 to have its effects:
        i. Vascular smooth muscle cells have endothelin A (ETA) receptors, which mediate vasoconstriction, proliferation, and fibrosis.
        ii. Endothelin B (ETB) receptors: Found on smooth muscle and endothelial cells, these receptors have two functions:
            - In endothelial cells: Promotes prostacyclin (PGI_2) and nitric oxide (NO), which results in vasodilation.
            - On smooth muscle cells: Causes proliferation and vasoconstriction, much like ETA activation.
            - The role of ET-1 in the aetiology of pulmonary hypertension:
            - In response to inflammatory mediators, shear stress, and hypoxia, endothelial cells produce ET-1 in the following ways: Using the endothelin-converting enzyme (ECE), PreproET-1 to Big ET-1 to ET-1 (active form).
            - ET-1 acts on ETA and ETB receptors after being released into the pulmonary circulation.
            - On pulmonary artery smooth muscle cells (PASMCs), ET-1 attaches itself to ETA receptors.
            - As a result, the Gq protein-coupled pathway is activated, which causes: Activation of phospholipase C (PLC) - ↑ Inositol triphosphate (IP_3) - ↑ Intracellular Ca2+- Smooth muscle contraction dependent on calcium - pulmonary vasoconstriction.

C. Smooth muscle growth results from the activation of mitogen-activated protein kinase (MAPK) pathways.

D. Vascular fibrosis is the result of fibroblast activation and extracellular matrix (ECM) deposition:

- In endothelial cells, ET-1 stimulates ETB receptors, resulting in the release of NO and PGI2, which encourages vasodilation (protective effect).
- On the other hand, ETB receptor activation raises Ca2+ influx on smooth muscle cells, which, like ETA, promotes vasoconstriction and proliferation.
- Prolonged vasoconstriction and vascular remodelling are caused by chronic ET-1 overexpression.
    i. Excessive collagen deposition brought on by fibroblast activation results in fibrosis and vascular stiffening.
    ii. An increase in right ventricular afterload results in right heart strain and failure.
- Both ETA and ETB receptors are blocked by Macitentan, a dual endothelin receptor antagonist.

2. **Blocking of ETB and ETA Receptors:** ETB receptor blockade lowers inflammation and endothelial cell dysfunction; ETA receptor blockade stops smooth muscle growth and vasoconstriction; and macitentan, in contrast to bosentan, has balanced ETA and ETB inhibition, which results in more successful prevention of vascular remodelling. Although ETB receptors on endothelial cells help promote vasodilation through the release of nitric oxide and prostacyclin, they are also found on smooth muscle cells, where they contribute to vasoconstriction and cell growth. In pulmonary arterial hypertension, the protective vasodilatory role of ETB is often diminished due to endothelial dysfunction, while the harmful effects on smooth muscle remain active. By blocking both ETA and ETB receptors, macitentan reduces these harmful pathways, leading to overall vasodilation and vascular protection despite the loss of some ETB-mediated vasodilation.
3. **Decrease in Pulmonary Vascular Resistance (PVR):** Macitentan improves right ventricular function by lowering PVR by inhibiting vasoconstriction and proliferation.
4. **Delaying the Progression of the Disease:** By blocking ET-1 signalling, hospitalisations and the worsening of PAH are avoided.

Key Pharmacokinetic Parameters: It is well absorbed orally, with peak plasma concentration (Tmax) of around 8 hours. It is highly lipophilic, allowing deep tissue penetration. Plasma protein binding is around 99%, predominantly to albumin. It is extensively metabolized in the liver by CYP3A4 (major) and CYP2C19 (minor). The active metabolite (10 times more potent than the parent drug) contributes to prolonged receptor blockade. It is partly excreted via urine and faeces.

Adverse Drug Reactions: Hepatotoxicity (requires liver monitoring), anaemia, oedema, nasal congestion and nasopharyngitis.

Uses: First-line PAH therapy to improve exercise capacity and delay disease progression.

Dose: 10 mg orally once daily.

5. Treprostinil

Introduction: An artificial prostacyclin analogue called treprostinil is used to treat pulmonary arterial hypertension (PAH, WHO Group 1). It has effects similar to those of prostacyclin (PGI_2), including vascular remodelling reduction, inhibition of platelet aggregation, and vasodilation.

Clinical Trial Phase / FDA-Approval: FDA-approved in 2020. Improved exercise capacity and haemodynamics were shown in the FREEDOM trials.

Mechanism of Action:

1. **Prostacyclin (IP) receptor activation and pulmonary artery vasodilation**
   - Vascular smooth muscle cells' (VSMCs') prostacyclin (IP) receptors are bound by prostacyclinil.
   - This stimulates adenylyl cyclase (AC) by activating the Gs protein-coupled receptor pathway.
   - ATP is changed into cyclic AMP (cAMP) by adenylyl cyclase.
   - Smooth muscle relaxation results from cAMP's inhibition of myosin light-chain kinase (MLCK).
   - Vasodilation of the pulmonary arteries results from decreased calcium influx in smooth muscle cells, which lowers right ventricular afterload and pulmonary vascular resistance (PVR).
2. **Inhibition of Platelet Aggregation:** Treprostinil lowers thromboxane A2 (TXA2) levels, which inhibits platelet aggregation and lessens thrombotic complications in PAH.
3. **Anti-Proliferative and Anti-Fibrotic Effects:** Treprostinil slows down vascular remodelling caused by PAHs by suppressing the proliferation of vascular smooth muscle. It also lessens endothelial dysfunction and fibrosis in pulmonary arteries.

Key Pharmacokinetic Parameters: Treprostinil has a flexible pharmacokinetic profile, allowing multiple routes of administration (i.v., s.c., inhaled, oral). It is highly plasma protein-bound (91%), mainly to albumin. It is metabolized primarily by the liver (CYP2C8 enzyme) and forms inactive metabolites. It is excreted in urine and faeces.

Adverse Drug Reactions: Flushing, jaw pain, nausea, diarrhoea, injection site pain (subcutaneous form), hypotension and hepatic enzyme elevation.

Uses: Used in advanced PAH as an alternative to i.v. prostacyclin therapy.

Dose: 1.25 ng/kg/min (s.c. or i.v. continuous infusion).

6. Other recent advances in the treatment of Pulmonary Arterial Hypertension (PAH):

Table 2: Current developments in the management of Pulmonary Arterial Hypertension (PAH)

Drug Name / Approach	Mechanism of Action	Clinical Trial Phase	Adverse Reactions	Distinctive / Salient Features
Anti-Inflammatory and Anti-Fibrotic Agents (e.g. Tocilizumab, Pirfenidone)*	Target inflammatory cytokines (IL-6) or fibrotic pathways to limit vascular remodelling in PAH.	Ongoing early-phase I/II trials.	May lead to immunosuppression, GI upset, liver function changes.	Multifactorial approach addressing inflammation-driven and fibrotic changes in pulmonary vasculature.
Stem Cell and Gene Therapy Approaches*	Use of progenitor cells or gene-editing methods to repair or replace dysfunctional endothelium and modulate pathways implicated in PH.	Early Phase I/II trial.	Potential for immune reactions, off-target effects, long-term safety unknown.	Highly experimental but could offer disease-modifying or curative approaches in the future.

Implantable Interatrial Shunt Devices	Placement of a shunt to decompress the right heart and limit RV failure progression by allowing controlled right-to-left atrial flow in advanced PH.	Phase I clinical trials.	Risk of paradoxical embolism, hypoxemia, arrhythmias.	Interventional procedure that can improve haemodynamics in carefully selected patients with severe RV dysfunction.

* Investigational therapies; still under evaluation for regulatory approvals in certain regions.

Key Therapeutic Targets & Strategies

1. **Refinement of Prostacyclin Pathway:** Selexipag's oral formulation ensures targeted stimulation of the prostacyclin (IP) receptor while avoiding some limitations associated with IV or subcutaneous prostanoids. It has demonstrated benefits in both functional capacity and survival metrics in PAH.
2. **Enhancement of cGMP-Mediated Vasodilation:** Riociguat uniquely augments guanylate cyclase activity, even in the absence of nitric oxide (NO). By complementing or replacing PDE-5 inhibitors, it offers an alternative route to sustain cGMP levels and promote vasodilation in patients who respond poorly or have contraindications to PDE-5 inhibitors.
3. **Targeting Inflammation and Remodelling:** Research increasingly recognizes inflammation, immune dysregulation, and fibrotic processes as central in PH pathogenesis. Agents such as tocilizumab (IL-6 inhibitor) are undergoing investigation to determine if modulating these pathways can arrest or reverse vascular remodelling.
4. **Gene & Cell Therapies:** Although still experimental, regenerative approaches aim to restore healthy pulmonary vasculature or correct genetic anomalies that predispose individuals to PAH. If validated, these therapies could be transformative, shifting management from symptom relief to actual reversal of pathologic changes.
5. **Interventional Cardiology / Surgical Options:** In chronic thromboembolic PH (CTEPH), surgical pulmonary endarterectomy can be curative. For inoperable cases, balloon pulmonary angioplasty and riociguat have shown promise. Beyond CTEPH, advanced catheter-based procedures and shunt devices are being explored to manage right heart overload in refractory PH.
6. **Combination Therapy:** Because PH involves multiple dysregulated pathways, combination regimens have become the standard of care for many PAH patients. Early aggressive use of targeted therapies—particularly if risk stratification indicates severe disease—can improve functional class, delay progression, and enhance survival.

Conclusion

Once a consistently fatal condition, pulmonary hypertension is now more controllable due to advanced interventions and targeted medications. Endothelin receptor antagonists, PDE-5 inhibitors, and prostacyclin analogues are examples of first-line targeted agents, oxygen therapy, and diuretics that are the mainstays of conventional management. But many patients' functional capacity, haemodynamics, and survival are significantly improved by the combination regimens used in many current therapeutic approaches, which address several pathogenic pathways at once. Current advancements highlight a persistent shift towards more targeted, mechanistically guided therapies, specifically refined endothelin antagonists, soluble guanylate cyclase stimulators, and selective IP receptor agonists. In addition, current studies on inflammation, cellular repair, and gene therapy could result in next-generation methods that can stop or reverse vascular remodelling, which would have a more significant effect on long-term results. Interventional cardiology has also extended beyond surgical pulmonary endarterectomy for CTEPH to include right heart support devices for different PH subtypes and balloon angioplasty. Despite the fact that there are still many obstacles to overcome, including early diagnosis, risk assessment, expense, and patient response variability, the direction of innovation in the treatment of pulmonary hypertension is unquestionably encouraging. Clinicians are able to provide more individualised treatments that prolong life and enhance quality of life in this complex disease by combining innovative therapies, precise phenotyping, and multidisciplinary care.

References

1. Mitchell G. Integration of primary care into the management of chronic pain. Pain: The person, the science, the clinical interface. 2015 Jan 1;1:278.
2. Guignabert C, Aman J, Bonnet S, Dorfmüller P, Olschewski AJ, Pullamsetti S, Rabinovitch M, Schermuly RT, Humbert M, Stenmark KR. Pathology and pathobiology of pulmonary hypertension: current insights and future directions. European Respiratory Journal. 2024 Oct 31;64(4).
3. Galie N, Torbicki A, Barst R, Dartevelle P, Haworth S, Higenbottam T, Olschewski H, Peacock A, Pietra G, Rubin LJ, Simonneau G. Guidelines on diagnosis and treatment of pulmonary arterial hypertension: The Task Force on Diagnosis and Treatment of Pulmonary Arterial Hypertension of the European Society of Cardiology. European heart journal. 2004 Dec 1;25(24):2243-78.
4. Bousseau S, Fais RS, Gu S, Frump A, Lahm T. Pathophysiology and new advances in pulmonary hypertension. BMJ medicine. 2023 Mar 23;2(1):e000137.
5. Pharmaceutical Journal. Pulmonary hypertension: recognition, diagnosis and management [Internet]. London: Royal Pharmaceutical Society; 2024 Mar [cited 2025 Jun 7]. Available from: https://pharmaceutical-journal.com/article/ld/pulmonary-hypertension-recognition-diagnosis-and-management.
6. Simonneau G, Montani D, Celermajer DS, Denton CP, Gatzoulis MA, Krowka M, Williams PG, Souza R. Haemodynamic definitions and updated clinical classification of pulmonary hypertension. European respiratory journal. 2019 Jan 24;53(1).
7. Hoeper MM, Humbert M, Souza R, Idrees M, Kawut SM, Sliwa-Hahnle K, Jing ZC, Gibbs JS. A global view of pulmonary hypertension. The Lancet Respiratory Medicine. 2016 Apr 1;4(4):306-22.
8. Thenappan T, Shah SJ, Rich S, Gomberg-Maitland M. A USA-based registry for pulmonary arterial hypertension: 1982–2006. European Respiratory Journal. 2007 Nov 30;30(6):1103-10.
9. Sitbon O, Channick R, Chin KM, Frey A, Gaine S, Galiè N, Ghofrani HA, Hoeper MM, Lang IM, Preiss R, Rubin LJ. Selexipag for the treatment of pulmonary arterial hypertension. New England Journal of Medicine. 2015 Dec 24;373(26):2522-33.
10. Price LC, Wort SJ, Perros F, Dorfmüller P, Huertas A, Montani D, Cohen-Kaminsky S, Humbert M. Inflammation in pulmonary arterial hypertension. Chest. 2012 Jan 1;141(1):210-21.
11. Kocken JM, da Costa Martins PA. Epigenetic regulation of pulmonary arterial hypertension-induced vascular and right ventricular remodeling: new opportunities?. International journal of molecular sciences. 2020 Nov 24;21(23):8901.
12. Galiè N, Channick RN, Frantz RP, Grünig E, Jing ZC, Moiseeva O, Preston IR, Pulido T, Safdar Z, Tamura Y, McLaughlin VV. Risk stratification and medical therapy of pulmonary arterial hypertension. European Respiratory Journal. 2019 Jan 24;53(1).
13. Sommer N, Ghofrani HA, Pak O, Bonnet S, Provencher S, Sitbon O, Rosenkranz S, Hoeper MM, Kiely DG. Current and future treatments of pulmonary arterial hypertension. British journal of pharmacology. 2021 Jan;178(1):6-30.
14. Schermuly RT, Janssen W, Weissmann N, Stasch JP, Grimminger F, Ghofrani HA. Riociguat for the treatment of pulmonary hypertension. Expert opinion on investigational drugs. 2011 Apr 1;20(4):567-76.
15. Humbert M, Sitbon O, Guignabert C, Savale L, Boucly A, Gallant-Dewavrin M, McLaughlin V, Hoeper MM, Weatherald J. Treatment of pulmonary arterial hypertension: recent progress and a look to the future. The Lancet Respiratory Medicine. 2023 Sep 1;11(9):804-19.
16. Shah AJ, Beckmann T, Vorla M, Kalra DK. New drugs and therapies in pulmonary arterial hypertension. International Journal of Molecular Sciences. 2023 Mar 19;24(6):5850.
17. Brunton LL, Hilal-Dandan R, Knollmann BC, editors. *Goodman & Gilman's: The Pharmacological Basis of Therapeutics*. 13th ed. New York: McGraw-Hill Education; 2018.
18. Katzung BG, Vanderah TW. *Basic & Clinical Pharmacology*. 15th ed. New York: McGraw-Hill Education; 2021.
19. Humbert M, Kovacs G, Hoeper MM, et al. 2022 ESC/ERS guidelines for the diagnosis and treatment of pulmonary hypertension. *Eur Respir J*. 2022;60(5):2200879.
20. McLaughlin VV, Lajoie AC, Barbeau C, et al. Long-term use of macitentan in pulmonary arterial hypertension: Insights from the SERAPHIN trial. *Eur Heart J*. 2020;41(17):1598–605.
21. Kang C. Sotatercept: first approval. Drugs. 2024 Jul;84(7):857-62.
22. Goren S, Kidwai N, Aronow WS, Lanier GM. The Role of Intravenous Selexipag in Managing PAH and Bridging Gaps in Oral Treatment: A Narrative Review. Therapeutics and Clinical Risk Management. 2025 Dec 31:55-60.

23. Rosenkranz S, Ghofrani HA, Hoeper MM, Langleben D, Hegab S, Rahner C, Richard JF, McLaughlin VV. Safety and efficacy of riociguat in patients with pulmonary arterial hypertension and cardiometabolic comorbidities: Data from interventional clinical trials. The Journal of Heart and Lung Transplantation. 2025 Feb 1;44(2):135-46.
24. Grünig E, Jansa P, Fan F, Hauser JA, Pannaux M, Morganti A, Rofael H, Chin KM. Randomized trial of macitentan/tadalafil single-tablet combination therapy for pulmonary arterial hypertension. Journal of the American College of Cardiology. 2024 Jan 30;83(4):473-84.
25. Nguyen T, Chang C, Cipolla D, Malinin V, Perkins W, Viramontes V, Zhou J, Corboz M. Treprostinil palmitil inhalation powder leverages endogenous lung enzymes to provide sustained treprostinil. Expert Opinion on Drug Delivery. 2024 Aug 2;21(8):1297-305.

Section 6

Rheumatology

Chapter 24

Recent Advances in the Management of Rheumatoid Arthritis

Author: Dr. Pranab Das

Introduction

Rheumatoid arthritis (RA) is a chronic autoimmune disease characterised by ongoing synovial inflammation, joint damage, and various extra-articular manifestations. Untreated rheumatoid arthritis results in considerable disability, diminished quality of life, and heightened mortality risk from cardiovascular issues. Recent advancements in the understanding of rheumatoid arthritis pathogenesis, particularly regarding the roles of cytokines such as TNF-α, IL-6, and IL-1, along with the interactions of B and T lymphocytes, have significantly transformed disease management. The treatment objective has transitioned from managing symptoms to implementing early, aggressive interventions focused on inducing remission or attaining low disease activity.

Conventional synthetic disease-modifying antirheumatic drugs (csDMARDs), including methotrexate, continue to serve as the first-line treatment. However, biologic DMARDs (bDMARDs) and targeted synthetic DMARDs (tsDMARDs), such as Janus kinase (JAK) inhibitors, have notably broadened the range of therapeutic alternatives. Current personalised approaches prioritise treat-to-target strategies and biomarker-guided decisions, thereby improving outcomes and reducing toxicity. Therapeutic advancements have not resolved all challenges, such as incomplete responses, long-term safety concerns, and access to advanced therapies. Current investigations into new targets, combination therapies, and immune modulation are transforming the treatment landscape for rheumatoid arthritis, providing prospects for more precise and sustained disease management.

Historical Perspective

Over the past century, rheumatoid arthritis (RA) treatment has undergone significant change. Salicylates and gold salts were the only available treatments in the early 20th century; they provided symptomatic relief but had no effect on the course of the disease. Corticosteroids were first introduced in the middle of the 20th century thanks to Philip Hench and associates at the Mayo Clinic. Hench won the Nobel Prize for their 1949 discovery that cortisone could significantly lower inflammation in RA. Because of its effectiveness and tolerability, methotrexate, which was developed in the 1980s, became the mainstay of traditional synthetic DMARD therapy, marking a significant turning point.

The first anti-TNF drug, infliximab, was introduced in the late 1990s, and it was followed by etanercept and adalimumab, which marked the beginning of a biologic revolution. By directly altering disease pathways, these treatments, which target important inflammatory cytokines, revolutionised the management of RA. The therapeutic arsenal was then expanded by biologics that target IL-6 (tocilizumab), B cells (rituximab), and T-cell co-stimulation (abatacept). Targeted synthetic DMARDs were introduced in the 2010s with the approval of Janus kinase (JAK) inhibitors such as tofacitinib and baricitinib, providing oral alternatives with a quick onset of action. As research now focusses on precision medicine, earlier intervention, and long-term remission in RA patients, the field is being reshaped by the increasing emphasis on treat-to-target strategies and biomarker-driven therapy.

Definition

Rheumatoid arthritis is clinically defined as a chronic inflammatory polyarthritis with hallmark features of symmetrical joint involvement, morning stiffness lasting more than one hour, and progressive joint damage detectable on imaging (e.g. erosions, joint space narrowing). The most recent classification criteria (2010 ACR/EULAR) incorporate joint involvement, serological markers (rheumatoid factor [RF] and anti-citrullinated protein antibodies [ACPA]), acute-phase reactants (C-reactive protein [CRP], erythrocyte sedimentation rate [ESR]), and symptom duration. These criteria facilitate early diagnosis, which is critical for timely therapeutic intervention to prevent irreversible joint damage.

Types

Although the term "rheumatoid arthritis" is often used universally, subtypes are sometimes defined based on serologic markers:

1. **Seropositive RA**
   - Presence of rheumatoid factor (RF) and/or anti-citrullinated protein antibodies (ACPA).
   - Commonly associated with more aggressive joint disease and extra-articular manifestations.
   - Represents the majority of RA cases.
2. **Seronegative RA**
   - RF and ACPA are absent.
   - May have a somewhat milder course but can still be erosive.
   - Diagnosis sometimes requires careful exclusion of other inflammatory arthritis.

Additionally, there is growing recognition of the importance of disease phenotype, comorbidities (e.g. cardiovascular disease), and genetic risk factors (e.g. shared epitope in HLA-DRB1) that may influence treatment response and prognosis.

Brief Note on Conventional Medicines

For many years, the backbone of RA treatment was anchored in non-biologic (conventional synthetic) DMARDs, with methotrexate (MTX) serving as the anchor drug. Below is a concise summary of these foundational therapies:

Table 1: Concise overview of conventional medications utilized in the management of Rheumatoid Arthritis

Drug Names	Mechanism of Action	Adverse Drug Reactions	Uses
Methotrexate			
(MTX)	Inhibits dihydrofolate reductase, affecting purine synthesis; also has anti-inflammatory effects.	Gastrointestinal upset, mucosal ulcers, hepatotoxicity, bone marrow suppression, teratogenicity.	First-line disease-modifying anti-rheumatic drug (DMARD); reduces joint inflammation and progression of RA.
Leflunomide	Inhibits dihydroorotate dehydrogenase, reducing pyrimidine synthesis and T-cell proliferation.	Diarrhoea, alopecia, hepatotoxicity, teratogenicity.	Used as an alternative to methotrexate; inhibits pyrimidine synthesis to reduce inflammation.
Sulfasalazine	Anti-inflammatory and immunomodulatory; exact mechanism in RA not fully defined.	GI discomfort, headaches, rash, reversible oligospermia, potential hypersensitivity reactions.	Used in combination with other DMARDs; anti-inflammatory and immunomodulatory effects.
Hydroxychloroquine	Interferes with antigen presentation and certain Toll-like receptor functions.	Retinal toxicity (regular eye exams needed), GI intolerance, skin hyperpigmentation.	Used in mild RA or in combination therapy; inhibits immune system overactivation.
Glucocorticoids (e.g. Prednisone)	Broad immunosuppressive and anti-inflammatory effects.	Weight gain, hyperglycaemia, osteoporosis, increased infection risk, adrenal suppression.	Used for short-term flare management and symptom relief.

These traditional DMARDs have demonstrated efficacy in controlling disease activity but often require 6–12 weeks for onset of action, and many patients do not achieve sustained remission on conventional therapy alone. Recognizing these limitations, biologic agents that selectively target key immune mediators and the more recent targeted synthetic DMARDs have become mainstays for moderate-to-severe or refractory RA.

Newer Drugs / Recent Advances

Over the past two decades, researches have improved our understanding of immune dysregulation in RA—particularly involving T cells, B cells, and proinflammatory cytokines such as tumour necrosis factor (TNF)-α, interleukin (IL)-6, and IL-17—has driven a paradigm shift in treatment. Below is a summarizing notable newer or emerging therapies, followed by a deeper exploration of each category.

1. Otilimab

Introduction: Otilimab is a monoclonal antibody that inhibits GM-CSF, a pro-inflammatory cytokine involved in the pathogenesis of RA. GM-CSF plays a critical role in the activation of macrophages, neutrophils, and synovial fibroblasts, leading to joint inflammation and destruction.

Clinical Trial Phase / FDA-Approval: Phase III trials completed but not yet FDA-approved. Investigated in the ContRAst Phase III trials, showing promising efficacy in patients with inadequate response to conventional DMARDs.

Mechanism of Action:

- Otilimab binds specifically to GM-CSF, a cytokine responsible for promoting the survival, proliferation, and activation of myeloid lineage immune cells like macrophages, neutrophils, and dendritic cells.
- GM-CSF normally interacts with its receptor (GM-CSFRα/β) present on monocytes, macrophages, and other immune cells.
- Otilimab prevents GM-CSF from binding to its receptor.
- Without GM-CSF activation, key inflammatory pathways, such as the JAK-STAT (Janus kinase/signal transducer and activator of transcription) and MAPK (mitogen-activated protein kinase) signalling, are downregulated.
- This leads to reduced transcription of pro-inflammatory genes and thereby reduces the release of cytokines such as TNF-α, IL-6, IL-1β, and chemokines like CCL17.
- These molecules are crucial mediators of inflammation, pain, and tissue destruction in diseases like rheumatoid arthritis and osteoarthritis.
- By lowering these cytokine levels, otilimab reduces the recruitment and activation of neutrophils, macrophages, and T-cells at inflammatory sites. This helps in mitigating chronic inflammation and tissue damage.
- GM-CSF also plays a role in osteoclast differentiation, contributing to bone erosion in inflammatory arthritis.
- Otilimab indirectly prevents bone and cartilage degradation by inhibiting osteoclast activation.

Key Pharmacokinetic Parameters: It is administered via subcutaneous (s.c.) injection and is degraded via proteolytic pathways, like other monoclonal antibodies. There is no evidence of hepatic or renal metabolism, minimizing drug-drug interactions. It is cleared via the reticuloendothelial system (monocyte/macrophage degradation).

Adverse Drug Reactions: Injection site reactions, upper respiratory tract infections, transient increase in liver enzymes and mild leukopenia.

Uses: Under investigation for moderate to severe rheumatoid arthritis and osteoporosis, particularly in DMARD-resistant patients.

Dose: 180 mg subcutaneous once weekly, used in Phase 2b and Phase 3 trials (NCT04134728).

2. Upadacitinib

Introduction: Upadacitinib is an oral JAK inhibitor, selectively inhibiting JAK1, which plays a crucial role in cytokine-mediated immune responses.

Clinical Trial Phase / FDA-Approval: FDA-approved for moderate-to-severe RA. Evaluated in SELECT Phase III trials, showing superior efficacy to methotrexate.

Mechanism of Action:

- In inflammatory diseases, pro-inflammatory cytokines (e.g., IL-6, IL-12, IL-23, IFN-γ) bind to their respective cell surface receptors on immune cells.
- These receptors are associated with Janus kinase (JAK) family proteins, including JAK1, JAK2, JAK3, and TYK2.

- Upon cytokine-receptor interaction, JAK proteins undergo phosphorylation and activate Signal Transducers and Activators of Transcription (STATs).
- Activated STATs translocate into the nucleus, promoting transcription of pro-inflammatory genes.
- Upadacitinib selectively inhibits JAK1, preventing phosphorylation of STAT proteins.
- This reduces the expression of inflammatory cytokines and interrupts the inflammatory signalling cascade.
- By blocking cytokine signalling, Upadacitinib decreases the activation of T-cells, macrophages, and other immune cells responsible for inflammation.
- The inhibition of JAK1 leads to decreased production of TNF-α, IL-6, and IFN-γ, reducing inflammation, joint damage (in RA), skin lesions (in AD), and gut inflammation (in IBD).

Key Pharmacokinetic Parameters: Rapidly absorbed orally with an oral bioavailability of 80%. It is widely distributed in tissues. It is primarily metabolized via CYP3A4 enzyme and is excreted mainly by faeces.

Adverse Drug Reactions: Headache, nausea, and fatigue, increased risk of serious infections, elevated liver enzymes and dyslipidaemia.

Uses: Approved for moderate to severe rheumatoid arthritis in patients unresponsive to methotrexate.

Dose: 15 mg once daily (oral).

3. Filgotinib

Introduction: Filgotinib is a highly selective JAK1 inhibitor, providing effective control of inflammation with fewer off-target effects.

Clinical Trial Phase/FDA-Approval: Approved in Europe and Japan but not FDA-approved due to concerns over testicular toxicity. Evaluated in FINCH Phase III trials, showing rapid onset of action.

Mechanism of Action:

- Inflammatory cytokines such as IL-6, IL-12, IL-23, IFN-γ, and GM-CSF bind to their respective receptors on immune cells.
- These receptors are linked to Janus kinase (JAK) proteins, which include JAK1, JAK2, JAK3, and TYK2.
- Upon cytokine binding, JAKs phosphorylate and activate Signal Transducers and Activators of Transcription (STATs), leading to gene transcription and the promotion of inflammatory responses.
- Filgotinib selectively inhibits JAK1, preventing its activation and blocking downstream STAT signalling.
- This leads to reduced expression of pro-inflammatory cytokines, thereby suppressing inflammation.
- Inhibition of JAK1 decreases the activation of macrophages, neutrophils, and T-cells, which are key players in autoimmune inflammation.
- This reduces joint damage (RA), skin inflammation (PsA, AD), and intestinal inflammation (UC, CD).
- By disrupting the JAK1 pathway, Filgotinib decreases the levels of TNF-α, IL-6, IL-17, and IL-23, which are involved in chronic inflammation.
- This results in symptom relief, improved joint function, and reduced disease progression.

Key Pharmacokinetic Parameters: Filgotinib is orally administered and reaches peak plasma concentration (Tmax) within 2-4 hours. It has a bioavailability of approximately 80%. The drug has moderate protein binding (55%). Filgotinib is metabolized primarily in the liver by carboxylesterase-2 (CES2) into its active metabolite GS-829845, which retains strong JAK1 inhibitory activity. It is mainly excreted by urine and partly by faeces.

Adverse Drug Reactions: Upper respiratory tract infections, headache, fatigue, gastrointestinal disturbances and venous thromboembolism.

Uses: Approved for moderate to severe rheumatoid arthritis (2020) in Europe and Japan.

Dose: 200 mg once daily.

4. Abrocitinib

Introduction: Abrocitinib is an oral JAK1 inhibitor, currently under clinical investigation for RA.

Clinical Trial Phase / FDA-Approval: Phase III clinical trials ongoing.

Mechanism of Action:

- In Rhematoid arthritis (RA), pro-inflammatory cytokines such as IL-6, IL-23, IL-12, IFN-γ, and GM-CSF bind to their receptors on immune cells (e.g., T cells, macrophages, synovial fibroblasts).
- These cytokine receptors activate Janus kinases (JAKs), a family of intracellular tyrosine kinases that include JAK1, JAK2, JAK3, and TYK2.
- The activation of JAK proteins leads to phosphorylation of Signal Transducers and Activators of Transcription (STATs), which translocate into the nucleus and promote transcription of inflammatory genes.
- Abrocitinib selectively binds to JAK1, preventing its phosphorylation and activation.
- This blocks the downstream activation of STAT proteins, thereby reducing the transcription of inflammatory genes.
- Unlike non-selective JAK inhibitors (e.g., tofacitinib, which inhibits JAK1 and JAK3), Abrocitinib spares JAK2 and JAK3, reducing hematologic and thromboembolic risks.
- JAK1 inhibition prevents the activation of macrophages, T-cells, and synovial fibroblasts, which are responsible for inflammation and joint destruction in RA.
- This leads to reduced synovial inflammation, joint swelling, and pain relief.
- Abrocitinib decreases levels of IL-6, TNF-α, IL-17, and IL-23, cytokines that drive inflammation and joint destruction in RA.
- As a result, the drug reduces joint damage and improves physical function.

Key Pharmacokinetic Parameters: Abrocitinib is rapidly absorbed following oral administration, reaching peak plasma concentration (Tmax) within 1–4 hours. It has an oral bioavailability of approximately 60-80%. The drug is highly distributed in body tissues. Abrocitinib is primarily metabolized in the liver via cytochrome P450 enzymes (CYP2C19 and CYP3A4), producing active metabolites that contribute to its pharmacologic effects. Its half-life (t½) is approximately 4-8 hours, allowing for once-daily dosing. The drug is eliminated via renal excretion (approximately 60%) and faecal excretion (approximately 30%), mostly in its metabolized form. Unlike non-selective JAK inhibitors, Abrocitinib's selectivity for JAK1 reduces its impact on hematopoiesis and erythropoiesis, minimizing some adverse effects commonly seen with JAK2 inhibition.

Adverse Drug Reactions: Upper respiratory tract infections, nausea, vomiting, diarrhoea and transient increase in liver enzymes.

Uses: Under investigation for rheumatoid arthritis and other autoimmune diseases like inflammatory bowel disease. Under investigation for use in osteoporosis.

Dose: 100 mg to 200 mg once daily (oral) used in early-phase trials.

5. Bimekizumab

Introduction: Bimekizumab is a monoclonal antibody targeting IL-17A and IL-17F, reducing inflammation in RA.

Clinical Trial Phase / FDA-Approval: Phase III trials ongoing.

Mechanism of Action:

- IL-17A and IL-17F are pro-inflammatory cytokines that play a central role in joint inflammation, cartilage degradation, and bone erosion in RA.
- These cytokines stimulate synovial fibroblasts, osteoclasts, and immune cells, leading to chronic joint inflammation and progressive joint destruction.
- High levels of IL-17 have been found in synovial fluid and tissues of RA patients, correlating with disease severity and joint damage.
- Unlike other IL-17 inhibitors (e.g., secukinumab, ixekizumab) that block only IL-17A, Bimekizumab inhibits both IL-17A and IL-17F, providing greater suppression of inflammation.
- This reduces synovial fibroblast activation, preventing excessive matrix metalloproteinase (MMP) production, which breaks down cartilage in RA.
- Bimekizumab also inhibits osteoclast activation, reducing bone resorption and joint damage.
- IL-17A and IL-17F work synergistically with TNF-α, IL-6, and IL-23, amplifying inflammation in RA.
- Bimekizumab disrupts this inflammatory cascade, leading to reduced cytokine production and immune cell activation.
- It reduces T-helper 17 (Th17) cell activity, which is a key driver of autoimmune inflammation in RA.
- It also decreases the recruitment of neutrophils and macrophages to synovial joints, reducing joint swelling and tenderness.

Key Pharmacokinetic Parameters: Bimekizumab is administered via subcutaneous injection and has a high bioavailability (approximately 70-80%). Following administration, it reaches peak plasma concentration (Tmax) in approximately 3–7 days. The drug has a large volume of distribution (Vd approximately 8 L), reflecting its extensive extracellular tissue penetration. Bimekizumab is metabolized via proteolytic degradation, like other monoclonal antibodies, and does not rely on hepatic CYP enzymes, minimizing drug-drug interactions. Bimekizumab has a long half-life (t½ approximately 20–30 days), allowing for monthly dosing regimens. It is eliminated slowly via the reticuloendothelial system and does not require renal or hepatic clearance, making it safe in patients with kidney or liver dysfunction.

Adverse Drug Reactions: Nasopharyngitis, headache, fatigue, Gi upset, increased risk of fungal reactions and hypersensitivity reactions.

Uses: Under investigation for use in rheumatoid arthritis and other inflammatory conditions.

Dose: 160 mg to 320 mg subcutaneously every 4 weeks (trial dosing).

6. Other recent advances in the treatment of rheumatoid arthritis:

Table 2: Recent innovations in managing the symptoms of Rheumatoid Arthritis

Drug / Strategy	Mechanism of Action	Clinical Trial Phase / Status	Adverse Reactions	Distinctive / Salient Features
TNF-α Inhibitors (e.g. Infliximab, Adalimumab, Etanercept)	Neutralize TNF-α activity, reducing inflammation and joint destruction.	FDA-approved, standard in moderate-to-severe RA.	Infection risk (TB reactivation), injection/ infusion site reactions, possible malignancy risk.	Transformative for RA management; typically combined with MTX for optimal efficacy.
IL-6 Inhibitors (e.g. Tocilizumab, Sarilumab)	Block IL-6 signalling, reducing synovial inflammation and systemic effects of RA (e.g. anaemia of chronic disease).	FDA-Approved for RA inadequately responding to TNF-α inhibitors or MTX.	Infection risk, hyperlipidaemia, elevated liver enzymes, GI perforation in rare cases.	Effective especially in systemic features and high CRP levels.
T-cell Co-stimulation Blockade (Abatacept)	Binds CD80/86 on antigen-presenting cells, preventing CD28-mediated T-cell activation.	FDA-Approved for moderate-to-severe RA.	Infection risk, infusion reactions, possible exacerbation of COPD.	Particularly beneficial in patients with high T-cell activation; more gradual onset of action.
B-cell Depletion (Rituximab)	Anti-CD20 monoclonal antibody depletes B cells, thereby reducing autoantibody production.	FDA-Approved for refractory RA, often used post-TNF failure.	Infusion reactions, infection risk, rare progressive multifocal leukoencephalopathy (PML).	Extended dosing intervals; can lead to long-lasting remission in some patients.
IL-17 / IL-23 Pathway Inhibitors (e.g. Secukinumab, Guselkumab)	Block IL-17 or IL-23 cytokines, reducing Th17-mediated inflammation.	More established in psoriatic arthritis; trials ongoing for RA.	Infection risk, possible exacerbation of inflammatory bowel disease in some cases.	Showed promise in RA subsets with overlap features (psoriasis, enthesitis).
Biosimilars (e.g. Infliximab-dyyb, Adalimumab-adbm, etc.)	Biologically similar versions of reference monoclonal antibodies, offering similar efficacy and safety at potentially lower cost.	FDA-Approved and increasingly used worldwide.	Similar to reference biologic: injection site reactions, infections.	Expand accessibility by reducing therapy costs; but must demonstrate equivalence in efficacy, safety, immunogenicity.

Precision Medicine and Other Emerging Concepts:

As multiple therapeutic options proliferate, a central challenge is identifying which patients will respond best to a given drug or combination. Precision medicine approaches leverage genetic, serologic, and molecular biomarkers to guide therapy selection. For example, certain HLA-DRB1 "shared epitope" alleles or high baseline ACPA titres may predict better responses to specific biologics. Similarly, emerging composite biomarkers (e.g. multi-biomarker disease activity tests) could provide real-time disease activity assessments, further personalizing treatment. Beyond targeting inflammation, research increasingly addresses the need for better management of comorbidities—particularly cardiovascular disease, which is a leading cause of morbidity and mortality in RA. Strategies range from aggressive lipid management and blood pressure control to routine screening for subclinical atherosclerosis. Integration of allied health interventions (e.g. physical therapy, occupational therapy) and patient education about smoking cessation, weight control, and exercise also play essential roles in a comprehensive RA management plan.

Conclusion

The management of rheumatoid arthritis has undergone significant advancement in the last twenty years, transitioning from primarily palliative care to a phase where remission or little disease activity is attainable for numerous individuals. Traditional synthetic DMARDs, especially methotrexate, continue to be fundamental. The advent of biologic DMARDs that target TNF, IL-6, T-cell co-stimulation, and B cells, along with oral JAK inhibitors, has expanded therapy options. These advances can significantly enhance long-term outcomes—preventing joint degradation, maintaining function, and minimising extra-articular problems. However, unaddressed needs persist. As many as one-third of patients may not achieve ideal responses to any specific therapy, and the costs of medications can be exorbitant. Progress in biomarker identification and precision medicine offers potential for more customised therapies and enhanced cost-efficiency by aligning patients with the most appropriate therapy from the beginning. Biosimilars are continually advancing, providing a method to enhance accessibility. In the future, we might anticipate innovative targets in immunomodulation and tailored techniques that enhance current treatment achievements, ultimately progressing towards a world when the debilitating effects of RA are significantly reduced or completely prevented.

References

1. Brown P, Pratt AG, Hyrich KL. Therapeutic advances in rheumatoid arthritis. Bmj. 2024 Jan 17;384.
2. Gao Y, Zhang Y, Liu X. Rheumatoid arthritis: pathogenesis and therapeutic advances. MedComm. 2024 Mar;5(3):e509.
3. Kathoke P, Thombre K, Gupta KR, Umekar MJ. Innovative therapies and strategies for rheumatoid arthritis. Current Rheumatology Reviews. 2025 Jan 27.
4. McInnes IB, Schett G. Pathogenetic insights from the treatment of rheumatoid arthritis. The Lancet. 2017 Jun 10;389(10086):2328-37.
5. Smolen JS, Landewé R, Bijlsma J, Burmester G, Chatzidionysiou K, Dougados M, Nam J, Ramiro S, Voshaar M, Van Vollenhoven R, Aletaha D. EULAR recommendations for the management of rheumatoid arthritis with synthetic and biological disease-modifying antirheumatic drugs: 2016 update. Annals of the rheumatic diseases. 2017 Jun 1;76(6):960-77.
6. Aletaha D, Neogi T, Silman AJ, Funovits J, Felson DT, Bingham III CO, Birnbaum NS, Burmester GR, Bykerk VP, Cohen MD, Combe B. 2010 rheumatoid arthritis classification criteria: an American College of Rheumatology/European League Against Rheumatism collaborative initiative. Arthritis & rheumatism. 2010 Sep;62(9):2569-81.
7. Viatte S, Plant D, Raychaudhuri S. Genetics and epigenetics of rheumatoid arthritis. Nature Reviews Rheumatology. 2013 Mar;9(3):141-53.
8. Singh JA, Saag KG, Bridges Jr SL, Akl EA, Bannuru RR, Sullivan MC, Vaysbrot E, McNaughton C, Osani M, Shmerling RH, Curtis JR. 2015 American College of Rheumatology guideline for the treatment of rheumatoid arthritis. Arthritis & rheumatology. 2016 Jan;68(1):1-26.
9. Feldmann M, Maini RN. Anti-TNF therapy, from rationale to standard of care: what lessons has it taught us?. The Journal of immunology. 2010 Jul 15;185(2):791-4.
10. Mohamed MEF, Bhatnagar S, Parmentier JM, Nakasato P, Wung P. Upadacitinib: Mechanism of action, clinical, and translational science. Clin Transl Sci. 2024 Jan;17(1):e13688.

11. Dougados M, van der Heijde D, Chen YC, Greenwald M, Drescher E, Liu J, Beattie S, Witt S, de la Torre I, Gaich C, Rooney T. Baricitinib in patients with inadequate response or intolerance to conventional synthetic DMARDs: results from the RA-BUILD study. Annals of the rheumatic diseases. 2017 Jan 1;76(1):88-95.
12. Kremer JM, Westhovens R, Leon M, Di Giorgio E, Alten R, Steinfeld S, Russell A, Dougados M, Emery P, Nuamah IF, Williams GR. Treatment of rheumatoid arthritis by selective inhibition of T-cell activation with fusion protein CTLA4Ig. New England Journal of Medicine. 2003 Nov 13;349(20):1907-15.
13. Edwards JC, Cambridge G. B-cell targeting in rheumatoid arthritis and other autoimmune diseases. Nature Reviews Immunology. 2006 May 1;6(5):394-403.
14. O'Shea JJ, Gadina M. Selective Janus kinase inhibitors come of age. Nature Reviews Rheumatology. 2019 Feb;15(2):74-5.
15. Smolen JS, Pangan AL, Emery P, Rigby W, Tanaka Y, Vargas JI, Zhang Y, Damjanov N, Friedman A, Othman AA, Camp HS. Upadacitinib as monotherapy in patients with active rheumatoid arthritis and inadequate response to methotrexate (SELECT-MONOTHERAPY): a randomised, placebo-controlled, double-blind phase 3 study. The Lancet. 2019 Jun 8;393(10188):2303-11.
16. Westhovens R, Rigby WF, van der Heijde D, Ching DW, Stohl W, Kay J, Chopra A, Bartok B, Matzkies F, Yin Z, Guo Y. Filgotinib in combination with methotrexate or as monotherapy versus methotrexate monotherapy in patients with active rheumatoid arthritis and limited or no prior exposure to methotrexate: the phase 3, randomised controlled FINCH 3 trial. Annals of the rheumatic diseases. 2021 Jun 1;80(6):727-38.
17. Genovese MC, Kalunian K, Gottenberg JE, Mozaffarian N, Bartok B, Matzkies F, et al. Filgotinib in combination with methotrexate in an active rheumatoid arthritis population with inadequate response to biologic DMARDs. *Rheumatology (Oxford)*. 2021;60(4):1517–25.
18. Wang F, Tang X, Zhu M, Mao H, Wan H, Luo F. Efficacy and safety of JAK inhibitors for rheumatoid arthritis: a meta-analysis. Journal of Clinical Medicine. 2022 Jul 30;11(15):4459.
19. Zhao MY, Zhang W, Rao GW. Targeting Janus kinase (JAK) for fighting diseases: the research of JAK inhibitor drugs. Current Medicinal Chemistry. 2022 Sep 1;29(29):5010-40.
20. Cheema KS, Mansour AB, Raychaudhuri SP. What's new on the horizon for rheumatoid arthritis management. Best Practice & Research Clinical Rheumatology. 2025 Feb 11:102038.
21. Blockmans D, Penn SK, Setty AR, Schmidt WA, Rubbert-Roth A, Hauge EM, Keen HI, Ishii T, Khalidi N, Dejaco C, Cid MC. A phase 3 trial of upadacitinib for giant-cell arteritis. New England Journal of Medicine. 2025 Apr 2.
22. Mease PJ, Gensler LS, Orbai AM, Warren RB, Bajracharya R, Ink B, Marten A, Massow U, Shende V, Manente M, Peterson L. Long-term safety of bimekizumab in adult patients with axial spondyloarthritis or psoriatic arthritis: pooled results from integrated phase IIb/III clinical studies. RMD open. 2025 Apr 1;11(2):e005026.
23. Buch MH, Walker D, Edwards CJ, Barry J, Akroyd L, Ekoka Omoruyi EV, Taylor PC. Efficacy and safety of filgotinib in patients with moderately active rheumatoid arthritis and an inadequate response to methotrexate. Rheumatology. 2025 Apr;64(4):1661-71.

Section 7

Endocrine System

Chapter 25

Recent Advances in the Management of Osteoporosis

Author: Dr. Pranab Das

Introduction

Osteoporosis is a systemic skeletal disorder defined by low bone mass and microarchitectural deterioration of bone tissue, leading to an increase in bone fragility and susceptibility to fractures. Often referred to as a "silent disease," osteoporosis typically remains asymptomatic until a fracture occurs. Globally, osteoporosis and osteopenia affect millions of people, representing a major source of morbidity, healthcare costs, and reduced quality of life—particularly in older adults. Hip, vertebral, and wrist fractures are among the most common osteoporotic fractures, with hip fractures often associated with significant morbidity and mortality.

Over the past several decades, the management of osteoporosis has expanded considerably beyond basic calcium and vitamin D supplementation. The discovery of key molecular pathways involved in bone remodelling—particularly the RANK-RANKL-OPG system, Wnt signalling, and sclerostin inhibition—has revolutionized pharmacotherapy, offering multiple lines of treatment. Yet challenges remain: poor medication adherence, side-effect profiles, underdiagnosis, and undertreatment of high-risk individuals continue to hinder progress in reducing osteoporotic fractures. Against this backdrop, research continues to focus on novel anti-osteoporotic agents, improved screening and diagnostic tools (e.g. refined imaging technologies, biomarkers) and personalized approaches. This chapter provides an overview of osteoporosis definition and classification, briefly summarizes conventional medications, and then delves into recent and emerging therapeutic strategies.

Historical Perspective

The pharmacological treatment of osteoporosis has advanced considerably since the mid-20th century, propelled by the increasing awareness of its contribution to age-related fractures and morbidity. The original comprehension of osteoporosis originated from Fuller Albright's research in the 1940s, which connected postmenopausal oestrogen insufficiency to bone loss, so establishing the basis for hormone replacement therapy (HRT) as a preliminary preventive measure. The introduction of etidronate in the 1980s initiated bisphosphonate therapy, subsequently succeeded by more potent drugs such as alendronate, developed by Merck and licensed in 1995, which emerged as a first-line treatment for postmenopausal osteoporosis due to its efficacy in inhibiting bone resorption.

The 1990s witnessed the emergence of selective oestrogen receptor modulators (SERMs), particularly raloxifene, which provided oestrogenic advantages for bone while minimising hazards to the breast and uterus. In the early 2000s, focus shifted to anabolic therapy. Teriparatide, a recombinant fragment of parathyroid hormone, received approval in 2002 for its role in encouraging new bone production, marking a significant shift in treatment methodology. Denosumab, a monoclonal antibody that inhibits RANKL to diminish osteoclast activity, was launched in 2010 and has subsequently emerged as a pivotal antiresorptive drug, especially in high-risk groups.

The recent introduction of romosozumab, a sclerostin inhibitor licensed in 2019, signifies an increasing interest in dual-action medicines that promote bone formation while simultaneously inhibiting resorption. The advancing therapeutic landscape currently emphasises personalised care, long-term safety, and sequencing tactics to optimise skeletal advantages while reducing risks. These advancements highlight a shift from merely preventing fractures to proactively reconstructing and maintaining bone health in ageing demographics.

Definition

Osteoporosis is characterized by diminished bone mineral density (BMD) and structural compromise of bone microarchitecture, resulting in increased bone fragility. The World Health Organization (WHO) operationally defines osteoporosis in postmenopausal women and men over 50 years old as a BMD T-score of ≤−2.5 at the lumbar spine, femoral neck, or total hip, measured by dual-energy X-ray absorptiometry (DXA). Patients with a T-score between −1.0 and −2.5 are classified as having osteopenia, reflecting low bone mass that raises future risk of osteoporosis. Other factors—such as age, previous fracture history, family history, glucocorticoid use, smoking, and comorbidities—further modulate individual fracture risk.

Types of Osteoporosis

Though osteoporosis is often thought of as a single entity, it encompasses multiple aetiologies:

1. **Primary Osteoporosis:**
   - Type I (Postmenopausal Osteoporosis): Often related to oestrogen deficiency in women after menopause, leading to rapid bone resorption and predominantly trabecular bone loss (e.g. vertebral fractures).
   - Type II (Age-Related Osteoporosis): Generally occurs in both men and women over 70, linked to a gradual decline in bone turnover, reduced osteoblast function, and decreased calcium absorption.
2. **Secondary Osteoporosis**
   - Arises from a broad spectrum of conditions or medications, including glucocorticoid therapy, hyperthyroidism, hyperparathyroidism, malabsorption syndromes (e.g. celiac disease), chronic kidney disease, and others.
   - Addressing the underlying cause is paramount for reversing or mitigating bone loss.

Understanding these subtypes helps guide both diagnostic and therapeutic decisions. For instance, identifying steroid-induced osteoporosis calls for distinct prophylactic or therapeutic regimens, such as earlier use of anti-resorptive drugs.

Brief Note on Conventional Medications

For many years, the mainstay of pharmacological management has centered on agents that either slow bone resorption or stimulate bone formation. Below is a concise summary of widely used conventional therapies.

Table 1: Concise overview of traditional pharmacotherapy for osteoporosis management.

Drug Class / Drug Names	Mechanism of Action	Adverse Drug Reactions	Uses
Bisphosphonates (e.g. Alendronate, Risedronate, Zoledronic Acid)	Binds to hydroxyapatite crystals in the bone matrix and inhibit osteoclast-mediated bone resorption.	GI upset (oral), osteonecrosis of the jaw (rare), atypical femur fractures (rare), acute flu-like reactions (i.v.).	First-line treatment to reduce fracture risk by inhibiting osteoclast-mediated bone resorption.
Selective Estrogen Receptor Modulators (SERMs) (e.g. Raloxifene)	Provide oestrogen-agonist effects on bone and antagonist effects on breast/uterine tissue.	Hot flashes, venous thromboembolism risk, leg cramps.	Prevent osteoporosis in postmenopausal women, reduce vertebral fracture risk.
Denosumab	Human monoclonal antibody to RANKL, preventing osteoclast formation/function.	Hypocalcaemia, rebound bone loss if discontinued abruptly, possible risk of infections, osteonecrosis of the jaw (rare).	Inhibits RANKL to reduce bone resorption, used in patients intolerant to bisphosphonates.
Teriparatide (PTH 1-34)	Anabolic agent that stimulates osteoblast activity and bone formation.	Hypercalcemia, leg cramps, dizziness, theoretical risk of osteosarcoma (seen in rats during clinical trials).	Stimulates bone formation in severe osteoporosis.
Hormone Replacement Therapy (HRT)	Estrogen/progesterone supplementation reduces bone turnover (osteoclastic activity) in postmenopausal women.	Increased risks of breast cancer, cardiovascular events, venous thromboembolism.	Used in postmenopausal women for osteoporosis prevention and symptom relief.
Calcium and Vitamin D Supplements	Provide necessary substrates for bone mineralization and support bone homeostasis.	GI discomfort, hypercalcemia (if excessive intake), kidney stones.	Essential for bone mineralization, usually combined with other therapies.

These therapies, when combined with lifestyle interventions (adequate calcium/vitamin D intake, weight-bearing exercises, smoking cessation, alcohol moderation), have significantly reduced osteoporotic fracture incidence in many populations. However, concerns over long-term safety (e.g. bisphosphonates and atypical fractures, denosumab and rebound phenomenon) and incomplete fracture risk reduction underscore the demand for new or adjunctive options.

Newer Drugs / Recent Advances

Recent progress in understanding bone remodelling and osteoimmunology has spurred the development of novel agents targeting specific regulatory pathways. Below is a summarizing notable, newer or emerging therapies, followed by a detailed discussion of each.

1. Romosozumab (Anti-Sclerostin Antibody)

Introduction: Sclerostin is a protein secreted primarily by osteocytes that inhibits the Wnt signalling pathway necessary for osteoblast function. Romosozumab is a monoclonal antibody that binds to sclerostin, thereby stimulating bone formation and, to some degree, reducing bone resorption. Clinical trials have demonstrated significant increase in bone mineral density (BMD) and reductions in vertebral fractures within 12 months.

Romosozumab is generally approved for use in postmenopausal women at high risk of fracture, typically for a limited duration (up to 12 months), after which a transition to another antiresorptive agent (e.g. bisphosphonates) is recommended to maintain gains.

Clinical Trial Phase / FDA-Approval: FDA-approved under the brand name Evenity. Evaluated in the FRAME, ARCH, and STRUCTURE trials, demonstrating significant fracture risk reduction.

Mechanism of Action:

A. **Sclerostin Inhibition and Wnt Signalling Activation**
   - Sclerostin is a natural inhibitor of the Wnt/β-catenin signalling pathway, which is essential for osteoblast differentiation and function.
   - Romosozumab binds to and neutralizes sclerostin, leading to enhanced Wnt signalling activation, resulting in:
     I. Increased osteoblast activity - More bone formation.
     II. Reduced osteoclast differentiation - Less bone resorption.
   - This dual effect makes romosozumab unique among osteoporosis treatments.

B. **Effects on Bone Formation and Resorption**
   - Increases osteoblast differentiation and function, leading to increased bone matrix production.
   - Reduces osteoclast-mediated bone resorption, leading to enhanced bone mass.
   - Bone mineral density enhancement are more rapid and pronounced compared to bisphosphonates or teriparatide.

C. **Clinical Effects on Bone Mineral Density and Fracture Risk**
   - Increases BMD by approximately 13% at the spine and approximately 6% at the hip over 12 months.
   - Reduces vertebral fractures by approximately 73% and hip fractures by approximately 38%.
   - First-line therapy for severe osteoporosis in postmenopausal women.

Key Pharmacokinetic Parameters: It is administered as a monthly subcutaneous (s.c.) injection at a dose of 210 mg. Peak serum concentration (Cmax) is achieved within 5–7 days. It exhibits approximately 81% bioavailability after s.c. administration. It is metabolized via proteolytic degradation into small peptides and amino acids, similar to other monoclonal antibodies. Plasma half-life is around 12.8 to 18 days, supporting monthly dosing.

Adverse Drug Reactions: Arthralgia, myalgia, injection-site reactions (pain, redness, swelling), hypocalcaemia and osteonecrosis of jaw.

Uses: Treatment of osteoporosis in postmenopausal women and patients at high fracture risk who fail to respond to bisphosphonates.

Dose: 210 mg subcutaneously once monthly for 12 months.

2. Abaloparatide (PTHrP Analog)

Introduction: Abaloparatide is an analogue of PTH-related peptide (PTHrP), which selectively activates the PTH1 receptor in a transient manner that favours bone formation over resorption. Clinical trials have shown that abaloparatide can significantly increase bone mineral density and reduce fracture risk (particularly vertebral fractures), offering an alternative to teriparatide. Common side effects include hypercalcemia and dizziness, often related to the anabolic effect on bone and transient changes in serum calcium.

Clinical Trial Phase/FDA-Approval: FDA-approved under the brand name Tymlos. Studied in the ACTIVE and ACTIVExtend trials, showing superior fracture risk reduction compared to teriparatide.

Mechanism of Action:

A. **PTH1R Binding and Activation**
   - Abaloparatide binds to PTH1R, which exists in two conformations:
     1. RG (G-protein-dependent conformation) → Anabolic signalling.
     2. R0 (non-G-protein-dependent conformation) → Catabolic effects.
   - Abaloparatide has a greater affinity for the RG conformation, leading to enhanced bone formation with reduced resorption.

B. **Stimulation of Osteoblast Activity**
   - Increases osteoblast differentiation and function, leading to greater bone matrix production.
   - Reduces osteoblast apoptosis - prolonging their bone-forming activity.
   - Unlike teriparatide, abaloparatide results in lower activation of osteoclasts, reducing bone resorption.

C. **Effects on Bone Mineral Density (BMD) and Fracture Risk**
   - Increases bone mineral density at the lumbar spine (approximately 12%) and total hip (approximately 6%) over 18 months.
   - Reduces vertebral fractures by 86% and non-vertebral fractures by 43%.
   - Has a rapid onset of action, with significant BMD gains within 3–6 months.

Key Pharmacokinetic Parameters: It is administered subcutaneously. It is metabolized into inactive fragments via proteolytic degradation. It's plasma half-life ($t^{1/2}$) is approximately around 1.7 hours (shorter than teriparatide). It is eliminated via the renal system, with no significant hepatic metabolism.

Adverse Drug Reactions: Hypercalcaemia, hypotension, dizziness and palpitations.

Uses: Severe osteoporosis with high fracture risk.

Dose: 80 mcg subcutaneously once daily for up to 18 months.

3. Cathepsin K Inhibitors (Odanacatib)

Introduction: Cathepsin K is a protease used by osteoclasts to degrade collagen within bone. Odanacatib, a highly selective cathepsin K inhibitor, showed promise in reducing bone resorption without severely impacting osteoclast viability or bone formation. However, its development was halted due to a higher incidence of stroke and other cardiovascular events in phase III trials, highlighting the complexity of selectively inhibiting bone-degrading enzymes without unintended systemic consequences.

Clinical Trial Phase/FDA-Approval: Discontinued in Phase III trial due to cardiovascular concerns. Studied in the LOFT trial, showing increased bone mineral density and fracture reduction.

Mechanism of Action:

A. **Inhibition of Cathepsin K in Osteoclasts**
   - Cathepsin K (CatK) is a cysteine protease expressed in osteoclasts and is responsible for collagen degradation in bone matrix.
   - Odanacatib selectively inhibits CatK, reducing collagen breakdown without impairing osteoclast viability.

- Unlike bisphosphonates, which cause osteoclast apoptosis, odanacatib allows osteoclasts to remain active but prevents them from degrading the bone matrix.

B. **Effects on Bone Remodelling**
   - Reduces bone resorption while maintaining osteoblast-mediated bone formation, leading to net BMD gains.
   - Increases cortical bone thickness and trabecular bone volume by inhibiting excessive bone turnover.
   - Long-term odanacatib use increases bone mass and strength in primate studies.

C. **Clinical Impact on Bone Mineral Density (BMD) and Fracture Risk**
   - Increased BMD at the spine (+9.2%) and hip (+5.8%) over 5 years.
   - Reduced vertebral fractures by 54% and hip fractures by 47%.
   - Maintained bone microarchitecture, unlike bisphosphonates, which sometimes lead to brittle bones.

Key Pharmacokinetic Parameters: It is administered orally once weekly. Oral bioavailability is 30-50%. It is highly bound to plasma protein albumin. It is metabolized by CYP3A4, with minor contributions from CYP2D6. It is excreted primarily via faeces.

Adverse Drug Reactions: Mild hypocalcaemia, musculoskeletal pain, diarrhoea and increase risk of stroke and atrial fibrillation (rare).

Uses: Was under investigation for postmenopausal osteoporosis but discontinued in phase III trial due to cardiovascular concerns.

Dose: 50 mg orally once weekly (investigational - discontinued).

4. Combination Therapy (Denosumab and high dose Teriparatide)

Introduction: Considering that anti-resorptives (e.g. bisphosphonates, denosumab) primarily reduce bone breakdown and anabolic agents (e.g. teriparatide, abaloparatide) stimulate new bone formation, researchers have explored whether combining these categories yields additive or synergistic effects. Trials such as the DATA study examined denosumab plus teriparatide, reporting greater increase in bone mineral density than either agent alone. However, cost and complexity of dual therapy, and limited long-term fracture data have tampered immediate adoption.

Clinical Trial Phase / FDA-Approval: Currently in Phase IV trial.

Mechanism of Action:

1. **Mechanism of Action of Denosumab**

   Denosumab is a monoclonal antibody that targets the receptor activator of nuclear factor-κB ligand (RANKL), an essential regulator of osteoclast formation and activity.

   a. **Inhibition of RANKL - Suppression of Osteoclast Activity**
      - RANKL binds to RANK (on osteoclast precursors), promoting their differentiation into mature bone-resorbing osteoclasts.
      - Denosumab blocks RANKL, preventing osteoclast formation, function, and survival.
      - This leads to decreased bone resorption and increased bone mineral density (BMD).

b. **Effects on Bone Turnover**
   - Rapid and profound suppression of bone resorption [decreases serum C-terminal telopeptide (CTX) levels within days].
   - Unlike bisphosphonates, denosumab does not get incorporated into bone, meaning its effects are reversible upon discontinuation.

c. **Clinical Outcomes**
   - Reduces vertebral fractures by approximately 68% and hip fractures by approximately 40% over 3 years.
   - Increases BMD by approximately 8-10% at the lumbar spine and approximately 6-7% at the hip joint.

2. **Mechanism of Action of Teriaparatide**

   Teriparatide is a recombinant human parathyroid hormone (PTH 1-34) that acts as an anabolic (bone-building) agent.

   a. **Intermittent PTH1R Activation - Stimulation of Osteoblasts**
      - PTH receptor type 1 (PTH1R) activation in osteoblasts leads to:
        1. Increased osteoblast differentiation and activity.
        2. Enhanced bone matrix production and mineralization.
        3. Reduced osteoblast apoptosis, prolonging bone formation.

   b. **Effects on Bone Turnover**
      - Intermittent PTH stimulation increases bone formation > resorption (anabolic effect).
      - Unlike denosumab, teriparatide stimulates bone turnover, leading to new bone growth.
      - Maximal bone mineral density (BMD) gains occur at the spine (approximately 10-14%) and hip (approximately 5-7%).

   c. **Clinical Outcomes**
      - Reduces vertebral fractures by approximately 65% and non-vertebral fractures by approximately 53%.
      - Used in severe osteoporosis or high-risk fracture patients.

Key Pharmacokinetic Parameters:

1. **Denosumab:** It is administered subcutaneously at a dose of 60 mg every 6 months. It is not metabolized by the liver and is eliminated via reticuloendothelial clearance.
2. **Teriparatide:** It is administered as a subcutaneous injection. It is rapidly cleared from plasma and mainly acts on PTH1R in osteoblasts. It is metabolized by hepatic and renal proteolysis into inactive fragments.

Adverse Drug Reactions:

1. Denosumab: Hypocalcaemia, musculoskeletal pain, skin infections, osteonecrosis of jaw and atypical femoral fractures.
2. Teriparatide: Nausea, headache, dizziness, hypercalcaemia, hypotension and syncope.

Uses: Postmenopausal osteoporosis, glucocorticoid-induced osteoporosis and patients with multiple osteoporotic fractures.

Dose: Denosumab: 60 mg subcutaneously every 6 months; Teriparatide: 20 mcg daily (standard-dose); High-dose Teriparatide (in DATA-HD trial): 40 mcg subcutaneously once daily.

5. Long-Acting PTH Analogues (TransCon PTH)

Introduction: Another approach aims to improve the convenience and efficacy of PTH-based treatments. TransCon PTH, for instance, is a sustained-release form designed to provide a steady background level of PTH—more closely mimicking physiologic hormone patterns than once-daily injections. Early clinical trials suggest favourable effects on bone mineral density and serum calcium homeostasis, potentially reducing the peaks and troughs that can lead to side effects or suboptimal bone outcomes. If proven safe and effective, these formulations could simplify anabolic therapy for patients requiring long-term or continuous bone-building approaches.

Clinical Trial Phase / FDA-Approval: Currently undergoing Phase III clinical trials.

Mechanism of Action:

A. **Prolonged PTH1R Activation and Bone Remodelling**
  - TransCon PTH is a sustained-release prodrug of PTH (1-34), which binds to the parathyroid hormone receptor type 1 (PTH1R).
  - Unlike teriparatide (PTH 1-34), which leads to spikes in PTH levels, TransCon PTH maintains continuous PTH exposure, mimicking natural PTH secretion.
  - PTH1R activation stimulates osteoblast differentiation and reduces osteoblast apoptosis, enhancing bone formation.

B. **Effects on Bone Formation and Resorption**
  - Enhances osteoblast proliferation and activity, leading to increased bone mineral density (BMD).
  - Prevents excessive osteoclast activation, reducing bone resorption compared to intermittent PTH therapy (e.g. teriparatide).
  - More favourable anabolic effects compared to conventional PTH therapy due to prolonged receptor activation.

C. **Clinical Effects on Bone Strength and Fracture Risk**
  - Increases BMD by approximately 13% at the lumbar spine and approximately 6% at the total hip over 12 months.
  - Reduces vertebral fractures by approximately 73% and nonvertebral fractures by approximately 40%.
  - Faster and more potent BMD gains compared to teriparatide.

Key Pharmacokinetic Parameters: It is administered as a once-daily subcutaneous (s.c.) injection. It is an extended-release prodrug—slowly releases active PTH 1-34 over 24 hours, mimicking endogenous PTH secretion. It is metabolized by proteolytic degradation in the bloodstream and is eliminated primarily via renal clearance.

Adverse Drug Reactions: Mild hypercalcaemia, injection-site reactions (pain, redness, swelling), headache, nausea, dizziness and hypercalciuria.

Uses: Osteoporosis and hyperparathyroidism.

Dose: 18–20 μg subcutaneously once daily.

6. Emerging Genetic / Cell Therapies

As the genetic underpinnings of bone metabolism become clearer, gene and cell-based interventions offer a potential frontier. Gene editing tools (e.g. CRISPR/Cas9) and stem cell therapies might one day selectively enhance osteoblast function, suppress excessive osteoclast activity, or correct monogenic disorders causing severe osteoporosis. Current research remains largely preclinical, focusing on safety, targeted delivery, and durability of effect. While it may be years before these therapies reach routine clinical practice, they exemplify the ongoing quest to move beyond symptomatic management toward root-cause modification of bone fragility.

Conclusion

The landscape of osteoporosis treatment is evolving with newer anabolic and antiresorptive agents. Romosozumab and abaloparatide are already FDA-approved, while combination therapies and long-acting PTH analogues are emerging as promising strategies. These advances provide better bone density improvement and fracture prevention, shaping the future of osteoporosis management.

References

1. Fuggle N, Laslop A, Rizzoli R, Al-Daghri N, Alokail M, Balkowiec-Iskra E, Beaudart C, Bruyère O, Bemden AB, Burlet N, Cavalier E. Treatment of osteoporosis and osteoarthritis in the oldest old. Drugs. 2025 Feb 19:1-8.
2. Shashidhara A, Tahir SH, Abbas Z, Lee J, Tahir H. An update on the pharmacotherapy of osteoporosis. Expert Opinion on Pharmacotherapy. 2025 Apr 5.
3. Zou L, Chen G, Rong Y, Tang C, Lv X, Fan Y. Three signalling pathways for iron overload in osteoporosis: a narrative review. Journal of Orthopaedic Surgery and Research. 2025 Feb 20;20(1):186.
4. Eastell R, Rosen CJ, Black DM, Cheung AM, Murad MH, Shoback D. Pharmacological management of osteoporosis in postmenopausal women: an Endocrine Society clinical practice guideline. The Journal of Clinical Endocrinology & Metabolism. 2019 May;104(5):1595-622.
5. Kanis JA, McCloskey EV, Johansson H, Cooper C, Rizzoli R, Reginster JY. European guidance for the diagnosis and management of osteoporosis in postmenopausal women. Osteoporosis international. 2013 Jan;24(1):23-57.
6. Cosman F, de Beur SJ, LeBoff MS, Lewiecki EM, Tanner B, Randall S, Lindsay R. Clinician's guide to prevention and treatment of osteoporosis. Osteoporosis international. 2014 Oct;25:2359-81.
7. Svedbom A, Hernlund E, Ivergård M, Compston J, Cooper C, Stenmark J, McCloskey EV, Jönsson B, Kanis JA, EU review panel of the IOF. Osteoporosis in the European Union: a compendium of country-specific reports. Archives of osteoporosis. 2013 Dec;8:1-218.
8. WHO Study Group on Assessment of Fracture Risk, its Application to Screening for Postmenopausal Osteoporosis. Assessment of fracture risk and its application to screening for postmenopausal osteoporosis: report of a WHO study group. World Health Organization; 1994.
9. Buckley L, Guyatt G, Fink HA, Cannon M, Grossman J, Hansen KE, Humphrey MB, Lane NE, Magrey M, Miller M, Morrison L. 2017 American College of Rheumatology guideline for the prevention and treatment of glucocorticoid-induced osteoporosis. Arthritis & rheumatology. 2017 Aug;69(8):1521-37.
10. Saag KG, Petersen J, Brandi ML, Karaplis AC, Lorentzon M, Thomas T, Maddox J, Fan M, Meisner PD, Grauer A. Romosozumab or alendronate for fracture prevention in women with osteoporosis. New England Journal of Medicine. 2017 Oct 12;377(15):1417-27.
11. Tsai JN, Lee H, David NL, Eastell R, Leder BZ. Combination denosumab and high dose teriparatide for postmenopausal osteoporosis (DATA-HD): a randomised, controlled phase 4 trial. The Lancet Diabetes & Endocrinology. 2019 Oct 1;7(10):767-75.
12. Cosman F, Crittenden DB, Adachi JD, Binkley N, Czerwinski E, Ferrari S, Hofbauer LC, Lau E, Lewiecki EM, Miyauchi A, Zerbini CA. Romosozumab treatment in postmenopausal women with osteoporosis. New England Journal of Medicine. 2016 Oct 20;375(16):1532-43.
13. Bone HG, Cosman F, Miller PD, Williams GC, Hattersley G, Hu MY, Fitzpatrick LA, Mitlak B, Papapoulos S, Rizzoli R, Dore RK. ACTIVExtend: 24 months of alendronate after 18 months of abaloparatide or placebo for postmenopausal osteoporosis. The Journal of Clinical Endocrinology & Metabolism. 2018 Aug;103(8):2949-57.
14. Leder BZ, Tsai JN, Uihlein AV, Burnett-Bowie SA, Zhu Y, Foley K, Lee H, Neer RM. Two years of Denosumab and teriparatide administration in postmenopausal women with osteoporosis (The DATA Extension Study): a randomized controlled trial. The Journal of Clinical Endocrinology & Metabolism. 2014 May 1;99(5):1694-700.
15. Reid IR, Billington EO. Drug therapy for osteoporosis in older adults. The Lancet. 2022 Mar 12;399(10329):1080-92.
16. Rauner M, Taipaleenmäki H, Tsourdi E, Winter EM. Osteoporosis treatment with anti-sclerostin antibodies—Mechanisms of action and clinical application. J Clin Med. 2021 Feb 16;10(4):787.

17. Händel MN, Cardoso I, Von Bülow C, Rohde JF, Ussing A, Nielsen SM, Christensen R, Body JJ, Brandi ML, Diez-Perez A, Hadji P. Fracture risk reduction and safety by osteoporosis treatment compared with placebo or active comparator in postmenopausal women: systematic review, network meta-analysis, and meta-regression analysis of randomised clinical trials. Bmj. 2023 May 2;381.
18. Cummings SR, Martin JS, McClung MR, Siris ES, Eastell R, Reid IR, Delmas P, Zoog HB, Austin M, Wang A, Kutilek S. Denosumab for prevention of fractures in postmenopausal women with osteoporosis. New England Journal of Medicine. 2009 Aug 20;361(8):756-65.
19. Tashjian AH, Gagel RF. Teriparatide [human PTH (1-34)] in osteoporosis. *J Clin Endocrinol Metab*.2006;91(2):709–15.
20. Elahmer NR, Wong SK, Mohamed N, Alias E, Chin KY, Muhammad N. Mechanistic insights and therapeutic strategies in osteoporosis: a comprehensive review. Biomedicines. 2024 Jul 23;12(8):1635.
21. Mäkinen VN, Sølling AS, McClung M, Langdahl BL. Romosozumab for the treatment of osteoporosis–a systematic review. Journal of Endocrinological Investigation. 2025 Mar;48(3):547-72.
22. Chen L, Ji B, Xia C. Efficacy and Safety of Abaloparatide, Denosumab, Teriparatide, Oral Bisphosphonates, and Intravenous Bisphosphonates in the Treatment of Male Osteoporosis: A Systematic Review and Bayesian Network Meta-Analysis. Frontiers in Endocrinology.;16:1558560.
23. Nguyen TT, Woo SM, Seo SU, Banstola A, Kim H, Duwa R, Vu AT, Hong IS, Kwon TK, Yook S. Enhanced anticancer efficacy of TRAIL-conjugated and odanacatib-loaded PLGA nanoparticles in TRAIL resistant cancer. Biomaterials. 2025 Jan 1;312:122733.

Chapter 26

Recent Advances in the Management of Diabetes Mellitus

Author: Dr. Pranab Das

Introduction

A chronic metabolic disease called diabetes mellitus is marked by hyperglycaemia brought on by either insulin resistance, insulin insufficiency, or both. The International Diabetes Federation reports that the prevalence of diabetes is still increasing worldwide, with significant effects on patient health and medical expenses. Early detection and effective management are crucial because diabetes can cause major complications such as cardiovascular disease, chronic kidney disease, retinopathy, and neuropathy. More specialised and efficient treatments have resulted from enormous advancements in our knowledge of the pathophysiology of diabetes over time, especially the interaction between insulin resistance, beta-cell dysfunction, and complex genetic and environmental factors.

Type 1 (T1DM) and Type 2 (T2DM) diabetes mellitus are generally distinguished by the autoimmune-mediated destruction of pancreatic beta cells in Type 1 and the progressive insulin resistance and beta-cell exhaustion in Type 2. Advanced insulin formulations, new non-insulin agents, and state-of-the-art technology for insulin delivery and glycaemic monitoring are also examples of recent therapeutic advancements. This chapter examines the definition and classification of diabetes, summarizes conventional management strategies, and delves into the latest advances reshaping diabetes care.

Historical Perspective

Over the past century, there has been a significant change in the treatment of diabetes mellitus, moving from simple insulin therapy to complex pharmacologic approaches based on mechanisms. Frederick Banting and Charles Best won a Nobel Prize in 1921 for their discovery of insulin, which transformed the management of type 1 diabetes. Until Marcel Janbon discovered sulfonylureas in the 1950s, the first oral hypoglycaemics for type 2 diabetes, insulin was the only effective treatment for decades. Metformin, which was first created in the 1920s but later improved, became widely used in the 1990s after its cardiovascular safety and effectiveness were established. Following the advent of incretin-based treatments, such as GLP-1 receptor agonists and DPP-4 inhibitors, which were based on Joel Habener and Daniel Drucker's ground-breaking research in gut hormone physiology, the early 2000s saw the rise of thiazolidinediones and meglitinides.

More recently, the EMPA-REG OUTCOME and DAPA-CKD trials have confirmed that sodium-glucose co-transporter 2 (SGLT2) inhibitors, such as empagliflozin and dapagliflozin, have revolutionised treatment by lowering cardiovascular and renal complications. The next step towards weight loss and metabolic optimisation in type 2 diabetes is the approval of dual agonists like tirzepatide, which targets both GLP-1 and GIP receptors. With an emphasis on early combination therapy, personalised medicine, and disease-modifying strategies, this advancement represents a larger movement away from glucose control alone and towards complete metabolic and organ protection.

Definition

Diabetes mellitus is clinically defined by persistent hyperglycaemia that can be diagnosed using the following criteria (as recommended by professional bodies such as the American Diabetes Association):

1. Fasting Plasma Glucose (FPG) ≥126 mg/dL, or
2. Postprandial Plasma Glucose (PPG) after two hours during an oral glucose tolerance test (OGTT) is ≥200 mg/dL, or
3. Haemoglobin A1C (HbA1c) ≥6.5%, or
4. Random Plasma Glucose ≥200 mg/dL (11.1 mmol/L) in the presence of classic hyperglycaemic symptoms or hyperglycaemic crisis.

In clinical practice, the diagnosis is confirmed by repeating the test on another day unless hyperglycaemic symptoms are evident. Once diagnosed, management goals centre around preventing acute complications (e.g. hyperglycaemic crises) and reducing long-term macrovascular (cardiovascular disease) and microvascular (retinopathy, nephropathy, neuropathy) complications.

Types of Diabetes Mellitus

1. **Type 1 Diabetes Mellitus (T1DM)**
   - Autoimmune destruction of pancreatic beta cells leading to absolute insulin deficiency.
   - Typically presents in childhood or adolescence but can occur at any age.
   - Patients require lifelong exogenous insulin therapy.
2. **Type 2 Diabetes Mellitus (T2DM)**
   - Characterized by insulin resistance and relative insulin deficiency.
   - Strongly associated with obesity, sedentary lifestyle, and genetic predisposition.
   - Treatment ranges from lifestyle modification and oral medications to injectable therapies (GLP-1 receptor agonists, insulin).
3. **Gestational Diabetes Mellitus (GDM)**
   - Hyperglycaemia first recognized during pregnancy.
   - Can increase the risk of adverse pregnancy outcomes and long-term maternal T2DM.
4. **Other Specific Types**
   - Monogenic forms (e.g. MODY—Maturity-Onset Diabetes of the Young).
   - Secondary causes (e.g. due to endocrinopathies, pancreatic diseases, medications like steroids).

   Understanding the aetiology helps tailor therapy to maintain near-normal glycaemic control, which remains the cornerstone for preventing complications.

Brief Note on Conventional Management

A. Non-Pharmacological Interventions

A foundation of diabetes management is lifestyle modification, which includes medical nutrition therapy, increased physical activity, and weight reduction for overweight or obese individuals. Often, structured programs led by dietitians or diabetes educators provide sustained benefits. Smoking cessation and psychosocial support are also critical, given the strong link between cardiovascular risk and poor glycaemic control.

B. Pharmacological Therapies

Table 1: Concise overview of classical pharmacotherapies for diabetes mellitus management

Drug Name & Class	Mechanism of Action	Key Pharmacokinetic Parameters	Adverse Drug Reactions	Uses
Metformin (Biguanide)	Reduces hepatic gluconeogenesis by inhibiting mitochondrial glycerophosphate dehydrogenase (mGPD). Increases insulin sensitivity by activating AMP-activated protein kinase (AMPK), leading to increased peripheral glucose uptake.	Oral bioavailability: 50–60%. Peak plasma time (Tmax): 2-3 hours. Excretion via urine (approximately 90% unchanged). Half-life: 4-8 hours.	GI upset (nausea, diarrhoea, bloating), lactic acidosis (rare but serious) and vitamin B12 deficiency.	First-line drug for Type 2 Diabetes Mellitus (T2DM). Also used in polycystic ovarian syndrome (PCOS).
Glipizide, Glyburide (Sulfonylureas)	Bind to sulfonylurea receptor (SUR1) on pancreatic β-cells, closing ATP-sensitive K+ channels. This depolarizes the cell membrane, leading to Ca2+ influx and insulin secretion.	Oral bioavailability: >80%. Metabolised in liver (CYP2C9). Half-life: 2-10 hours (drug-dependent). Excreted via urine.	Hypoglycaemia (especially in elderly) and weight gain.	Type 2 diabetes.
Repaglinide, Nateglinide (Meglitinides)	Act on ATP-sensitive K+ channels in β-cells, similar to sulfonylureas, but with a shorter duration of action. Rapidly stimulate postprandial insulin release, reducing meal-related glucose spikes.	Rapidly absorbed orally (Tmax approximately 1 hour). Short half-life: 1-2 hours. Metabolized in liver (CYP3A4, CYP2C8). Excreted via faeces mainly.	Hypoglycaemia (less than sulfonylureas), weight gain and hepatic enzyme elevation (rare).	Postprandial glucose control in T2DM.
Pioglitazone, Rosiglitazone (Thiazolidinediones - TZDs)	Activate peroxisome proliferator-activated receptor gamma (PPAR-γ), increasing glucose uptake in muscle & adipose tissue. Suppress hepatic gluconeogenesis. Improve insulin sensitivity by modulating adipokines.	High oral bioavailability. Metabolized in liver (CYP2C8, CYP3A4) Half-life: 3-7 hours. Excreted via faeces & urine.	Fluid retention (oedema), heart failure exacerbation and risk of bladder cancer (pioglitazone).	Type 2 diabetes (esp. in insulin resistance). NAFLD/NASH (off-label use).
Acarbose, Miglitol (α-Glucosidase Inhibitors)	Inhibit α-glucosidase enzymes in the small intestine, delaying carbohydrate breakdown & glucose absorption. Reduces postprandial hyperglycaemia.	Minimal systemic absorption. It is metabolized by gut bacteria. Excreted unchanged in faeces.	GI upset (flatulence, bloating, diarrhoea) and abdominal cramps.	Postprandial glucose control in T2DM. Used in pre-diabetes to prevent progression.

Insulin (Rapid-acting, Short-acting, Intermediate, Long-acting)	Activates insulin receptors, increasing glucose uptake in muscle and fat while inhibiting hepatic glucose production.	Rapid-acting (Lispro, Aspart): Onset is within 15 min and duration is 4 hours. Short-acting (Regular insulin): Onset is within 30 min and duration is 6-8 hours. Long-acting (Glargine, Detemir): Duration is 24 hours.	Hypoglycaemia, weight gain and lipodystrophy (at injection sites)	Type 1 & Type 2 diabetes. Diabetic ketoacidosis (DKA) & Hyperosmolar Hyperglycaemic State (HHS) management.

Despite these conventional treatments, many individuals remain sub-optimally controlled, especially those with long-standing disease or multiple comorbidities. Additionally, cardiovascular and renal complications remain a major burden. As such, recent therapeutic developments aim to offer not only superior glycaemic control but also cardiometabolic and renal protective benefits.

Newer Drugs / Recent Advances

1. Dapagliflozin

Introduction: An SGLT2 inhibitor called dapagliflozin improves glucose excretion through the urine, lowering blood sugar levels and having positive effects on cardiac function.

Clinical Trial Phase / FDA-Approval: Originally FDA-approved for Type 2 Diabetes Mellitus (T2DM), its indication has been expanded to include Heart Failure with Reduced Ejection Fraction (HFrEF) and Chronic Kidney Disease (CKD).

Mechanism of Action:

1. **Inhibition of SGLT2 in the Proximal Renal Tubule**

   Dapagliflozin exerts its primary effect by selectively inhibiting the sodium-glucose co-transporter 2 (SGLT2), which is located in the proximal convoluted tubule (PCT) of the nephron. Under normal physiology, SGLT2 is responsible for reabsorbing approximately 90% of filtered glucose. In individuals with diabetes, SGLT2 expression is upregulated, exacerbating glucose reabsorption and contributing to persistent hyperglycaemia. By blocking this transporter, dapagliflozin promotes urinary glucose excretion (glucosuria), thereby reducing plasma glucose levels. This results in an average HbA1c reduction of approximately 0.5-1.2%, depending on baseline glycaemia.

2. **Insulin-Independent Glucose Lowering**

   Dapagliflozin lowers blood glucose levels through a mechanism that is independent of insulin secretion or insulin receptor signalling. This makes it effective in patients with insulin resistance as well as those with progressive Œ≤-cell failure, a common scenario in advanced Type 2 Diabetes Mellitus (T2DM).

3. **Reduction of Glucotoxicity and Preservation of Œ≤-Cell Function**

   Chronic hyperglycaemia imposes a toxic burden on pancreatic Œ≤-cells, impairing their function and promoting apoptosis. By improving glycaemic control through enhanced urinary glucose loss, dapagliflozin reduces glucotoxic stress and contributes to the preservation of endogenous insulin production.

4. **Metabolic Effects: Weight Loss and Improved Insulin Sensitivity**

   The loss of glucose through urine-estimated at 70-80 grams/day-translates into a caloric deficit of approximately 280-320 kcal/day. This negative energy balance promotes modest weight loss (about 2-3 kg over six months) and has been associated with improvements in insulin sensitivity, likely secondary to reduced adiposity and improved metabolic homeostasis.

5. **Cardiovascular and Renal Protective Effects**

   Dapagliflozin also exhibits haemodynamic benefits through natriuresis and osmotic diuresis, which result in modest reductions in systolic blood pressure (approximately 4-5 mmHg). These effects reduce cardiac preload and afterload, offering clinical benefit in patients with heart failure with reduced ejection fraction (HFrEF).In the kidneys, dapagliflozin attenuates glomerular hyperfiltration and intraglomerular hypertension, reducing albuminuria and slowing the progression of chronic kidney disease (CKD).

Key Pharmacokinetic Parameters: After oral administration, dapagliflozin is quickly absorbed, reaching its peak plasma concentration (Tmax) in 1-2 hours. Because of its roughly 78% oral bioavailability, it can be taken once daily. About 90% of plasma proteins bind to the drug, mostly albumin. Through the action of UDP-glucuronosyltransferase (UGT1A9), dapagliflozin is metabolised in the liver to produce an inactive glucuronide metabolite that is ultimately removed. With a half-life (t½) of roughly 12–13 hours, the effect is guaranteed to last for 24 hours. About 25% are eliminated in faeces, and the majority (roughly 75%) are eliminated through the renal route as metabolites. Mild-to-moderate renal or hepatic impairment does not necessitate major dose adjustments; however, severe renal dysfunction (eGFR <45 mL/min/1.73 m2) warrants caution due to diminished drug efficacy.

Adverse Drug Reactions: Urinary tract infections (UTIs), genital mycotic infections, hypotension, acute kidney injury and dehydration.

Uses: Approved for Type 2 diabetes, heart failure with reduced ejection fraction, and chronic kidney disease.

Dose: 10 mg orally once daily.

2. Canagliflozin

Introduction: Canagliflozin is a potent SGLT2 inhibitor that lowers glucose levels through renal glucose loss.

Clinical Trial Phase / FDA-Approval: FDA-approved for T2DM; shown cardiovascular and renal benefit in the CANVAS trial.

Mechanism of Action:

1. **Inhibition of SGLT2 in the Proximal Renal Tubule**

   Canagliflozin selectively inhibits the sodium-glucose cotransporter 2 (SGLT2), a high-capacity transporter located in the proximal convoluted tubule (PCT) of the kidney. Under normal physiological conditions, SGLT2 is responsible for reabsorbing approximately 90% of the filtered glucose load. In individuals with Type 2 Diabetes Mellitus (T2DM), upregulation of SGLT2 contributes to excessive glucose reabsorption and persistent hyperglycaemia. By blocking this transporter, canagliflozin significantly increases urinary glucose excretion-typically in the range of 70-100 g/day-thereby reducing plasma glucose concentrations, lowering HbA1c by 0.6-1.2%, and improving overall glycaemic control. This also contributes to enhanced insulin sensitivity.

2. **Insulin-Independent Glucose Lowering**

   Unlike insulin secretagogues or exogenous insulin, canagliflozin acts independently of pancreatic B-cell function. It does not stimulate insulin secretion, making it particularly effective in patients with insulin resistance or insulin deficiency. Importantly, the risk of hypoglycaemia is minimal when used as monotherapy, though it may increase when combined with insulin or sulfonylureas.

3. **Reduction of Glucotoxicity and Preservation of B-Cell Function**

   Chronic hyperglycaemia exerts a toxic effect on B-cells, known as glucotoxicity, leading to impaired insulin secretion. By lowering blood glucose levels and reducing the glycaemic burden, canagliflozin helps preserve B-cell integrity and function, thereby supporting endogenous insulin production over time.

4. **Additional Metabolic Benefits: Weight Loss and Lipid Profile Improvement**

   The glucose loss induced by canagliflozin results in a caloric deficit of approximately 300 kcal/day, leading to modest but consistent weight reduction (~2-3 kg over six months). The drug has also been associated with a reduction in visceral adiposity and favourable changes in lipid profile, including increased HDL and a shift in LDL particle size towards a less atherogenic pattern.

5. **Cardiovascular and Renal Protective Effects**

   Canagliflozin reduces renal sodium reabsorption, promoting osmotic diuresis and natriuresis, which contribute to a modest blood pressure reduction (4-6 mmHg). These haemodynamic effects decrease cardiac preload and afterload, leading to reduced rates of heart failure hospitalisation-a benefit observed even in non-diabetic populations. Additionally, the drug exerts renoprotective effects by decreasing intraglomerular pressure, reducing hyperfiltration, mitigating albuminuria, and limiting tubulointerstitial fibrosis, thereby slowing the progression of chronic kidney disease (CKD).

Key Pharmacokinetic Parameters: After oral administration, canagliflozin is rapidly absorbed, with peak plasma concentrations (Tmax) reached within 1 to 2 hours. Its moderate oral bioavailability (~65%) supports once-daily dosing. The drug is highly bound to plasma proteins, primarily albumin (~99%), facilitating widespread systemic distribution. Metabolism occurs predominantly via the hepatic enzymes UGT1A9 and UGT2B4, which convert the drug into inactive glucuronide metabolites. A smaller proportion (~7%) undergoes oxidative metabolism through cytochrome P450 isoenzymes CYP3A4 and CYP2C8. The elimination half-life ranges between 10 and 13 hours, allowing for sustained therapeutic activity over a 24-hour period. Excretion is mainly via the faeces (41%) and urine (33%), with a portion excreted unchanged in the urine. In patients with moderate to severe renal impairment (eGFR <45 mL/min/1.73 m^2), reduced efficacy and an increased risk of adverse effects necessitate clinical caution.

Adverse Drug Reactions: Urinary tract infections, mild dehydration, polyuria, Fournier's gangrene and hypotension.

Uses: Approved for Type 2 diabetes, with cardiovascular and renal protection.

Dose: 100 mg orally once daily before the first meal.

3. Teplizumab

Introduction: Teplizumab is a monoclonal antibody that delays the onset of Type 1 diabetes by preserving pancreatic beta-cell function.

Clinical Trial Phase / FDA-Approval: FDA-approved (2022) for delaying Type 1 diabetes in at-risk individuals. Studied in the TN-10 trial, showing significant delay in diabetes onset.

Mechanism of Action:

1. **CD3 Binding and Induction of Immune Tolerance**

   Type 1 Diabetes Mellitus (T1DM) is an autoimmune condition marked by progressive destruction of pancreatic B-cells by autoreactive T lymphocytes. Cytotoxic CD8+ T cells directly attack B-cells, while CD4+ helper T cellsamplify this response, exacerbating B-cell loss. Teplizumab is a humanized monoclonal antibody that selectively binds to the CD3Œµ subunit of the T-cell receptor (TCR) complex, thereby inhibiting T-cell activation and clonal expansion. This downregulates autoreactive T-cell activity-particularlythat of CD8+ cytotoxic T cells-reducing their destructive effects on pancreatic B-cells.

2. **Expansion of Regulatory T Cells (Tregs)**

   Teplizumab promotes the development and proliferation of regulatory T cells (Tregs), including CD4+ Tregs, which function to suppress autoimmune responses. These cells inhibit the activation of effector T cells and reduce the production of pro-inflammatory cytokines such as interleukin-2 (IL-2), interferon-Œ≥ (IFN-Œ≥), and tumor necrosis factor-Œ± (TNF-Œ±). The result is decreased B-cell inflammation and apoptosis.

3. **Induction of T-Cell Exhaustion and Anergy**

   Teplizumab induces a hyporesponsive state in autoreactive T cells, often referred to as T-cell exhaustion or anergy. In this state, T cells become functionally inactive when re-exposed to B-cell antigens, thereby limiting their capacity to perpetuate autoimmunity. This contributes to a delay in disease progression and preserves remaining B-cell mass.

4. **Modulation of Antigen-Presenting Cells (APCs)**

   Teplizumab also affects dendritic cells and macrophages, diminishing their ability to present B-cell antigens to na√Øve T cells. This dampens the initiation of additional autoimmune responses and helps maintain immune tolerance within the pancreatic microenvironment.

5. **Preservation of Endogenous Insulin Secretion**

   By attenuating immune-mediated B-cell destruction, teplizumab helps preserve residual endogenous insulin production. This is reflected in sustained C-peptide levels, improved glycaemic control, and a reduced need for exogenous insulin in individuals at early stages of T1DM.

Key Pharmacokinetic Parameters: Teplizumab is administered intravenously over a 14-day period using a gradual dose-escalation protocol to reduce the risk of immune-related adverse events. Following administration, the drug exhibits a biphasic distribution pattern, initially dispersing into both vascular and interstitial fluid compartments. As a monoclonal antibody, it demonstrates high plasma protein binding. Its terminal elimination half-life is approximately 5 to 8 days, enabling sustained immunomodulatory effects beyond the treatment window. Teplizumab is degraded by proteolytic enzymes, similar to endogenous immunoglobulins, and is primarily cleared via the reticuloendothelial system. It does not undergo significant renal or hepatic elimination, and no notable drug–drug interactions have been identified.

Adverse Drug Reactions: Transient lymphopenia, rash, increased risk of upper respiratory tract infections, cytokine release syndrome, reactivation of latent viral infections and hypersensitivity reactions.

Uses: Approved for delaying Type 1 diabetes onset in at-risk patients.

Dose: 14-day IV infusion regimen - Starting at 65 µg/m^2, gradually titrated to a maximum of 1,030 µg/m^2/day (based on body surface area).

4. Tirzepatide

Introduction: Tirzepatide is a dual GLP-1 and GIP receptor agonist, promoting insulin secretion, weight loss, and glycemic control.

Clinical Trial Phase / FDA-Approval: FDA-approved (2022) for Type 2 diabetes. Evaluated in SURPASS trials, demonstrating superior glycaemic control.

Mechanism of Action:

1. **Dual GIP and GLP-1 Receptor Agonism**

   Tirzepatide acts as a dual agonist at the receptors for glucose-dependent insulinotropic polypeptide (GIP) and glucagon-like peptide-1 (GLP-1)-both incretin hormones secreted postprandially by the gut. These hormones enhance glucose-dependent insulin secretion; however, GIP additionally supports lipid metabolism and promotes pancreatic B-cell survival. In individuals with Type 2 Diabetes Mellitus (T2DM), this incretin effect is blunted, contributing to hyperglycaemia, insulin resistance, and B-cell dysfunction.

   Tirzepatide's concurrent activation of both receptors results in a synergistic enhancement of insulin secretion, surpassing the glycaemic efficacy of GLP-1 receptor agonists alone.

   GIP effects: Amplifies insulin release and improves lipid handling.

   GLP-1 effects: Suppresses glucagon, slows gastric emptying, and reduces appetite.

2. **Stimulation of Insulin Secretion and Improvement in Insulin Sensitivity**

   Tirzepatide stimulates cAMP-mediated insulin release via both GIP and GLP-1 receptors on pancreatic B-cells, augmenting both postprandial and fasting insulin levels. GIP receptor activation also promotes insulin sensitivity in skeletal muscle and adipose tissue, thereby lowering peripheral insulin resistance.

3. **Glucagon Suppression and Reduction of Hepatic Glucose Output**

   By inhibiting glucagon secretion from pancreatic Œ±-cells, Tirzepatide reduces hepatic glucose production. This leads to improved fasting glycaemia and attenuates the risk of postprandial hyperglycaemic surges.

4. **Delayed Gastric Emptying and Appetite Regulation**

   GLP-1 receptor activation in the gastrointestinal tract slows gastric emptying, helping to control postprandial glucose spikes. Additionally, Tirzepatide influences central appetite regulation by acting on hypothalamic pathways, leading to substantial weight loss-approximately 10-15% of body weight in clinical trials.

5. **Cardiometabolic Advantages**

   Tirzepatide has been associated with improvements in several cardiometabolic parameters, including reductions in blood pressure, serum triglycerides, and LDL cholesterol. Furthermore, it exhibits anti-inflammatory and antioxidative properties, contributing to its therapeutic potential in cardiovascular disease and non-alcoholic fatty liver disease (NAFLD).

Key Pharmacokinetic Parameters: Tirzepatide is administered as a once-weekly subcutaneous injection due to its long elimination half-life (approximately 5 days). After administration, the peak plasma concentration (Tmax) is reached in approximately 24–72 hours. The drug has an absolute bioavailability of approximately 80%, facilitating efficient systemic absorption. It exhibits high plasma protein binding (approximately 99%), ensuring a prolonged duration of action. Tirzepatide undergoes proteolytic degradation by catabolic enzymes rather than cytochrome P450 metabolism, reducing potential drug-drug interactions. It is eliminated primarily via the liver (approximately 60%) and kidneys (approximately 30%), with no significant impact of renal impairment on drug clearance. The pharmacokinetics of tirzepatide are not significantly altered by mild-to-moderate hepatic impairment, making dose adjustments unnecessary.

Adverse Drug Reactions: Nausea ,vomiting, hypoglycaemia (when combined with insulin or sulfonylureas), pancreatitis, reduced appetite and weight loss.

Uses: Approved for Type 2 diabetes with additional weight-loss benefits.

Dose: 2.5 mg subcutaneously once weekly.

5. Retatrutide

Introduction: Retatrutide is a triple agonist (GLP-1, GIP, and glucagon receptor agonist), under investigation for Type 2 diabetes and obesity management.

Clinical Trial Phase / FDA-Approval: Phase III clinical trials ongoing.

Mechanism of Action:

1. **GLP-1 Receptor Activation – Enhancement of Insulin Secretion and Glucagon Suppression**

   Retatrutide activates GLP-1 receptors located on pancreatic B-cells, thereby enhancing glucose-dependent insulin secretion. Concurrently, it suppresses glucagon release, leading to reduced hepatic glucose output and improved fasting glycaemia. Additionally, GLP-1 receptor stimulation delays gastric emptying, which helps attenuate postprandial glucose excursions.

2. **GIP Receptor Activation – Improvement in Insulin Sensitivity**

   Stimulation of GIP receptors further augments insulin secretion while simultaneously alleviating B-cell stress, thus supporting pancreatic function. GIP signalling also promotes glucose uptake in skeletal muscle and adipose tissue, thereby improving insulin sensitivity and reducing peripheral insulin resistance.

3. **Glucagon Receptor Activation – Augmentation of Energy Expenditure**

   Unlike traditional incretin-based therapies, Retatrutide also targets glucagon receptors, resulting in enhanced lipid metabolism and increased energy expenditure. This mechanism contributes to substantial weight loss-reported to be approximately 20-25% in clinical trials-surpassing the efficacy of GLP-1 monotherapy. Moreover, glucagon receptor activation may favourably influence hepatic lipid turnover, offering potential benefits in non-alcoholic fatty liver disease (NAFLD).

4. **Appetite Regulation and Weight Reduction**

   By engaging both GLP-1 and GIP receptors within hypothalamic appetite-regulating centres, Retatrutide reduces hunger and food intake. This appetite suppression contributes to a negative energy balance, further enhancing glycaemic control and promoting metabolic health.

5. **Cardiometabolic and Hepatic Benefits**

   Retatrutide has demonstrated potential to improve multiple cardiometabolic parameters, including reductions in blood pressure, serum triglycerides, and LDL cholesterol. In addition, it may reduce hepatic fat content, offering therapeutic promise for individuals with NAFLD and metabolic syndrome.

Key Pharmacokinetic Parameters: Retatrutide is administered once weekly via subcutaneous injection, a regimen supported by its prolonged half-life and sustained receptor activity. Peak plasma concentrations are typically achieved within 24 to 72 hours, allowing for extended therapeutic coverage. Owing to its peptide-based structure—comparable to that of GLP-1 receptor agonists—the drug demonstrates high bioavailability and efficient systemic absorption. Approximately 90% of Retatrutide is bound to plasma proteins, which contributes to its stability and prolonged duration of action. It is primarily metabolised through proteolytic degradation by endogenous enzymes in the liver and kidneys, bypassing significant involvement of the cytochrome P450 system, thus minimising the potential for drug–drug interactions. The elimination half-life is around 6 days, permitting convenient weekly dosing. Clearance occurs mainly through hepatic and renal pathways, with minimal elimination via the gastrointestinal tract.

Adverse Drug Reactions: Nausea, vomiting, diarrhoea, dizziness, hypoglycaemia, pancreatitis and thyroid C-cell hyperplasia.

Uses: Under investigation for Type 2 diabetes and obesity.

Dose: 1 mg to 12 mg subcutaneously once weekly (trial dosing).

6. Newer Insulin Formulations:

Mechanism of action of Insulin in Diabetes Mellitus:

1. **Insulin Binding to Insulin Receptors (IRs)**
   - Insulin binds to the insulin receptor (IR), a transmembrane tyrosine kinase receptor, found in skeletal muscle, adipose tissue, and liver cells.
   - The insulin receptor consists of two α-subunits (extracellular, insulin-binding site) and two β-subunits (intracellular, tyrosine kinase domain).
2. **Activation of Intracellular Signalling Pathways**

   Once insulin binds to the IR, it triggers autophosphorylation of tyrosine residues in the receptor's β-subunits, leading to the activation of two key intracellular pathways:

   A. PI3K-Akt Pathway
   - Phosphoinositide-3-kinase (PI3K) activation leads to phosphorylation of Akt (Protein Kinase B), which mediates several metabolic effects:
     1. **Glucose Transport:**
        - Akt stimulates GLUT4 (glucose transporter-4) translocation to the cell membrane, facilitating glucose uptake into skeletal muscle and adipose cells.
     2. **Glycogen Synthesis:**
        - Akt inactivates Glycogen Synthase Kinase-3 (GSK-3), allowing glycogen synthase activation, which promotes glucose storage as glycogen in the liver and muscles.
     3. **Inhibition of Gluconeogenesis & Lipolysis:**
        - Suppresses gluconeogenic enzymes (PEPCK, G6Pase) in the liver, reducing hepatic glucose output.
        - Inhibits hormone-sensitive lipase (HSL) in adipose tissue, preventing fat breakdown (lipolysis).

   B. MAPK Pathway (Growth & Gene Expression)
   - Mitogen-Activated Protein Kinase (MAPK) pathway is activated, leading to:
   - Increased cell growth and differentiation.
   - Enhanced lipogenesis and protein synthesis.

3. **Regulation of Blood Glucose Levels**
   - Insulin facilitates glucose clearance from the bloodstream by promoting:
     1. Glycogen storage in the liver and muscles.
     2. Fat storage (lipogenesis) in adipose tissue.
     3. Protein synthesis by stimulating amino acid uptake into muscle cells.
        - In the absence of insulin (T1DM) or insulin resistance (T2DM), glucose cannot enter cells efficiently, leading to persistent hyperglycaemia.

1. Ultra-Rapid Lispro (URLi; Insulin lispro-aabc)

Introduction: Ultra-Rapid Lispro (URLi), commercially known as Lyumjev, is a modified formulation of insulin lispro developed to enhance postprandial glycaemic control. By incorporating absorption-enhancing excipients, it achieves a faster onset of action and accelerated absorption, more closely mimicking physiological insulin release following meals.

Clinical Trial Phase / FDA-Approval: Ultra-Rapid Lispro was approved by the FDA in 2020 for the management of both Type 1 and Type 2 diabetes mellitus. Its efficacy and safety were evaluated in the PRONTO-T1D and PRONTO-T2D clinical trials, where it demonstrated superior postprandial glucose control compared to conventional insulin lispro, without compromising overall glycaemic management.

Characteristics:

- Contains treprostinil and citrate, accelerating subcutaneous absorption.
- Reduces postprandial glucose spikes, mimicking physiological insulin secretion.

Key Pharmacokinetic Parameters:

- Onset of action: approximately 1–2 minutes.
- Peak action: 30–60 minutes.
- Duration of action: approximately 4 hours.

Adverse Drug Reactions: Hypoglycaemia and injection site reactions.

Uses: Approved for Type 1 and Type 2 diabetes, enhancing postprandial glucose control.

Dose: Individualized based on patient needs; typically administered immediately before meals or within 20 minutes after starting a meal. Dose equivalent to U-100 insulin lispro, but faster onset and absorption

2. Insulin Icodec

Introduction: Insulin Icodec is a once-weekly basal insulin analogue developed to reduce the burden of daily injections while providing sustained and consistent basal insulin coverage. Its pharmacokinetic profile is designed to maintain stable glycaemic control over a full week with a single subcutaneous dose.

Clinical Trial Phase / FDA-Approval: It is currently undergoing evaluation in Phase III ONWARDS clinical trials, where it has shown comparable efficacy and safety to once-daily basal insulin formulations in individuals with Type 2 diabetes.

Characteristics:

- Slowly absorbed due to strong albumin binding, allowing once-weekly dosing.
- Provides steady basal insulin levels, reducing fluctuations in glucose levels.

Key Pharmacokinetic Parameters:

- Half-life: approximately 196 hours (8 days).
- Onset of action: Slow and prolonged.

Adverse Drug Reactions: Hypoglycaemia (less frequent than daily basal insulins) and mild injection site reactions.

Uses: Under investigation for Type 2 diabetes, offering a convenient once-weekly dosing option.

Dose: 70 units subcutaneously once weekly (fixed dose in clinical trials).

3. Insulin Glargine U-300

Introduction: Insulin Glargine U-300 (Toujeo) is a concentrated, longer-acting formulation of insulin glargine, providing a more stable and prolonged insulin release.

Clinical Trial Phase / FDA-Approval: FDA-approved for Type 1 and Type 2 diabetes. Evaluated in EDITION trials, showing lower risk of nocturnal hypoglycaemia.

Characteristics:

- Forms microprecipitates at the injection site, allowing slow and continuous insulin release.
- Key Pharmacokinetic Parameters:
- Duration: >36 hours.
- Peak action: Minimal, providing a flat glucose-lowering effect.

Adverse Drug Reactions: Hypoglycaemia and weight gain.

Uses: Approved for Type 1 and Type 2 diabetes, reducing hypoglycaemia risk.

Dose: 0.2 units/kg once daily; adjusted based on fasting plasma glucose and clinical response.

4. Insulin Degludec

Introduction: Insulin Degludec is an ultra-long-acting basal insulin, providing stable glucose control for over 42 hours.

Clinical Trial Phase / FDA-Approval: FDA-approved for Type 1 and Type 2 diabetes.

Characteristics:

- Forms multi-hexamer complexes, allowing gradual insulin release.

Key Pharmacokinetic Parameters:

- Half-life: approximately 25 hours.

Adverse Drug Reactions: Hypoglycaemia, lipodystrophy and injection site reactions.

Uses: Approved for basal insulin therapy.

Dose: 0.2–0.4 units/kg/day for insulin-naive patients.

5. Insulin AspartFiasp

Introduction: Insulin AspartFiasp is a faster-acting formulation of insulin aspart, designed for rapid mealtime glucose control.

Clinical Trial Phase / FDA-Approval: FDA-approved for Type 1 and Type 2 diabetes.

Characteristics:

- Contains niacinamide, enhancing absorption speed.

Key Pharmacokinetic Parameters:

- Onset of action: approximately 2–5 minutes.

Adverse Drug Reactions: Hypoglycaemia, peripheral oedema and injection-site reactions.

Uses: Approved for postprandial glucose control.

Dose: Dosed immediately before meals or within 20 minutes after starting a meal. Dosing is individualized and similar in unit-for-unit conversion with other rapid insulins.

6. Novel Approaches and Future Directions

- **Cell-Based Therapies:** Stem cell–derived beta cells or islet transplantation could offer curative potential, though challenges include graft rejection, immunosuppression, and sustainability of function.
- **Gene Editing:** CRISPR-based strategies might one day repair genetic mutations underlying monogenic diabetes or confer insulin-producing capacity in alternative cells, though these remain in early experimental stages.
- **Precision Medicine:** Genetic and biomarker profiling (e.g. autoantibody panels, insulin secretion phenotypes) can refine diagnosis and optimize therapy selection, matching patients to the most effective drugs and regimens.
- **Digital Health:** Telemedicine platforms, smartphone apps, and wearable tech empower patients with real-time data, remote clinician support, and personalized behavioural interventions—trends accelerated by the COVID-19 pandemic.

Insulin Resistance

Definition: According to the American Diabetes Association (ADA) and World Health Organization (WHO), insulin resistance is defined as:

- Reduced glucose uptake by tissues despite normal or elevated insulin levels.
- Homeostatic Model Assessment for Insulin Resistance (HOMA-IR) >2.5.

Causes of Insulin Resistance

A. **Genetic Factors**
   1. Mutations in INSR (insulin receptor gene).
   2. Polymorphisms in IRS-1, IRS-2 (insulin receptor substrate genes).

B. **Lifestyle & Environmental Factors**
   1. Obesity – Increased visceral fat leads to adipokine imbalance (↑ TNF-α, IL-6, ↓ adiponectin).
   2. Physical Inactivity – Reduces GLUT4 expression in muscles, impairing glucose uptake.

3. Diets High in Saturated Fats & Processed Carbs - Leads to lipotoxicity and inflammation.
4. Chronic Stress & Sleep Deprivation - Raises cortisol levels, promoting insulin resistance.

C. Pathophysiological Causes

1. Inflammation - Cytokines (TNF-α, IL-6) impair insulin signaling.
2. Mitochondrial Dysfunction - Leads to oxidative stress, worsening insulin resistance.
3. Non-Alcoholic Fatty Liver Disease (NAFLD) - Causes hepatic insulin resistance.

Diagnostic Criteria for Insulin Resistance

Table 2: Criteria for Diagnosing Insulin Resistance

Test	Criteria for Insulin Resistance
Fasting Insulin	>10 μU/mL (Hyperinsulinemia)
HOMA-IR Index (HOMA-IR = [Fasting insulin (μU/mL) × Fasting glucose (mg/dL)] / 405)	>2.5

Newer Drugs for Insulin Resistance

Table 3: Development of Novel Pharmacological Agents for Managing Insulin Resistance

Drug Name	Mechanism of Action	Adverse Drug Reactions	Clinical Trial Phase / FDA-Approval
Tirzepatide	Dual GLP-1/GIP receptor agonist, enhances insulin secretion and reduces glucose levels.	Nausea, vomiting, mild GI discomfort.	FDA Approved (2022) for Type 2 Diabetes.
Bexagliflozin	SGLT2 inhibitor, increases glucose excretion via urine, reducing insulin demand.	UTIs, ketoacidosis, mild dehydration.	Approved in Japan and China. Currently in Phase III trials in the U.S. and Europe.
Efpeglenatide	Long-acting GLP-1 receptor agonist, stimulates insulin release and suppresses glucagon.	Nausea, weight loss, risk of pancreatitis.	Phase III trials.
Lanifibranor	PPAR α/δ/γ agonist, improves insulin signalling and reduces liver fat (NAFLD/NASH).	Weight gain, oedema, increased risk of CHF.	Phase III trials.
Imeglimin	Targets mitochondrial dysfunction, enhances insulin sensitivity.	GI side effects, mild hypoglycaemia.	Approved in Japan (2021). Currently in Phase III trials in the U.S. and Europe.

Conclusion

The management of diabetes mellitus, encompassing both Type 1 and Type 2, has progressed significantly in the last decade, driven by enhanced pathophysiological insights and technology innovations. Conventional lifestyle interventions and well-established therapies (metformin, sulfonylureas, basal-bolus insulin) remain foundational. However, the advent of incretin-based drugs (GLP-1 RAs, dual GIP/GLP-1 agonists), SGLT2 inhibitors, and advanced insulin formulations has expanded therapeutic options—offering not only improved glycaemic control but also notable benefits in weight reduction, cardiovascular protection, and renal preservation. In parallel, diabetes technology—continuous glucose monitoring, automated insulin delivery systems, and digital health solutions—has revolutionized self-management, reducing glycaemic variability and the burden on patients. These innovations hold particular promise for Type 1 diabetes, yet also increasingly apply to insulin-treated T2DM. Looking to the future, ongoing research in immunotherapy, cell-based therapies, and precision medicine has the potential to shift paradigms again—possibly leading to disease-modifying or curative approaches. Until then, optimizing current therapies through patient-centred, individualized regimens and robust care models remains the key to mitigating diabetes complications and preserving patients' quality of life.

References

1. American Diabetes Association. Classification and diagnosis of diabetes: Standards of Medical Care in Diabetes—2023. Diabetes Care. 2023;46(Suppl 1):S19–40.
2. Subramanian S, Khan F, Hirsch IB. New advances in type 1 diabetes. Bmj. 2024 Jan 26;384.
3. Jaiswal R, Ahmad S, Pandey S, Ali A, Jaiswal R, Yadav R, Yadav R, Ahsan R, Dwivedi T. Innovative Approaches to Eczema Treatment: A Review of Fevipiprant and Its Potential as a New Therapeutic Agent. Prostaglandins & Other Lipid Mediators. 2024 Dec 29:106946.
4. Chong K, Chang JK, Chuang LM. Recent advances in the treatment of type 2 diabetes mellitus using new drug therapies. The Kaohsiung Journal of Medical Sciences. 2024 Mar;40(3):212-20.
5. Ntentakis DP, Correa VS, Ntentaki AM, Delavogia E, Narimatsu T, Efstathiou NE, Vavvas DG. Effects of newer-generation anti-diabetics on diabetic retinopathy: a critical review. Graefe's Archive for Clinical and Experimental Ophthalmology. 2024 Mar;262(3):717-52.
6. Bliss M. The Discovery of Insulin. Chicago: University of Chicago Press; 1982.
7. Saeedi P, Petersohn I, Salpea P, Malanda B, Karuranga S, Unwin N, Colagiuri S, Guariguata L, Motala AA, Ogurtsova K, Shaw JE. Global and regional diabetes prevalence estimates for 2019 and projections for 2030 and 2045: Results from the International Diabetes Federation Diabetes Atlas. Diabetes research and clinical practice. 2019 Nov 1;157:107843.
8. Davies MJ, D'Alessio DA, Fradkin J, Kernan WN, Mathieu C, Mingrone G, Rossing P, Tsapas A, Wexler DJ, Buse JB. Management of hyperglycemia in type 2 diabetes, 2018. A consensus report by the American Diabetes Association (ADA) and the European Association for the Study of Diabetes (EASD). Diabetes care. 2018 Oct 5;41(12):2669.
9. Handelsman Y, Bloomgarden ZT, Grunberger G, Umpierrez G, Zimmerman RS, Bailey TS, Blonde L, Bray GA, Cohen AJ, Dagogo-Jack S, Davidson JA. American Association of Clinical Endocrinologists and American College of Endocrinology–clinical practice guidelines for developing a diabetes mellitus comprehensive care plan–2015—executive summary. Endocrine Practice. 2015 Apr 1;21(4):413-37.
10. Pratley R, Amod A, Hoff ST, Kadowaki T, Lingvay I, Nauck M, Pedersen KB, Saugstrup T, Meier JJ. Oral semaglutide versus subcutaneous liraglutide and placebo in type 2 diabetes (PIONEER 4): a randomised, double-blind, phase 3a trial. The Lancet. 2019 Jul 6;394(10192):39-50.
11. Singh JS, Neal CP, Gulsin GS, McCann GP, Sattar N, McMurray JJV, et al. Mechanisms of cardiovascular benefit of sodium glucose co-transporter 2 (SGLT2) inhibitors. Heart. 2021 Jul;107(13):1032–1038. Available from: https://heart.bmj.com/content/107/13/1032.
12. Zinman B, Wanner C, Lachin JM, Fitchett D, Bluhmki E, Hantel S, Mattheus M, Devins T, Johansen OE, Woerle HJ, Broedl UC. Empagliflozin, cardiovascular outcomes, and mortality in type 2 diabetes. New england journal of medicine. 2015 Nov 26;373(22):2117-28.
13. Frías JP, Davies MJ, Rosenstock J, Pérez Manghi FC, Fernández Landó L, Bergman BK, Liu B, Cui X, Brown K. Tirzepatide versus semaglutide once weekly in patients with type 2 diabetes. New England Journal of Medicine. 2021 Aug 5;385(6):503-15.
14. Giorgi MA, Litwak LE, Sanabria H, Lavalle Cobo A, Musso C, Salmeri E, Álvarez J, Aranguren F, Belcastro F, Brites F, Buso C. Consenso de manejo del paciente con diabetes mellitus y patología cardiovascular. Sociedad Argentina de Cardiología (SAC)-Sociedad Argentina de Diabetes (SAD). Revista de la Sociedad Argentina de Diabetes. 2021 Mar;55:3-70.
15. Lind M, Polonsky W, Hirsch IB, Heise T, Bolinder J, Dahlqvist S, Schwarz E, Ólafsdóttir AF, Frid A, Wedel H, Ahlén E. Continuous glucose monitoring vs conventional therapy for glycemic control in adults with type 1 diabetes treated with multiple daily insulin injections: the GOLD randomized clinical trial. Jama. 2017 Jan 24;317(4):379-87.
16. Neal B, Perkovic V, Mahaffey KW, De Zeeuw D, Fulcher G, Erondu N, Shaw W, Law G, Desai M, Matthews DR. Canagliflozin and cardiovascular and renal events in type 2 diabetes. New England Journal of Medicine. 2017 Aug 17;377(7):644-57.
17. Wiviott SD, Raz I, Bonaca MP, Mosenzon O, Kato ET, Cahn A, Silverman MG, Zelniker TA, Kuder JF, Murphy SA, Bhatt DL. Dapagliflozin and cardiovascular outcomes in type 2 diabetes. New England Journal of Medicine. 2019 Jan 24;380(4):347-57.
18. Chatzianagnostou K, Gaggini M, Suman Florentin A, Simonini L, Vassalle C. New molecules in type 2 diabetes: advancements, challenges and future directions. International Journal of Molecular Sciences. 2024 Jun 5;25(11):6218.

19. Jastreboff AM, Kaplan LM, Frías JP, Wu Q, Du Y, Gurbuz S, Coskun T, Haupt A, Milicevic Z, Hartman ML. Triple-hormone-receptor agonist retatrutide for obesity—a phase 2 trial. New England Journal of Medicine. 2023 Aug 10;389(6):514-26.
20. Campbell JE, Müller TD, Finan B, DiMarchi RD, Tschöp MH, D'Alessio DA. GIPR/GLP-1R dual agonist therapies for diabetes and weight loss—chemistry, physiology, and clinical applications. Cell metabolism. 2023 Sep 5;35(9):1519-29.
21. Haddad F, Dokmak G, Bader M, Karaman R. A comprehensive review on weight loss associated with anti-diabetic medications. Life. 2023 Apr 14;13(4):1012.
22. Li T, Liu H, Li S, Yu H, Li J, Tan H, Yu Y. The effect of BMI on pharmacokinetic and pharmacodynamic parameters of insulin Degludec: results from an euglycemic glucose clamp study. Clinical Pharmacokinetics. 2023 Mar;62(3):449-56.
23. DeFronzo RA, Ferrannini E. Insulin resistance: a multifaceted syndrome responsible for NIDDM, obesity, hypertension, dyslipidemia, and atherosclerotic cardiovascular disease. Diabetes care. 1991 Mar 1;14(3):173-94.
24. Kosmalski M, Deska K, Bąk B, Różycka-Kosmalska M, Pietras T. Pharmacological support for the treatment of obesity—present and future. InHealthcare 2023 Feb 2 (Vol. 11, No. 3, p. 433). MDPI.
25. Pinnaro CT, Tansey MJ. The evolution of insulin administration in type 1 diabetes. Journal of diabetes mellitus. 2021 Nov 17;11(5):249.
26. Russell-Jones D, Bode BW, De Block C, Franek E, Heller SR, Mathieu C, Philis-Tsimikas A, Rose L, Woo VC, Østerskov AB, Graungaard T. Fast-acting insulin aspart improves glycemic control in basal-bolus treatment for type 1 diabetes: results of a 26-week multicenter, active-controlled, treat-to-target, randomized, parallel-group trial (onset 1). Diabetes Care. 2017 Jul 1;40(7):943-50.
27. Haahr H, Heise T. Fast-acting insulin aspart: a review of its pharmacokinetic and pharmacodynamic properties and the clinical consequences. Clinical Pharmacokinetics. 2020 Feb;59(2):155-72.

Chapter 27

Newer Contraceptives

Author: Dr. Pranab Das

Introduction

Contraception is an essential aspect of reproductive health, enabling people and couples to plan and spacing pregnancies, decrease unplanned pregnancies, and enhance maternal and child health outcomes. In recent decades, innovative contraceptive methods and formulations have emerged to overcome the shortcomings of older drugs, enhance adherence, and provide greater autonomy. Although oral contraceptive pills (OCPs) and barrier methods (such as condoms and diaphragms) have traditionally been the primary forms of contraception, there is an increasing interest in longer-acting, user-friendly, and more efficacious alternatives, including transdermal patches, implants, injectables, intrauterine devices (IUDs), vaginal rings, and potential male contraceptive methods.

The increasing demand for personalised contraceptive techniques signifies broader cultural changes, including postponed childbirth, a preference for discreet options, and recognition of varied reproductive needs among diverse communities. This chapter delineates the notion of contraception, succinctly outlines traditional methods, and emphasises current advancements, including novel hormonal delivery systems, long-acting reversible contraceptives (LARCs), non-hormonal innovations, and upcoming male contraceptive technologies. These modern contraceptives seek to augment alternatives.

Historical Perspective

The evolution of contraceptive techniques has paralleled progress in hormonal science, reproductive biology, and societal consciousness. The contemporary contraceptive period commenced in the 1950s, when Dr. Gregory Pincus and Dr. John Rock created the inaugural oral contraceptive pill, Enovid, which received FDA approval in 1960. It integrated synthetic oestrogen and progestin to inhibit ovulation, signifying a crucial advancement in reproductive autonomy. The following decades witnessed the development of combination tablets featuring reduced hormone dosages and enhanced safety characteristics. The 1990s saw the emergence of third-generation progestins such as desogestrel and gestodene, formulated to mitigate androgenic effects and cardiovascular concerns. Subsequent non-oral administration systems, such as the transdermal patch and vaginal ring, enhance adherence. The advent of long-acting reversible contraceptives (LARCs)—specifically levonorgestrel-releasing intrauterine systems and subdermal implants—revolutionized global contraceptive approaches by providing prolonged effectiveness with minimal user intervention.

Recent advancements have concentrated on selective progesterone receptor modulators, ultra-low-dose hormonal alternatives, and non-hormonal approaches such as pH modulators and male contraceptive gels. Novel agents such as drospirenone-only pills and combined estrogen/progestin regimens utilising estetrol, a foetal oestrogen with a distinctive safety profile, signify the advancement of contraceptive options. Moreover, investigations on male hormonal contraception utilising testosterone analogues and progestins have advanced to late-stage clinical studies. These advancements signify a continuous transition towards safer, more user-centric, and individualised contraception for both women and men, integrating reproductive science with changing societal demands.

Definition

Contraception encompasses all methods, medications, and devices employed to prevent pregnancy by interfering with the normal process of ovulation, fertilization, or implantation. Broadly, contraceptive methods can be classified into:

1. Hormonal methods: Use synthetic hormones (oestrogen and/or progestin) to prevent ovulation, thicken cervical mucus, or alter the endometrium.
2. Barrier methods: Physically block sperm from reaching the egg (e.g. male/female condoms, diaphragms).
3. Intrauterine devices (IUDs): Inserted into the uterine cavity, either releasing hormones or creating a local inflammatory environment to prevent implantation.
4. Sterilization: Permanent methods for men (vasectomy) or women (tubal ligation).
5. Natural or fertility awareness-based methods: Tracking fertility signs (e.g. basal body temperature, cervical mucus) and abstaining or using barrier methods during fertile windows.

Recent emphasis has been on developing methods that are highly effective, easily reversible, safe, and require minimal user intervention. Such characteristics are vital for reducing method failure rates and improving real-world efficacy.

Brief Note on Conventional Methods

Many existing contraceptive options have well-established track records but may exhibit drawbacks in terms of side effects, adherence requirements, or variable efficacy. Below is a concise summary table of common conventional contraceptive methods:

Table 1: Concise overview of standard contraceptive methods

Method	Mechanism of Action	Common Dosage Forms	Typical Side Effects / Limitations
Combined Oral Contraceptives (COCs)	Contain oestrogen + progestin: prevent ovulation, thicken cervical mucus.	Oral pills, taken daily for 21 consecutive days.	Need for daily adherence; potential side effects (headache, nausea, etc.); contraindications in smokers >35 years.
Progestin-Only Pills (POPs)	Primarily thicken cervical mucus, may partially inhibit ovulation.	Oral pills, taken daily.	Strict adherence to timing; less forgiving if doses missed, potential for irregular bleeding.
Injectables (e.g. DMPA)	Depot medroxyprogesterone acetate prevents ovulation, thickens cervical mucus.	Intramuscular or subcutaneous injection every 3 months.	Irregular bleeding, potential weight gain, possible delayed fertility return.
Intrauterine Devices (IUDs) (Copper or Levonorgestrel)	Copper IUD creates a local inflammatory reaction toxic to sperm; LNG-IUD releases levonorgestrel.	T-shaped device inserted in uterus.	Cramping, heavier periods (copper IUD), irregular/light bleeding (LNG-IUD), risk of expulsion, skilful insertion needed.
Implants (e.g. Etonogestrel implant)	Slowly release progestin, inhibiting ovulation and thickening cervical mucus.	Rod implanted subdermally in the medial aspect of upper arm.	Irregular bleeding, must be inserted/ removed by trained provider, but high effectiveness and convenience.

Barrier Methods (Condoms, Diaphragms)	Physically block sperm from entering the cervical canal.	Male latex condom, female condom, diaphragm, etc.	Can fail due to improper use or breakage; typically less effective than hormonal or LARC methods.
Sterilization	Permanent interruption, ligation or removal of the reproductive tract (e.g. tubal ligation, vasectomy).	Surgical procedure	Not intended to be reversible; requires specialized procedures or minor surgery.

While these methods provide a spectrum of choices, they may not suit every individual's lifestyle or health profile. This reality underscores the importance of continuous innovation to expand contraceptive choices, address adverse effects, and simplify use.

Newer Contraceptives / Recent Advances

1. **Novel Oral Formulations and Extended Regimens**

   Extended-cycle or continuous-use pills have gained popularity as a means to reduce withdrawal bleeding frequency. Traditional COCs offer 21 days of active hormones followed by a 7-day hormone-free interval. Extended regimens (e.g. 84 days of active pills followed by a short placebo interval) limit menstrual bleeding to only four times a year, appealing to those seeking fewer periods. Some women prefer continuous pills (365 days of active pills), eliminating scheduled bleeding entirely. These approaches can improve compliance and may reduce dysmenorrhea, migraines, and other hormone-withdrawal symptoms, although some experience breakthrough spotting initially.

2. **Transdermal Patches and Vaginal Rings**

   A. **Transdermal Contraceptive Patch**

   - **Mechanism:** Delivers a combination of oestrogen and progestin through the skin into systemic circulation. It works by inhibiting the hypothalamic-pituitary-ovarian (HPO) axis, preventing the release of follicle-stimulating hormone (FSH) and luteinizing hormone (LH), which are essential for ovulation.
     1. **Estrogen (Ethinylestradiol) Effect:**
        a. Provides negative feedback to the hypothalamus and anterior pituitary.
        b. Reduces the release of gonadotropin-releasing hormone (GnRH) from the hypothalamus.
        c. This lowers FSH secretion, preventing follicular recruitment and maturation in the ovary.
     2. **Progestin Effect:**
        a. Suppresses LH secretion, preventing the LH surge, which is essential for ovulation.
        b. Without this LH peak, ovulation (release of an egg) does not occur.
   - **Examples:** Norelgestromin/ethinyl oestradiol patch (applied weekly for three weeks, followed by one patch-free week).
   - **Advantages:** Simplifies dosing to once a week instead of daily; consistent hormone delivery.
   - **Disadvantages:** Potential skin irritation, reduced efficacy in women above certain weight thresholds (approximately 90 kg), and slightly elevated risk of thrombotic events due to overall higher oestrogen exposure than low-dose COCs.

B. Vaginal Ring

- **Mechanism:** Releases a combination of etonogestrel and ethinyl oestradiol (e.g. NuvaRing®) or segesterone acetate and ethinyl oestradiol (Annovera™) when placed intravaginally.
- **Advantages:** Monthly or yearly insertion/usage cycles (Annovera ring can be reused for up to 13 cycles), good cycle control, user-controlled.
- **Disadvantages:** Vaginal discomfort, rare expulsion, potential side effects similar to other combined hormonal methods.

These methods cater to individuals desiring predictable bleeding patterns and simpler dosing regimens, bridging the gap between daily oral pills and long-acting methods.

3. Updated Long-Acting Reversible Contraceptives (LARCs)

LARCs are revered for their high efficacy and user independence (i.e., once placed, they do not require daily or weekly attention). Recent developments focus on refining existing LARC methods or exploring novel sustained-release systems:

- **New Intrauterine Systems (IUS):** Lower-dose levonorgestrel-releasing intrauterine systems, such as the 13.5 mg or 19.5 mg LNG-IUS, reduce local hormone exposure while maintaining contraceptive effectiveness for 3–5 years. Some women experience lighter or absent bleeding, while side effects like cramping are generally mild.
- **Second-Generation Implants:** Etonogestrel implants (e.g. Nexplanon®) provide up to 3 years of contraception. Efforts to minimize irregular bleeding or extend the duration of action remain areas of active research. The development of radiopaque implants aids in detection if insertion location is uncertain.

4. Self-Administered Injectable Contraceptives

Depot medroxyprogesterone acetate (DMPA) has historically been administered intramuscularly by healthcare professionals every 3 months. More recently, subcutaneous DMPA (DMPA-SC) formulations enable self-injection at home, improving accessibility and reducing clinic visits. Studies show that self-injection fosters higher continuation rates due to user autonomy. Minimal training is required, and discrete administration may benefit populations with limited healthcare access or privacy concerns. Side effects remain similar to IM DMPA (menstrual irregularities, possible weight gain, delayed return to fertility).

5. Non-Hormonal Innovations

Copper IUD Modifications

While the Copper T 380A IUD has served as a highly effective non-hormonal method for decades, research explores modifications to reduce side effects (e.g. heavier periods, dysmenorrhea). For instance, smaller frame copper IUDs with reduced copper surface area (e.g. Mini Cu T) aim to mitigate bleeding, though real-world data on comparative outcomes is evolving.

6. Vaginal pH Regulators

Investigational vaginal gels or rings that maintain an acidic vaginal pH environment offer a non-hormonal contraceptive effect by hindering sperm motility. Some formulations also protect against sexually transmitted infections (STIs). Such approaches are appealing to those wishing to avoid systemic hormones or device insertions. Clinical trials indicate moderate efficacy, though not at the level of IUDs or implants.

7. **Emerging Male Contraceptive Methods**

Contraceptive responsibility has disproportionately fallen on women. Consequently, interest in male-centric options beyond condoms or vasectomy is high. Innovations under investigation include:

- **Hormonal Male Contraception:** Combinations of progestins (to suppress gonadotropins) with testosterone (to maintain androgenic function) in the form of injectables, implants, or topical gels. Preliminary trials demonstrate promising efficacy, but occasional side effects (acne, mood changes) remain a concern.
- **Non-Hormonal Agents:** E.g. Adjudin (impairs sperm maturation), vas-occlusive devices (e.g. RISUG/Vasalgel), and gene-silencing technologies targeting spermatogenesis.
- **Thermoregulation / Ultrasound:** Exploring the possibility of testicular heat application or ultrasound to transiently reduce sperm production. Feasibility and user acceptance remain to be demonstrated.

Male contraceptive development faces challenges: finding the right balance of efficacy, reversibility, and minimal side effects while also achieving widespread acceptance. Nonetheless, successes could dramatically broaden the contraceptive landscape, promoting gender equity in reproductive responsibility.

8. **Digital Fertility Monitors and Apps**

Fertility-awareness methods have been modernized through smartphone apps and wearable sensors that track basal body temperature, heart rate variability, and other physiological parameters. Users receive daily updates on their fertility window, enabling them to avoid intercourse or use barrier protection on fertile days. While appealing to those avoiding hormones or devices, real-world efficacy depends on strict adherence to guidelines and careful interpretation of data. Certain apps have received regulatory approvals [e.g. CE (Conformité Européenne) marking in Europe] as medical devices for contraception. Nevertheless, controversy persists regarding over-reliance on technology, and some women may require backup methods or more robust forms of contraception for reliable protection.

Several newer contraceptives are discussed below:

1. Norgestrel

Introduction: Opill (Norgestrel) is a progestin-only pill (POP) that provides effective contraception without estrogen, making it suitable for women at risk of oestrogen-related complications.

Clinical Trial Phase/FDA-Approval: FDA-approved (2023) as the first over-the-counter (OTC) contraceptive pill in the U.S.

Mechanism of Action:

1. **Suppression of Ovulation**
   - Norgestrel inhibits the release of gonadotropins (FSH & LH) from the anterior pituitary gland.
   - Prevents the mid-cycle LH surge, thereby blocking ovulation.
   - Unlike combination pills, progestin-only contraceptives (like norgestrel) do not always suppress ovulation completely but reduce ovulatory frequency.
2. **Thickening of Cervical Mucus**
   - Increases the viscosity of cervical mucus, making it impermeable to sperm.
   - Reduces sperm motility and penetration into the uterus, preventing fertilization.

3. **Endometrial Alteration and Prevention of Implantation**
   - Induces atrophic changes in the endometrial lining, making it less receptive to implantation.
   - Prevents proliferation of endometrial cells, reducing the chances of successful embryo attachment.
4. **Slowing of Fallopian Tube Motility**
   - Alters the contractility of the fallopian tubes, delaying ovum transport and preventing fertilization.
5. **Reduction in Sperm Capacitation**
   - Affects capacitation (biochemical changes in sperm required for fertilization), further reducing sperm function.

Key Pharmacokinetic Parameters: After oral administration, norgestrel is rapidly absorbed from the gastrointestinal tract. The peak plasma concentration (Tmax) is reached within 1–2 hours. It exhibits high plasma protein binding (approximately 97%), primarily to sex hormone-binding globulin (SHBG) and albumin. Norgestrel undergoes hepatic metabolism via the cytochrome P450 (CYP3A4) enzyme system, resulting in hydroxylated and conjugated metabolites that are eventually excreted through urine and faeces. The elimination half-life ($t^{1/2}$) is approximately 10–24 hours, supporting once-daily dosing in oral contraceptive formulations. In IUDs or implants, controlled release allows for extended duration of action over several years.

Adverse Drug Reactions: Irregular bleeding, breast tenderness, headaches, mood changes, depression and mild acne.

Uses: Over the counter oral contraceptive, recommended for all reproductive-age women.

Dose: 0.075 mg (75 mcg) once daily, taken at the same time each day.

2. Dapivirine-Levonorgestrel Vaginal Ring

Introduction: The dual-purpose vaginal ring is an innovative biomedical intervention that combines two active agents: levonorgestrel, a well-established hormonal contraceptive, and dapivirine, an antiretroviral drug used for HIV prevention. Designed for intravaginal use, this ring offers a long-acting, female-controlled method to simultaneously prevent unintended pregnancy and reduce the risk of HIV acquisition. It represents a promising solution for addressing two major global public health concerns—unintended pregnancies and sexually transmitted infections—especially in regions with high HIV prevalence and limited access to reproductive healthcare (Figure 1).

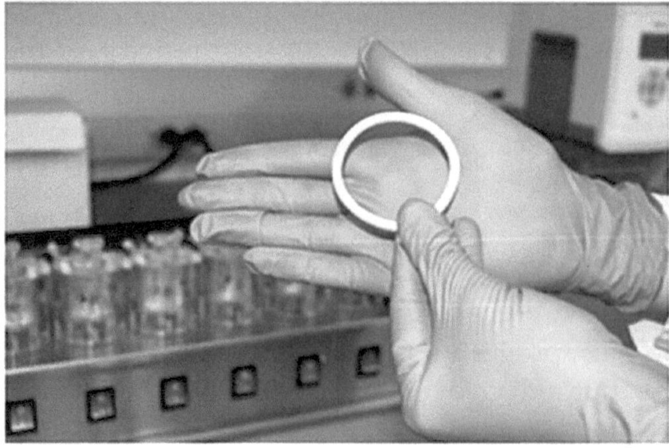

Figure 1: The Vaginal Ring of Dapivirine-Levonorgestrel for HIV Prevention and Contraception (Source: Population Council. The dapivirine-levonorgestrel vaginal ring for HIV prevention and contraception).

Clinical Trial Phase/FDA-Approval: Currently in Phase III clinical development, the agent has been evaluated in the MTN-044 and DREAM studies, where it demonstrated dual efficacy in providing contraception and preventing HIV acquisition, highlighting its potential as a long-acting multipurpose prevention technology.

Mechanism of Action:

1. **Levonorgestrel – Progestin-Based Contraceptive Effect**

   Levonorgestrel is a synthetic progestin that prevents pregnancy through a combination of endocrine and local mechanisms:

   A. Suppression of Ovulation

   Levonorgestrel inhibits the release of gonadotropins, particularly follicle-stimulating hormone (FSH) and luteinizing hormone (LH), thereby suppressing follicular development and preventing the LH surge required for ovulation.

   B. Cervical Mucus Thickening

   The hormone increases the viscosity of cervical mucus, creating a physical barrier that restricts sperm penetration and motility within the cervical canal, thereby reducing the likelihood of fertilisation.

   C. Endometrial Alteration

   Levonorgestrel induces atrophic changes in the endometrium, making it less receptive to embryo implantation, further contributing to its contraceptive efficacy.

2. **Dapivirine – Localised Antiretroviral Action for HIV Prevention**

   Dapivirine is a non-nucleoside reverse transcriptase inhibitor (NNRTI) formulated for intravaginal delivery, providing targeted prevention against HIV infection:

   A. Inhibition of Viral Replication

   Dapivirine binds to HIV-1 reverse transcriptase, inhibiting its activity and blocking the conversion of viral RNA into DNA. This prevents the virus from integrating into host cell genomes and replicating within the vaginal mucosa.

   B. Localised Protective Effect

   Delivered via the vaginal ring, dapivirine maintains high concentrations in the local mucosal tissue with minimal systemic absorption, ensuring effective HIV prophylaxis at the site of potential exposure. Clinical trials have shown a reduction in HIV acquisition risk by approximately 50%.

Key Pharmacokinetic Parameters: Levonorgestrel is a synthetic progestin used in various contraceptive formulations, including oral pills, intrauterine devices (IUDs), and emergency contraception (EC). It is rapidly absorbed after oral administration, reaching peak plasma concentration (Tmax) in approximately 1.5 hours. The oral bioavailability is approximately 100%, as it undergoes minimal first-pass metabolism. It is highly protein-bound (approximately 98%), primarily to sex hormone-binding globulin (SHBG) and albumin. Levonorgestrel is metabolized in the liver via cytochrome P450 (CYP3A4), producing inactive metabolites excreted mainly in urine (approximately 50%) and faeces (approximately 20%). The elimination half-life ($t½$) is approximately 24–32 hours, making it suitable for once-daily use in combination contraceptives or extended release in IUDs.

Adverse Drug Reactions: Menstrual irregularities, headache, nausea, venous thromboembolism, acne, mood disturbances and breast tenderness..

Uses: Under investigation for contraception and HIV prevention.

Dose: 200 mg dapivirine + 320 mg levonorgestrel, releasing 4 mg/day dapivirine and 20 mcg/day levonorgestrel over 90 days (investigational dose).

3. Segesterone acetate and Ethinyl oestradiol (Annovera)

Introduction: Annovera is a reusable, long-acting vaginal contraceptive system that delivers a combination of segesterone acetate (a novel progestin) and ethinyl estradiol for one full year of contraception. It offers a user-controlled, non-daily hormonal option with a convenient cyclic use pattern.

Clinical Trial Phase / FDA-Approval: Annovera has been approved by the FDA for long-term hormonal contraception in women of reproductive age.

Mechanism of Action:

1. **Inhibition of Ovulation**

   Segesterone acetate functions as a progestin receptor agonist, inhibiting the secretion of follicle-stimulating hormone (FSH) and luteinizing hormone (LH) from the anterior pituitary. This suppression prevents follicular maturation and inhibits the mid-cycle LH surge, thereby effectively blocking ovulation.

2. **Thickening of Cervical Mucus**

   Segesterone acetate also increases the viscosity of cervical mucus, creating a hostile environment for sperm. This impedes sperm penetration and migration through the cervical canal, reducing the likelihood of fertilisation even if ovulation were to occur.

3. **Endometrial Changes**

   The hormonal components induce endometrial thinning, reducing the likelihood of implantation. The endometrial lining becomes less receptive to embryo attachment, thereby providing an additional contraceptive mechanism.

4. **Extended Hormonal Release**

   The ring is designed for continuous, low-dose release of hormones over a 21-day cycle. This maintains consistent systemic hormone levels, avoiding the peaks and troughs often seen with daily oral contraceptives. The result is a stable contraceptive effect with fewer hormonal side effects.

Key Pharmacokinetic Parameters: Segesterone acetate (SA) and ethinyl estradiol (EE) are efficiently absorbed through the vaginal mucosa, enabling a sustained and consistent release of hormones over a 21-day period. This steady-state delivery supports effective contraceptive coverage without the need for daily administration. SA is primarily metabolised in the liver via hydrolysis and reduction, while EE undergoes hepatic metabolism through cytochrome P450 3A4 (CYP3A4), followed by conjugation via glucuronidation and sulfation. The metabolites are eliminated mainly through biliary and renal excretion. The Annovera ring is designed for cyclic use: it is inserted intravaginally for 21 consecutive days, followed by a 7-day ring-free interval, during which withdrawal bleeding may occur. This cycle is repeated monthly, and a single ring is reusable for up to 13 cycles, providing approximately one year of contraceptive protection.

Adverse Drug Reactions: Vaginal discharge, breast tenderness, nausea, headache and irregular menstrual bleeding.

Uses: Approved for Long-acting reversible contraception (LARC): one-year contraception, requiring monthly removals.

Dose: 103 mg of segesterone acetate and 17.4 mg of ethinyl oestradiol per ring. Administers 150 mcg/day of segesterone acetate and 13 mcg/day of ethinyl oestradiol. Utilised cyclically for 13 cycles (1 year): Inserted for 21 days, withdrawn for 7 days, and thereafter reused.

4. 17alpha-ethynylestradiol and Levonorgestrel Transdermal Patch (Twirla)

Introduction: Twirla is a low-dose, transdermal contraceptive patch designed to deliver levonorgestrel (a progestin) and ethinyl oestradiol (an oestrogen) in a controlled manner. It provides effective hormonal contraception with the benefits of improved cycle regulation and lower systemic oestrogen exposure compared to some traditional oral contraceptives.

Clinical Trial Phase / FDA-Approval: Twirla is approved by the FDA for use as a combined hormonal contraceptive in reproductive-age women.

Mechanism of Action:

1. **Suppression of Ovulation via Hypothalamic-Pituitary-Ovarian (HPO) Axis Inhibition**

   Twirla prevents ovulation through negative feedback on the HPO axis:

   i. Levonorgestrel (Progestin Component)
      - Suppresses luteinizing hormone (LH) secretion, preventing the mid-cycle LH surge required for ovulation.
      - Inhibits follicular maturation, making ovulation unlikely.

   ii. Ethinyl Oestradiol (Oestrogen Component)
      - Suppresses follicle-stimulating hormone (FSH) secretion, preventing the development of a dominant follicle.
      - Enhances tissue sensitivity to progestins, augmenting ovulation inhibition.

2. **Cervical Mucus Modification**

   Levonorgestrel increases the viscosity of cervical mucus, forming a physical barrier that inhibits sperm penetration and motility, thereby reducing the likelihood of fertilisation.

3. **Endometrial Alteration**

   Levonorgestrel induces endometrial atrophy, making the uterine lining less receptive to embryo implantation. Concurrently, ethinyl oestradiol stabilises the endometrium, reducing the risk of irregular or breakthrough bleeding.

4. **Advantages of Transdermal Hormone Delivery**

   Twirla provides continuous systemic hormone release via transdermal absorption, bypassing first-pass hepatic metabolism. This results in stable plasma hormone concentrations, reducing fluctuations that are often associated with adverse effects such as nausea, mood changes, or hormonal withdrawal symptoms.

Key Pharmacokinetic Parameters: Transdermal absorption bypasses first-pass hepatic metabolism, providing more consistent plasma hormone levels than oral contraceptives. Steady-state concentrations are achieved within 48 hours of the first patch application. Highly protein-bound (approximately 98%), mainly to albumin and sex hormone-binding globulin (SHBG). Levonorgestrel is metabolized in the liver via CYP3A4, forming inactive glucuronide and sulphate conjugates. Ethinyl oestradiol undergoes hepatic hydroxylation and conjugation, excreted via bile and urine.

Adverse Drug Reactions: Skin irritation, breakthrough bleeding, weight gain and hepatic dysfunction (rare).

Uses: Approved for weekly contraceptive use.

Dose: Delivers 30 mcg/day ethinyl estradiol and 120 mcg/day levonorgestrel. Applied once weekly for 3 weeks, followed by 1 patch-free week.

5. Drospirenone-only pill (Sylnd)

Introduction: Slynd is a progestin-only oral contraceptive that stands out from traditional progestin-only pills (POPs) due to its extended missed-dose window, offering more flexibility for users. This makes it a more forgiving option in daily contraceptive routines.

Clinical Trial Phase / FDA-Approval: Slynd has successfully undergone clinical evaluation and is approved by the FDA for use as a contraceptive.

Mechanism of Action:

1. **Inhibition of Ovulation**

   Drospirenone, the active ingredient in Slynd, functions as a progestin receptor agonist. By acting on the hypothalamic-pituitary-ovarian (HPO) axis, it suppresses the release of key gonadotropins-follicle-stimulating hormone (FSH) and luteinizing hormone (LH). This interference halts follicular development and blocks the LH surge that would typically trigger ovulation. When taken consistently, Slynd's ovulation suppression is about 98% effective.

2. **Thickening of Cervical Mucus**

   One of Slynd's key contraceptive actions is increasing the thickness of cervical mucus. This creates a physical barrier that impedes sperm movement and survival, effectively preventing sperm from reaching and fertilizing an egg.

3. **Endometrial Modifications**

   Slynd also works by altering the endometrium. It promotes endometrial atrophy, which reduces the likelihood of successful embryo implantation. These changes in the endometrial lining make it less receptive, further contributing to contraceptive efficacy.

4. **Anti-mineralocorticoid and Anti-androgenic Effects**

   Derived from spironolactone, drospirenone also has mild anti-mineralocorticoid properties. This helps reduce fluid retention and bloating-common concerns for many users. In addition, its ability to act as a competitive inhibitor of androgen receptors can be beneficial in managing hormonal imbalances, especially in conditions like polycystic ovary syndrome (PCOS).

Key Pharmacokinetic Parameters: After oral administration, Slynd (drospirenone) is absorbed quickly into the bloodstream. Its oral bioavailability is around 76%, which means some of the drug is lost during the first pass through the liver — a common process known as first-pass hepatic metabolism. Once in circulation, drospirenone binds extensively to plasma proteins, primarily albumin, with about 95–97% of the drug bound. Importantly, it does not significantly bind to sex hormone-binding globulin (SHBG). This low affinity for SHBG helps minimize androgenic side effects, which can be a concern with other hormonal contraceptives. In the liver, drospirenone is extensively metabolized, primarily by the enzyme CYP3A4, resulting in inactive metabolites. Before the drug is excreted, it undergoes glucuronidation and sulfation — two chemical processes that prepare substances for elimination from the body. The drug has a plasma half-life of approximately 30 to 34 hours, which means it remains active in the body long enough to support once-daily dosing — adding to its convenience and reliability as a contraceptive option.

Adverse Drug Reactions: Irregular bleeding, nausea, bloating, breast tenderness, mood changes and hyperkalaemia.

Uses: Approved for oral contraception.

Dose: 4 mg drospirenone once daily, in 24 active + 4 inert pill format.

Conclusion

Recent contraceptive technologies and delivery mechanisms have broadened the range of family planning alternatives, providing enhanced ease, effectiveness, and autonomy. Innovations such as extended-use pills, patches, vaginal rings, and long-acting reversible contraceptives address diverse requirements, while self-injectables enhance accessibility in underdeveloped regions. Current investigations into non-hormonal approaches and male contraceptive options demonstrate a dedication to diversity and individualised treatment. The emergence of digital fertility technologies introduces novel, data-driven options, yet necessitating careful utilisation. Guaranteeing affordability and accessibility, in conjunction with ongoing clinical assessment, will be essential for optimising the worldwide influence of these advancements and promoting reproductive health and autonomy.

References

1. Barton BE, Erickson JA, Allred SI, Jeffries JM, Stephens KK, Hunter MI, Woodall KA, Winuthayanon W. Reversible female contraceptives: historical, current, and future perspectives. Biology of Reproduction. 2024 Jan;110(1):14-32.
2. Asubiaro J. The impact of hormonal contraceptives on the incidence and progression of cardiovascular diseases in women: a systematic review. Cureus. 2024 Jul 25;16(7).
3. Gandhi AB, Supe PA. Evolution of Oral Contraceptive Pills. The Journal of Obstetrics and Gynecology of India. 2024 Apr;74(2):109-12.
4. Polis CB, Bradley SE, Bankole A, Onda T, Croft TN, Singh S. Contraceptive failure rates in the developing world: an analysis of demographic and health survey data in 43 countries. *Contraception.* 2016;94(1):11–7.
5. Darroch JE, Woog V, Bankole A, Ashford LS. Adding it up: The costs and benefits of investing in sexual and reproductive health 2017—estimation methodology. *Guttmacher Institute* [Internet]. 2018 [cited 2024 Mar 25]. Available from: https://www.guttmacher.org.
6. Arendsen LP, Thakar R, Sultan AH. The use of copper as an antimicrobial agent in health care, including obstetrics and gynecology. Clinical microbiology reviews. 2019 Sep 18;32(4):10-128.
7. Ilani N, Liu PY, Swerdloff RS, McLachlan RI, Bremner WJ, Nieschlag E, et al. Male hormonal contraception: progress and prospects. *Curr Opin Endocrinol Diabetes Obes.* 2019;26(3):193–9.
8. Duane M, Schliep KC, Green A, Bouchard T, Stanford JB. Modern fertility awareness-based methods: the efficacy and application of smartphone apps for fertility tracking. *Curr OpinObstet Gynecol.* 2020;32(6):453–8.
9. Bahamondes L, Bahamondes MV. The Advantages of LARC Methods. Female and Male Contraception. 2021:101-14.
10. Shim JY, Garbo G, Grimstad FW, Scatoni A, Barrera EP, Boskey ER. Use of the drospirenone-only contraceptive pill in adolescents with endometriosis. Journal of Pediatric and Adolescent Gynecology. 2024 Aug 1;37(4):402-6.
11. Palacios S, Colli E, Regidor PA. Efficacy and cardiovascular safety of the new estrogen-free contraceptive pill containing 4 mg drospirenone alone in a 24/4 regime. BMC Women's Health. 2020 Dec;20:1-9.
12. Population Council. The dapivirine-levonorgestrel vaginal ring for HIV prevention and contraception [Internet]. New York: Population Council; [cited 2025 Jun 7]. Available from: https://popcouncil.org/project/the-dapivirine-levonorgestrel-vaginal-ring-for-hiv-prevention-and-contraception/.
13. Regidor PA, Richter WH, Koytchev R, Kirkov V, Colli E. Evaluation of the food effect on a drospirenone only contraceptive containing 4 mg administered with and without high-fat breakfast in a randomised trial. BMC Women's Health. 2022 Sep 19;22(1):381.
14. Cameron NA, Blyler CA, Bello NA. Oral contraceptive pills and hypertension: a review of current evidence and recommendations. Hypertension. 2023 May;80(5):924-35.
15. Fleurant E, Mokashi M, Simon MA. Over-the-Counter Progestin-Only Oral Contraceptives. JAMA. 2023 Nov 14;330(18):1810.
16. Blakely KK. A new year-long combination hormonal contraceptive. Nursing for Women's Health. 2019 Apr 1;23(2):172-6.

Section 8

Gastrointestinal System

Chapter 28

Recent Advances in the Management of Peptic Ulcer

Author: Dr. Pranab Das

Introduction

Peptic ulcer disease (PUD) comprises ulcers in the stomach (gastric ulcer) or duodenum (duodenal ulcer), typically arising from an imbalance between the aggressive factors (e.g. acid, pepsin, Helicobacter pylori) and the protective mechanisms of the mucosa (e.g. mucus, bicarbonate, prostaglandins). Although the incidence of peptic ulcer disease has declined in some high-income countries—partly due to improved sanitary conditions and widespread Helicobacter pylori eradication—PUD remains a major global health concern. Traditionally, peptic ulcers have been primarily linked to H. pylori infection and nonsteroidal anti-inflammatory drug (NSAID) use. The understanding of peptic ulcer pathophysiology and management greatly advanced with the discovery of H. pylori and the development of proton pump inhibitors (PPIs).

Although major advances in treatment have greatly lowered complication rates and improved healing outcomes for peptic ulcers, several challenges still remain. These include the growing threat of antibiotic-resistant Helicobacter pylori strains, inconsistent adherence to treatment regimens, and the recurrence of ulcers even after therapy. Additionally, there are increasing concerns about the long-term use of proton pump inhibitors (PPIs), especially regarding their safety over extended periods. This chapter takes a comprehensive look at how peptic ulcers are defined and classified, reviews the standard approaches to management, and highlights the latest developments in drug therapy and diagnostic techniques. It also discusses emerging strategies aimed at enhancing healing, preventing complications, and confronting the critical issue of antibiotic resistance in ulcer treatment.

Historical Perspective

The management of peptic ulcer disease has significantly evolved due to important pharmacological advancements and a deeper comprehension of stomach physiology. During the early 20th century, therapeutic options were confined to bland diets and surgical interventions, resulting in elevated rates of recurrence and morbidity. The development of antacids and the inaugural histamine H2-receptor antagonist, cimetidine, by James Black in the 1970s marked a tremendous advancement, substantially decreasing acid output and accelerating ulcer healing time. This was succeeded by the emergence of proton pump inhibitors (PPIs), particularly omeprazole in the late 1980s, which provided more effective and prolonged acid control. In 1982, Barry Marshall and Robin Warren made a ground-breaking discovery by identifying Helicobacter pylori as a primary cause of most peptic ulcers, transforming the therapeutic approach from only acid suppression to antibiotic-based eradication therapies. The "triple therapy" regimen—consisting of a proton pump inhibitor, clarithromycin, and either amoxicillin or metronidazole—established itself as the standard of care. Recent advancements have concentrated on refining eradication tactics in response to increasing antibiotic resistance, incorporating bismuth-based quadruple therapy and innovative acid blockers like vonoprazan, a potassium-competitive acid blocker (P-CAB), which improves efficacy. Advancements in the comprehension of NSAID-induced ulcers include the utilisation of selective COX-2 inhibitors and proton pump inhibitor co-therapy as preventive measures. These milestones highlight the shift from symptomatic alleviation to curative strategies in the therapy of peptic ulcers.

Definition

Peptic ulcer disease is characterized by mucosal erosions equal to or deeper than 5 mm in the stomach or duodenum that typically extend through the muscularis mucosae. Peptic ulcer disease (PUD) often presents with epigastric pain or general dyspepsia, but in some cases, it may first appear through serious complications such as gastrointestinal bleeding, perforation, or gastric outlet obstruction.

There are two primary causes behind most cases of PUD:

1. **Helicobacter pylori infection:** This gram-negative bacterium colonizes the gastric mucosa, triggering chronic inflammation that can lead to ulcer formation.
2. **Use of Nonsteroidal Anti-inflammatory Drugs (NSAIDs):** These drugs interfere with prostaglandin synthesis, which in turn reduces mucosal blood flow and bicarbonate secretion. This weakens the stomach's protective lining, making it more vulnerable to damage.

   In rarer cases, peptic ulcers may result from stress-related mucosal injury, Zollinger-Ellison syndrome (a gastrin-secreting tumor), or other less common conditions.

   The main goal in managing PUD is to identify and treat the root cause-whether it's H. pylori infection or NSAID use-while also promoting ulcer healing, preventing recurrence, and minimizing the risk of serious complications.

Types of Peptic Ulcer

Although gastric and duodenal ulcers share many of the same risk factors, there are key differences between the two that are important for diagnosis and management:

1. **Gastric Ulcer**
   - Typically linked to normal or even reduced levels of stomach acid.
   - Pain often worsens with eating, as food stimulates both acid secretion and gastric distention, irritating the ulcer.
   - Pain often worsens with eating, as food stimulates both acid secretion and gastric distention, irritating the ulcer.
2. **Duodenal Ulcer**
   - More often associated with excess acid production.
   - Pain, often described as "hunger pain," usually improves after eating or with the use of antacids.
   - They are more commonly linked to Helicobacter pylori infection compared to gastric ulcers.

An accurate diagnosis (via endoscopy and biopsy if needed) helps guide appropriate therapy, from eradicating H. pylori to adjusting acid suppression and lifestyle modifications.

Brief Note on Conventional Management

Conventional therapy for peptic ulcers hinges on three major pillars:

1. Eradication of H. pylori (if present).
2. Acid Suppression (to facilitate ulcer healing).
3. Discontinuation or Reduction of Ulcerogenic Agents (especially NSAIDs).

Eradication of H. pylori

The standard first-line treatment for Helicobacter pylori infection has traditionally been triple therapy, which includes a proton pump inhibitor (PPI) such as lansoprazole, combined with clarithromycin and amoxicillin.

For patients with a penicillin allergy, metronidazole is used instead of amoxicillin. This regimen is typically prescribed for 7 to 14 days.

However, in recent years, the effectiveness of triple therapy has declined, especially in areas with high clarithromycin resistance. As a result, several alternative treatment options have been developed:

i. **Bismuth-Based Quadruple Therapy:** This regimen combines a PPI, bismuth subcitrate, tetracycline, and metronidazole, and is especially useful in regions with high antibiotic resistance.

ii. **Concomitant Therapy:** All four drugs-PPI, clarithromycin, amoxicillin, and metronidazole-are taken simultaneously, providing a broader antibacterial spectrum.

iii. **Sequential Therapy:** This approach starts with PPI and amoxicillin for the first 5 days, followed by a second phase of PPI, clarithromycin, and metronidazole for another 5 days, aiming to improve eradication rates by minimizing resistance development.

Table 1: Concise overview of classical management of peptic ulcer

Drug Name / Drug Class	Mechanism of Action	Adverse Drug Reactions	Uses
Omeprazole, Esomeprazole, Pantoprazole (Proton Pump Inhibitors - PPIs)	Irreversibly inhibit H^+/K^+-ATPase (proton pump) in gastric parietal cells, leading to long-lasting suppression of gastric acid secretion.	Common: Headache, nausea, diarrhoea, abdominal pain. Serious: Hypomagnesemia, osteoporosis, Clostridium difficile GI infection, gastric polyps with long-term use.	First-line treatment for peptic ulcer disease (PUD), gastroesophageal reflux disease (GERD), Zollinger-Ellison syndrome, and H. pylori eradication therapy (in combination with antibiotics).
Ranitidine, Famotidine (H_2 Receptor Antagonists - H_2RAs)	Block histamine H_2 receptors on gastric parietal cells, reducing mainly basal gastric acid secretion and pepsin activity.	Common: Dizziness, headache, constipation, diarrhoea. Serious: Gynecomastia (ranitidine), hepatotoxicity (rare).	Used for mild PUD, stress ulcer prophylaxis, and GERD. Less effective than PPIs.
Misoprostol (Prostaglandin E1 Analog)	Stimulates prostaglandin receptors in gastric mucosa, enhancing mucus and bicarbonate secretion while reducing acid production.	Common: diarrhoea, abdominal cramps. Serious: Uterine contractions (contraindicated in pregnancy).	Prevention of NSAID-induced ulcers.
Bismuth Subsalicylate (Mucosal Protective Agent)	Coats the ulcer site, enhances mucus and bicarbonate secretion, and has antimicrobial activity against H. pylori.	Common: Black stools, darkened tongue. Serious: Reye's syndrome (in children).	Used in H. pylori eradication therapy (bismuth-based quadruple therapy).

Recent Advances in the Management of Peptic Ulcer Disease

1. Vonoprazan

Introduction: Vonoprazan is a potassium-competitive acid blocker (PCAB) that offers rapid and sustained suppression of stomach acid. It works by directly blocking the H^+/K^+-ATPase enzyme in gastric parietal cells—the final step in acid production. Compared to traditional proton pump inhibitors (PPIs), vonoprazan acts faster and provides stronger acid control, improving healing in conditions like peptic ulcer disease and GERD.

Clinical Trial Phase / FDA-Approval: Approved by the FDA in 2022 for use in H. pylori eradication and erosive esophagitis, following positive results in PHALCON-EE and PHALCON-HP trials.

Mechanism of Action:

1. **Inhibition of H^+/K^+-ATPase (Proton Pump) in Gastric Parietal Cells**
   - Vonoprazan reversibly binds to the potassium binding site of H^+/K^+-ATPase (proton pump) in gastric parietal cells, blocking the final step of acid secretion.
   - Unlike PPIs, which require acid activation and irreversible binding, vonoprazan binds directly in a potassium-competitive manner, providing a faster onset of action.
   - This results in stronger and more prolonged gastric acid suppression, helping in peptic ulcer healing and prevention.
2. **Rapid and Sustained Acid Suppression**
   - Vonoprazan inhibits acid secretion within 2 hours of administration, compared to PPIs, which take 2–3 days for full effect.
   - Long duration of action: It remains active for 24 hours, blocking acid secretion both during the day and night.
   - Stronger acid suppression helps prevent NSAID-induced ulcers and recurrent bleeding ulcers.
3. **Stability in Acidic pH**
   - Vonoprazan remains stable even at low gastric pH (approximately 1–2), whereas PPIs degrade at acidic pH.
   - This property allows vonoprazan to exert sustained acid suppression without requiring acid activation.
4. **Potentiation of H. pylori Eradication Therapy**
   - Vonoprazan increases the efficacy of H. pylori eradication regimens by maintaining a higher gastric pH, which enhances antibiotic stability and effectiveness.
   - It has higher eradication rates than PPI-based triple therapy.

Key Pharmacokinetic Parameters: It is rapidly absorbed after oral administration, reaching peak plasma concentration (Cmax) within 1–2 hours. It has a high oral bioavailability (80%). It is primarily metabolized in the liver via CYP3A4, forming inactive metabolites. It undergoes minimal first-pass metabolism, leading to high systemic exposure. It is eiminated via faeces (65%) and urine (35%).

Adverse Drug Reactions: Headache, nausea, diarrhoea, hypergastrinemia with long-term use and increased risk of Clostridium Difficile infection due to reduced acid barrier.

Uses: H. pylori eradication therapy (combined with antibiotics), peptic ulcer disease and gastroesophageal reflux disease (GERD).

Dose: 20 mg orally once daily.

2. Tegoprazan

Introduction: Tegoprazan is another PCAB designed to rapidly and reversibly suppress acid secretion. It's gaining attention as a fast-acting alternative to PPIs with long-lasting benefits.

Clinical Trial Phase / FDA-Approval: Approved in South Korea and China for peptic ulcers and GERD. Ongoing Phase III trials are evaluating its use in the U.S..

Mechanism of Action:

1. **Inhibition of H^+/K^+-ATPase (Proton Pump) in Gastric Parietal Cells**
   - Tegoprazan reversibly binds to the potassium binding site and inhibits the H^+/K^+-ATPase enzyme, which is responsible for the final step of gastric acid secretion.
   - Unlike PPIs, which require activation in an acidic environment, tegoprazan directly inhibits the proton pump in a potassium-competitive manner.
   - This results in strong and prolonged acid suppression, promoting rapid ulcer healing and symptom relief.
2. **Rapid and Sustained Acid Suppression**
   - Tegoprazan achieves peak inhibition of gastric acid within 2 hours of administration, compared to PPIs, which take 2–3 days for full effect.
   - Long half-life (approximately 8–12 hours) ensures continuous acid suppression throughout the day and night.
   - More effective than PPIs in preventing NSAID-induced ulcers and recurrent bleeding ulcers.
3. **Stability in Acidic pH**
   - Tegoprazan remains stable in acidic pH (approximately 1–2), whereas PPIs degrade in acidic conditions.
   - This stability allows faster onset of action and eliminates the need for enteric coating or delayed-release formulations.
4. **Enhancement of H. pylori Eradication Therapy**
   - Tegoprazan maintains a high gastric pH for a longer duration, improving H. pylori eradication rates by enhancing the stability and effectiveness of antibiotics.
   - Used in dual, triple, and quadruple therapy regimens for H. pylori infection.

Key Pharmacokinetic Parameters: It is rapidly absorbed after oral administration. Peak plasma concentration (Cmax) is reached within 1–2 hours. Oral bioavailability is high and unaffected by food intake. It is primarily metabolized in the liver via CYP3A4, forming inactive metabolites. It undergoes minimal first-pass metabolism, leading to high systemic exposure. It is eliminated via faeces and urine.

Adverse Drug Reactions: Diarrhoea, mild nausea, dizziness, hypomagnesemia, hypergastrinemia and increased risk of Clostridium Difficile infections.

Uses: Peptic ulcer disease, H. Pylori Eradication Therapy and GERD.

Dose: 50 mg orally once daily.

3. Rebamipide

Introduction: Rebamipide is a mucosal-protective agent that doesn't suppress acid directly but instead promotes gastric healing by enhancing the natural defenses of the stomach lining.

Clinical Trial Phase / FDA-Approval: Approved in Japan, China, and South Korea for gastric mucosal protection.

Mechanism of Action:

1. **Enhancement of Gastric Mucosal Defense**
   - Rebamipide stimulates the production of prostaglandins (PGE2 and PGI2) in the gastric mucosa.
   - Prostaglandins enhance mucus and bicarbonate secretion, forming a protective barrier against gastric acid and pepsin.
   - This effect increases mucosal resistance to injury and accelerates ulcer healing.
2. **Promotion of Gastric Mucosal Repair**
   - Rebamipide promotes angiogenesis and epithelial regeneration in the ulcerated mucosa.
   - It upregulates cyclooxygenase-2 (COX-2) expression, which facilitates wound healing and gastric epithelial proliferation.
   - It stimulates epidermal growth factor (EGF) and fibroblast growth factor (FGF), further aiding in tissue repair.
3. **Antioxidant and Anti-Inflammatory Effects**
   - Rebamipide scavenges free radicals and reduces oxidative stress, preventing further damage to the gastric lining.
   - It inhibits neutrophil infiltration and reduces pro-inflammatory cytokines (TNF-α, IL-8), mitigating mucosal inflammation.
   - This effect helps protect the gastric mucosa from NSAID-induced injury and H. pylori-associated gastritis.
4. **Modulation of Tight Junction Proteins**
   - Rebamipide strengthens gastric epithelial cell junctions, reducing increased permeability and back-diffusion of hydrogen ions.
   - This stabilizes the gastric mucosal barrier, further protecting against acid-related damage.

Key Pharmacokinetic Parameters: Oral bioavailability is low (approximately 10–15%) due to limited gastrointestinal absorption. Peak plasma concentration (Cmax) is reached within 2–3 hours after oral administration. Plasma protein binding is approximately 98%, leading to a low free drug concentration in circulation. It undergoes minimal hepatic metabolism and remains mostly unchanged in circulation. Not metabolized via the cytochrome P450 (CYP) enzyme system, reducing the risk of drug interactions.

Adverse Drug Reactions: Mild nausea, constipation, slight elevation in liver enzymes and hypersensitivity reactions.

Uses: NSAID-induced ulcers, peptic ulcer and gastric mucosal protection.

Dose: 100 mg orally three times daily (TID).

4. Lafutidine

Introduction: Lafutidine is a second-generation H_2-receptor antagonist (H_2RA) that not only reduces acid but also enhances gastric mucosal protection. It offers broader protection than older H_2 blockers like ranitidine or famotidine.

Clinical Trial Phase / FDA-Approval: Approved in Japan for GERD and peptic ulcers.

Mechanism of Action:

1. **H_2 Receptor Antagonism**

   Gastric acid secretion is regulated by histamine, acetylcholine, and gastrin. Histamine binds to H_2 receptors on gastric parietal cells, stimulating adenylyl cyclase and cAMP, leading to activation of the H^+/K^+ ATPase (proton pump), which secretes HCl into the stomach. Lafutidine blocks histamine H_2 receptors on gastric parietal cells, thereby reducing gastric acid secretion. This suppression of acid helps prevent further damage to the ulcerated mucosa and promotes healing.

2. **Stimulation of Gastroprotective Factors**

   Unlike other H_2RAs, lafutidine stimulates endogenous protective mechanisms, including:

   - Mucus and bicarbonate secretion: It enhances mucus production by activating gastric sensory afferent neurons.
   - Increased gastric mucosal blood flow: The drug stimulates calcitonin gene-related peptide (CGRP) release, leading to improved microcirculation and ulcer healing.

3. **Anti-Inflammatory and Antioxidant Effects**

   Lafutidine reduces inflammation by inhibiting interleukin-8 (IL-8) production, which is linked to Helicobacter pylori (H. pylori)-induced gastritis. This action reduces oxidative stress and enhances mucosal defense.

4. **Capsaicin-Sensitive Sensory Neuron Activation**

   A unique feature of lafutidine is its ability to stimulate capsaicin-sensitive sensory neurons, which promotes mucosal healing independent of acid suppression. This leads to:

   - Increased prostaglandin E_2 (PGE_2) levels, which protect the gastric lining.
   - Nitric oxide (NO)-mediated vasodilation, improving gastric mucosal integrity.

5. **Protection Against NSAID-Induced Ulcers**

   Non-steroidal anti-inflammatory drugs (NSAIDs) often cause gastric ulcers. Lafutidine counteracts NSAID-induced damage by:

   - Preventing oxidative stress in the gastric mucosa.
   - Enhancing mucosal resistance via capsaicin-sensitive neurons and NO release.

Key Pharmacokinetic Parameters: Food delays absorption but does not significantly affect overall bioavailability. Gastric acid suppression is enhanced when taken postprandially due to increased CGRP (calcitonin gene-related peptide) release. It undergoes hepatic metabolism via CYP450 enzyme. Plasma half-life is 2.5-3.5 hours. It is mainly excreted by urine.

Adverse Drug Reactions: Dizziness, mild nausea, hepatotoxicity, and hypersensitivity reactions.

Uses: Peptic ulcer disease and GERD treatment.

Dose: 10 mg orally twice daily.

5. Ilaprazole

Introduction: Ilaprazole is a long-acting proton pump inhibitor (PPI) that provides stronger and longer-lasting acid suppression than many of the traditional PPIs. It's particularly effective in managing acid-related conditions such as peptic ulcers and gastroesophageal reflux disease (GERD) due to its extended duration of action.

Clinical Trial Phase / FDA-Approval: Ilaprazole is currently approved for clinical use in China and South Korea.

Mechanism of Action:

1. **Absorption and Activation**

   Ilaprazole is a prodrug—it's absorbed in the small intestine and transported through the bloodstream to the parietal cells in the stomach.

2. **Activation in Acidic Environment**

   Once it reaches the acidic canaliculi of the gastric parietal cells, ilaprazole undergoes a pH-dependent transformation. At the low pH levels typical of this environment (around 1.5), the drug is converted into its active form.

3. **Irreversible Binding to Proton Pumps**

   The active form of ilaprazole binds covalently to the H^+/K^+-ATPase enzyme—specifically to cysteine residues Cys813 and Cys822. This irreversible binding effectively shuts down the final step in acid production.

4. **Prolonged Acid Suppression**

   With a half-life of 5–8 hours and slow metabolic breakdown, ilaprazole provides sustained inhibition of acid secretion, often maintaining control for up to 24 hours.

5. **Gastroprotective Properties**

   In addition to reducing acid, ilaprazole indirectly boosts mucus and bicarbonate secretion, offering added protection to the gastric mucosa.

Key Pharmacokinetic Parameters: Ilaprazole offers higher bioavailability than many other proton pump inhibitors, meaning a greater proportion of the drug reaches the bloodstream and exerts its effect. It also has a longer duration of acid suppression, with a half-life of 5 to 8 hours, compared to just 1 to 2 hours for omeprazole. A key advantage of ilaprazole is that, unlike omeprazole—which is extensively metabolized by the CYP2C19 enzyme—its metabolism is less influenced by genetic variations. This means ilaprazole works more consistently across different patient populations, regardless of their CYP2C19 genotype. Its potent acid-suppressing effect can last up to 24 hours, helping to reduce the risk of ulcer recurrence with once-daily dosing. The drug is primarily eliminated through the urine.

Adverse Drug Reactions: Nausea, dizziness, increased fracture risk and acute interstitial nephritis (rare).

Uses: Peptic ulcer and GERD.

Dose: 10–20 mg orally once daily.

6. Other recent advances in the treatment of Peptic Ulcer:

a. **Novel H. pylori Eradication Regimens**

Tailored or Personalized Therapy:

- Instead of empirical triple or quadruple therapy, some centres perform antibiotic susceptibility testing prior to treatment. Cultured H. pylori isolates identify resistance patterns, guiding antibiotic choice. While more resource-intensive, this method can significantly improve eradication rates.

Rescue Therapies:

- For patients failing first- or second-line therapy, new regimens—like rifabutin-based triple therapy (PPI + rifabutin + amoxicillin)—may offer improved salvage treatment success if resistance to clarithromycin and metronidazole is high.

High-Dose Dual Therapy:

- High-dose PPI plus amoxicillin for 14 days has emerged as an alternative in areas with prevalent clarithromycin or metronidazole resistance. The concept is to maintain intragastric pH above 6 for extended periods, enhancing amoxicillin's bactericidal activity. Preliminary studies reveal encouraging eradication rates with fewer side effects.

b. Probiotics and Microbiome-Oriented Approaches

Growing recognition of the gut microbiome's role in GI health has propelled interest in probiotics as adjunct therapy. Certain strains (e.g. Lactobacillus, Bifidobacterium) may:

- Improve H. pylori eradication rates by reducing local inflammation and enhancing antibiotic efficacy.
- Mitigate antibiotic-associated side effects (e.g. diarrhoea, dysbiosis).

However, data on the optimal probiotic strains, dosing, and duration remain somewhat inconsistent. Trials suggest modest incremental benefits, indicating that probiotic supplementation can be a supportive measure alongside standard therapy.

c. Endoscopic Innovations in Bleeding Ulcers

For peptic ulcers complicated by haemorrhage, endoscopic intervention (e.g. injection of epinephrine, thermal coagulation, clipping) is the mainstay. Recent technological advances:

- Haemostatic Powders (e.g. TC-325): Sprayed onto the bleeding site to form a mechanical barrier, particularly useful in diffuse oozing or lesions challenging to treat with conventional modalities.
- Newer Endoscopic Clips: Over-the-scope clips and specialized devices providing stronger compression and improved grip.
- Endoscopic Ultrasound (EUS)-guided therapy: Allows targeted injection of substances (e.g. cyanoacrylate) in complex vascular lesions or pseudoaneurysms associated with ulcer bleeding.

These tools augment standard endoscopic treatment, reducing re-bleeding risk and enhancing salvage for difficult bleeds. PPIs post-endoscopy (high-dose IV or oral) remain crucial for promoting clot stability and healing.

d. Enhanced Surveillance and Risk Stratification

Risk stratification models (e.g. Glasgow-Blatchford score, Rockall score) guide clinical decision-making for upper GI bleeding—essentially determining urgent endoscopy vs. outpatient management. Meanwhile, non-invasive breath tests (e.g. 13C-urea breath test) and stool antigen tests have improved H. pylori detection and post-treatment confirmation of eradication. Some centres incorporate genetic analysis or molecular diagnostics (PCR-based) to detect antibiotic resistance mutations directly from gastric biopsies or stool samples, enabling real-time tailored therapy.

e. Alternative Approaches and Future Prospects

- Vaccines Against H. pylori: Though experimental, prophylactic or therapeutic vaccines targeting key bacterial antigens hold promise for controlling infection in high-prevalence regions. Trials have faced challenges with immunogenicity and safety but remain under investigation.

- Muco-Protective Agents: Ongoing interest in novel mucosal protectants (e.g. rebamipide analogues) or growth factor-based therapies that bolster mucosal defense, reduce inflammation, and accelerate ulcer healing.
- Gut-Brain Axis Insights: Some research explores how stress-related neurohormonal changes affect gastric mucosal defenses, suggesting mind-body interventions or novel pharmacologic targets. However, these remain more exploratory.

Conclusion

The management of peptic ulcer disease has evolved considerably over the last few decades, marked by landmark discoveries (H. pylori) and transformative therapies (PPIs). Yet challenges persist, such as escalating antibiotic resistance that undermines classical triple therapy, complicated ulcer disease in elderly or comorbid patients using NSAIDs, and concerns about the long-term safety of potent acid suppression. Recent advances address these hurdles through personalized H. pylori eradication (guided by resistance testing or new regimens like high-dose P-CAB triple therapy), next-generation acid blockers (vonoprazan) offering rapid and consistent gastric pH control, and novel endoscopic hemostatic techniques for managing bleeding ulcers. Complementary strategies, including probiotics to support eradication and refined diagnostic tools, further enhance care. In the near future, emergent concepts like H. pylori vaccination, advanced mucosal protectants, and microbiome modulation may usher in additional breakthroughs. For current clinical practice, vigilant antibiotic stewardship, routine post-treatment testing to confirm H. pylori eradication, and careful selection of acid suppression regimens remain fundamental. By integrating these advances with appropriate lifestyle modifications (e.g. limiting NSAIDs, reducing alcohol or smoking) and targeted prevention (especially for high-risk groups), we can continue to reduce the burden of peptic ulcer disease and its potentially life-threatening complications.

References

1. Almadi MA, Lu Y, Alali AA, Barkun AN. Peptic ulcer disease. The Lancet. 2024 Jul 6;404(10447):68-81.
2. Sapkota B, Pandey B, Sapkota B, Dhakal K, Aryal B. A systematic review and meta-analysis on pharmacist-led interventions for the management of peptic ulcer disease. PloS one. 2025 Mar 25;20(3):e0320181.
3. Mal S, Das TK, Pradhan S, Ghosh K. Probiotics as a Therapeutic Approach for Non-Infectious Gastric Ulcer Management: A Comprehensive Review. Probiotics and Antimicrobial Proteins. 2025 Feb;17(1):393-418.
4. Tassone D, Kazi S, Lee T, Gilmore R, Ding N. Systematic review and meta-analysis of endoscopic versus medical management of peptic ulcers with adherent clots. Journal of Gastroenterology and Hepatology. 2024 Oct;39(10):2031-42.
5. Black JW, Duncan WA, Durant CJ, Ganellin CR, Parsons EM. Definition and antagonism of histamine H2-receptors. Nature. 1972;236(5347):385–390.
6. Sung JJ, Kuipers EJ, El-Serag HB. Systematic review: the global incidence and prevalence of peptic ulcer disease. Alimentary pharmacology & therapeutics. 2009 May;29(9):938-46.
7. Kinoshita Y, Ishimura N, Ishihara S. Review article: potassium-competitive acid blockers for the treatment of acid-related disorders. ResearchGate [Internet]. 2021 [cited 2025 Jun 7]. Available from: https://www.researchgate.net/publication/349376970_Review_article_potassium-competitive_acid_blockers_for_the_treatment_of_acid-related_disorders.
8. Chey WD, Wong BC, Practice Parameters Committee of the American College of Gastroenterology. American College of Gastroenterology guideline on the management of Helicobacter pylori infection. Official journal of the American College of Gastroenterology | ACG. 2007 Aug 1;102(8):1808-25.
9. Graham DY, Lee YC, Wu MS. Rational Helicobacter pylori therapy: evidence-based medicine rather than medicine-based evidence. Clinical Gastroenterology and Hepatology. 2014 Feb 1;12(2):177-86.
10. Liou JM, Chen CC, Chen MJ, Chen CC, Chang CY, Fang YJ, Lee JY, Hsu SJ, Luo JC, Chang WH, Hsu YC. Sequential versus triple therapy for the first-line treatment of Helicobacter pylori: a multicentre, open-label, randomised trial. The Lancet. 2013 Jan 19;381(9862):205-13.
11. Sakurai Y, Mori Y, Okamoto H, Nishimura A, Komura E, Araki T, Shiramoto M. Acid-inhibitory effects of vonoprazan 20 mg compared with esomeprazole 20 mg or rabeprazole 10 mg in healthy adult male subjects-a randomised open-label cross-over study. Alimentary pharmacology & therapeutics. 2015 Sep;42(6):719-30.
12. Szajewska H, Horvath A, Piwowarczyk A. Meta-analysis: the effects of Saccharomyces boulardii supplementation on Helicobacter pylori eradication rates and side effects during treatment. Alimentary pharmacology & therapeutics. 2010 Nov;32(9):1069-79.

13. Gravina AG, Zagari RM, De Musis C, Romano L, Loguercio C, Romano M. Helicobacter pylori and extragastric diseases: A review. World journal of gastroenterology. 2018 Aug 7;24(29):3204.
14. De Bortoli N, Martinucci I, Giacchino M, Blandizzi C, Marchi S, Savarino V, Savarino E. The pharmacokinetics of ilaprazole for gastro-esophageal reflux treatment. Expert Opinion on Drug Metabolism & Toxicology. 2013 Oct 1;9(10):1361-9.
15. Pu J, Wang F, Tang W, Zhu M. Biotransformation of ilaprazole in human liver microsomes and human: role of CYP3A4 in ilaprazole clearance and drug-drug interaction. Drug Metabolism and Disposition. 2018 Oct 1;46(10):1453-61.
16. Ihara E, Hata Y, Ogino H. Can personalized optimization of acid suppression dosage and duration improve the management of artificial ulcers after gastric endoscopic submucosal dissection?. Journal of Gastroenterology. 2025 Feb 9:1-2.
17. Pathak R, Chandra P. Bioactive Compounds from Myrica esculenta: Antioxidant Insights and Docking Studies on H+ K+-ATPase and H2 Receptor Targets. Medicinal Chemistry. 2025 Feb 4.
18. Mohanto N, Mondal H, Park YJ, Jee JP. Therapeutic delivery of oxygen using artificial oxygen carriers demonstrates the possibility of treating a wide range of diseases. Journal of Nanobiotechnology. 2025 Jan 18;23(1):25.
19. Park JK. Optimal Use of Proton Pump Inhibitors and Potassium-competitive Acid Blockers. The Korean Journal of Helicobacter and Upper Gastrointestinal Research. 2023 Sep 8;23(3):180-7.
20. Zhang Z, Liu F, Ai F, Chen X, Liu R, Zhang C, Fang N, Fu T, Wang X, Tang A. The efficacy and mechanism of vonoprazan-containing triple therapy in the eradication of Helicobacter pylori. Frontiers in Pharmacology. 2023 May 5;14:1143969.
21. Scarpignato C, Hunt RH. Acid suppressant therapy: a step forward with potassium-competitive acid blockers. Current Treatment Options in Gastroenterology. 2021 Mar;19:94-132.
22. Kak M. Rebamipide in gastric mucosal protection and healing: An Asian perspective. World Journal of Gastrointestinal Pharmacology and Therapeutics. 2025 Mar 5;16(1):101753.
23. Sagar S, Srinivas L. Bio-analytical Method Development for Pharmacokinetic Study of Novel Lafutidine Formulation in Rabbit Plasma Using RP-HPLC. Indian journal of pharmaceutical education and research. 2024 Jan 1;58(1):S224-31.
24. Castus HI, Priyadharshini A. Ilaprazole: Distinctive Pharmacokinetic and Pharmacodynamic Properties Among Proton Pump Inhibitors. Gastroenterology & Endoscopy. 2025 Apr 9.

Chapter 29

Recent Advances in the Management of Irritable Bowel Syndrome (IBS)

Author: Dr. Pranab Das

Introduction

Irritable Bowel Syndrome (IBS) is a common functional gastrointestinal (GI) disorder marked by abdominal pain or discomfort in combination with changes in bowel habits, which may include diarrhoea, constipation, or a mix of both. Affecting an estimated 10–15% of adults worldwide, IBS places a considerable burden not only on healthcare systems but also on patients' daily lives and overall well-being. One of the main challenges with IBS is that symptoms are often chronic and relapsing, yet no clear structural abnormalities are detected during diagnostic testing. This can make both diagnosis and treatment more complex, often requiring a process of exclusion. Traditionally, the management of IBS has focused on symptom relief through measures like dietary modifications—particularly low-FODMAP diets—as well as pharmacologic treatments such as antispasmodics, laxatives, and anti-diarrheal agents, depending on the patient's predominant symptoms.

However, our understanding of IBS has grown well beyond the idea of simple gut motility disturbances. Current research highlights a complex interplay involving the gut-brain axis, intestinal microbiota, immune system dysregulation, and visceral hypersensitivity—a heightened response to pain or discomfort from internal organs. These deeper insights have opened the door to new therapeutic approaches. In addition to traditional treatments, options now include:

- Neuromodulators that target central and peripheral pain pathways,
- Advanced probiotics tailored to influence gut flora balance,
- And gut-directed therapies that address both GI and central nervous system (CNS) involvement in symptom perception.

This chapter provides a comprehensive review of the definition and subtypes of IBS, outlines standard treatment strategies, and explores emerging advances in areas such as pharmacotherapy, dietary interventions, and microbiome- or CNS-focused therapies—all aiming to offer more personalized and effective care for IBS patients.

Historical Perspective

The advancement of irritable bowel syndrome (IBS) care illustrates the increasing comprehension of its intricate pathophysiology, which includes modified motility, visceral hypersensitivity, and dysfunction of the gut–brain axis. Initially regarded as a psychosomatic condition, IBS acquired clinical recognition in the 1970s with the establishment of diagnostic criteria, subsequently formalised by the Rome criteria, first published in 1990. Initial therapies concentrated on alleviating symptoms by the administration of antispasmodics, laxatives, and fibre supplements. The emergence of serotonergic drugs in the 1990s represented a significant milestone. Alosetron, a 5-HT3 receptor antagonist created by GlaxoSmithKline for the treatment of IBS with diarrhoea (IBS-D), received approval in 2000; nevertheless, safety concerns restricted its application.

Tegaserod, a 5-HT4 agonist for irritable bowel syndrome with constipation (IBS-C), was developed by Novartis and was briefly available in the early 2000s.

Subsequent pharmacological advancements were influenced by an improved comprehension of gastrointestinal neurotransmission, culminating in the approval of linaclotide (2012) and plecanatide (2017), both guanylate cyclase-C agonists that augment fluid secretion and alleviate pain in IBS-C. Rifaximin, a non-absorbable antibiotic, received FDA approval in 2015 for IBS-D following significant research by Mark Pimentel that elucidated the role of gut flora. Eluxadoline, a combined μ-opioid receptor agonist and δ-antagonist, was developed for IBS-D, providing clinical relief with a reduced risk of constipation. Recent advancements have investigated the influence of nutrition (e.g., low-FODMAP therapies), microbiome modification, and gut-brain neuromodulators such as ibodutant and neuromodulatory peptides. This indicates a transition from exclusively symptom-focused treatment to precision approaches aimed at addressing underlying processes and individual phenotypes.

Definition

Irritable Bowel Syndrome (IBS) is a functional gastrointestinal (GI) disorder defined by chronic abdominal pain and changes in bowel habits such as constipation, diarrhoea, or a combination of both. It is most commonly classified based on bowel habit patterns, using the Rome IV diagnostic criteria – an internationally accepted standard for identifying functional GI disorders.

According to the Rome IV criteria, a diagnosis of IBS requires that a patient has experienced recurrent abdominal pain, on average, at least one day per week over the past three months. This pain must be associated with two or more of the following features:

i. Related to defecation.
ii. Associated with a change in frequency of stool.
iii. Associated with a change in form (appearance) of stool.

These symptoms should begin at least six months prior to diagnosis. Although IBS does not cause lasting damage or increase mortality, its persistent symptoms and impact on daily functioning justify extensive research into better diagnostic and therapeutic methods.

Types of Irritable Bowel Syndrome

According to the Rome IV criteria, the classification of Irritable Bowel Syndrome (IBS) subtypes is based primarily on the predominant stool pattern observed:

1. **IBS with Predominant Constipation (IBS-C):**
   - Hard or lumpy stools are present at least 25% of the time.
   - Loose or watery stools occur less than 25% of the time.
2. **IBS with Predominant Diarrhoea (IBS-D):**
   - Loose or watery stools are experienced 25% of the time or more.
   - Hard or lumpy stools are present less than 25% of the time.
3. **IBS with Mixed Bowel Habits (IBS-M):**
   - Both hard or lumpy stools and loose or watery stools are observed at least 25% of the time.
4. **IBS Unclassified (IBS-U):**
   - Stool consistency changes are insufficient to meet the diagnostic thresholds for IBS-C, IBS-D, or IBS-M.

Recognizing the specific subtype of IBS is crucial for directing appropriate management strategies. For instance, treatments aimed at IBS-D typically focus on slowing intestinal transit and minimizing fluid secretion, whereas therapies for IBS-C emphasize promoting laxation and stool softening. In cases where symptoms overlap or fluctuate between patterns, combination therapies or adaptive treatment approaches may be necessary to achieve optimal symptom control.

Brief Note on Conventional Management

Historically, IBS management has centred on:

1. **Lifestyle and Dietary Interventions**
   - Low-FODMAP Diet: Restricting the intake of fermentable oligosaccharides, disaccharides, monosaccharides, and polyols has been shown to significantly reduce bloating and abdominal discomfort in many individuals with IBS.
   - Fiber Supplementation: Incorporating soluble fiber, such as psyllium, can help regulate bowel movements. However, it is important to note that insoluble fiber may worsen symptoms in certain patients.
2. **Symptomatic Pharmacotherapy**
   - Antispasmodic Agents (e.g., hyoscine, mebeverine): These medications act by relaxing the smooth muscle of the gut, thereby relieving abdominal cramping.
   - Laxatives for IBS-C (e.g., polyethylene glycol, lactulose): Utilized to promote bowel movements in patients with constipation-predominant IBS.
   - Anti-diarrheal Medications for IBS-D (e.g., loperamide): Help to reduce stool frequency and improve stool consistency in diarrhoea-predominant cases.
   - Bile Acid Sequestrants (e.g., cholestyramine): Particularly beneficial for patients whose diarrhoea is associated with bile acid malabsorption.
3. **Psychological Approaches**
   - Cognitive Behavioural Therapy (CBT) and gut-directed hypnotherapy have demonstrated efficacy in reducing symptom severity and improving quality of life, highlighting the gut-brain axis component.
   - Antidepressants (e.g. low-dose tricyclics, SSRIs) often used for pain modulation and to address comorbid depression/anxiety.

   While many patients achieve partial improvement with these strategies, variable response rates and ongoing symptom flares indicate a need for more targeted and effective therapies.

Recent Advances in IBS Management

1. Novel Pharmacological Agents

A. IBS-C: Secretagogues and Prokinetics

1. Linaclotide:

Introduction: Guanylate cyclase-C (GC-C) agonists are a class of medications that stimulate the secretion of chloride and bicarbonate into the intestinal lumen. This action increases the fluid content of the stool and accelerates intestinal transit. Beyond their effects on motility, GC-C agonists also help reduce visceral pain by modulating sensory pathways. Among them, linaclotide has emerged as a cornerstone treatment for moderate-to-severe IBS-C, consistently demonstrating significant improvements in both bowel habits and abdominal pain.

Clinical Trial Phase / FDA-Approval: Linaclotide has been approved by the U.S. Food and Drug Administration (FDA) for the treatment of irritable bowel syndrome with constipation (IBS-C) and chronic idiopathic constipation (CIC). Clinical trials, including the Linzess IBS-C studies, have shown marked improvements in stool consistency and reductions in abdominal pain, reinforcing its role as a key therapeutic option.

Mechanism of Action: Linaclotide exerts its effects by activating guanylate cyclase-C (GC-C) receptors located on the luminal surface of intestinal epithelial cells. Upon activation, there is an increase in cyclic guanosine monophosphate (cGMP) production, which regulates intestinal fluid secretion, motility, and nociceptive (pain-related) pathways.

Mechanisms Underlying Linaclotide's Effects in IBS-C:

1. **Binding to GC-C Receptors:** Linaclotide binds specifically to GC-C receptors expressed on the epithelial cells lining the small intestine and colon. These receptors are naturally activated by endogenous peptides such as guanylin and uroguanylin, which help maintain intestinal fluid balance.
2. **Elevation of cGMP Levels:** Activation of GC-C leads to the conversion of guanosine triphosphate (GTP) into cyclic GMP (cGMP).
   - Intracellular cGMP stimulates the cystic fibrosis transmembrane conductance regulator (CFTR), promoting the secretion of chloride and bicarbonate ions into the intestinal lumen.
   - Extracellular cGMP acts on sensory neurons, reducing pain signalling.
3. **Chloride and Bicarbonate Secretion via CFTR Activation:** Activation of CFTR channels results in the secretion of chloride and bicarbonate ions into the lumen, creating an osmotic gradient that draws water into the intestine. This hydration softens stools and enhances bowel movement frequency and consistency.
4. **Inhibition of Sodium-Hydrogen Exchanger 3 (NHE3):** Linaclotide also inhibits NHE3, a transporter responsible for sodium absorption. By limiting sodium uptake, it further promotes water retention in the intestinal lumen, thus improving stool hydration and facilitating transit.
5. **Visceral Pain Modulation via Extracellular cGMP:** Elevated levels of extracellular cGMP attenuate nociceptor activity in colonic afferent neurons. This mechanism leads to:
   - A reduction in visceral hypersensitivity.
   - Diminished abdominal pain.
   - Inhibition of pain signals traveling from the gut to the central nervous system (CNS).
6. **Potential Effects on Gut Microbiota:** Emerging evidence suggests that linaclotide may also influence the gut microbiota, contributing to improved intestinal homeostasis and a reduction in mucosal inflammation.

Key Pharmacokinetic Parameters: Linaclotide has poor oral bioavailability (less than 1%) and is minimally absorbed into systemic circulation, making systemic side effects rare. After oral administration, linaclotide is rapidly degraded in the stomach and small intestine into its active metabolite (MM-419447), which retains GC-C agonist activity. The drug and its metabolite are excreted in faeces with no significant renal clearance.

Adverse Drug Reactions: Diarrhoea (most common), abdominal pain, bloating and allergic reactions.

Uses: IBS-C and chronic idiopathic constipation (CIC).

Dose: 290 mcg once daily, taken 30 minutes before the first meal of the day.

2. Lubiprostone:

Introduction: Lubiprostone is a chloride channel activator that enhances fluid secretion in the intestines, thereby softening stools and alleviating constipation. While clinical studies have shown a modest reduction in abdominal pain, its principal value lies in treating IBS-C, particularly among adult women.

Clinical Trial Phase/FDA-Approval: Lubiprostone has received FDA approval for the treatment of irritable bowel syndrome with constipation (IBS-C). In clinical evaluations, including the Amitiza IBS-C trials, the drug demonstrated notable improvements in bowel movement frequency and a significant reduction in straining during defecation.

Mechanism of Action: The primary mechanism by which lubiprostone exerts its therapeutic effects involves the activation of type-2 chloride channels (ClC-2) in the gastrointestinal epithelium. This activation enhances intestinal fluid secretion and promotes motility, independent of cyclic nucleotide pathways such as cGMP or cAMP.

Mechanisms Underlying Lubiprostone's Effects in IBS-C

1. **Activation of ClC-2 Channels**

   Lubiprostone directly binds to and activates ClC-2 channels located on the apical membrane of intestinal epithelial cells. Unlike agents such as linaclotide, lubiprostone does not act through guanylate cyclase-C (GC-C) or secondary messenger systems like cGMP.

2. **Chloride Secretion and Osmotic Water Movement**

   Activation of ClC-2 channels leads to secretion of chloride ions into the intestinal lumen. This creates an osmotic gradient, pulling sodium and water into the lumen, increasing stool moisture and facilitating smoother bowel movements.

3. **Inhibition of Sodium Absorption**

   Lubiprostone inhibits the activity of the sodium-hydrogen exchanger 3 (NHE3), reducing sodium reabsorption and promoting water retention within the stool. This mechanism supports the maintenance of softer stool consistency.

4. **Stimulation of Prostaglandin Receptors (EP4 Subtype)**

   Additionally, lubiprostone activates prostaglandin EP4 receptors, which further augment chloride secretion and enhance gastrointestinal motility.

5. **Acceleration of Intestinal Transit**

   The combined effects of enhanced fluid secretion and diminished sodium absorption result in faster intestinal transit, effectively relieving constipation.

6. **Visceral Pain Reduction and Anti-Inflammatory Effects**

   Beyond its prosecretory action, lubiprostone may also play a role in modulating visceral pain by reducing intestinal inflammation and normalizing gut sensory signaling. These effects are particularly beneficial for IBS-C patients who experience significant abdominal discomfort and bloating.

Key Pharmacokinetic Parameters: Lubiprostone has poor systemic bioavailability (<10%), as it acts locally in the intestine. Metabolized via carbonyl reductase in the stomach and intestine to its active metabolite M3. Does not undergo CYP450 metabolism, reducing the risk of drug-drug interactions. Primarily excreted in faeces (>90%), with minimal renal elimination.

Adverse Drug Reactions: Nausea, diarrhoea, headache and abdominal distension.

Uses: IBS-C, opioid-induced constipation and chronic idiopathic constipation (CIC).

Dose: 8 mcg twice daily with food and water.

3. Tegaserod (5-HT4 receptor agonist):

Introduction: Tegaserod is approved for the treatment of IBS-C in women under 65 years of age who do not have significant cardiovascular risk factors. It functions by accelerating gastrointestinal (GI) transit and may also reduce abdominal pain through modulation of serotonin-mediated gut motility and sensation. However, clinical use requires caution due to previous concerns regarding potential cardiac events associated with the drug.

Clinical Trial Phase / FDA-Approval: Tegaserod has been granted FDA approval specifically for women under the age of 65 with IBS-C. Its approval is supported by clinical trials demonstrating benefits in improving bowel symptoms, although careful patient selection remains important to minimize cardiovascular risks.

Mechanism of Action: Tegaserod acts as a selective agonist at 5-hydroxytryptamine 4 (5-HT4) receptors, which are predominantly located on enteric neurons within the gastrointestinal tract. These receptors are key regulators of intestinal motility, fluid secretion, and visceral pain perception.

Mechanism of Tegaserod in IBS-C:

1. **Activation of 5-HT4 Receptors on Enteric Neurons**

   Tegaserod selectively binds to 5-HT4 receptors on presynaptic neurons within the myenteric plexus. This binding stimulates the release of neurotransmitters such as acetylcholine (ACh), calcitonin gene-related peptide (CGRP), and nitric oxide (NO) — all crucial mediators that drive intestinal peristalsis.

2. **Enhancement of Gastrointestinal Motility**

   The release of ACh and CGRP promotes smooth muscle contraction, thereby enhancing peristaltic activity and improving colonic transit. Concurrently, nitric oxide contributes to the relaxation of intestinal muscles, ensuring coordinated movement and smoother passage of stool.

3. **Increase in Intestinal Fluid Secretion**

   Tegaserod activates submucosal secretomotor neurons, leading to increased secretion of chloride and bicarbonate ions. This enhances stool hydration and consistency, facilitating easier and more regular bowel movements.

4. **Modulation of Visceral Pain Sensitivity**

   By activating 5-HT4 receptors, tegaserod diminishes afferent pain signaling from the gut to the central nervous system. This action reduces visceral hypersensitivity and provides relief from hallmark IBS-C symptoms such as abdominal pain and bloating.

5. **Anti-Inflammatory and Epithelial Repair Effects**

   Tegaserod has demonstrated the ability to reduce levels of pro-inflammatory cytokines, including tumor necrosis factor-alpha (TNF-α), interleukin-6 (IL-6), and interleukin-8 (IL-8). This contributes to maintaining gut homeostasis and mitigating intestinal inflammation.

6. **No Effect on 5-HT3 Receptors (Avoidance of Nausea and Vomiting)**

   Unlike some other serotonergic agents, such as cisapride, tegaserod does not interact with 5-HT3 receptors. As a result, it avoids side effects commonly associated with 5-HT3 modulation, such as nausea, vomiting, and diarrhea.

Key Pharmacokinetic Parameters: It is rapidly absorbed after oral administration, with a peak plasma concentration (Tmax) of 1 hour. Oral bioavailability is 10%, reduced by first-pass metabolism. It shows moderate plasma protein binding, mainly to albumin. Extensively metabolized in the liver via oxidation and glucuronidation. It is excreted mainly in faeces.

Adverse Drug Reactions: Diarrhoea, abdominal pain, nausea and allergic reactions.

Uses: IBS-C and chronic idiopathic constipation (CIC).

Dose: 6 mg twice daily before meals.

B. IBS-D: Antidiarrheal and Peripheral Modulators

1. Eluxadoline:

Introduction: Eluxadoline is a mixed μ-opioid receptor agonist and δ-opioid receptor antagonist designed to decrease bowel motility. It is indicated for the treatment of IBS-D in adults who do not have a history of biliary disorders or pancreatitis. Eluxadoline effectively reduces stool frequency and improves stool consistency; however, it carries a risk of constipation and, in susceptible individuals, can cause sphincter of Oddi spasm.

Clinical Trial Phase / FDA-Approval: Eluxadoline has been approved by the FDA for the management of diarrhea-predominant irritable bowel syndrome (IBS-D). Clinical studies have validated its efficacy in decreasing diarrhea symptoms while maintaining an acceptable safety profile when used in appropriately selected patients.

Mechanism of Action:

Eluxadoline acts as a peripherally acting opioid receptor modulator, employing a unique triple mechanism that confers both antidiarrheal and visceral analgesic benefits without inducing the severe constipation often associated with traditional opioids.

Opioid Receptor Modulation in the Gut:

1. μ-Opioid Receptor (MOR) Agonism: Activation of μ-opioid receptors in the enteric nervous system (ENS) reduces intestinal motility and secretion. This leads to slower colonic transit and decreased stool frequency, thereby addressing the hallmark diarrheal symptoms of IBS-D.
2. δ-Opioid Receptor (DOR) Antagonism: While δ-opioid receptor activation in the gut typically promotes motility and amplifies nociceptive signaling, eluxadoline counteracts these effects by blocking δ-opioid receptors. This antagonism results in further reductions in intestinal motility and attenuation of visceral pain.
3. κ-Opioid Receptor (KOR) Agonism: Activation of κ-opioid receptors by eluxadoline provides significant visceral analgesia, helping to alleviate abdominal pain and discomfort commonly experienced in IBS-D. This is particularly beneficial for patients who suffer from heightened visceral hypersensitivity, a common feature of the condition.

Effects on the Enteric Nervous System and Gut Function:

- Eluxadoline decreases the peristaltic reflex, preventing excessive contractions that contribute to IBS-D symptoms.
- The drug inhibits hypersecretion of fluid into the intestinal lumen, further reducing diarrhoea.
- It modulates afferent sensory pathways, reducing pain perception from distension and irritation in the gut.

Absence of Significant Central Opioid Effects:

- Due to its poor CNS penetration, eluxadoline does not cause sedation, respiratory depression, or addiction, which are common concerns with systemic opioids.

Key Pharmacokinetic Parameters: Peak plasma concentration (Tmax) occurs within 1.5 hours of oral administration. Bioavailability is low (approximately 1%), indicating minimal systemic absorption. It is highly bound to plasma proteins (81%), mainly albumin. It is metabolized via hepatic glucuronidation (UGT1A3 and UGT2B7). Primary elimination is via faeces.

Adverse Drug Reactions: Nausea, abdominal pain, constipation and pancreatitis (rare, but serious ADR).

Uses: IBS-D.

Dose: 100 mg twice daily with food. 75 mg twice daily for those:

i. Without gallbladder
ii. Unable to tolerate 100 mg
iii. Taking OATP1B1 inhibitors

2. Rifaximin

Introduction: A poorly absorbed antibiotic targeting small intestinal bacterial overgrowth (SIBO) or dysbiosis implicated in IBS-D pathogenesis. Rifaximin can reduce bloating and diarrhoea; repeated courses may be used for symptom relapse. However, data on long-term safety and resistance patterns require ongoing vigilance.

Clinical Trial Phase / FDA-Approval: FDA-approved for IBS-D.

Mechanism of Action:

Rifaximin exerts its therapeutic effects in IBS-D through multiple mechanisms, including altering gut microbiota, reducing bacterial overgrowth, and modulating immune responses and intestinal permeability.

Mechanism of Rifaximin in IBS-D

1. **Modulation of Gut Microbiota (Primary Mechanism)**
   - Rifaximin binds to the β-subunit of bacterial DNA-dependent RNA polymerase, preventing transcription.
   - This leads to inhibition of bacterial RNA synthesis, ultimately blocking bacterial replication and growth.
   - Rifaximin selectively alters the composition of gut microbiota without significantly disrupting beneficial bacteria.
2. **Reduction of Bacterial Overgrowth in Small Intestinal Bacterial Overgrowth (SIBO)**
   - Many IBS-D patients have SIBO, characterized by an excessive number of bacteria in the small intestine.
   - Rifaximin targets gram-positive and gram-negative bacteria, reducing bacterial fermentation and gas production that contribute to bloating, diarrhoea, and cramping.
3. **Decreasing Intestinal Inflammation**
   - Rifaximin lowers levels of pro-inflammatory cytokines (TNF-α, IL-6, IL-8), reducing gut inflammation and immune activation.

- This helps restore gut barrier function, preventing leaky gut syndrome, which is common in IBS-D.

4. **Reduction of Bile Acid Malabsorption (BAM)**
   - In some IBS-D patients, excess bile acids reach the colon, stimulating fluid secretion and worsening diarrhoea.
   - Rifaximin modulates bile acid metabolism, improving bile acid reabsorption and reducing diarrhoea severity.
5. **Improvement of Gut Motility**
   - Gut bacteria produce lipopolysaccharides (LPS), which can disrupt serotonin (5-HT) pathways, leading to dysregulated motility.
   - By reducing bacterial overgrowth, rifaximin normalizes serotonin signalling, improving peristalsis and reducing diarrhoea episodes.
6. **Modulation of the Gut-Brain Axis**
   - Emerging evidence suggests that rifaximin reduces visceral hypersensitivity by modulating gut-derived neurotransmitters.
   - This leads to a reduction in abdominal pain and bloating, which are key symptoms of IBS-D.

Key Pharmacokinetic Parameters: Rifaximin has extremely poor systemic absorption (<0.4%), ensuring it remains localized in the gut. Food slightly increases systemic absorption but remains clinically insignificant. Due to its minimal systemic absorption, rifaximin does not accumulate in the plasma or other organs. Instead, it achieves high luminal concentrations in the small intestine and colon, where it exerts its antimicrobial effects. Rifaximin undergoes minimal hepatic metabolism, largely remaining unchanged in the gastrointestinal tract. No significant CYP450 enzyme interactions, making it safe for polypharmacy patients. 97% of rifaximin is excreted unchanged in faeces, confirming its gut-selective action.

Adverse Drug Reactions: Nausea, flatulence, headache, abdominal pain and Clostridium Difficile infection.

Uses: IBS-D, Traveller's diarrhoea and hepatic encephalopathy.

Dose: 400-550 mg three times daily for 14 days

3. Alosetron (5-HT3 receptor antagonist):

Introduction: Indicated for severe IBS-D in women who have failed other therapies. Alosetron reduces peristalsis and visceral sensitivity but is limited by a risk of ischemic colitis, mandating careful patient selection and restricted prescribing programs in some regions.

Clinical Trial Phase / FDA-Approval: Phase II clinical trials ongoing.

Mechanism of Action:

Alosetron works by blocking 5-HT3 receptors located in the gastrointestinal tract and central nervous system. These receptors play a crucial role in gut motility, secretion, and pain perception.

Mechanism of Alosetron in IBS-D:

1. **Inhibition of 5-HT3 Receptors on Enteric Neurons**
   - 5-HT3 receptors are ligand-gated ion channels found on enteric neurons of the gut.
   - Increased serotonin (5-HT) levels in IBS-D patients lead to accelerated colonic transit and diarrhoea.
   - Alosetron selectively blocks 5-HT_3 receptors, reducing neuronal excitability and gut hyperactivity.

2. **Reduction of Colonic Motility and Slowed Transit Time**
   - IBS-D is characterized by rapid colonic transit, leading to frequent, loose stools.
   - By inhibiting serotonergic signalling, alosetron prolongs colonic transit time, allowing for more water absorption and improved stool consistency.
3. **Modulation of Visceral Pain Perception**
   - The 5-HT3 receptor plays a role in visceral pain transmission from the gut to the brain.
   - Alosetron reduces afferent sensory signalling, alleviating abdominal pain and discomfort.
4. **Reduction of Excessive Intestinal Secretion**
   - In IBS-D, serotonin stimulates excessive chloride and water secretion, exacerbating diarrhoea.
   - Alosetron inhibits secretomotor activity, reducing fluid accumulation in the intestines.
5. **Central Nervous System (CNS) Effects**
   - Alosetron modifies CNS processing of pain signals, contributing to its analgesic effects in IBS-D.

Key Pharmacokinetic Parameters: Alosetron has a moderate bioavailability (50-60%) after oral administration, with peak plasma concentrations occurring within 1–1.5 hours. It undergoes extensive hepatic metabolism via cytochrome P450 enzymes (CYP1A2, CYP3A4, and CYP2C19), leading to multiple metabolites with minimal activity. Due to its metabolism via CYP1A2, strong CYP1A2 inhibitors (e.g. fluvoxamine) significantly increase alosetron levels, necessitating dose adjustments. The drug exhibits low protein binding (approximately 82%), reducing its risk for drug interactions. The elimination half-life is approximately 1.5 hours, but its pharmacodynamic effects last much longer (12–24 hours) due to high receptor affinity. Alosetron is primarily excreted via urine (approximately 74%), with a smaller proportion eliminated in faeces (approximately 11%). Since alosetron metabolism is sex-dependent, plasma levels are higher in women (since Alosetron is primarily metabolized by CYP1A2 and CYP3A4 in the liver and men have higher CYP1A2 activity, leading to faster drug metabolism and clearance, whereas, women have lower CYP1A2 activity, resulting in higher plasma drug levels and prolonged drug action.), which may contribute to its preferential use in female IBS-D patients.

Adverse Drug Reactions: Constipation, nausea, abdominal pain, flatulence, headache, dry mouth and ischaemic colitis (rare, but serious ADR).

Uses: IBS-D.

Dose: 0.5 mg twice daily, may increase to 1 mg twice daily after 4 weeks if tolerated.

2. Microbiome-Oriented Therapies

A. **Probiotics:** Specific strains like Bifidobacterium infantis and certain multi-strain formulations have shown potential to reduce global IBS symptoms, bloating, and pain. However, results are strain-dependent and may not generalize to all probiotic products.

B. **Faecal Microbiota Transplantation (FMT):** FMT involves transferring stool from a healthy donor to a patient to restore a beneficial microbial ecosystem. While robust evidence supports FMT for recurrent Clostridioides difficile infection, its role in IBS remains investigational. Early small trials yield mixed results—some demonstrating improvement in IBS symptoms, others showing no significant benefit. Ongoing research aims to clarify optimal donor selection, processing methods, and subpopulations most likely to respond.

C. **Prebiotics and Synbiotics:** Prebiotics (fermentable fibers, inulin-type fructans) selectively fuel beneficial gut microbes, potentially improving IBS symptom severity. Combining prebiotics with probiotic strains (synbiotics) is also being explored, though standardization of dosages and product formulations remains a challenge.

3. Neuromodulation and Central Nervous System Approaches

Emerging therapies underscore the contribution of altered pain processing and heightened CNS sensitivity in IBS:

- **Central Neuromodulators:** Low-dose tricyclic antidepressants (amitriptyline, desipramine) or SSRIs (paroxetine, citalopram) have been used, but novel agents like SNRIs (duloxetine) or alpha-2-delta ligands (pregabalin, gabapentin) may confer enhanced visceral analgesia with fewer side effects. Trials are ongoing to determine optimal regimens and patient subsets.
- **Gut-Brain Behavioural Therapies:** Remote, app-based CBT or digital therapeutics targeting GI symptom management have gained traction, leveraging telemedicine to expand access. Studies show these structured programs can significantly reduce IBS symptom burden and associated anxiety.
- **Transcutaneous Vagus Nerve Stimulation (tVNS):** Vagus nerve stimulation influences the parasympathetic tone and may modulate the gut-brain axis. Preliminary data suggest possible improvement in visceral pain thresholds and autonomic balance. Larger controlled studies are awaited to confirm its efficacy and cost-effectiveness.

4. Personalized Nutrition and Dietetics

While the low-FODMAP diet remains a gold standard for many IBS patients, emerging refinements aim to personalize dietary recommendations:

- **Carbohydrate-Specific Interventions:** Some focus on specific subgroups of FODMAPs or non-celiac gluten sensitivity.
- **Precision Microbiome Profiling:** Tests that assess gut microbiota composition to predict dietary tolerance or identify potential IBS phenotypes (e.g. methane-dominant SIBO).
- **Elimination-Rechallenge Protocols:** Systematic reintroduction of foods helps determine individualized triggers while avoiding overly restrictive, unsustainable diets.

Moreover, mobile apps and telehealth dietitian consults offer ongoing support and tracking, improving compliance and outcomes.

5. Emerging Diagnostic Tools

Although IBS remains a clinical diagnosis per Rome IV criteria, new biomarkers and imaging modalities strive to detect subtle pathophysiologic changes:

- **Serological Biomarkers:** Anti-vinculin and anti-CdtB antibodies, associated with post-infectious IBS, may help confirm IBS-D in certain contexts. These markers, however, are not universally validated.
- **Transcriptomic and Proteomic Profiles:** Exploratory studies examine intestinal mucosal gene expression patterns distinguishing IBS subtypes from other functional GI disorders.
- **Low-Cost Technologies:** Breath testing (hydrogen, methane) to detect SIBO or carbohydrate malabsorption can guide targeted therapies like rifaximin or dietary adjustments. Yet, standardization of testing protocols remains variable.

6. Complementary and Alternative Approaches

Increasing patient interest in non-pharmacologic solutions has spurred exploration of:

- **Peppermint Oil:** A known antispasmodic effect through calcium-channel blockade in smooth muscle. Enteric-coated formulations can reduce abdominal pain and bloating in mild-to-moderate IBS.
- **Acupuncture:** Some trials suggest modest benefits in IBS symptom relief, potentially via neuromodulatory effects, though robust, high-quality evidence is mixed.
- **Herbal Remedies:** Formulations such as STW 5 (Iberogast®) or multi-component Chinese herbal mixtures have garnered interest. However, variation in composition and lack of standardized clinical trials hamper widespread recommendations.

Given IBS's multifactorial aetiology, a multimodal approach harnessing dietary modification, targeted pharmacotherapy, gut-brain behavioural interventions, and (where indicated) complementary therapies can optimize patient outcomes.

Conclusion

Thanks to growing knowledge of gut-brain interactions, microbiome dynamics, and neuromodulatory mechanisms, the treatment of irritable bowel syndrome has entered a new era. IBS care is still based on traditional therapies, such as dietary modifications, symptom-focused medications, and psychological support. The shift towards precision medicine for IBS is highlighted by the development of new pharmacological targets (such as GC-C agonists and opioid receptor modulators), microbiome interventions (such as probiotics and FMT), and sophisticated neuromodulation techniques. Clinically speaking, individualised treatment entails a thorough evaluation of the patient's microbiome profile, possible dietary triggers, comorbid conditions (such as anxiety or fibromyalgia), and IBS subtype. Patient-centered, integrated care may be made easier by the growing acceptance of digital interventions and telehealth. Notwithstanding these advancements, there are still issues, chief among them being the variability of IBS, the large range of individual reactions, and the high rates of placebo response that are characteristic of functional gastrointestinal disorders. Methods will be optimised and standardised with the aid of additional large-scale trials, biomarker discovery, and mechanistic research. Providing safe, effective, and tolerable treatments that reduce the psychosocial burden of this complex disorder, improve quality of life, and ease IBS symptoms is the ultimate goal that has not changed as the field has developed.

References

1. Camilleri M. Diagnosis and treatment of irritable bowel syndrome: a review. Jama. 2021 Mar 2;325(9):865-77.
2. Bonetto S, Fagoonee S, Battaglia E, Grassini M, Saracco GM, Pellicano R. Recent advances in the treatment of irritable bowel syndrome. Pol Arch Intern Med. 2021 Aug 30;131(7-8):709-15.
3. Sommermeyer H, Piątek J. Synbiotics as Treatment for Irritable Bowel Syndrome: A Review. Microorganisms. 2024 Jul 21;12(7):1493.
4. Nybacka S, Törnblom H, Josefsson A, Hreinsson JP, Böhn L, Frändemark Å, Weznaver C, Störsrud S, Simrén M. A low FODMAP diet plus traditional dietary advice versus a low-carbohydrate diet versus pharmacological treatment in irritable bowel syndrome (CARIBS): a single-centre, single-blind, randomised controlled trial. The Lancet Gastroenterology & Hepatology. 2024 Jun 1;9(6):507-20.
5. Shah ED, Kim HM, Schoenfeld PS. Efficacy and tolerability of pharmacologic therapies for IBS with constipation: Systematic review and network meta-analysis. Am J Gastroenterol. 2018;113(1):49–60.
6. Layer P, Stanghellini V. Review article: Linaclotide for the management of irritable bowel syndrome with constipation. Aliment Pharmacol Ther. 2014 Feb;39(4):371–84. Available from: https://doi.org/10.1111/apt.12604
7. Camilleri M, Boeckxstaens G. Irritable bowel syndrome: treatment based on pathophysiology and biomarkers. Gut. 2023 Mar 1;72(3):590-9.
8. Drossman DA. Functional gastrointestinal disorders: history, pathophysiology, clinical features, and Rome IV. Gastroenterology. 2016 May 1;150(6):1262-79.
9. Canavan C, West J, Card T. The economic impact of the irritable bowel syndrome. Alimentary pharmacology & therapeutics. 2014 Nov;40(9):1023-34.

10. Rao S, Lembo AJ, Shiff SJ, Lavins BJ, Currie MG, Jia XD, Shi K, MacDougall JE, Shao JZ, Eng P, Fox SM. A 12-week, randomized, controlled trial with a 4-week randomized withdrawal period to evaluate the efficacy and safety of linaclotide in irritable bowel syndrome with constipation. Official journal of the American College of Gastroenterology | ACG. 2012 Nov 1;107(11):1714-24.
11. Lembo AJ, Lacy BE, Zuckerman MJ, Schey R, Dove LS, Andrae DA, Davenport JM, McIntyre G, Lopez R, Turner L, Covington PS. Eluxadoline for irritable bowel syndrome with diarrhea. New England Journal of Medicine. 2016 Jan 21;374(3):242-53.
12. Pimentel M, Lembo A, Chey WD, Zakko S, Ringel Y, Yu J, Mareya SM, Shaw AL, Bortey E, Forbes WP. Rifaximin therapy for patients with irritable bowel syndrome without constipation. New england journal of medicine. 2011 Jan 6;364(1):22-32.
13. Halkjær SI, Christensen AH, Lo BZ, Browne PD, Günther S, Hansen LH, Petersen AM. Faecal microbiota transplantation alters gut microbiota in patients with irritable bowel syndrome: results from a randomised, double-blind placebo-controlled study. Gut. 2018 Dec 1;67(12):2107-15.
14. Khanna R, MacDonald JK, Levesque BG. Peppermint oil for the treatment of irritable bowel syndrome: a systematic review and meta-analysis. Journal of clinical gastroenterology. 2014 Jul 1;48(6):505-12.
15. McQuaid KR. Drugs used in the treatment of gastrointestinal diseases. Basic & clinical pharmacology. 2018;12.
16. Zarowitz BJ. Pharmacologic consideration of commonly used gastrointestinal drugs in the elderly. Gastroenterology Clinics. 2009 Sep 1;38(3):547-62.
17. Liu R, Staller K. Update on eluxadoline for the treatment of irritable bowel syndrome with diarrhea: patient selection and perspectives. Drug Design, Development and Therapy. 2020 Apr 9:1391-400.
18. Barshop K, Staller K. Eluxadoline in irritable bowel syndrome with diarrhea: rationale, evidence and place in therapy. Therapeutic advances in chronic disease. 2017 Nov;8(11):153-60.
19. Chey WD, Shah ED, DuPont HL. Mechanism of action and therapeutic benefit of rifaximin in patients with irritable bowel syndrome: a narrative review. Therapeutic Advances in Gastroenterology. 2020 Jan;13:1756284819897531.
20. Harris LA, Chang L. Alosetron: an effective treatment for diarrhea-predominant irritable bowel syndrome. Women's Health. 2007 Jan;3(1):15-27.
21. Chang L, Tong K, Ameen V. Ischemic colitis and complications of constipation associated with the use of alosetron under a risk management plan: clinical characteristics, outcomes, and incidences. Official journal of the American College of Gastroenterology | ACG. 2010 Apr 1;105(4):866-75.
22. Munjal A, Dedania B, Cash BD. Current and emerging pharmacological approaches for treating diarrhea-predominant irritable bowel syndrome. Expert Opinion on Pharmacotherapy. 2020 Jan 2;21(1):63-71.

Chapter 30

Recent Advances in the Management of Inflammatory Bowel Disease (IBD)

Author: Dr. Pranab Das

Introduction

Inflammatory bowel disease (IBD) principally includes two chronic, relapsing-remitting conditions—Crohn's disease (CD) and ulcerative colitis (UC)—marked by inappropriate mucosal immune activation and a dysregulated immune response to the intestinal flora. In recent decades, the prevalence of inflammatory bowel disease (IBD) has increased globally, especially in newly industrialised nations. Previously deemed incurable, advancements in the comprehension of IBD's pathogenesis have resulted in enhanced disease management and results. Modern treatment strategies focus on achieving mucosal healing, decreasing dependence on corticosteroids, and preventing structural bowel damage, hence reducing problems and enhancing quality of life.

Conventional treatments have encompassed aminosalicylates, corticosteroids, immunomodulators (such as thiopurines and methotrexate), and biologics that target tumour necrosis factor (TNF). Nonetheless, not all patients exhibit sufficient responsiveness to these medications, and some may experience diminished efficacy over time or notable adverse effects. In recent years, the therapeutic repertoire has broadened to encompass innovative biologics with distinct mechanisms (e.g. anti-integrins, anti-IL-12/23) and oral small molecules (e.g. JAK inhibitors, sphingosine-1-phosphate receptor modulators). This chapter delineates the diagnosis and subcategories of IBD, succinctly reviews traditional management approaches, and emphasises current advancements in pharmacology, individualised treatment techniques, and emerging concepts such as the significance of the microbiome and therapeutic drug monitoring.

Historical Perspective

From empirical therapies to highly targeted biologic and small-molecule agents, the treatment of Inflammatory Bowel Disease (IBD), which includes Crohn's disease and ulcerative colitis, has drastically changed. The first pharmacologic breakthrough in ulcerative colitis occurred in the 1950s when Dr. Nanna Svartz introduced sulfasalazine in Sweden. This medication combined antimicrobial and anti-inflammatory properties. Dr. Derek Jewell and others made important contributions to defining the effectiveness of corticosteroids and immunomodulators like azathioprine in IBD during the 1970s and 1980s. These medications were adapted from transplant medicine. Tolerability and localised anti-inflammatory action were enhanced by the introduction of 5-aminosalicylic acid (5-ASA) formulations in the 1980s, particularly by Dr. Stephen Hanauer.

When infliximab, a chimeric anti-TNF monoclonal antibody created by Drs. Jan Vilček and Teresa Tarrant, was approved in 1998 as the first biologic treatment for Crohn's disease, a significant paradigm shift got underway. Other anti-TNF medications like golimumab, certolizumab pegol, and adalimumab (approved in 2007) came next, increasing the range of treatment options for Crohn's disease and ulcerative colitis. Vedolizumab, a gut-selective anti-integrin monoclonal antibody developed by Takeda Pharmaceuticals, was introduced in the early 2010s. It offers enhanced safety by preventing systemic immunosuppression. A novel cytokine-targeting strategy was provided by ustekinumab, an anti-IL-12/23 monoclonal antibody created by Janssen that was approved in 2016 for Crohn's disease and later expanded to ulcerative colitis.

Most recently, oral small molecules have emerged as strong substitutes for biologics, as evidenced by the approval of Janus kinase (JAK) inhibitors like tofacitinib (approved in 2018 for ulcerative colitis), upadacitinib, and filgotinib. These developments, which bring the field closer to personalised care strategies, are fuelled by a deeper comprehension of the immunopathogenesis of IBD and the creation of precision therapeutics.

Definition

Inflammatory bowel disease (IBD) refers to chronic inflammatory disorders of the GI tract:

- Ulcerative Colitis (UC): Limited to the colon and rectum, with continuous mucosal inflammation beginning in the rectum and extending proximally to a variable extent.
- Crohn's Disease (CD): Can affect any segment of the GI tract from mouth to anus, often in a discontinuous (skip) pattern. Inflammation may be transmural, leading to complications such as strictures, fistulas, and abscesses.

  The clinical presentation of IBD varies widely. Patients may experience chronic diarrhoea, rectal bleeding, abdominal pain, weight loss, and extraintestinal manifestations (e.g. arthritis, uveitis). Disease severity typically waxes and wanes; however, uncontrolled or undertreated IBD can substantially degrade health-related quality of life and increase the risk of complications, including colorectal cancer.

Types and Clinical Subtypes

Ulcerative Colitis

- Proctitis: Inflammation confined to the rectum.
- Left-Sided Colitis: Extends from the rectum up to the splenic flexure.
- Pancolitis: Involves the entire colon.

Crohn's Disease

- Ileal (Terminal Ileum) Crohn's: Most common location, can lead to right lower quadrant pain, strictures, or fistulas.
- Colonic Crohn's: May mimic ulcerative colitis but often with patchy involvement, perianal disease, or deeper ulcerations.
- Gastroduodenal or Jejunoileal Crohn's: Less common, presenting with upper GI involvement.

  Classification systems like the Montreal Classification categorize disease behaviour (inflammatory, stricturing, penetrating) and location, which influences therapy selection.

Brief Note on Conventional Management

Table 1: Concise overview of the conventional method management of Inflammatory Bowel Disease

Drug Class / Drug Names	Mechanism of Action	Key Pharmacokinetic Parameters	Adverse Drug Reactions	Uses
Aminosalicylates (5-ASA) (e.g. Mesalamine, Sulfasalazine, Balsalazide, Olsalazine)	Anti-inflammatory action in the colon: Inhibits prostaglandins and leukotrienes, reduces cytokine production, and scavenges free radicals. Also inhibits NF-κB activation, reducing immune response.	Limited systemic absorption - localized colonic action. Sulfasalazine is metabolized in the colon by azoreductase to mesalamine and sulphapyridine. Eliminated via faeces and urine.	Gastrointestinal symptoms (nausea, diarrhoea, dyspepsia), hypersensitivity reactions and nephrotoxicity (rare).	First-line therapy for mild-to-moderate ulcerative colitis. Less effective in Crohn's disease.
Corticosteroids (e.g. Prednisone, Budesonide, Hydrocortisone, Methylprednisolone)	Potent anti-inflammatory effects via inhibition of phospholipase A2, reducing prostaglandin and leukotriene synthesis. Suppresses cytokines (IL-1, IL-6, TNF-α) and decreases T-cell activation.	Rapid GI absorption. Hepatic metabolism via CYP3A4. Excreted via urine.	Cushingoid features (weight gain, moon face, osteoporosis), hypertension, hyperglycaemia, adrenal suppression and withdrawal symptoms and increased infection risk.	Acute flares of both Crohn's disease and ulcerative colitis. Short-term use only to induce remission.
Immunomodulators (e.g. Azathioprine, 6-Mercaptopurine)	Immunosuppressive agents inhibiting T-cell proliferation by blocking purine synthesis. Converted to active 6-thioguanine nucleotides (6-TGNs), which are incorporated into DNA, leading to apoptosis of inflammatory cells.	Oral bioavailability is approximately 50%. Hepatic metabolism is via thiopurine methyltransferase (TPMT). Excreted via urine.	Myelosuppression (leukopenia, anaemia, thrombocytopenia), hepatotoxicity, increased risk of lymphoma and skin cancer and pancreatitis.	Maintenance therapy in steroid-dependent IBD. Used in combination with biologics to prevent antibody formation.

While many patients respond well to these treatments, a subset remains refractory or intolerant, prompting exploration of novel drug targets and personalized therapeutic approaches.

Recent Advances in IBD Management

1. Vedolizumab

Introduction: Vedolizumab is a humanized monoclonal antibody targeting α4β7 integrin, a key molecule involved in the migration of T-lymphocytes to the intestinal mucosa. It is a gut-selective biologic therapy, reducing systemic immunosuppression risks.

Clinical Trial Phase / FDA-Approval: FDA-approved for moderate-to-severe Crohn's disease and ulcerative colitis. GEMINI I & II trials demonstrated superior remission rates compared to placebo.

Mechanism of Action: Vedolizumab is a humanized IgG1 monoclonal antibody that selectively binds to the α4β7 integrin, a key adhesion molecule involved in gut-specific immune responses.

1. **Inhibition of Gut-Directed Lymphocyte Trafficking**
   - α4β7 integrin is expressed on gut-homing T lymphocytes.
   - These lymphocytes interact with MAdCAM-1 (mucosal addressin cell adhesion molecule-1), which is found on intestinal endothelial cells.
   - Vedolizumab blocks α4β7 integrin, preventing lymphocytes from adhering to MAdCAM-1 and migrating into inflamed gut tissue.
2. **Reduction of Intestinal Inflammation**
   - By preventing lymphocyte infiltration, vedolizumab limits the release of pro-inflammatory cytokines (TNF-α, IL-6, IL-12, IL-23).
   - This leads to a localized reduction in inflammation without systemic immunosuppression.
3. **No Systemic Immune Suppression**
   - Unlike TNF-α inhibitors (e.g. infliximab, adalimumab), vedolizumab does not interfere with systemic immune function, reducing the risk of serious infections.
   - This gut-specific action makes vedolizumab safer than systemic immunosuppressants.

Key Pharmacokinetic Parameters: Vedolizumab is administered as via intravenous route. It has a bioavailability of 100% when given intravenously and follows non-linear pharmacokinetics. After administration, vedolizumab rapidly binds to α4β7 integrin on circulating lymphocytes, reducing gut inflammation. It has a long elimination half-life (approximately 25 days), allowing dosing every 8 weeks during maintenance therapy. Metabolism occurs via proteolytic degradation into peptides and amino acids, with no hepatic or renal excretion, making it safe for patients with liver or kidney dysfunction. Vedolizumab does not interact with cytochrome P450 enzymes, reducing the risk of drug interactions. Steady-state concentrations are reached after third or fourth dose, ensuring sustained suppression of gut inflammation.

Adverse Drug Reactions: Nasopharyngitis, headache, joint pain and Progressive Multifocal Leukoencephalopathy (rare).

Uses: Moderate-to-severe UC and CD, particularly in patients unresponsive to TNF inhibitors.

Dose: 300 mg IV at weeks 0, 2, and 6, then every 8 weeks thereafter

2. Ustekinumab

Introduction: Ustekinumab is a fully human monoclonal antibody that targets IL-12 and IL-23, cytokines involved in Th1 and Th17 immune responses.

Clinical Trial Phase / FDA-Approval: FDA-approved for Crohn's disease, and ulcerative colitis. UNITI-1, UNITI-2, and IM-UNITI trials confirmed high clinical remission rates in IBD.

Mechanism of Action: Ustekinumab works by blocking the IL-12/IL-23 pathway, which is central to chronic inflammation in IBD.

1. **Inhibition of IL-12 and IL-23 Cytokines**
   - IL-12 and IL-23 are pro-inflammatory cytokines that drive Th1 and Th17 immune responses, respectively.
   - IL-12 promotes Th1 cell differentiation, leading to the release of interferon-gamma (IFN-γ) and TNF-α, which worsens gut inflammation.
   - IL-23 is critical for Th17 cell survival, which secretes IL-17 and IL-22, contributing to epithelial barrier dysfunction.
   - Ustekinumab inhibits both IL-12 and IL-23, thereby reducing gut inflammation and epithelial barrier dysfunction.
2. **Suppression of Th1 and Th17 Inflammatory Pathways**
   - Th1 cells play a key role in Crohn's disease, while Th17 cells contribute to both Crohn's disease and ulcerative colitis.
   - Ustekinumab binds to the shared p40 subunit of IL-12 and IL-23, preventing their interaction with the IL-12Rβ1 receptor on immune cells.
   - This results in reduced differentiation and activation of Th1 and Th17 cells, leading to decreased inflammation in the intestinal mucosa.
3. **Restoration of Gut Barrier Integrity**
   - By reducing IL-17 and IL-22, ustekinumab prevents excessive epithelial damage and improves mucosal healing.
   - This reduces intestinal permeability, preventing further immune activation.
4. **No Systemic Immunosuppression**
   - Unlike TNF-α inhibitors, ustekinumab does not suppress the entire immune system, leading to a lower risk of infections.

Key Pharmacokinetic Parameters: Ustekinumab is available as intravenous (i.v.) and subcutaneous (s.c.) formulations. The i.v. formulation is used for induction therapy, while s.c. injections are used for maintenance. Following i.v. administration, peak plasma concentrations are reached within 1–2 hours, whereas s.c. injections result in a delayed peak at 7–14 days due to absorption kinetics. The drug has a long elimination half-life (approximately 19–29 days), allowing maintenance dosing every 8–12 weeks. Ustekinumab undergoes proteolytic degradation, with no hepatic or renal clearance, making it safe for patients with liver or kidney dysfunction. The drug's pharmacokinetics are influenced by body weight, with higher doses required in heavier patients to achieve optimal drug levels. Antibodies to ustekinumab (anti-drug antibodies) are rare but may affect drug efficacy in some patients.

Adverse Drug Reactions: Nasopharyngitis, arthralgia, headache and upper respiratory tract infections.

Uses: Moderate-to-severe Ulcerative colitis and Crohn's disease, particularly in patients unresponsive to TNF inhibitors.

Dose: Single weight-based IV dose (induction dose):

i. <55 kg: 260 mg
ii. 55–85 kg: 390 mg
iii. 85 kg: 520 mg

Maintenance dose: 90 mg subcutaneously every 8 weeks, starting 8 weeks after IV dose.

3. Risankizumab

Introduction: Risankizumab is a selective IL-23 inhibitor, offering more targeted immune suppression than ustekinumab.

Clinical Trial Phase / FDA-Approval: FDA-approved (2022) for Crohn's disease; Phase III trials for UC ongoing. ADVANCE and MOTIVATE trials showed high remission rates in Crohn's patients.

Mechanism of Action:

1. **Role of IL-23 in Immune-Mediated Diseases**
   - L-23 is a pro-inflammatory cytokine secreted by dendritic cells and macrophages.
   - It promotes the differentiation and survival of Th17 cells, leading to the release of IL-17, IL-22, and TNF-α, which drive chronic inflammation.
   - Dysregulated IL-23 signalling is implicated in psoriasis, psoriatic arthritis, and Crohn's disease.
2. **Selective Targeting of IL-23p19 by Risankizumab**
   - Risankizumab selectively binds to the p19 subunit of IL-23, preventing its interaction with the IL-23 receptor on T cells.
   - Unlike ustekinumab, which targets both IL-12 and IL-23 (p40 subunit), risankizumab is more selective for IL-23 inhibition.
3. **Downregulation of Th17-Mediated Inflammation**

Blocking IL-23 reduces Th17 cell differentiation and IL-17 production, leading to:

1. Decreases intestinal inflammation by reducing TNF-α, IFN-γ, and IL-6 levels.
2. Restores gut epithelial barrier integrity, promoting mucosal healing.
3. Reduces neutrophil infiltration, lowering colonic damage in IBD patients.

Key Pharmacokinetic Parameters: Risankizumab is available as intravenous (i.v.) and subcutaneous (s.c.) formulations. The i.v. formulation is used for induction therapy, while s.c. injections are used for maintenance. It is degraded by proteolysis without hepatic metabolism, primarily eliminated via reticuloendothelial system. Plasma half-life (t1/2) is around 28 days, allowing for extended dosing intervals.

Adverse Drug Reactions: Nasopharyngitis, headache, arthralgia, elevation of liver enzymes and hypersensitivity reactions.

Uses: Moderate-to-severe Crohn's disease, with trials ongoing for Ulcerative colitis.

Dose: Induction dose: 600 mg IV at weeks 0, 4, and 8; maintenance dose: 360 mg subcutaneously every 8 weeks, starting at week 12.

4. Upadacitinib

Introduction: Upadacitinib is an oral Janus kinase (JAK) inhibitor, modulating cytokine-mediated inflammation in IBD.

Clinical Trial Phase / FDA-Approval: FDA-approved (2022) for ulcerative colitis; Phase III trials for Crohn's disease ongoing. U-ACHIEVE and U-ACCOMPLISH trials demonstrated superior remission rates.

Mechanism of Action:

1. **Inhibition of the JAK-STAT Signalling Pathway**
   - The JAK (Janus kinase) family consists of JAK1, JAK2, JAK3, and TYK2, which mediate cytokine signalling.
   - In IBD, excessive activation of JAK1-dependent pathways leads to chronic inflammation, epithelial barrier dysfunction, and immune overactivation.
   - Upadacitinib selectively inhibits JAK1, preventing downstream activation of signal transducer and activator of transcription (STAT) proteins, reducing inflammatory gene expression.
2. **Reduction of Pro-Inflammatory Cytokine Signalling**
   - Upadacitinib suppresses the activity of IL-6, IL-12, IL-23, and IFN-γ, key cytokines involved in the Th1 and Th17 inflammatory responses in IBD.
   - Unlike non-selective JAK inhibitors (e.g. tofacitinib, which inhibits JAK1/JAK3), upadacitinib preserves JAK2-mediated erythropoiesis, reducing hematologic side effects.
3. **Suppression of Gut Inflammation and Restoration of Barrier Integrity**
   - The JAK-STAT pathway contributes to epithelial cell apoptosis, worsening mucosal damage in IBD.
   - By reducing IL-6 and IL-23 signalling, upadacitinib enhances epithelial healing, restoring gut barrier function

Key Pharmacokinetic Parameters: Upadacitinib is rapidly absorbed after oral administration, reaching peak plasma concentrations within 2–4 hours. It has a high oral bioavailability (approximately 75%), allowing once-daily dosing. The drug is extensively metabolized in the liver via CYP3A4, with minor contributions from CYP2D6. Due to its metabolism by CYP3A4, strong CYP3A4 inhibitors (e.g. ketoconazole) increase upadacitinib levels, while CYP3A4 inducers (e.g. rifampin) decrease its efficacy. Upadacitinib has a long half-life (approximately 12–16 hours), maintaining steady-state concentrations with once-daily dosing. The drug is primarily eliminated via faeces (approximately 80%), with a smaller proportion excreted in urine (approximately 20%). Unlike biologics, no dose adjustment is needed in mild-to-moderate renal or hepatic impairment.

Adverse Drug Reactions: Nasopharyngitis, headache, dyslipidaemia, thrombosis risk and risk of opportunistic infections.

Uses: Moderate-to-severe ulcerative colitis, with trials ongoing for Crohn's disease.

Dose: Induction dose: 45 mg orally once daily for 8 weeks; maintenance dose: 15 mg or 30 mg orally once daily, based on response and tolerability.

5. Ozanimod

Introduction: Ozanimod is an oral sphingosine-1-phosphate (S1P) receptor modulator, reducing lymphocyte migration.

Clinical Trial Phase / FDA-Approval: FDA-approved for ulcerative colitis; Phase III trials for Crohn's disease ongoing. TRUE NORTH trials demonstrated significant remission rates.

Mechanism of Action:

1. **Modulation of the Sphingosine-1-Phosphate (S1P) Receptor**
   - Ozanimod is a selective S1P receptor modulator that targets S1P1 and S1P5 receptors.
   - The S1P1 receptor is essential for lymphocyte egress from lymphoid tissues into circulation.
   - By binding to S1P1, ozanimod induces receptor internalization and degradation, blocking lymphocyte exit from lymph nodes.
2. **Reduction of Inflammatory Lymphocyte Trafficking in the Gut**
   - In IBD, excessive T-cell migration into intestinal tissues contributes to chronic inflammation.
   - Ozanimod reduces the number of circulating lymphocytes, decreasing immune cell infiltration into the gut mucosa.
   - This results in local immune suppression without significant systemic immunosuppression, lowering the risk of infections.
3. **Preservation of Protective Immunity**
   - Unlike non-selective S1P modulators (e.g. fingolimod), ozanimod does not affect S1P3 and S1P4 receptors, reducing cardiovascular and immunological side effects.
   - S1P5 activation may contribute to neuroprotective effects, suggesting potential CNS benefits.
4. **Improvement of Intestinal Barrier Function**
   - Inflammation in IBD disrupts intestinal epithelial integrity.
   - Ozanimod indirectly improves epithelial repair by reducing pro-inflammatory T-cell infiltration.

Key Pharmacokinetic Parameters: Ozanimod has high oral bioavailability and follows linear pharmacokinetics. After oral administration, it undergoes slow absorption, reaching peak plasma concentrations in 6–8 hours. The drug is extensively metabolized in the liver by cytochrome P450 enzymes (CYP2C8 and CYP3A4), producing two major active metabolites (CC112273 and CC1084037) that contribute to its prolonged efficacy. Ozanimod has a half-life of approximately 21 hours, but due to its active metabolites, its effective half-life extends to approximately 11 days, allowing for once-daily dosing. The drug is primarily eliminated via hepatic metabolism, with minimal renal excretion, making it safe in patients with mild-to-moderate renal impairment. Food does not significantly affect its pharmacokinetics, ensuring consistent drug exposure.

Adverse Drug Reactions: Bradycardia, hypertension, nasopharyngitis and elevated liver enzymes.

Uses: Moderate-to-severe ulcerative colitis, with trials ongoing for Crohn's disease.

Dose: 0.23 mg orally once daily on Days 1–4; 0.46 mg orally once daily on Days 5–7; 0.92 mg orally once daily from Day 8.

6. Personalized and Combination Strategies

The concept of treat-to-target—achieving and maintaining objective markers of remission, like endoscopic mucosal healing—has driven the development of:

- **Therapeutic Drug Monitoring (TDM):** Measuring drug trough levels and anti-drug antibodies (especially for biologics like infliximab or adalimumab) to optimize dosing, reduce secondary loss of response, and limit immunogenicity.

- **Combination Biologic Therapy:** Investigations into combining different biologics (e.g. anti-TNF plus anti-integrin or anti-IL-23) or biologics with small molecules (e.g. vedolizumab + tofacitinib) in refractory cases. Early studies indicate possible synergistic effects but raise concerns about infection risk and cost.
- **Precision Medicine Approaches:** Profiling genetic risk variants, serologic markers, and microbiome signatures to predict responsiveness to specific drugs, thereby reducing trial-and-error prescribing.

The Role of the Microbiome

Increasingly, the gut microbiome is implicated in IBD pathogenesis—perturbations in microbial diversity and functionality can drive or perpetuate intestinal inflammation. Recent interventions include:

- **Faecal Microbiota Transplantation (FMT):** Mixed success in UC, with some trials demonstrating remission induction, whereas results in CD are less consistent. Future refinements may entail standardized donor screening, targeted bacterial consortia, or repeated administrations to sustain microbial shifts.
- **Microbiome-based adjuncts:** Probiotic cocktails, prebiotics (dietary fibers fuelling beneficial microbes), or postbiotics (metabolites produced by commensals) might complement standard treatments, though robust, large-scale data are lacking.

Endoscopic and Surgical Innovations

Deep Remission increasingly emphasizes endoscopic healing. Advances include:

- **Enhanced Endoscopic Imaging:** Techniques like confocal laser endomicroscopy or chromoendoscopy can detect subtle inflammation or dysplasia, guiding precise therapy escalation.
- **Stricture Management:** Endoscopic balloon dilation or stent placement may prevent repeated surgeries in Crohn's strictures, especially for short fibrotic lesions.
- **Minimally Invasive Surgery:** Laparoscopic and robotic approaches reduce post-operative complications and expedite recovery in cases requiring resection. Progress in organ-sparing techniques (strictureplasty, minimal resection) helps preserve bowel length and function.

Emerging Concepts and Future Directions

- **CRISPR and Gene Therapy:** Early-stage investigations explore whether gene editing might modulate immune dysregulation in IBD. The feasibility, safety, and targeting specificity remain to be determined.
- **Dietary Modifications and Exclusive Enteral Nutrition (EEN)**: Already integral in paediatric Crohn's to induce remission, more adult trials investigate partial enteral diets or specialized formulas as bridging therapies, possibly shaping the gut microbiome and immune response.
- **Cellular Therapies:** Mesenchymal stem cells (MSCs) have shown promise in perianal fistulizing Crohn's disease. Allogeneic MSC injections can promote fistula closure and tissue regeneration, offering an alternative when medical therapy fails.
- **Psychological Interventions:** Recognizing the gut-brain axis role, integrated mental health support (cognitive-behavioural therapy, stress management) can improve symptom severity and adherence. Digital health solutions and telemedicine-based care models further reduce barriers to specialist input.

Conclusion

The management of inflammatory bowel disease has undergone a major evolution, transitioning from a reactive approach to a proactive, treat-to-target strategy prioritizing mucosal healing and steroid-free remission. While aminosalicylates, corticosteroids, and classic immunomodulators remain foundational in mild to moderate cases, complex or refractory disease now benefits from an expanding array of targeted therapies. Biologics beyond TNF antagonism (e.g. vedolizumab, ustekinumab, IL-23 inhibitors) and oral small molecules (JAK inhibitors, S1P modulators) deliver more individualized care. In parallel, the blossoming fields of therapeutic drug monitoring, combination therapy, and microbiome manipulation are refining disease control and improving long-term outcomes. Even so, many challenges persist: heterogeneous disease phenotypes, primary or secondary nonresponse to treatments, safety concerns (infection risk, malignancy), and cost barriers. Ongoing research in precision medicine—integrating genetic, serologic, and microbiome-based tools—seeks to match patients with the most effective therapies and reduce trial-and-error prescribing. Meanwhile, endoscopic and surgical innovations, along with supportive measures like nutritional interventions and mental health support, increasingly enable holistic care. As science illuminates IBD's pathogenesis further, the ultimate goal remains consistent: to maximize clinical and endoscopic remission, preserve gut integrity, and enhance patients' quality of life.

References

1. Cai Z, Wang S, Li J. Treatment of inflammatory bowel disease: a comprehensive review. Frontiers in medicine. 2021 Dec 20;8:765474.
2. Roy S, Dhaneshwar S. Role of prebiotics, probiotics, and synbiotics in management of inflammatory bowel disease: Current perspectives. World Journal of Gastroenterology. 2023 Apr 14;29(14):2078.
3. D'Haens GR, van Deventer S. 25 years of anti-TNF treatment for inflammatory bowel disease: lessons from the past and a look to the future. Gut. 2021 Jul 1;70(7):1396-405.
4. Chaparro M, Garre A, Núñez Ortiz A, Diz-Lois Palomares MT, Rodríguez C, Riestra S, Vela M, Benítez JM, Fernández Salgado E, Sánchez Rodríguez E, Hernández V. Incidence, clinical characteristics and management of inflammatory bowel disease in Spain: large-scale epidemiological study. Journal of clinical medicine. 2021 Jun 29;10(13):2885.
5. Svartz N. Salazopyrin, a new sulfanilamide preparation. A. Therapeutic Results in Rheumatic Polyarthritis. B. Therapeutic Results in Ulcerative Colitis. C. Toxic Manifestations in Treatment with Sulfanilamide Preparations. Acta Medica Scandinavica. 1942 Jan 12;110(6):577-98.
6. Kaplan GG, Ng SC. Globalisation of inflammatory bowel disease: perspectives from the evolution of inflammatory bowel disease in the UK and China. The lancet Gastroenterology & hepatology. 2016 Dec 1;1(4):307-16.
7. Gros B, Kaplan GG. Ulcerative colitis in adults: a review. Jama. 2023 Sep 12;330(10):951-65.
8. Feagan BG, Greenberg GR, Wild G, Fedorak RN, Paré P, McDonald JW, et al. Vedolizumab in the treatment of ulcerative colitis: an evidence-based review of safety, efficacy, and place of therapy. Core Evid. 2020;15:57–71.
9. Sandborn WJ, Feagan BG, Rutgeerts P, Hanauer S, Colombel JF, Sands BE, Lukas M, Fedorak RN, Lee S, Bressler B, Fox I. Vedolizumab as induction and maintenance therapy for Crohn's disease. New England Journal of Medicine. 2013 Aug 22;369(8):711-21.
10. Sandborn WJ, Gasink C, Gao LL, Blank MA, Johanns J, Guzzo C, Sands BE, Hanauer SB, Targan S, Rutgeerts P, Ghosh S. Ustekinumab induction and maintenance therapy in refractory Crohn's disease. New England Journal of Medicine. 2012 Oct 18;367(16):1519-28.
11. Sandborn WJ, Su C, Sands BE, D'Haens GR, Vermeire S, Schreiber S, Danese S, Feagan BG, Reinisch W, Niezychowski W, Friedman G. Tofacitinib as induction and maintenance therapy for ulcerative colitis. New England Journal of Medicine. 2017 May 4;376(18):1723-36.
12. Sandborn WJ, Feagan BG, D'Haens G, Wolf DC, Jovanovic I, Hanauer SB, Ghosh S, Petersen A, Hua SY, Lee JH, Charles L. Ozanimod as induction and maintenance therapy for ulcerative colitis. New England Journal of Medicine. 2021 Sep 30;385(14):1280-91.
13. Papamichael K, Cheifetz AS, Melmed GY, Irving PM, Vande Casteele N, Kozuch PL, Raffals LE, Baidoo L, Bressler B, Devlin SM, Jones J. Appropriate therapeutic drug monitoring of biologic agents for patients with inflammatory bowel diseases. Clinical Gastroenterology and Hepatology. 2019 Aug 1;17(9):1655-68.
14. Panés J, García-Olmo D, Van Assche G, Colombel JF, Reinisch W, Baumgart DC, Dignass A, Nachury M, Ferrante M, Kazemi-Shirazi L, Grimaud JC. Long-term efficacy and safety of stem cell therapy (Cx601) for complex perianal fistulas in patients with Crohn's disease. Gastroenterology. 2018 Apr 1;154(5):1334-42.
15. Peyrin-Biroulet L, Sandborn W, Sands BE, Reinisch W, Bemelman W, Bryant RV, D'Haens G, Dotan I, Dubinsky M, Feagan B, Fiorino G. Selecting therapeutic targets in inflammatory bowel disease (STRIDE): determining therapeutic goals for treat-to-target. Official journal of the American College of Gastroenterology | ACG. 2015 Sep 1;110(9):1324-38.
16. Wetwittayakhlang P, Bessissow T, Lakatos PL. Novel and emerging drugs for the treatment of Crohn's disease: a review of phase II and III trials. Expert Opinion on Emerging Drugs. 2024 Jan 2;29(1):19-34.

17. Bots S, Gecse K, Barclay M, D'Haens G. Combination immunosuppression in IBD. Inflammatory bowel diseases. 2018 Feb 16;24(3):539-45.
18. Diez-Martin E, Hernandez-Suarez L, Muñoz-Villafranca C, Martin-Souto L, Astigarraga E, Ramirez-Garcia A, Barreda-Gómez G. Inflammatory bowel disease: a comprehensive analysis of molecular bases, predictive biomarkers, diagnostic methods, and therapeutic options. International Journal of Molecular Sciences. 2024 Jun 27;25(13):7062.
19. Sun XL, Chen SY, Tao SS, Qiao LC, Chen HJ, Yang BL. Optimized timing of using infliximab in perianal fistulizing Crohn's disease. World Journal of Gastroenterology. 2020 Apr 14;26(14):1554.
20. Sulz MC, Burri E, Michetti P, Rogler G, Peyrin-Biroulet L, Seibold F. Treatment algorithms for Crohn's disease. Digestion. 2020 Sep 29;101(Suppl. 1):43-57.
21. Catanzaro R, Marotta F, Yazdani A, Sciuto M. Inflammatory Bowel Disease Therapies and Acute Liver Injury. Toxics. 2024 Jun 8;12(6):421.
22. Sands BE, Peyrin-Biroulet L, Loftus Jr EV, Danese S, Colombel JF, Törüner M, Jonaitis L, Abhyankar B, Chen J, Rogers R, Lirio RA. Vedolizumab versus adalimumab for moderate-to-severe ulcerative colitis. New England Journal of Medicine. 2019 Sep 26;381(13):1215-26.
23. Feagan BG, Sandborn WJ, Gasink C, Jacobstein D, Lang Y, Friedman JR, Blank MA, Johanns J, Gao LL, Miao Y, Adedokun OJ. Ustekinumab as induction and maintenance therapy for Crohn's disease. New England journal of medicine. 2016 Nov 17;375(20):1946-60.
24. Ernest-Suarez K, Panaccione R. Update on the role of upadacitinib in the treatment of adults with moderately to severely active ulcerative colitis. Therapeutic Advances in Gastroenterology. 2023 Mar;16:17562848231158235.
25. Tandon P, Natt N, Malhi G, Wong EC, Matthews P, Reinisch W, Narula N. Clinical remission in paired phase two and three studies in inflammatory bowel disease: a systematic review with meta-analysis. European Journal of Gastroenterology & Hepatology. 2023 Mar 1;35(3):231-40.
26. Rubin D, Danese S, Irving P, Nakase H, Wolf DC, Sinh P, Cree BA, Alekseeva O, Lublin FD, Santiago NR, Liu Z. S3 Integrated Long-Term Safety of Ozanimod Across Two Different Indications: Results from Clinical Trials in Patients With Moderately to Severely Active Ulcerative Colitis or Relapsing Multiple Sclerosis. Official journal of the American College of Gastroenterology | ACG. 2024 Dec 1;119(12S):S1.

Section 9

Antimicrobial Agents

Chapter 31

Newer Beta-Lactam Antibiotics

Author: Dr. Pranab Das

Introduction

Beta-lactam antibiotics (BLAs) represent one of the most important and widely used classes of antimicrobials, primarily due to their efficacy and generally favourable safety profiles. They include penicillins, cephalosporins, carbapenems, and monobactams, all sharing the beta-lactam ring responsible for inhibiting bacterial cell wall synthesis.

However, the rise of antimicrobial resistance (AMR) — especially among Gram-negative bacteria producing extended-spectrum beta-lactamases (ESBLs), AmpC beta-lactamases, carbapenemases, and other resistance mechanisms — has increasingly challenged the utility of many established BLAs. In response, pharmaceutical research has developed a new wave of beta-lactams and beta-lactam/beta-lactamase inhibitor (BLI) combinations to combat multidrug-resistant (MDR) pathogens. This chapter provides an overview of beta-lactam antibiotics, briefly reviews classical agents, and highlights the newest members of this class, focusing on their spectrum of activity against resistant organisms, clinical applications, and emerging therapeutic roles. By expanding clinicians' therapeutic arsenal and optimizing usage of these novel agents, we can address the evolving landscape of antibiotic resistance while striving to preserve the efficacy of established compounds.

Historical Classification

The advancement of beta-lactam antibiotics represents a significant milestone in contemporary medicine. The voyage commenced with Alexander Fleming's discovery of penicillin in 1928, but it was not until the 1940s that Howard Florey and Ernst Chain facilitated its mass manufacture and clinical use. In subsequent decades, penicillin resistance led to the development of semi-synthetic penicillins, such as methicillin in the late 1950s, created by British scientists to withstand β-lactamase enzymes. Cephalosporins were developed to combat developing Gram-negative bacteria, with cephalothin being therapeutically utilised for the first time in 1964, following the ground-breaking research of Giuseppe Brotzu, who identified Cephalosporium acremonium from a Sardinian sewage in 1945.

The identification of carbapenems represented a significant breakthrough. Thienamycin, the progenitor molecule, was identified by Merck researchers in 1976 and served as the foundation for imipenem, which received approval in the 1980s, distinguished by its extensive spectrum and resistance to β-lactamase. The monobactam class, spearheaded by aztreonam, was introduced in the early 1980s, specifically targeting aerobic Gram-negative bacilli while exhibiting negligible cross-reactivity in individuals sensitive to penicillin.

The 21st century introduced novel beta-lactams designed explicitly to combat multidrug-resistant pathogens. Ceftaroline, authorised in 2010, was the inaugural β-lactam exhibiting MRSA action owing to its strong affinity for PBP2a, a resistance factor in Staphylococcus aureus. Ceftolozane-tazobactam, launched in 2014, integrates a sophisticated cephalosporin with a β-lactamase inhibitor to combat Pseudomonas aeruginosa. Ceftazidime-avibactam, introduced in 2015, constituted an innovative combination of a third-generation cephalosporin and avibactam, a non-β-lactam β-lactamase inhibitor effective against KPC and certain OXA enzymes. Recently, meropenem-vaborbactam and imipenem-relebactam have augmented the carbapenem-based armament against carbapenemase-producing Enterobacterales. These drugs exemplify the ongoing struggle against resistance and the persistent enhancement of β-lactam chemistry to address contemporary antimicrobial concerns.

Definition and Classification

Beta-lactam antibiotics are defined by a beta-lactam ring in their molecular structure, which irreversibly binds to penicillin-binding proteins (PBPs). This leads to the inhibition of bacterial cell wall synthesis, ultimately causing cell lysis in actively dividing bacteria. Classic beta-lactam categories include:

1. Penicillins (natural penicillins, aminopenicillins, carbenicillins, etc.).
2. Cephalosporins (1st to 5th generations).
3. Carbapenems (imipenem, meropenem, ertapenem, doripenem).
4. Monobactams (aztreonam).

Over decades, multiple structural modifications and combination strategies with beta-lactamase inhibitors have broadened beta-lactam coverage against resistant bacteria. Yet, new resistance mechanisms necessitate continual innovation.

Brief Note on Conventional Beta-Lactam Antibiotics

Table 1: Concise overview of standard beta-lactam antibiotics

Drug Class / Drug Name	Mechanism of Action	Adverse Drug Reactions	Uses
Penicillins (e.g. Penicillin G, Amoxicillin, Ampicillin)	Inhibits bacterial cell wall synthesis by binding to penicillin-binding proteins (PBPs), preventing peptidoglycan cross-linking and leading to bacterial lysis.	Hypersensitivity reactions (rash, anaphylaxis), GI disturbances (diarrhoea, nausea), nephrotoxicity (high doses) and seizures (in renal impairment patients).	Gram-positive infections *(Streptococcus, Enterococcus, Listeria)*, respiratory tract infections, syphilis, endocarditis and skin & soft-tissue infections.
Cephalosporins (e.g. Cefazolin, Ceftriaxone, Cefepime)	Inhibits PBPs, blocking bacterial cell wall synthesis. More resistant to beta-lactamases than penicillins. Classified into five generations, each with broader Gram-negative coverage.	Allergic reactions (cross-reactivity with penicillins approximately 5%), neurotoxicity (Cefepime-associated seizures).	Broad-spectrum use for sepsis, pneumonia, UTIs, meningitis. Cefepime (4th gen) for *Pseudomonas* infections.
Carbapenems (e.g. Meropenem, Imipenem)	Inhibits bacterial PBPs, leading to cell wall disruption. Resistant to most beta-lactamases, making them effective against multidrug-resistant (MDR) bacteria.	Seizures (especially with Imipenem in renal failure patients), GI upset (nausea, diarrhoea).	Severe hospital-acquired infections (HAP, VAP, sepsis). Resistant Gram-negative infections (ESBL-producing bacteria).

Monobactams (e.g. Aztreonam)	Selectively inhibits Gram-negative bacterial PBPs, inhibiting cell wall synthesis. No cross-reactivity with penicillins or cephalosporins.	Minimal cross-allergenicity. Occasional GI upset, rash.	Gram-negative infections *(Pseudomonas, Enterobacteriaceae)*. Used in penicillin-allergic patients.
Beta-lactamase Inhibitors (e.g. Clavulanic Acid)	Bind irreversibly to beta-lactamase enzymes, preventing the hydrolysis of beta-lactam antibiotics. Enhance the spectrum of beta-lactams against resistant bacteria.	GI disturbances (diarrhoea, nausea), hepatotoxicity (rare, associated with Clavulanic acid) and hypersensitivity reactions.	Used in combination with penicillins (e.g. Amoxicillin-Clavulanate, Piperacillin-Tazobactam) for resistant bacterial infections, nosocomial pneumonia, complicated UTIs and intra-abdominal infections.

Despite these established agents, increasing incidence of ESBLs, carbapenemases, and other resistant phenotypes underscores the need for novel beta-lactams and combination therapies.

Recent Advances in Beta-Lactam Antibiotics

A. New Beta-Lactam/Beta-Lactamase Inhibitor Combinations

1. Ceftazidime-Avibactam (Beta-Lactam/BLI Combination)

Introduction: Ceftazidime-Avibactam is a combination of a third-generation cephalosporin (ceftazidime) and a novel beta-lactamase inhibitor (avibactam), offering activity against carbapenem-resistant Enterobacterales (CRE) and multidrug-resistant (MDR) Gram-negative bacteria.

Clinical Trial Phase / FDA-Approval: FDA-approved for complicated intra-abdominal infections (cIAI), urinary tract infections (cUTI), and hospital-acquired pneumonia (HAP).

Mechanism of Action:

1. **Ceftazidime: Inhibition of Bacterial Cell Wall Synthesis**
    - Ceftazidime crosses the bacterial outer membrane via porin channels (OmpF, OmpC in Gram-negative bacteria).
    - Hydrophilic nature allows rapid diffusion into Gram-negative bacteria, including *Pseudomonas aeruginosa*.
    - PBPs are essential enzymes in bacterial cell wall synthesis.
    - Ceftazidime has a high affinity for PBP3, a key enzyme in peptidoglycan cross-linking in Gram-negative bacteria.
    - Ceftazidime prevents the final transpeptidation step required for forming a rigid bacterial cell wall.
    - This leads to the accumulation of unlinked peptidoglycan precursors, weakening the bacterial structure.
    - Bacterial cell wall loses structural integrity, leading to increased permeability.
    - Osmotic pressure increases, causing water influx into the bacterial cell.
    - Cell rupture occurs due to high osmotic pressure.
    - Bacteria lose viability and cannot recover, ensuring a bactericidal effect.

2. **Avibactam: Inhibition of beta-lactamase Enzymes**

   Beta-lactamases degrades beta-lactam antibiotics, making bacteria resistant. Avibactam binds irreversibly to beta-lactamases (Class A, C, and some Class D), restoring ceftazidime's activity against resistant pathogens. Unlike older inhibitors (e.g. clavulanic acid), avibactam is not a beta-lactam and does not induce beta-lactamase expression, preventing resistance development.

3. **Spectrum of Activity**

   Ceftazidime-Avibactam is effective against:

   - Carbapenem-resistant Enterobacterales (CRE) *(Klebsiella pneumoniae, Escherichia coli).*
   - Multidrug-resistant *Pseudomonas aeruginosa.*
   - Extended-spectrum Beta-lactamase (ESBL)-producing bacteria.
   - Lacks activity against *Acinetobacter baumannii* and *Stenotrophomonas maltophilia.*

Key Pharmacokinetic Parameters: Ceftazidime and avibactam are both administered intravenously and exhibit linear pharmacokinetics. Ceftazidime achieves peak plasma concentrations within 1 hour of infusion, while avibactam reaches steady-state levels rapidly. Both drugs distribute mainly in extracellular fluid, including the lungs, peritoneal fluid, and cerebrospinal fluid (CSF). Neither ceftazidime nor avibactam undergoes hepatic metabolism, making them safe in patients with liver disease. Elimination occurs primarily via the kidneys (approximately 85%), with a half-life of approximately 2 hours for both components. Dose adjustments are necessary in renal impairment, but there are no significant drug-drug interactions.

Adverse Drug Reactions: Hypersensitivity, diarrhoea, nausea, headache, hypokalaemia and elevated liver enzymes.

Uses: MDR Gram-negative infections, including CRE and ESBL-producing bacteria.

Dose: 2.5 g (ceftazidime 2 g + avibactam 0.5 g) infused IV over 2 hours and given every 8 hourly.

2. Meropenem-Vaborbactam (Beta-Lactam/BLI Combination)

Introduction: Meropenem-Vaborbactam is a carbapenem/BLI combination with broad-spectrum activity against KPC *(Klebsiella pneumoniaecarbapenemase)*-producing Enterobacterales.

Clinical Trial Phase / FDA-Approval: FDA-approved for complicated UTI (cUTI), HAP, and bloodstream infections.

Mechanism of Action:

Meropenem-vaborbactam combines a carbapenem antibiotic (meropenem) with a novel, non-β-lactam β-lactamase inhibitor (vaborbactam) to overcome β-lactamase-mediated resistance.

1. **Meropenem: Inhibition of Bacterial Cell Wall Synthesis**
   - Meropenem is a β-lactam carbapenem antibiotic that binds to penicillin-binding proteins (PBPs), which are essential for bacterial cell wall synthesis.
   - It inhibits peptidoglycan cross-linking, leading to cell wall rupture and bacterial death.
   - Meropenem has bactericidal activity and demonstrates time-dependent killing.
2. **Vaborbactam: Inhibition of β-Lactamase Enzymes**
   - β-lactamases degrade β-lactam antibiotics, making bacteria resistant to carbapenems.
   - Vaborbactam is a boronic acid-based β-lactamase inhibitor that binds irreversibly to serine β-lactamases (KPC, Class A, and some Class C enzymes).

- It restores meropenem's activity against carbapenem-resistant Enterobacterales (CRE) by inhibiting KPC enzymes, which are responsible for carbapenem resistance.
- Unlike older β-lactamase inhibitors (e.g. tazobactam), vaborbactam does not induce β-lactamase expression.

3. **Spectrum of Activity**
   - Carbapenem-resistant Enterobacterales (CRE) *(Klebsiella pneumoniae, Escherichia coli, Enterobacter spp.).*
   - Multidrug-resistant *Pseudomonas aeruginosa.*
   - Extended-spectrum β-lactamase (ESBL)-producing bacteria.
   - Lacks activity against *Acinetobacter baumannii* and *Stenotrophomonas maltophilia.*
4. **Advantages Over Other β-Lactamase Inhibitors**
   - Stronger inhibition of KPC carbapenemases than avibactam.
   - More potent against CRE than ceftazidime-avibactam.
   - Lower resistance emergence compared to colistin-based therapies.

Key Pharmacokinetic Parameters: Meropenem-vaborbactam is administered intravenously (i.v.) and exhibits linear pharmacokinetics. Meropenem achieves peak plasma concentrations within 1 hour of infusion, while vaborbactam has a longer half-life (approximately 2.2 hours), allowing for prolonged β-lactamase inhibition. Both drugs distribute widely in extracellular fluids, including lungs, soft tissues, and urine. Shows minimal protein binding (approximately 2%). Neither meropenem nor vaborbactam undergoes hepatic metabolism, making the combination safe in liver disease. Renal clearance is the primary elimination route, with 85–95% of the dose excreted unchanged in urine. Dose adjustments are necessary in renal impairment, but no significant drug-drug interactions have been observed. Unlike colistin, meropenem-vaborbactam does not require therapeutic drug monitoring (TDM).

Adverse Drug Reactions: Hypokalaemia, diarrhoea and elevated liver enzymes and seizures (rare).

Uses: Carbapenem-resistant Enterobacterales (CRE) infections and complicated UTI.

Dose: 4 g (meropenem 2 g + vaborbactam 2 g) infused IV over 3 hours and given every 8 hourly.

3. Imipenem-Cilastatin-Relebactam (Beta-Lactam/BLI Combination)

Introduction: A novel triple combination designed for carbapenem-resistant Pseudomonas aeruginosa and ESBL-producing Enterobacterales.

Clinical Trial Phase / FDA-Approval: FDA-approved for complicated UTI (cUTI), complicated intra-abdominal infections (cIAI), and HAP/VAP.

Mechanism of Action:

Imipenem-Cilastatin-Relebactam is a three-component combination:

- Imipenem: A broad-spectrum carbapenem β-lactam antibiotic.
- Cilastatin: A renal dehydropeptidase-I (DHP-I) inhibitor, preventing imipenem degradation.
- Relebactam: A β-lactamase inhibitor that restores imipenem's activity against resistant bacteria.

1. **Imipenem: Inhibition of Bacterial Cell Wall Synthesis**
   - Imipenem binds to penicillin-binding proteins (PBPs), which are essential for bacterial cell wall synthesis.

- It inhibits peptidoglycan cross-linking, causing cell wall rupture and bacterial lysis.
- It is bactericidal and exhibits time-dependent killing.

2. **Cilastatin: Prevention of Imipenem Degradation**
   - Imipenem is rapidly degraded in the kidney by dehydropeptidase-I (DHP-I).
   - Cilastatin blocks DHP-I, increasing imipenem's half-life and effectiveness.
3. **Relebactam: Inhibition of β-Lactamase Enzymes**
   - β-lactamases degrade carbapenems, leading to bacterial resistance.
   - Relebactam is a diazabicyclooctane β-lactamase inhibitor that binds irreversibly to KPC, ESBL, and AmpC β-lactamases.
   - This restores imipenem's activity against carbapenem-resistant Enterobacterales (CRE) and MDR Pseudomonas.
4. **Spectrum of Activity**
   - Carbapenem-resistant Enterobacterales (CRE) *(Klebsiella pneumoniae, Escherichia coli, Enterobacter spp.).*
   - Multidrug-resistant *Pseudomonas aeruginosa.*
   - ESBL-producing bacteria.
   - No activity against *Acinetobacter baumannii* or metallo-β-lactamase-producing bacteria.

Key Pharmacokinetic Parameters: Imipenem-Cilastatin-Relebactam is administered intravenously (IV) and exhibits linear pharmacokinetics. Imipenem and relebactam achieve peak plasma concentrations within 1 hour after infusion. The drug is widely distributed in extracellular fluids, including lungs, urine, soft tissues, and CSF. Minimal hepatic metabolism occurs, making it safe in patients with liver disease. Elimination is primarily renal (approximately 80%), requiring dose adjustments in renal impairment. The half-life of imipenem and relebactam is approximately 1.2 hours, necessitating frequent dosing (every 6 hours). Unlike colistin, it does not require therapeutic drug monitoring (TDM).

Adverse Drug Reactions: CNS toxicity (seizures), nephrotoxicity and elevated liver enzymes.

Uses: CRE (Carbapenem-Resistant Enterobacterales), MDR *Pseudomonas* infections, complicated UTI (cUTI), complicated intra-abdominal infections (cIAI), and HAP/VAP.

Dose: 1.25 g (imipenem 500 mg + cilastatin 500 mg + relebactam 250 mg) infused IV over 30 minutes and administered every 6 hourly.

4. Cefepime-Enmetazobactam (Beta-Lactam/BLI Combination)

Introduction: A novel fourth-generation cephalosporin (cefepime) combined with enmetazobactam, a new beta-lactamase inhibitor targeting ESBLs and KPC-producing bacteria.

Clinical Trial Phase / FDA-Approval: FDA-approved (2024) for complicated UTI (cUTI).

Mechanism of Action:

Cefepime-Enmetazobactam is a combination of:

- Cefepime: A fourth-generation cephalosporin β-lactam antibiotic.
- Enmetazobactam: A novel penicillanic acid sulfone β-lactamase inhibitor that extends cefepime's spectrum.

1. **Cefepime: Inhibition of Bacterial Cell Wall Synthesis**
   - Cefepime binds to penicillin-binding proteins (PBPs), which are essential for bacterial cell wall synthesis.
   - It inhibits peptidoglycan cross-linking, causing bacterial cell lysis and death.
   - Cefepime has a broad spectrum, covering Gram-negative and Gram-positive bacteria with bactericidal activity.
   - It is less affected by AmpC β-lactamases compared to earlier cephalosporins.
2. **Enmetazobactam: Inhibition of β-Lactamase Enzymes**
   - β-lactamases degrade β-lactam antibiotics, leading to bacterial resistance.
   - Enmetazobactam is a β-lactamase inhibitor that targets ESBLs (e.g. CTX-M), KPC *(Klebsiella pneumoniae*carbapenemase), and some AmpC enzymes.
   - It restores cefepime's activity against β-lactamase-producing bacteria, especially ESBL-producing Enterobacterales.
   - Unlike earlier β-lactamase inhibitors (e.g. tazobactam), enmetazobactam has a higher binding affinity for ESBLs, making it more potent.
3. **Spectrum of Activity**
   - ESBL-producing Enterobacterales *(Klebsiella pneumoniae, Escherichia coli, Enterobacter spp.).*
   - Carbapenem-resistant Enterobacterales (CRE).
   - No activity against *Acinetobacter baumannii* or metallo-β-lactamase (MBL)-producing bacteria.

Key Pharmacokinetic Parameters: Cefepime-Enmetazobactam is administered intravenously (i.v.) and follows linear pharmacokinetics. Cefepime achieves peak plasma concentrations within 1 hour, while enmetazobactam maintains prolonged β-lactamase inhibition. The drug is widely distributed in extracellular fluids, including lungs, urine, soft tissues, and cerebrospinal fluid (CSF). Minimal hepatic metabolism occurs, making it safe in patients with liver disease. Renal clearance (approximately 85%) is the primary elimination route, requiring dose adjustments in renal impairment. The half-life of cefepime is approximately 2 hours, and enmetazobactam's half-life is around 1-2 hours, necessitating dosing every 8 hours.

Adverse Drug Reactions: Hypersensitivity, GI upset, *C. difficile* gut infection and elevated liver enzymes.

Uses: Complicated UTIs.

Dose: 2 g cefepime + 0.5 g enmetazobactam infused IV over 2 hours and administered every 8 hourly.

5. Cefiderocol (Newer Cephalosporin)

Introduction: Cefiderocol is a siderophore cephalosporin with activity against carbapenem-resistant Gram-negative bacteria.

Clinical Trial Phase / FDA-Approval: FDA-approved for complicated UTI (cUTI), HAP, VAP.

Mechanism of Action: Cefiderocol's mechanism of action combines the β-lactam activity of cephalosporins with a novel iron transport system.

1. **Siderophore-Mediated Active Transport into Bacteria**
   - Unlike conventional β-lactam antibiotics, cefiderocol acts as a siderophore, meaning it binds to iron and uses bacterial iron transport systems to enter the periplasmic space.
   - This circumvents porin mutations, which are a major mechanism of carbapenem resistance in Gram-negative bacteria.

- The iron-bound cefiderocol is actively transported into bacterial cells, leading to high intracellular antibiotic concentrations.

2. **Inhibition of Bacterial Cell Wall Synthesis**
   - Once inside the periplasmic space, cefiderocol binds to penicillin-binding proteins (PBPs), particularly PBP3.
   - This prevents cross-linking of peptidoglycan chains, leading to bacterial cell wall disruption and bactericidal activity.
   - It exhibits time-dependent killing.

3. **Resistance Avoidance**
   - Cefiderocol is stable against β-lactamases, including KPC, AmpC, OXA, and some metallo-β-lactamases (NDM, VIM, IMP).
   - The siderophore-mediated entry bypasses porin channel mutations, which often cause resistance to carbapenems.

4. **Spectrum of Activity**
   - Carbapenem-resistant Enterobacterales (CRE) *(Klebsiella pneumoniae, Escherichia coli, Enterobacter spp.).*
   - Multidrug-resistant *Pseudomonas aeruginosa.*
   - *Acinetobacter baumannii* (including carbapenem-resistant strains).
   - *Stenotrophomonas maltophilia.*
   - Metallo-β-lactamase (MBL)-producing bacteria (NDM, VIM, IMP).
   - Limited activity against Gram-positive bacteria and anaerobes.

Key Pharmacokinetic Parameters: Cefiderocol is administered intravenously (i.v.) and follows linear pharmacokinetics. It achieves peak plasma concentration within 1–2 hours post-infusion. The drug has low protein binding (approximately 58%), allowing effective distribution in lungs, urine, and soft tissues. It is not metabolized by the liver, making it safe in hepatic impairment. Cefiderocol is eliminated primarily by the kidneys (approximately 90%), with an elimination half-life of approximately 2–3 hours. Renal dose adjustments are necessary for patients with renal impairment. Unlike aminoglycosides or colistin, therapeutic drug monitoring (TDM) is not required.

Adverse Drug Reactions: Neurotoxicity, injection-site reactions, nausea and vomiting.

Uses: MDR Gram-negative infections, including Acinetobacter and Pseudomonas, HAP/VAP, complicated UTI and CRE infections.

Dose: 2 g IV every 8 hours (infused over 3 hours).

6. Ceftobiprole (Newer Cephalosporin)

Introduction: Ceftobiprole is a 5th-generation cephalosporin with broad Gram-positive and Gram-negative coverage.

Clinical Trial Phase / FDA-Approval: FDA approved for CAP and HAP (but not VAP).

Mechanism of Action:

Ceftobiprole targets bacterial cell wall synthesis by binding to multiple penicillin-binding proteins (PBPs), making it effective against resistant pathogens.

1. **Inhibition of Peptidoglycan Synthesis**
   - Ceftobiprole is a β-lactam antibiotic that binds to PBPs, enzymes essential for peptidoglycan cross-linking in bacterial cell walls.
   - This prevents bacterial cell wall synthesis, leading to cell lysis and death.
   - Ceftobiprole exhibits bactericidal activity and follows time-dependent killing.
2. **High Affinity for Key PBPs**
   - In Staphylococcus aureus, including MRSA:
     - Ceftobiprole binds strongly to PBP2a, the enzyme responsible for methicillin resistance.
     - This allows ceftobiprole to effectively kill MRSA, unlike older cephalosporins.
   - In Streptococcus pneumoniae:
     - Binds PBP2x, inhibiting strains that are penicillin-resistant.
   - In Enterobacterales *(E. coli, Klebsiella pneumoniae, Enterobacter spp.):*
     - Binds PBP2 and PBP3, inhibiting cell division and elongation.
3. **Stability Against β-Lactamases**
   - Ceftobiprole has moderate stability against AmpC β-lactamases but is not active against extended-spectrum β-lactamases (ESBLs) or carbapenemases.
   - It retains high activity against non-β-lactamase-producing Gram-negative bacteria.
4. **Spectrum of Activity**
   - Methicillin-resistant *Staphylococcus aureus* (MRSA).
   - Penicillin-resistant *Streptococcus pneumoniae.*
   - Gram-negative bacteria *(E. coli, Pseudomonas aeruginosa, Klebsiella spp.).*
   - Limited activity against ESBL-producing and carbapenem-resistant Enterobacterales.
   - No activity against *Acinetobacter baumannii* or anaerobes.

Key Pharmacokinetic Parameters: Ceftobiprole is administered intravenously (iv.) as its water-soluble prodrug, ceftobiprole medocaril, which is rapidly hydrolyzed into active ceftobiprole in plasma. It follows linear pharmacokinetics and achieves peak plasma concentration within 1 hour post-infusion. It distributes extensively into extracellular fluids, including lungs, skin, and soft tissues, but has limited penetration into cerebrospinal fluid (CSF). Protein binding is low (approximately 16%), ensuring effective tissue penetration. Ceftobiprole is not metabolized by the liver and is excreted unchanged via the kidneys (approximately 85%), requiring dose adjustment in renal impairment. The elimination half-life is approximately 3 hours, necessitating dosing every 8–12 hours.

Adverse Drug Reactions: Hypersensitivity, C. difficile infection and hepatotoxicity.

Uses: HAP, CAP and MRSA infections.

Dose: 500 mg IV every 8 hours (Infused over 2 hours).

7. Razupenem (Novel Carbapenem)

Introduction: Razupenem is a novel carbapenem designed for ESBL and carbapenem-resistant infections.

Clinical Trial Phase / FDA-Approval: Completed Phase II trials ongoing.

Mechanism of Action: Razupenem is a β-lactam carbapenem antibiotic that inhibits bacterial cell wall synthesis, leading to cell lysis and bacterial death.

1. **Inhibition of Peptidoglycan Synthesis**
    - Razupenem binds to penicillin-binding proteins (PBPs), which are essential for bacterial cell wall synthesis.
    - It has high affinity for PBP2 and PBP3, which play a crucial role in cell elongation and division.
    - By inhibiting PBPs, razupenem prevents peptidoglycan cross-linking, leading to bacterial cell wall instability and eventual cell lysis.
2. **Enhanced Activity Against MRSA and ESBL-Producers**
    - Unlike earlier carbapenems, razupenem binds strongly to PBP2a, the enzyme responsible for methicillin resistance in MRSA.
    - It remains stable against ESBL enzymes (e.g. CTX-M, TEM, SHV), making it effective against β-lactamase-producing Enterobacterales.
3. **Resistance Avoidance**
    - Razupenem is resistant to hydrolysis by most β-lactamases, including AmpC and ESBLs.
    - However, it is not effective against metallo-β-lactamase (MBL)-producing bacteria.
4. **Spectrum of Activity**
    - Methicillin-resistant *Staphylococcus aureus* (MRSA).
    - ESBL-producing Enterobacterales *(E. coli, Klebsiella pneumoniae, Enterobacter spp.).*
    - Penicillin-resistant *Streptococcus pneumoniae.*
    - *Pseudomonas aeruginosa.*
    - Limited activity against metallo-β-lactamase (MBL)-producing bacteria.
    - No activity against *Acinetobacter baumannii.*

Key Pharmacokinetic Parameters: Razupenem is administered intravenously (i.v.) and exhibits linear pharmacokinetics. It achieves peak plasma concentration within 1 hour of administration. The drug is widely distributed in extracellular fluids, including lungs, urine, and soft tissues, but has limited cerebrospinal fluid (CSF) penetration. Minimal hepatic metabolism occurs, making it safe in patients with liver disease. It is primarily excreted by the kidneys (85%), necessitating dose adjustments in renal impairment. The plasma half-life of razupenem is approximately 1.3 hours, requiring frequent dosing (every 8 hours). No significant drug-drug interactions have been observed.

Adverse Drug Reactions: Seizures (rare, but serious), nausea, hypokalaemia, nephrotoxicity and elevated liver enzymes.

Uses: Under investigation for use in MDR Gram-negative infections (complicated UTI, HAP/VAP and MRSA infections).

Dose: Phase II trials administered 500 mg to 1 g intravenously every 8 hours.

8. Clinical Implications and Best Practices

A. Appropriate Use and Stewardship

- Antimicrobial Stewardship: Ensuring these new agents are reserved for confirmed or highly suspected resistant infections. Indiscriminate use drives resistance and wastes precious therapeutic resources.
- Rapid Diagnostics: Techniques like multiplex PCR or whole-genome sequencing of bacterial isolates facilitate timely detection of specific beta-lactamase genes, guiding therapy selection.

B. **Therapeutic Drug Monitoring (TDM)**
   - TDM for beta-lactams is evolving to optimize pharmacokinetic/pharmacodynamic (PK/PD) targets, especially in critically ill patients with altered volume of distribution or augmented renal clearance. Achieving optimal time above the minimum inhibitory concentration can enhance efficacy.

C. **Combination Therapy vs. Monotherapy**
   - In certain scenarios (e.g. severe Pseudomonas infections, carbapenem-resistant Enterobacterales), combining new beta-lactam/BLI agents with other synergistic antibiotics may enhance bacterial kill or prevent resistance. However, data are mixed, and stewardship principles caution against routine combination if monotherapy suffices.

Future Directions and Emerging Concerns

- Metallo-Beta-Lactamase Inhibitors: BLI scaffolds that effectively block NDM, VIM, IMP, and other MBLs remain a pressing research priority. Aztreonam/avibactam offers partial coverage, but pan-effective MBL inhibitors are not yet clinically available.
- Global Access and Cost: Many novel agents carry high price tags, potentially limiting availability in low-resource settings where MDR pathogens often proliferate. Advocacy for equitable access and strategies to contain cost are vital.
- Resistance Evolution: Pathogens adapt rapidly, and new resistance genes or variants inevitably emerge. Continuous surveillance and readiness to develop 2nd or 3rd generation modifications of these new Beta-lactam antibiotics (BLAs) will be crucial.

Conclusion

The escalating challenge of antibiotic resistance in Gram-negative bacteria has revitalised the development of beta-lactam antibiotics. Novel combinations of beta-lactams and beta-lactamase inhibitors (e.g., ceftolozane/tazobactam, ceftazidime/avibactam, meropenem/vaborbactam, imipenem/relebactam) and innovative agents such as cefiderocol enhance treatment alternatives for doctors addressing ESBL- and carbapenemase-producing infections. While these medications signify considerable progress, their efficacy depends on prudent application guided by antimicrobial stewardship, fast diagnostic testing, and pharmacokinetic/pharmacodynamic optimisation. Future advancements in addressing metallo-beta-lactamases and enhancing coverage of challenging species, such as carbapenem-resistant Acinetobacter and Pseudomonas, are imperative. Furthermore, exorbitant costs and restricted worldwide accessibility present obstacles to practical implementation. Nonetheless, these novel beta-lactams provide an essential defence against contemporary multidrug-resistant pathogens, upholding the beta-lactam class's heritage as a fundamental component of current antimicrobial therapy.

References

1. Oliver A, Arca-Suárez J, Gomis-Font MA, González-Pinto L, López-Causapé C. Emerging resistance mechanisms to newer β-lactams in Pseudomonas aeruginosa. Clinical Microbiology and Infection. 2025 Mar 20.
2. Sargianou M, Stathopoulos P, Vrysis C, Tzvetanova ID, Falagas ME. New β-Lactam/β-Lactamase Inhibitor Combination Antibiotics. Pathogens. 2025 Mar 24;14(4):307.
3. Hsu AJ, Chiotos K, Heil EL, Shields RK, Tamma PD. The effectiveness of newer beta-lactams for the treatment of antimicrobial-resistant gram-negative meningitis. Clinical Infectious Diseases. 2025 Feb 20:ciaf071.
4. Fleming A. On the antibacterial action of cultures of a Penicillium, with special reference to their use in the isolation of B. influenzae. Br J Exp Pathol. 1929;10(3):226–236.
5. Chain E, Florey HW, Gardner AD, et al. Penicillin as a chemotherapeutic agent. Lancet. 1940;236(6104):226–228.
6. Blomquist KC, Nix DE. A critical evaluation of newer β-lactam antibiotics for treatment of Pseudomonas aeruginosa infections. Annals of Pharmacotherapy. 2021 Aug;55(8):1010-24.

7. Bush K, Bradford PA. Interplay between β-lactamases and new β-lactamase inhibitors. Nature Reviews Microbiology. 2019 May;17(5):295-306.
8. Zhanel GG, Chung P, Adam H, Zelenitsky S, Denisuik A, Schweizer F, Lagacé-Wiens PR, Rubinstein E, Gin AS, Walkty A, Hoban DJ. Ceftolozane/tazobactam: a novel cephalosporin/β-lactamase inhibitor combination with activity against multidrug-resistant gram-negative bacilli. Drugs. 2014 Jan;74:31-51.
9. Van Duin D, Bonomo RA. Ceftazidime/avibactam and ceftolozane/tazobactam: second-generation β-lactam/β-lactamase inhibitor combinations. Clinical Infectious Diseases. 2016 Jul 15;63(2):234-41.
10. Motsch J, Murta de Oliveira C, Stus V, Köksal I, Lyulko O, Boucher HW, Kaye KS, File Jr TM, Brown ML, Khan I, Du J. RESTORE-IMI 1: a multicenter, randomized, double-blind trial comparing efficacy and safety of imipenem/relebactam vs colistin plus imipenem in patients with imipenem-nonsusceptible bacterial infections. Clinical Infectious Diseases. 2020 Apr 15;70(9):1799-808.
11. Ito A, Sato T, Ota M, Takemura M, Nishikawa T, Toba S, Kohira N, Miyagawa S, Ishibashi N, Matsumoto S, Nakamura R. In vitro antibacterial properties of cefiderocol, a novel siderophore cephalosporin, against Gram-negative bacteria. Antimicrobial agents and chemotherapy. 2018 Jan;62(1):10-128.
12. Karlowsky JA, Lob SH, Kazmierczak KM, Young K, Motyl MR, Sahm DF. In-vitro activity of imipenem/relebactam and key β-lactam agents against Gram-negative bacilli isolated from lower respiratory tract infection samples of intensive care unit patients–SMART Surveillance United States 2015–2017. International journal of antimicrobial agents. 2020 Jan 1;55(1):105841.
13. Yahav D, Giske CG, Grāmatniece A, Abodakpi H, Tam VH, Leibovici L. New β-lactam–β-lactamase inhibitor combinations. Clinical microbiology reviews. 2020 Dec 16;34(1):10-128.
14. Livermore DM, Warner M, Mushtaq S, Doumith M, Zhang J, Woodford N. What remains against carbapenem-resistant Enterobacteriaceae? Evaluation of chloramphenicol, ciprofloxacin, colistin, fosfomycin, minocycline, nitrofurantoin, temocillin and tigecycline. International journal of antimicrobial agents. 2011 May 1;37(5):415-9.
15. Tamma PD, Aitken SL, Bonomo RA, Mathers AJ, Van Duin D, Clancy CJ. Infectious Diseases Society of America guidance on the treatment of AmpC β-lactamase–producing Enterobacterales, carbapenem-resistant Acinetobacter baumannii, and Stenotrophomonas maltophilia infections. Clinical infectious diseases. 2022 Jun 15;74(12):2089-114.
16. Rodríguez-Baño J, Gutiérrez-Gutiérrez B, Machuca I, Pascual A. Treatment of infections caused by extended-spectrum-beta-lactamase-, AmpC-, and carbapenemase-producing Enterobacteriaceae. Clinical microbiology reviews. 2018 Apr;31(2):10-128.
17. Bush K, Bradford PA. β-Lactams and β-lactamase inhibitors: an overview. Cold Spring Harbor perspectives in medicine. 2016 Aug 1;6(8):a025247.
18. Drawz SM, Bonomo RA. Three decades of β-lactamase inhibitors. Clinical microbiology reviews. 2010 Jan;23(1):160-201.
19. Waśko I, Kozińska A, Kotlarska E, Baraniak A. Clinically relevant β-lactam resistance genes in wastewater treatment plants. International Journal of Environmental Research and Public Health. 2022 Oct 24;19(21):13829.
20. Lim S, Yoo YM, Kim KH. No more tears from surgical site infections in interventional pain management. The Korean Journal of Pain. 2023 Jan 1;36(1):11-50.
21. Fratoni AJ, Gethers ML, Nicolau DP, Kuti JL. Non-KPC Attributes of Newer β-lactam/β-lactamase Inhibitors, Part 1: Enterobacterales and Pseudomonas aeruginosa. Clinical Infectious Diseases. 2024 Jul 15;79(1):33-42.
22. Lagacé-Wiens P, Walkty A, Karlowsky JA. Ceftazidime-avibactam: an evidence-based review of its pharmacology and potential use in the treatment of gram-negative bacterial infectionsinfections. Core evidence. 2014 Jan 1:13-25.
23. Darlow CA, Hope W, Dubey V. Cefepime/Enmetazobactam: a microbiological, pharmacokinetic, pharmacodynamic, and clinical evaluation. Expert opinion on drug metabolism & toxicology. 2025 Feb 1;21(2):115-23.
24. Wang H, Palasik B. Combating antimicrobial resistance with cefiderocol for complicated infections involving the urinary tract. Ther Adv Urol. 2022 Jan;14:17562872211065570.
25. Matesanz M, Mensa J. Ceftazidime-avibactam. Revista Española de Quimioterapia. 2021 Sep 30;34(Suppl1):38.
26. Bucataru A, Turcu-Stiolica A, Calina D, Balasoiu AT, Zlatian OM, Osman A, Balasoiu M, Ghenea AE. Systematic review and meta-analysis of clinical efficacy and safety of meropenem-vaborbactam versus best-available therapy in patients with carbapenem-resistant Enterobacteriaceae infections. International Journal of Molecular Sciences. 2024 Sep 4;25(17):9574.
27. Keam SJ. Cefepime/enmetazobactam: first approval. Drugs. 2024 Jun;84(6):737-44.
28. Sansone P, Giaccari LG, Di Flumeri G, Pace MC, Pota V, Coppolino F, Brunetti S, Aurilio C. Imipenem/Cilastatin/Relebactam for Complicated Infections: A Real-World Evidence. Life. 2024 May 10;14(5):614.

Chapter 32

Newer Antifungals

Author: Dr. Pranab Das

Introduction

Fungal infections have emerged as a significant cause of morbidity and mortality, especially among immunocompromised populations—such as patients undergoing organ transplantation, those receiving intensive chemotherapy, and individuals living with HIV/AIDS or other immune-deficient states. Conventional antifungal therapies, including polyenes (amphotericin B), azoles (fluconazole, itraconazole, voriconazole, posaconazole), and echinocandins (caspofungin, micafungin, anidulafungin), have long served as the cornerstone for managing invasive fungal diseases. However, increasing antifungal resistance (e.g. in Candida auris, certain Aspergillus species) alongside dose-limiting toxicities (particularly nephrotoxicity with amphotericin B) highlight the pressing need for novel agents.

Recent years have seen the advent of new antifungal molecules, novel delivery systems, and expanded roles for existing agents—each aiming to broaden spectrum, improve safety, and better address resistance patterns. This chapter outlines the spectrum of pathogenic fungal organisms, provides a brief overview of conventional antifungals, and delves into the latest developments in antifungal therapy, focusing on new drug classes, re-engineered molecules, and emerging strategies. By integrating these newer agents into thoughtful antifungal stewardship, clinicians can help mitigate resistance and optimize outcomes for patients with life-threatening fungal infections.

Historical Perspective

The advancement and development of antifungal treatment have been influenced by the growing awareness of invasive fungal infections in immunocompromised individuals. The contemporary antifungal period commenced with the advent of amphotericin B in 1958, extracted from Streptomyces nodosus by researchers at Squibb Laboratories, notably Gold, Hazen, and Brown. Although amphotericin B exhibits significant antifungal efficacy, its use is constrained by nephrotoxicity, leading to initiatives aimed at creating safer alternatives. In the late 1980s, the triazole class was introduced with fluconazole, developed by Ryder and associates at Pfizer, providing broad-spectrum efficacy, superior oral bioavailability, and central nervous system penetration.

The 1990s saw the proliferation of azole derivatives, notably itraconazole and voriconazole, the latter identified by Pfizer researchers and sanctioned in 2002 for invasive aspergillosis, establishing itself as a cornerstone in antifungal therapy. The advent of echinocandins in the early 2000s, namely caspofungin (Merck), micafungin (Astellas), and anidulafungin (Pfizer), signified a mechanistic advancement by inhibiting β-(1,3)-D-glucan production in the fungal cell wall—an strategy initially recognised by Douglas and associates.

In reaction to developing resistance and restricted effectiveness against moulds, the last ten years have introduced a novel class of antifungals. Isavuconazole, authorised in 2015, integrates a wide antifungal range with reduced medication interactions and enhanced pharmacokinetics. Rezafungin, an innovative echinocandin with a longer half-life facilitating weekly administration, was developed by Cidara Therapeutics and has demonstrated potential in recent phase III trials. Ibrexafungerp, sanctioned in 2021 and developed by Scynexis, emerged as the inaugural oral glucan synthase inhibitor distinct from echinocandins, exhibiting efficacy against Candida auris and azole-resistant strains. Fosmanogepix, a pioneering Gwt1 inhibitor developed by Amplyx Pharmaceuticals, is in advanced clinical trials and introduces a unique method aimed at fungal cell wall glycosylation.

These improvements signify the persistent demand for antifungals that are both effective and broad-spectrum, while also overcoming pharmacological constraints and increasing resistance. The pipeline currently features medicines with novel mechanisms, superior oral bioavailability, and improved safety profiles, signifying a new era in mycology and infectious disease therapies.

Definition and Burden of Fungal Infections

Fungi are eukaryotic organisms that can adopt yeast-like or filamentous (mould) forms. Clinically significant infections range from superficial mycoses (e.g. dermatophytosis) to invasive mycoses (e.g. invasive candidiasis, aspergillosis, mucormycosis), posing a critical threat to patients with diminished immune function. Common fungal pathogens include:

- Candida species (e.g. C. albicans, C. glabrata, C. auris).
- Aspergillus species (e.g. A. fumigatus).
- Cryptococcus neoformans (meningoencephalitis in immunocompromised).
- Mucorales (Mucormycosis, a fulminant infection).
- Endemic mycoses (e.g. Histoplasma, Blastomyces, Coccidioides).

Invasive fungal infections (IFIs) are notorious for high mortality rates when diagnosis or treatment is delayed. Adherence to effective prophylaxis and empirical or pre-emptive strategies are often paramount in high-risk settings, such as hematologic malignancies or transplant units. Nonetheless, the emergence of multidrug-resistant strains (e.g. Candida auris) and the complex pharmacokinetics and toxicity profiles of older antifungals have spurred the search for safer, broader-spectrum, and more resistance-resilient therapies.

Overview of Conventional Antifungal Agents

Table 1: Summary of traditional antifungal agents

Drug Names / Drug Class	Mechanism of Action	Adverse Drug Reactions	Uses
Amphotericin B (Polyene)	Binds to ergosterol in fungal membranes, creating pores that lead to ion leakage and fungal cell death.	Nephrotoxicity (hypokalaemia, renal failure), infusion-related reactions (fever, chills, hypotension) and electrolyte disturbances (hypokalaemia, hypomagnesemia).	Severe systemic mycoses (aspergillosis, cryptococcosis, histoplasmosis, candidiasis).
Fluconazole (Azole)	Inhibits lanosterol 14α-demethylase, blocking ergosterol synthesis, leading to fungal cell death.	Hepatotoxicity, QT prolongation, GI disturbances (nausea, vomiting).	Candidiasis (oral, oesophageal, systemic), cryptococcal meningitis.
Caspofungin (Echinocandin)	Inhibits β-glucan synthase, disrupting fungal cell wall synthesis, leading to cell lysis.	Histamine-related reactions (flushing, rash), elevated liver enzymes.	Invasive candidiasis, candidemia, salvage therapy for invasive aspergillosis.
Terbinafine (Allylamine)	Inhibits squalene epoxidase, blocking ergosterol synthesis and leading to toxic squalene accumulation.	Hepatotoxicity, taste disturbances	Onychomycosis (nail fungus), tinea infections (ringworm, athlete's foot)
Griseofulvin (Mitotic Inhibitor)	Binds microtubules, inhibiting fungal mitosis.	Hepatotoxicity, photosensitivity and teratogenicity.	Tinea infections (scalp, skin, nails).

Despite the expanded use of these classes, limitations persist: azole resistance in certain Candida and Aspergillus, potential toxicity of amphotericin B, intravenous-only routes for echinocandins, and evolving pharmaco-resistance patterns underscore the need for new strategies.

Newer Antifungal Agents

1. Ibrexafungerp

Introduction: Ibrexafungerp is the first oral glucan synthase inhibitor, providing an alternative to echinocandins for Candida infections.

Clinical Trial Phase / FDA-Approval: FDA-approved for vulvovaginal candidiasis (VVC). Being evaluated for invasive candidiasis and azole-resistant infections.

Mechanism of Action: Ibrexafungerp inhibits (1,3)-β-D-glucan synthase, a key enzyme in fungal cell wall biosynthesis.

1. **Inhibition of Fungal Cell Wall Synthesis**
   - Ibrexafungerp targets (1,3)-β-D-glucan synthase, which is crucial for synthesizing β-glucan, a major component of the fungal cell wall.
   - By inhibiting this enzyme, ibrexafungerp causes structural defects in the fungal cell wall, leading to increased permeability and fungal cell lysis.

- This results in fungal cell death, making ibrexafungerp fungicidal against Candida species and fungistatic against Aspergillus species.

2. **Broad-Spectrum Antifungal Activity**
   - Active against Candida species, including fluconazole-resistant strains and echinocandin-resistant isolates.
   - Effective against Aspergillus species., but with reduced potency compared to azoles.
   - Limited activity against Cryptococcus species and Mucorales fungi.

Key Pharmacokinetic Parameters: Ibrexafungerp is administered orally, making it the first oral glucan synthase inhibitor. It exhibits non-linear pharmacokinetics with moderate bioavailability (approximately 30%). Peak plasma concentrations are achieved within 4 hours of administration, and the drug is highly protein-bound (99%). Unlike azoles, ibrexafungerp does not require gastric acid for absorption, allowing it to be taken with or without food. It undergoes extensive hepatic metabolism via CYP3A4, necessitating dose adjustments when used with strong CYP3A4 inhibitors or inducers. The primary route of elimination is biliary excretion, with a half-life of around 20 hours, allowing twice-daily dosing. It does not require renal dose adjustments and has minimal drug interactions compared to azoles.

Adverse Drug Reactions: GI disturbances (nausea, diarrhoea), headache, dizziness and hepatotoxicity.

Uses: FDA-approved for vulvovaginal candidiasis (VVC). Investigational for invasive candidiasis, resistant Candida infections.

Dose: 300 mg orally twice daily for 1 day (total of 600 mg).

2. Oteseconazole

Introduction: Oteseconazole is a novel oral tetrazole antifungal designed to be more selective for fungal CYP51, reducing toxicity.

Clinical Trial Phase / FDA-Approval: FDA-approved for recurrent vulvovaginal candidiasis (RVVC).

Mechanism of Action: Oteseconazole works by inhibiting lanosterol 14α-demethylase (CYP51), a key enzyme in the ergosterol biosynthesis pathway.

1. **Inhibition of Ergosterol Biosynthesis**
   - Fungal cell membranes require ergosterol for integrity and function.
   - Oteseconazole inhibits CYP51, preventing the conversion of lanosterol to ergosterol.
   - This leads to accumulation of toxic sterol intermediates, causing membrane dysfunction, permeability loss, and fungal cell death.
2. **Selectivity for Fungal CYP51 Over Human CYP51**
   - Unlike older azoles (fluconazole, itraconazole), oteseconazole has higher binding affinity for fungal CYP51 and minimal inhibition of human CYP enzymes.
   - This reduces drug-drug interactions and hepatotoxicity, making oteseconazole safer than fluconazole.
3. **Potent Activity Against Fluconazole-Resistant Candida Strains**
   - Oteseconazole retains activity against fluconazole-resistant Candida species, including C. albicans, C. glabrata, and C. parapsilosis.
   - However, it has limited activity against Aspergillus species and Cryptococcus species.

Key Pharmacokinetic Parameters: Oteseconazole is administered orally and exhibits non-linear pharmacokinetics. It has high bioavailability (around 90%), allowing once-weekly or even less frequent dosing. Peak plasma concentrations are reached within 5 to 8 hours post-dose, and it is highly protein-bound (99%). Unlike fluconazole, which is renally excreted, oteseconazole undergoes hepatic metabolism and biliary excretion, reducing the need for dose adjustments in renal impairment. Its half-life is approximately 130 hours, making it ideal for long-term suppression therapy in recurrent infections. Minimal cytochrome P450 enzyme inhibition means fewer drug-drug interactions, a major advantage over traditional azoles.

Adverse Drug Reactions: Headache, nausea, dry mouth, QT prolongation and hepatotoxicity.

Uses: FDA-approved for recurrent vulvovaginal candidiasis (RVVC) and under investigation for Fluconazole-resistant Candida infections.

Dose: Loading Phase: 600 mg on Day 1 (as two 150 mg capsules twice); 450 mg on Day 2 (150 mg TID). Maintenance Phase: 150 mg once weekly for 11 weeks.

3. Rezafungin

Introduction: Rezafungin is a long-acting echinocandin with improved pharmacokinetics and stability compared to caspofungin.

Clinical Trial Phase / FDA-Approval: FDA-approved for candidemia and invasive candidiasis.

Mechanism of Action: Rezafungin inhibits (1,3)-β-D-glucan synthase, a key enzyme in fungal cell wall biosynthesis.

1. **Inhibition of Fungal Cell Wall Synthesis**
   - The fungal cell wall is composed of β-glucans, chitin, and mannoproteins.
   - Rezafungin specifically targets and inhibits (1,3)-β-D-glucan synthase, an enzyme crucial for β-glucan production.
   - This results in defective cell wall integrity, osmotic instability, and fungal cell death.
2. **Broad-Spectrum Antifungal Activity**
   - Highly active against Candida species, including azole-resistant and echinocandin-resistant strains.
   - Active against Aspergillus species, but not superior to voriconazole or amphotericin B.
   - Limited activity against Cryptococcus species and Mucorales fungi.
3. **Extended Half-Life Compared to Other Echinocandins**
   - Rezafungin has a longer half-life (110-130 hours) compared to caspofungin (9 hours) and micafungin (14 hours).
   - This allows once-weekly dosing, improving patient adherence and reducing hospital stay.

Key Pharmacokinetic Parameters: Rezafungin is administered intravenously (i.v.) and follows linear pharmacokinetics. It has a high protein-binding capacity (98%), which extends its elimination half-life (130 hours), allowing once-weekly dosing. Unlike micafungin and caspofungin, rezafungin undergoes minimal hepatic metabolism, reducing the risk of drug-drug interactions. It is eliminated primarily via faecal excretion (90%), with only minor renal clearance (10%), making it suitable for patients with renal dysfunction. No renal or hepatic dose adjustments are required, which is a major advantage over other echinocandins.

Adverse Drug Reactions: Infusion-related reactions, hepatic enzyme elevation, hypokalaemia and hypersensitivity reactions.

Uses: FDA-approved for candidemia and invasive candidiasis. Under investigation for invasive aspergillosis.

Dose: 400 mg IV on Day 1, followed by 200 mg IV once weekly.

4. Olorofim

Introduction: Olorofim is a novel antifungal targeting dihydroorotate dehydrogenase (DHODH), distinct from existing antifungals.

Clinical Trial Phase/FDA-Approval: Phase III trials ongoing for invasive aspergillosis and mould infections.

Mechanism of Action: Olorofim inhibits dihydroorotate dehydrogenase (DHODH), an essential enzyme in pyrimidine biosynthesis, leading to fungal cell death.

1. **Inhibition of Pyrimidine Biosynthesis**
   - Fungal cells require pyrimidines for DNA and RNA synthesis.
   - Olorofim targets and inhibits fungal dihydroorotate dehydrogenase (DHODH), the enzyme responsible for converting dihydroorotate to orotate.
   - This disrupts de novo pyrimidine biosynthesis, leading to nucleic acid depletion and fungal cell death.
2. **High Selectivity for Fungal DHODH**
   - Olorofim is highly selective for fungal DHODH and does not inhibit human DHODH, reducing off-target toxicity.
   - This selectivity makes it safer than traditional antifungals, such as azoles, which inhibit human cytochrome P450 enzymes.
3. **Fungicidal Against Aspergillus and Rare Moulds**
   - Olorofim is fungicidal against Aspergillus species, Fusarium species, Scedosporium species, and Lomentospora species, which are often resistant to azoles and echinocandins.
   - It is not effective against Candida spp. or Cryptococcus spp.

Key Pharmacokinetic Parameters: Olorofim is available in both oral and intravenous (i.v.) formulations. It exhibits linear pharmacokinetics with high oral bioavailability (90%). Peak plasma concentrations are reached within 2–4 hours post-administration, and the drug is highly protein-bound (99%). Unlike azoles, olorofim does not require gastric acid for absorption, allowing it to be taken with or without food. It undergoes hepatic metabolism via non-CYP pathways, which minimizes drug-drug interactions. The primary route of elimination is hepatic, with faecal excretion, and minimal renal clearance (5%), reducing the risk of nephrotoxicity. The half-life of 24–36 hours supports once-daily dosing, making it a convenient alternative to existing antifungals.

Adverse Drug Reactions: Infusion site reactions, hepatic toxicity, headache, and GI upset.

Uses: Under investigation for invasive aspergillosis and resistant fungal infections.

Dose: 150 mg orally twice daily (clinical trial dose).

5. Fosmanogepix

Introduction: Fosmanogepix is a novel antifungal inhibiting GPI-anchor biosynthesis, affecting fungal cell wall formation.

Clinical Trial Phase / FDA-Approval: Phase III trials ongoing for invasive mould and Candida infections.

Mechanism of Action: Fosmanogepix inhibits Glycosylphosphatidylinositol (GPI) biosynthesis, a critical process for fungal cell wall integrity.

1. **Inhibition of Gwt1 Enzyme**
    - The Gwt1 enzyme (GPI-anchored wall transfer protein 1) is required for the maturation and transport of GPI-anchored proteins, which are essential for fungal cell wall stability.
    - Fosmanogepix inhibits Gwt1, blocking the attachment of mannoproteins to the fungal cell wall.
2. **Disruption of Fungal Cell Membrane**
    - Without proper mannoprotein attachment, fungal cell wall integrity is lost, leading to membrane instability and fungal cell death.
    - This unique mechanism is fungicidal against Candida species and fungistatic against Aspergillus species.
3. **Broad-Spectrum Activity**
    - Highly active against Candida species, including fluconazole-resistant and echinocandin-resistant strains.
    - Effective against Aspergillus species, including strains with azole resistance.
    - Active against rare moulds (e.g. Fusarium species, Scedosporium species).
    - Limited activity against Cryptococcus species and Mucorales fungi.

Key Pharmacokinetic Parameters: Fosmanogepix is available in both oral and intravenous (i.v.) formulations. It exhibits linear pharmacokinetics with high oral bioavailability (80%), making it a suitable alternative to i.v. antifungals. Peak plasma concentrations are reached within 2–4 hours post-administration, and the drug is highly protein-bound (90%). Unlike azoles, fosmanogepix does not require gastric acid for absorption, allowing it to be taken with or without food. It undergoes hepatic metabolism via non-CYP pathways, minimizing drug-drug interactions. The primary route of elimination is hepatic (faecal excretion is around 85%), with minimal renal clearance (10%), reducing the risk of nephrotoxicity. Its half-life is approximately around 20–30 hours, supporting once-daily dosing.

Adverse Drug Reactions: GI disturbances, hepatic enzyme elevation and hypersensitivity reactions.

Uses: Under investigation for invasive fungal infections, including resistant Candida and Aspergillus.

Dose: Clinical trial dosing: 1000 mg IV twice on Day 1 (loading dose), then 600 mg IV once daily thereafter oral conversion: 700 mg orally twice daily.

6. New Formulations of Existing Agents

- **Liposomal Amphotericin B Variants:** Efforts to refine lipid formulations for targeted tissue penetration or reduced toxicity. Some novel formulations incorporate substances like phosphatidylcholine to lessen renal damage.
- **Submicron Formulations:** Submicron particle itraconazole and other "nano-formulations" aim to improve bioavailability, reduce GI side effects, and achieve stable plasma concentrations.

7. Combination Therapies and Synergistic Strategies

Drug synergy can enhance fungal clearance or circumvent resistance. Combinations under investigation include:

- **Echinocandins + Polyenes:** Particularly for severe or refractory Candida or Aspergillus infections. Some evidence suggests decreased mortality rates, albeit at the expense of higher toxicity and cost.
- **Azoles + Echinocandins:** For difficult Aspergillus or azole-resistant Candida. Trials yield mixed results, emphasizing the complexity of in vivo synergy.
- **Ibrexafungerp + Azoles or Echinocandins:** Preliminary data demonstrate potential synergy, notably for echinocandin-resistant C.auris.
- **Immunomodulators:** Agents that boost host immunity (e.g. GM-CSF, interferon-γ) combined with antifungals may aid in salvage scenarios for severely immunosuppressed patients with persistent infections.

Approaches to combination therapy remain individualized, guided by local susceptibility patterns, infection severity, and host factors. Randomized controlled trials are limited, making stewardship input and consultation with infectious disease specialists critical.

Expanding Approaches to Antifungal Stewardship

Amid the growing complexity of available antifungals, antifungal stewardship programs (AFSP) have emerged to optimize drug selection, dosing, and duration. Core components include:

1. **Diagnostic Stewardship:** Utilizing rapid diagnostics (e.g. beta-D-glucan, galactomannan, PCR-based assays) to distinguish fungal from bacterial or viral causes and identify specific pathogens earlier.
2. **Therapeutic Drug Monitoring (TDM):** Applied to triazoles (e.g. voriconazole, posaconazole) to maintain therapeutic concentrations while minimizing toxicity or resistance.
3. **De-Escalation Strategies:** Shifting from broad-spectrum or combination regimens to narrower-spectrum or single-agent therapy once susceptibilities are clarified.
4. **Infection Control Measures:** Preventing healthcare-associated fungal outbreaks (e.g. Candida auris) via rigorous disinfection, screening, and cohorting in institutions.

These measures can extend the lifespan of new antifungals and reduce iatrogenic complications in vulnerable patient populations.

Clinical Implications of Emerging Resistance

1. **Candida auris:** First identified just over a decade ago, C. auris rapidly gained notoriety for multidrug resistance (MDR) to azoles, echinocandins, and even polyenes in some isolates. Outbreaks in long-term care facilities have highlighted C. auris's capacity for skin colonization and environmental persistence. Novel agents such as ibrexafungerp or combination regimens are crucial for tackling echinocandin-resistant strains.

2. **Aspergillus fumigatus Azole Resistance:** In certain geographic regions, A. fumigatus has developed resistance to triazoles, often linked to agricultural fungicide use. Alternative therapies—such as liposomal amphotericin B, echinocandins, or novel antifungals in development—may be required. Combination therapies (e.g. voriconazole plus an echinocandin) have been investigated for resistant aspergillosis, though data on definitive benefits remain limited.

3. **Mucorales and Other Moulds:** Mucormycosis has seen a global uptick, partly associated with uncontrolled diabetes and COVID-19–related immunosuppression. While liposomal amphotericin B remains first-line, posaconazole and isavuconazole are second-line or salvage options. Ongoing research seeks to clarify the role of combination or new antifungals (e.g. fosmanogepix) for salvage therapy.

Future Directions and Research Frontiers

1. **Pan-Fungal Diagnostics:** Rapid broad-based molecular assays capable of detecting multiple fungi and identifying resistance markers (e.g. T2Candida, next-generation sequencing).
2. **Adjunctive Immunotherapies:** Agents that modulate the host immune system to enhance fungal clearance, potentially reducing fungal burden more swiftly or preventing relapse.
3. **Vaccines:** Investigational vaccines for Candida, Cryptococcus, or other pathogens remain conceptual but could transform prophylaxis in immunocompromised populations if proven effective.
4. **Precision Medicine:** Leveraging host genomics, fungal genotyping, and machine-learning algorithms to predict drug response, resistance emergence, and adverse effects, thereby guiding individualized therapy.
5. **Delivery Innovations:** Inhaled or topical formulations targeting fungal pneumonia or mucosal infections, minimizing systemic toxicity. Nanoparticle-based carriers could facilitate site-specific drug release and improve absorption.

Conclusion

Next-generation echinocandins (rezafungin), broad-spectrum agents with distinct targets (fosmanogepix), and ibrexafungerp (a novel orally active glucan synthesis inhibitor) are examples of innovations in antifungal therapy that are essential additions to the antifungal arsenal. These treatments tackle the problems caused by azole-resistant Aspergillus, emerging pathogens (like C. auris), and the scarcity of treatments for invasive or refractory fungal diseases. The growing selection of antifungals has the potential to lower morbidity and mortality in high-risk patients in addition to improved azole solubility and lipid amphotericin B variants, as well as potential synergy-based regimens. Antifungal stewardship, which includes infection control procedures, TDM, and quick diagnostics, is still crucial, though. Future success depends on continued research, international cooperation, and the prudent use of these valuable antifungal resources as resistant strains multiply and immunocompromised populations increase. In an era of growing fungal threats, clinicians can better combat invasive mycoses and save lives by combining novel agents with stewardship principles.

References

1. Logan A, Wolfe A, Williamson JC. Antifungal resistance and the role of new therapeutic agents. Current Infectious Disease Reports. 2022 Sep;24(9):105-16.
2. Bouz G, Doležal M. Advances in antifungal drug development: an up-to-date mini review. Pharmaceuticals. 2021 Dec 16;14(12):1312.
3. Stewart AG, Paterson DL. How urgent is the need for new antifungals?. Expert Opinion on Pharmacotherapy. 2021 Sep 22;22(14):1857-70.
4. Hazen EL, Brown R. Antibiotic substances from Streptomyces nodosus: I. Amphotericin A and B. AntibiotChemother. 1957;7(4):302–309.
5. Bongomin F, Gago S, Oladele RO, Denning DW. Global and multi-national prevalence of fungal diseases—estimate precision. Journal of fungi. 2017 Oct 18;3(4):57.
6. Pfaller MA, Pappas PG, Wingard JR. Invasive fungal pathogens: current epidemiological trends. Clinical Infectious Diseases. 2006 Aug 1;43(Supplement_1):S3-14.
7. Puumala E, Fallah S, Robbins N, Cowen LE. Advancements and challenges in antifungal therapeutic development. Clinical Microbiology Reviews. 2024 Mar 14;37(1):e00142-23.
8. Sofjan AK, Musgrove RJ, Garey KW. Impact of new diagnostic approaches for invasive candidiasis on antifungal stewardship. Current Fungal Infection Reports. 2016 Jun;10:68-77.
9. Cortegiani A, Misseri G, Fasciana T, Giammanco A, Giarratano A, Chowdhary A. Epidemiology, clinical characteristics, resistance, and treatment of infections by Candida auris. Journal of intensive care. 2018 Dec;6:1-3.
10. Cornely OA, Alastruey-Izquierdo A, Arenz D, Chen SC, Dannaoui E, Hochhegger B, Hoenigl M, Jensen HE, Lagrou K, Lewis RE, Mellinghoff SC. Global guideline for the diagnosis and management of mucormycosis: an initiative of the European

Confederation of Medical Mycology in cooperation with the Mycoses Study Group Education and Research Consortium. The Lancet infectious diseases. 2019 Dec 1;19(12):e405-21.
11. Arendrup MC, Patterson TF. Multidrug-resistant Candida: epidemiology, molecular mechanisms, and treatment. The Journal of infectious diseases. 2017 Aug 15;216(suppl_3):S445-51.
12. Pappas PG, Kauffman CA, Andes D, Benjamin Jr DK, Calandra TF, Edwards Jr JE, Filler SG, Fisher JF, Kullberg BJ, Ostrosky-Zeichner L, Reboli AC. Clinical practice guidelines for the management of candidiasis: 2009 update by the Infectious Diseases Society of America. Clinical infectious diseases: an official publication of the Infectious Diseases Society of America. 2009 Mar 1;48(5):503.
13. Hoenigl M, Arastehfar A, Arendrup MC, Brüggemann R, Carvalho A, Chiller T, Chen S, Egger M, Feys S, Gangneux JP, Gold JA. Novel antifungals and treatment approaches to tackle resistance and improve outcomes of invasive fungal disease. Clinical Microbiology Reviews. 2024 Jun 13;37(2):e00074-23.
14. Mudenda S. Global Burden of fungal infections and antifungal resistance from 1961 to 2024: Findings and future implications. Pharmacology & Pharmacy. 2024 Apr 12;15(4):81-112.
15. Satora M, Grunwald A, Zaremba B, Frankowska K. Treatment of vulvovaginal candidiasis—An overview of guidelines and the latest treatment methods. J Clin Med. 2023 Aug;12(16):5376.
16. Bhattacharya PK, Chakrabarti A, Sinha S, Pande R, Gupta S, Kumar AA, Mishra VK, Kumar S, Bhosale S, Reddy PK. ISCCM Position Statement on the Management of Invasive Fungal Infections in the Intensive Care Unit. Indian Journal of Critical Care Medicine: Peer-reviewed, Official Publication of Indian Society of Critical Care Medicine. 2024 Aug 10;28(Suppl 2):S20.
17. Osset-Trénor P, Pascual-Ahuir A, Proft M. Fungal drug response and antimicrobial resistance. Journal of Fungi. 2023 May 12;9(5):565.
18. Kow CS, Ramachandram DS, Hasan SS, Thiruchelvam K. Ibrexafungerp for the treatment of vulvovaginal candidiasis: a systematic review and meta-analysis of placebo-controlled trials. Journal of Medical Mycology. 2025 Jan 16:101534.
19. Bhosale VB, Koparde AA, Thorat VM. Vulvovaginal Candidiasis-An Overview of Current Trends and the Latest Treatment Strategies. Microbial Pathogenesis. 2025 Feb 5:107359.
20. Bassetti M, Stewart A, Bartalucci C, Vena A, Giacobbe DR, Roberts J. Rezafungin acetate for the treatment of candidemia and invasive candidiasis: a pharmacokinetic evaluation. Expert Opinion on Drug Metabolism & Toxicology. 2025 Feb 1;21(2):125-32.
21. Wiederhold NP, Patterson HP, Ferrer D, Garcia V, Thompson GR, Patterson TF. Olorofim demonstrates in vitro activity against Coccidioides species, including isolates against which fluconazole has reduced activity. Antimicrobial agents and chemotherapy. 2025 Jan 31;69(1):e00988-24.
22. Almajid A, Bazroon A, Al-Awami HM, Albarbari H, Alqahtani I, Almutairi R, Alsuwayj A, Alahmadi F, Aljawad J, Alnimer R, Asiri N. Fosmanogepix: the novel anti-fungal agent's comprehensive review of in vitro, in vivo, and current insights from advancing clinical trials. Cureus. 2024 Apr 28;16(4).

Chapter 33

Newer Antiviral Drugs

Author: Dr. Pranab Das

Introduction

With diseases ranging from seasonal influenza and respiratory viruses to chronic infections like hepatitis B and C, as well as new threats like novel coronaviruses and haemorrhagic fever viruses (like Ebola), viral infections continue to be a major global health concern. Rapid rates of mutation, immune evasion tactics, and zoonotic spillovers highlight the necessity of a diverse and ever-evolving arsenal of antiviral drugs.

Significant developments in molecular virology and drug development technologies in recent years have fuelled the development of new antivirals that are more effective, more well-tolerated, and able to target previously elusive stages of viral replication. New antiviral medications have surfaced, frequently with enhanced pharmacokinetics and increased activity against resistant strains, even though traditional agents (such as ribavirin for some RNA viruses, oseltamivir for influenza, and acyclovir for herpesviruses) continue to be mainstays of treatment. At the same time, new approaches to viral diagnostics and treatment plans for illnesses like hepatitis C and HIV have successfully transformed some once-fatal conditions into chronic illnesses that can be managed. The established antiviral classes are reviewed in this chapter, along with a brief overview of traditional treatments and new advancements in the treatment of influenza, coronaviruses, hepatitis viruses, and other important viral pathogens.

Historical Perspective

The advancement of antiviral therapy has been one of the most dynamic fields in contemporary medicine, propelled by the onset of viral pandemics and the necessity for specific treatments. The antiviral period commenced with William Prusoff's discovery of idoxuridine in the early 1960s, which was utilised topically for herpes simplex virus (HSV) keratitis. Acyclovir, a specific inhibitor of HSV DNA polymerase identified by Gertrude Elion in the late 1970s, subsequently established the basis for nucleoside analogue therapy. The global HIV/AIDS epidemic spurred antiviral innovation, resulting in the launch of zidovudine (AZT) in 1987 and the subsequent development of highly active antiretroviral therapy (HAART) in the mid-1990s.

The early 2000s saw the emergence of direct-acting antivirals (DAAs) aimed at the hepatitis C virus (HCV), resulting in a transformative shift in treatment. Significant developments encompassed sofosbuvir, a nucleotide polymerase inhibitor created by Michael Sofia and sanctioned in 2013, facilitating interferon-free treatments with effectiveness rates above 95%. This signified a transition to oral, abbreviated treatment protocols for persistent viral infections. Concurrently, tenofovir alafenamide (TAF) and entecavir established themselves as the standard for hepatitis B virus (HBV) suppression, exhibiting enhanced safety profiles.

The COVID-19 pandemic significantly expedited antiviral research. Remdesivir, initially created by Gilead Sciences for the Ebola virus, was repurposed and authorised in 2020 for SARS-CoV-2. Subsequently, molnupiravir, a ribonucleoside analogue created by Emory University and Merck, along with nirmatrelvir/ritonavir (Paxlovid), produced by Pfizer, received emergency use authorisations for the early outpatient treatment of COVID-19, specifically targeting viral polymerase and protease, respectively. These oral antivirals exhibited the practicality of swift implementation against emerging diseases.

Recent additions encompass maribavir for refractory cytomegalovirus (CMV) infections, baloxavirmarboxil for influenza (approved in 2018), and the ongoing development of antivirals for respiratory syncytial virus (RSV), including bemnifosbuvir and presatovir, signifying a transition towards host-targeted and highly specific mechanisms. Antiviral therapy is advancing towards precision, reduced treatment durations, and broad viral application in response to developing resistance and new threats.

Overview of Conventional Antiviral Therapies

Table 1: Synopsis of traditional antiviral treatments

Drug Name / Drug Class	Mechanism of Action	Adverse Drug Reactions	Uses
Acyclovir (Nucleoside Analogue)	Acyclovir is phosphorylated by viral thymidine kinase into acyclovir monophosphate, which is then converted to its active triphosphate form. Acyclovir triphosphate inhibits viral DNA polymerase, incorporating into the viral DNA chain and causing premature termination of viral replication.	Nephrotoxicity (crystalluria), neurotoxicity (hallucinations, seizures), nausea & vomiting.	Herpes simplex virus (HSV-1, HSV-2), Varicella-zoster virus (VZV) infections, HSV encephalitis.
Foscarnet (Non-Nucleoside DNA Polymerase Inhibitor)	Directly inhibits viral DNA polymerase and reverse transcriptase by binding to the pyrophosphate-binding site, without requiring activation by viral kinases.	Nephrotoxicity, hypocalcaemia, seizures.	Acyclovir-resistant HSV and CMV infections.
Ribavirin (RNA Polymerase Inhibitor, Guanosine Analogue)	Ribavirin is phosphorylated inside host cells, where it inhibits inosine monophosphate dehydrogenase (IMPDH), leading to depletion of GTP, required for viral RNA synthesis.	Haemolytic anaemia, flu-like symptoms and neuropsychiatric effects (insomnia, depression).	Respiratory syncytial virus (RSV), Hepatitis C virus (when combined with interferon), viral haemorrhagic fevers.
Oseltamivir (Neuraminidase Inhibitor)	Oseltamivir blocks neuraminidase, an enzyme required for viral release from infected host cells. This prevents viral spread and replication.	Nausea, vomiting, neuropsychiatric effects (delirium, hallucinations).	Influenza A & B (treatment and prophylaxis).
Efavirenz (Non-Nucleoside Reverse Transcriptase Inhibitor, NNRTI)	Directly binds and inhibits HIV reverse transcriptase, preventing viral RNA from being converted into DNA.	CNS toxicity (vivid dreams, depression), hepatotoxicity.	HIV infection.

While these categories remain fundamental, resistance, suboptimal efficacy in severe disease, and adverse effects drive the search for next-generation agents.

Recent Advances: Key Viral Targets and Novel Agents

1. Newer Anti-Influenza Drug

A. Baloxavir Marboxil

Introduction: Baloxavir marboxil is a first-in-class cap-dependent endonuclease inhibitor developed for the treatment of influenza A & B. Unlike traditional neuraminidase inhibitors (oseltamivir, zanamivir), baloxavir targets viral mRNA transcription, making it effective earlier in the influenza replication cycle.

Clinical Trial Status / FDA-Approval: FDA approved for acute influenza treatment. Ongoing trials are evaluating its efficacy in high-risk populations and oseltamivir-resistant strains.

Mechanism of Action: Baloxavir marboxil is a prodrug that is rapidly converted in the body to its active form, baloxavir acid. It targets the influenza virus replication process by inhibiting the cap-dependent endonuclease (CEN), a critical enzyme in viral RNA synthesis (Figure 1).

1. **Cap-Snatching Mechanism of Influenza Virus**
   - Influenza viruses lack a capping enzyme to initiate viral mRNA synthesis.
   - Instead, they use cap-snatching, where the viral polymerase complex (PA, PB1, and PB2 subunits) cleaves host pre-mRNA caps and attaches them to viral RNA for transcription.
   - This process occurs in the nucleus of infected cells and is essential for viral replication.
2. **Baloxavir Acid's Role in Inhibiting Replication**
   - Baloxavir acid specifically inhibits the PA subunit of the viral polymerase complex.
   - It blocks endonuclease activity, preventing cap-snatching and subsequent viral mRNA synthesis.
   - This leads to inhibition of viral replication, making it different from neuraminidase inhibitors (e.g. oseltamivir), which act later in the viral life cycle.
3. **Spectrum of Activity**
   - Effective against both influenza A and B viruses.
   - Demonstrates activity against oseltamivir-resistant strains.
   - Reduces viral replication more rapidly than neuraminidase inhibitors.

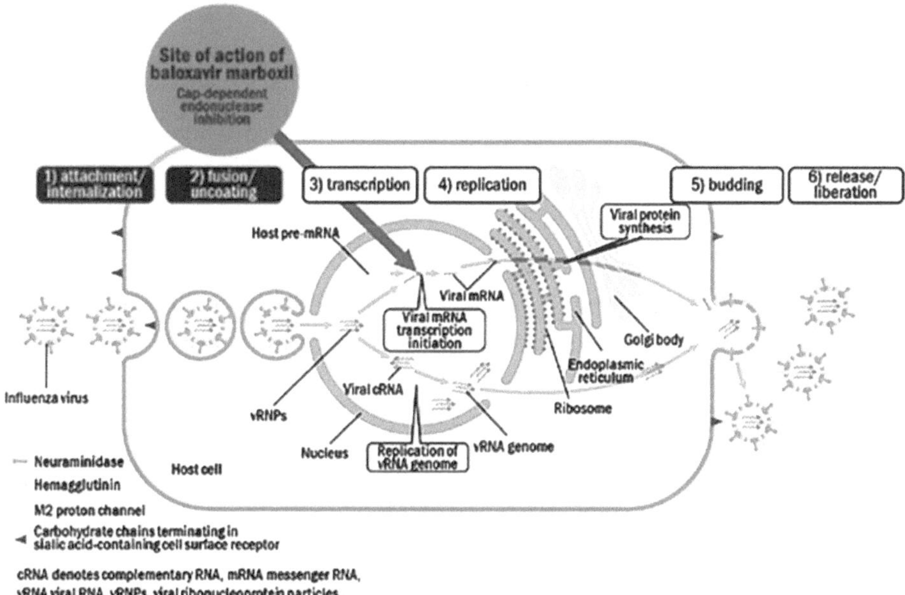

Figure 1: Mechanism of action of Baloxavirmarboxil (Source: Noshi T et al.).

Key Pharmacokinetic Parameters: Peak plasma concentration (Tmax) of baloxavir acid is reached 3-4 hours post-administration. Bioavailability is significantly reduced when taken with calcium-containing products, magnesium, or iron. Baloxavir acid has a large volume of distribution, suggesting extensive tissue penetration. Metabolized primarily by UDP-glucuronosyltransferase (UGT1A3) and minor contributions from CYP3A4. The drug has a half-life of approximately 79 hours, allowing single-dose administration. It is excreted primarily in faeces.

Adverse Drug Reactions: Diarrhoea, nausea, headache, nasopharyngitis, neuropsychiatric effects (hallucinations, behavioural changes) and hypersensitivity reactions.

Uses: Influenza A & B treatment (within 48 hours of symptom onset).

Dose: Single oral dose based on body weight: 40–<80 kg: 40 mg once and for ≥80 kg: 80 mg once. Administer within 48 hours of symptom onset or exposure.

2. Newer Anti-COVID Drugs

A. Molnupiravir

Introduction: Molnupiravir is an oral prodrug that induces viral error catastrophe, preventing SARS-CoV-2 replication. Unlike remdesivir, it is orally bioavailable, making it suitable for outpatient COVID-19 treatment.

Clinical Trial Status / FDA-Approval: FDA Emergency Use Authorization (EUA) granted in 2021.

Mechanism of Action: Molnupiravir is a broad-spectrum antiviral that acts by introducing mutations into the viral RNA of SARS-CoV-2, leading to viral replication failure. It is a prodrug of N4-hydroxycytidine (NHC) and functions as a ribonucleoside analogue, targeting the RNA-dependent RNA polymerase (RdRp) of SARS-CoV-2.

1. **Conversion to Active Form:**
   - Molnupiravir is orally administered and rapidly absorbed.
   - It undergoes hydrolysis in plasma to release NHC (N4-hydroxycytidine), its active metabolite.
   - Inside human cells, NHC is phosphorylated into its triphosphate form (NHC-TP), which is incorporated into viral RNA.
2. **Incorporation into Viral RNA:**
   - NHC-TP competes with natural cytidine (C) and uridine (U) during viral RNA replication.
   - The SARS-CoV-2 RNA polymerase (RdRp) mistakenly incorporates NHC-TP into the growing RNA strand instead of cytidine or uridine.
3. **Lethal Mutagenesis ("Error Catastrophe"):**
   - Once incorporated, NHC-TP induces base-pair mismatches by mimicking both cytidine and uridine, leading to G to A and C to U mutations in viral RNA.
   - This excessive mutation rate results in non-functional viral proteins, rendering the virus incapable of replication.
4. **Comparison with Other Antivirals:**
   - Unlike remdesivir, which acts as a chain terminator to stop viral replication, molnupiravir promotes excessive mutations leading to viral extinction.
   - Unlike monoclonal antibodies (e.g. sotrovimab), molnupiravir does not rely on the spike protein, making it effective against variant strains.

Key Pharmacokinetic Parameters: It is rapidly absorbed in the gastrointestinal tract following oral administration. High oral bioavailability (80%). It is widely distributed in plasma, respiratory tissues, and immune cells. Crosses the blood-brain barrier (BBB), making it a potential candidate for treating neuroinvasive viral infections. Molnupiravir is a prodrug and undergoes rapid hydrolysis to NHC in the plasma. The active metabolite (NHC) is not metabolized by cytochrome P450 enzymes (CYP450), reducing drug-drug interactions. It is excreted primarily via urine.

Adverse Drug Reactions: Diarrhoea, nausea, headache and potential teratogenic effects.

Uses: Mild to moderate COVID-19 in high-risk non-hospitalized patients.

Dose: 800 mg orally every 12 hours for 5 days.

B. Remdesivir

Introduction: Severe acute respiratory syndrome coronavirus 2 (SARS-CoV-2) is the causative agent of coronavirus disease 2019 (COVID-19), which is a respiratory disease that is capable of progressing to viral pneumonia and acute respiratory distress syndrome (ARDS); COVID-19 can be fatal. Like other RNA viruses, SARS-CoV-2 depends on an RNA-dependent RNA polymerase (RdRp) enzyme complex for genomic replication, which can be inhibited by a class of drugs known as nucleoside analogues. Remdesivir (GS-5734) is an adenosine triphosphate analogue first described in the literature in 2016 as a potential treatment for Ebola. Broad antiviral activity of remdesivir is suggested by its mechanism of action, and to date, it has demonstrated in vitro activity against the Arenaviridae, Flaviviridae, Filoviridae, Paramyxoviridae, Pneumoviridae, and Coronaviridae viral families. Remdesivir activity against the Coronaviridae family was first demonstrated in 2017, leading to considerable interest in remdesivir as a possible treatment for COVID-19. Remdesivir was confirmed as a non-obligate chain terminator of RdRp from SARS-CoV-2 and the related SARS-CoV and MERS-CoV, and has been investigated in multiple COVID-19 clinical trials. After initially being granted an FDA Emergency Use Authorization (EUA) on May 1st, 2020, remdesivir was fully approved by the FDA for the treatment of COVID-19 on October 22, 2020. Remdesivir is currently marketed under the trademark name VEKLURY by Gilead Sciences Inc. Remdesivir was also approved by the European Commission on July 3, 2020. Remdesivir for the treatment of COVID-19, was granted an FDA Emergency Use Authorization on November 19, 2020.

Clinical Trial Status / FDA-Approval: FDA approved in 2020 for COVID-19 treatment.

Mechanism of Action:

1. **Conversion to Active Form:**
   - Remdesivir is administered intravenously and rapidly converted into GS-441524, an active nucleoside monophosphate.
   - Inside human cells, GS-441524 undergoes phosphorylation to form the active triphosphate (GS-443902).
2. **Incorporation into Viral RNA:**
   - The viral RdRp enzyme incorporates remdesivir triphosphate (GS-443902) into the nascent viral RNA strand, mistaking it for natural ATP.
   - Once incorporated, remdesivir prevents further RNA chain elongation, leading to premature termination of viral RNA synthesis.
3. **Delayed Chain Termination and Viral Inhibition:**
   - Unlike classical chain terminators, remdesivir allows the addition of a few more nucleotides before halting RNA synthesis.

- This delayed termination disrupts viral genome replication, preventing the virus from producing infectious particles.

4. **Selectivity and Resistance:**
   - Remdesivir specifically targets SARS-CoV-2 RdRp and shows minimal effects on human polymerases.
   - Resistance mutations in RdRp (e.g. E802D mutation) can reduce its efficacy but remain rare in clinical settings.

Key Pharmacokinetic Parameters: Remdesivir is designed for intravenous administration due to its poor oral bioavailability. It accumulates rapidly in infected tissues, particularly the lungs, which are the primary site of SARS-CoV-2 replication. It is extensively distributed in plasma and lung tissues. Accumulates in immune cells, enhancing antiviral activity and is metabolized intracellularly to its active triphosphate form (GS-443902). Primarily undergoes hydrolysis by esterases, followed by phosphorylation in hepatocytes. Plasma half-life is 1 hour for remdesivir; GS-441524 has a longer half-life (25 hours). It is excreted mainly in urine.

Adverse Drug Reactions: Hepatic enzyme elevation, nausea, vomiting, bradycardia, nephrotoxicity and hypotension.

Uses: Severe COVID-19 requiring hospitalization.

Dose: Day 1: 200 mg IV once; days 2–5: 100 mg IV once daily.

3. Newer Anti-HBV Drug

A. Besifovir (BSV)

Introduction: Besifovir is a nucleotide analogue reverse transcriptase inhibitor (NtRTI) with lower nephrotoxicity than tenofovir.

Clinical Trial Status / FDA-Approval: Phase III trials indicate strong HBV suppression with fewer renal side effects.

Mechanism of Action: Besifovir is a prodrug that is metabolized into its active form, besifovir diphosphate, inside hepatocytes. Its antiviral action primarily involves inhibition of the HBV DNA polymerase, which is essential for HBV replication.

1. Conversion to Active Form: After oral administration, besifovir undergoes enzymatic hydrolysis and phosphorylation within liver cells to produce besifovir diphosphate.
2. Inhibition of HBV DNA Polymerase: Besifovir diphosphate competes with natural deoxyadenosine triphosphate (dATP) for incorporation into the growing viral DNA chain.
3. Once incorporated into HBV DNA, besifovir lacks the necessary 3′-hydroxyl (-OH) group, which is required for further nucleotide addition.
4. This leads to premature termination of DNA synthesis, effectively stopping HBV replication.

Selectivity for HBV Polymerase:

Besifovir selectively targets viral HBV polymerase, with minimal impact on host DNA polymerases, reducing the risk of mitochondrial toxicity.

Key Pharmacokinetic Parameters: Well absorbed after oral administration. Rapid uptake into hepatocytes, the primary site of HBV replication. High intracellular concentration of the active diphosphate form, ensuring sustained antiviral effect. Besifovir is metabolized in hepatocytes to its active form via phosphorylation. Unlike tenofovir disoproxil fumarate (TDF), besifovir does not require renal tubular secretion, reducing nephrotoxicity risks. It is primarily eliminated via hepatic metabolism with minimal renal clearance.

Adverse Drug Reactions: Fatigue, nausea, lactic acidosis, hepatotoxicity and bone mineral density loss.

Uses: Chronic Hepatitis B infection.

Dose: 150 mg orally once daily.

4. Newer Anti-HIV Drugs

A. Lenacapavir

Introduction: Lenacapavir is a drug that has been approved by the U.S. Food and Drug Administration (FDA) under the brand name Sunlenca for the treatment of HIV. Lenacapavir is also being studied as an investigational drug to prevent HIV infection. Lenacapavir belongs to a group of HIV drugs called capsid inhibitors. Capsid inhibitors interfere with HIV capsid, a protein shell that protects HIV's genetic material and enzymes needed for replication. Capsid inhibitors can disrupt HIV capsid during multiple stages of the viral life cycle. This prevents HIV from multiplying and can reduce the amount of HIV in the body. Lenacapavir may work against HIV strains that are resistant to other HIV drugs.

Clinical Trial Status / FDA-Approval: FDA approved in 2022 for multidrug-resistant HIV.

Mechanism of Action: Lenacapavir acts by targeting the HIV-1 capsid protein (CA), which plays a crucial role in viral replication, nuclear transport, and assembly.

1. **Capsid Binding and Inhibition of Viral Uncoating**
   - HIV-1 capsid is an essential protein shell that encases the viral RNA genome and key enzymes.
   - After viral entry, Lenacapavir binds to a pocket in the HIV-1 capsid hexamer, stabilizing the capsid structure and preventing uncoating.
   - This blocks reverse transcription, preventing the formation of proviral DNA.
2. **Disruption of Nuclear Import**
   - Normally, HIV-1 capsid interacts with nuclear transport proteins (Nup153, TNPO3) to deliver viral DNA into the host nucleus.
   - Lenacapavir inhibits nuclear import, preventing integration of HIV-1 DNA into the host genome.
3. **Inhibition of Viral Assembly and Maturation**
   - At later stages, HIV-1 capsid is required for assembly of new virions.
   - Lenacapavir disrupts capsid assembly, resulting in the production of non-infectious virus particles.

Key Pharmacokinetic Parameters: It is administered as oral tablets (for initial loading dose) followed by subcutaneous injection. Bioavailability of the oral formulation is low. It rapidly accumulates in lymphoid tissues, ensuring sustained antiviral activity. It shows slow hepatic metabolism via CYP3A4 and UGT1A1 enzymes. It is not significantly affected by renal clearance, making it safer in kidney-impaired patients. It is eliminated primarily in faeces.

Adverse Drug Reactions: Injection-site reactions, weight gain (on long-term use), hepatic dysfunction, headache, nausea, dizziness and immune reconstitution inflammatory syndrome (IRIS).

Uses: Multidrug-resistant HIV-1.

Dose: 600 mg orally on Day 1 followed by 600 mg orally on day 2.

B. Islatravir

Introduction: Islatravir is an investigational drug that is being studied to treat and prevent HIV infection. Islatravir belongs to a group of HIV drugs called nucleoside reverse transcriptase translocation inhibitors (NRTTIs). NRTTIs use several different methods to block an HIV enzyme called reverse transcriptase. By blocking reverse transcriptase, NRTTIs prevent HIV from multiplying and can reduce the amount of HIV in the body. Islatravir may be effective against certain HIV strains that are resistant to other HIV drugs.

Clinical Trial Status / FDA-Approval: Phase III trials for HIV treatment and PrEP.

Mechanism of Action:

1. **Prodrug Activation:**
   - Islatravir is orally administered and undergoes intracellular phosphorylation to its active form, islatravir-triphosphate (ISL-TP).
2. **Inhibition of Reverse Transcriptase via Multiple Mechanisms:**
   - Immediate Chain Termination:
     I. Once incorporated into the growing HIV DNA chain, ISL-TP prevents further nucleotide additions due to the absence of a 3'-hydroxyl (-OH) group.
     II. This terminates viral DNA synthesis early, blocking viral replication.
   - Translocation Inhibition:
     I. If the HIV reverse transcriptase enzyme attempts to add another nucleotide after ISL-TP incorporation, it fails to shift the DNA primer-template for the next nucleotide addition.
     II. This prevents correct positioning of subsequent nucleotides, further halting viral replication.
3. **Increased Potency and High Barrier to Resistance:**
   - Islatravir binds tightly to reverse transcriptase, making it more effective at lower concentrations than traditional NRTIs.
   - Demonstrates activity against drug-resistant HIV strains, including those resistant to tenofovir and lamivudine.

Key Pharmacokinetic Parameters: It is well absorbed after oral administration. It is highly concentrated in lymphoid tissues, which are key sites of HIV replication. High intracellular levels of islatravir-triphosphate (active form) allow for long-lasting antiviral effects. Primarily phosphorylated intracellularly to ISL-TP. It undergoes minimal metabolism by cytochrome P450 enzymes (CYP450), reducing drug-drug interactions. It has an extremely long intracellular half-life (128 hours), allowing for once-weekly or even once-monthly dosing. It is excreted mainly via the kidneys as unchanged drug.

Adverse Drug Reactions: Headache, nausea, diarrhoea, hepatotoxicity, lymphopenia and hypersensitivity reactions.

Uses: HIV-1 PrEP& treatment.

Dose: Oral 0.75 mg daily in combination with other agents.

Other Notable Developments

Hepatitis C Virus (HCV)

Over the last decade, HCV treatment has been revolutionized by direct-acting antivirals (DAAs), allowing >95% cure rates with minimal side effects. Key developments include:

- **Pan-Genotypic Combinations:** Glecaprevir/pibrentasvir, sofosbuvir/velpatasvir, and sofosbuvir/velpatasvir/voxilaprevir achieve high cure rates across HCV genotypes, including previously difficult-to-treat ones.
- **Shortened Therapy Durations:** Some regimens require just 8–12 weeks. Trials investigate 6-week or even 4-week ultra-short courses in select patients.
- **Real-World Impact:** These new-generation DAAs have transformed HCV into a curable infection, motivating efforts for global HCV elimination by 2030.

Cytomegalovirus (CMV)

- **Letermovir:** Targets CMV terminase complex, inhibiting viral DNA processing and packaging. Approved for prophylaxis in CMV-seropositive hematopoietic stem cell transplant recipients. Exhibits fewer side effects than ganciclovir or foscarnet.
- **Maribavir:** An investigational antiviral inhibiting the UL97 protein kinase, shows promise in refractory or resistant CMV infections. Recently approved in some regions for post-transplant CMV.

Ebola and Emerging Viruses

- Favipiravir, Remdesivir, Monoclonal Antibodies (e.g. mAb114, REGN-EB3) have been studied for Ebola. For Marburg, Nipah, and other emerging viruses, experimental therapies focus on broad-spectrum antivirals, host factor modulators, or prophylactic monoclonal antibodies.
- Filovirus-specific mAbs: Provide post-exposure prophylaxis or treatment in outbreak settings with high mortality rates. Ongoing expansions of monoclonal cocktails aim to mitigate resistance.

Respiratory Syncytial Virus (RSV)

- Monoclonal Antibody (Palivizumab) is well known for prophylaxis in high-risk infants.
- Fusion Inhibitors (e.g. Presatovir), small-molecule RSV polymerase inhibitors, and new prophylactic mAbs (nirsevimab) aim to fill gaps in RSV management. Some are already licensed or in late-stage trials.

Antiviral Stewardship and Resistance

A. Early Diagnostics and Genotypic Testing

- Rapid molecular assays (PCR, next-generation sequencing) identify specific viruses and detect resistance mutations, guiding targeted therapy.
- Example: HCV genotype testing historically guided DAA choice, though newer pan-genotypic regimens reduce the need. HIV integrase inhibitor or NRTI resistance testing can refine salvage regimens.

B. Rational Combination Therapy

- Many viruses rapidly mutate under selective drug pressure. Combination regimens (e.g. HIV cART, HCV DAAs) reduce resistance emergence and improve cure or suppression rates.

- For SARS-CoV-2 and influenza, combination therapy is still debated but may be beneficial in certain immunocompromised or severely ill patients to prevent suboptimal virologic response.

C. **Proactive Monitoring and Global Surveillance**

- WHO and CDC (Centers for Disease Control and Prevention) track resistance patterns for influenza, HIV, HBV, and emerging pathogens.
- Real-time data inform vaccine composition (influenza) and recommended first-line regimens (HIV, HBV, HCV).
- Ensuring equitable access to novel antivirals globally remains an unresolved challenge.

Expanding Horizons: Future Perspectives

1. **Host-Targeted Therapies**
   - Identify and inhibit host factors essential for viral replication, potentially reducing direct resistance pressure on the virus. Examples include CCR5 antagonists in HIV, or inhibitors of host proteases that cleave viral proteins.
2. **CRISPR-Based Antiviral Strategies**
   - While mostly preclinical, gene-editing tools may excise latent viral genomes (e.g. HIV provirus) or disrupt viral entry pathways. Obstacles include delivery, off-target effects, and incomplete editing.
3. **Broad-Spectrum Antivirals**
   - Agents like favipiravir or ribavirin have partial success, but more potent and less toxic broad-spectrum molecules remain a holy grail to rapidly address novel or re-emerging pathogens.
4. **Therapeutic Vaccines**
   - Vaccines that can treat chronic infections (e.g. HIV, HBV) by boosting host immunity. Research continues into T-cell–based immunogens, but robust clinical success is elusive.
5. **Non-traditional Modalities**
   - Monoclonal antibody cocktails, microRNA inhibitors, and small interfering RNA (siRNA) therapies are under exploration for a range of viruses, with potential synergy in combination regimens.

Conclusion

Treatment options for serious viral infections have changed as a result of recent developments in antiviral medication development. The changing landscape shows how molecular insights can change clinical outcomes, from a single-dose influenza treatment (baloxavir) and powerful combination regimens that cure hepatitis C to innovative broad-spectrum approaches for SARS-CoV-2 and growing prophylaxis for RSV. Furthermore, new classes of coronaviruses, like oral protease inhibitors and capsid assembly modulators for HBV, open the door to shorter, more efficient treatment courses. Viral resistance, exorbitant drug prices, restricted worldwide access, and the continuous emergence of new infections are enduring obstacles that highlight the necessity of careful antiviral stewardship and ongoing innovation. Strategic combination therapy and quick diagnostics continue to be essential tactics for preventing resistance. Antiviral care may be further expanded in the future by the promise of host-directed therapies, gene-editing technologies, and universal prophylactic agents. Clinicians can more effectively contain current viral threats and react quickly to future pandemics by adopting these innovative therapies while implementing strong stewardship practices.

References

1. Kar B, Dehury B, Singh MK, Pati S, Bhattacharya D. Identification of phytocompounds as newer antiviral drugs against COVID-19 through molecular docking and simulation based study. Journal of Molecular Graphics and Modelling. 2022 Jul 1;114:108192.
2. Valencia Deray KG, Danziger-Isakov LA, Downes KJ. Current and emerging antiviral agents in the prevention and treatment of cytomegalovirus in pediatric transplant recipients. Journal of the Pediatric Infectious Diseases Society. 2024 Feb 1;13(Supplement_1):S14-21.
3. Van Brummelen R, Van Brummelen AC. The potential role of resveratrol as supportive antiviral in treating conditions such as COVID-19–a formulator's perspective. Biomedicine & Pharmacotherapy. 2022 Apr 1;148:112767.
4. De Clercq E, Li G. Approved antiviral drugs over the past 50 years. Clinical microbiology reviews. 2016 Jul;29(3):695-747.
5. Hayden FG, Sugaya N, Hirotsu N, Lee N, de Jong MD, Hurt AC, Ishida T, Sekino H, Yamada K, Portsmouth S, Kawaguchi K. Baloxavirmarboxil for uncomplicated influenza in adults and adolescents. New England Journal of Medicine. 2018 Sep 6;379(10):913-23.
6. Hammond J, Leister-Tebbe H, Gardner A, Abreu P, Bao W, Wisemandle W, Baniecki M, Hendrick VM, Damle B, Simón-Campos A, Pypstra R. Oral nirmatrelvir for high-risk, nonhospitalized adults with Covid-19. New England Journal of Medicine. 2022 Apr 14;386(15):1397-408.
7. Noshi T, Kitano M, Taniguchi K, Yamamoto A. In vitro characterization of baloxavir acid, a first-in-class cap-dependent endonuclease inhibitor of the influenza virus polymerase PA subunit. Antiviral Res. 2018 Oct;160:109–117.
8. Feld JJ, Ward JW. Key elements on the pathway to HCV elimination: lessons learned from the AASLD HCV special interest group 2020. Hepatology Communications. 2021 Jun;5(6):911-22.
9. Ison MG, Portsmouth S, Yoshida Y, Shishido T, Mitchener M, Tsuchiya K, Uehara T, Hayden FG. Early treatment with baloxavirmarboxil in high-risk adolescent and adult outpatients with uncomplicated influenza (CAPSTONE-2): a randomised, placebo-controlled, phase 3 trial. The Lancet Infectious Diseases. 2020 Oct 1;20(10):1204-14.
10. Jayk Bernal A, Gomes da Silva MM, Musungaie DB, Kovalchuk E, Gonzalez A, Delos Reyes V, Martín-Quirós A, Caraco Y, Williams-Diaz A, Brown ML, Du J. Molnupiravir for oral treatment of Covid-19 in nonhospitalized patients. New England Journal of Medicine. 2022 Feb 10;386(6):509-20.
11. Beigel JH, Tomashek KM, Dodd LE, Mehta AK, Zingman BS, Kalil AC, Hohmann E, Chu HY, Luetkemeyer A, Kline S, Lopez de Castilla D. Remdesivir for the treatment of Covid-19. New England Journal of Medicine. 2020 Nov 5;383(19):1813-26.
12. Yim HJ, Kim W, Ahn SH, Yang JM, Jang JY, Kweon YO, Cho YK, Kim YJ, Hong GY, Kim DJ, Jung YK. Besifovirdipivoxil maleate 144-week treatment of chronic hepatitis B: an open-label extensional study of a phase 3 trial. Official journal of the American College of Gastroenterology | ACG. 2020 Aug 1;115(8):1217-25.
13. Ogbuagu O, Segal-Maurer S, Ratanasuwan W, Trottier B, Brunetta J, Shirasaka T, Koenig EL, Wang H, Margot NA, Dvory-Sobol H, Rhee MS. 1585. Efficacy and safety of long-acting subcutaneous lenacapavir in heavily treatment-experienced people with multi-drug resistant HIV: week 52 results. InOpen Forum Infectious Diseases 2022 Dec 15 (Vol. 9, No. Suppl 2, pp. ofac492-108).
14. Brunton LL, Knollmann BC, Hilal-Dandan R. *Goodman & Gilman's: The Pharmacological Basis of Therapeutics*.13th ed. New York: McGraw-Hill; 2018.
15. Katzung BG, Vanderah TW, Trevor AJ. *Basic & Clinical Pharmacology*. 15th ed. New York: McGraw-Hill; 2021.
16. Fairhead C, Levi J, Hill A. Challenges for Novel Antiretroviral Development in an Era of Widespread tenofovir-disoproxil/ lamivudine (or emtricitabine)/dolutegravir availability (TLD) Availability. Clinical Infectious Diseases. 2025 Feb 15;80(2):434-43.
17. Fujii A, Oishi T, Kondo E, Morihara Z, Ikeda Y, Sumida H, Ninomiya Y, Uesugi S, Okazaki K, Yoshioka D, Kobayashi M. Efficacy of baloxavirmarboxil as a prophylactic against influenza among in-patients and analysis of influenza virus mutations in their isolates at a Japanese hospital during the 2023–2024 flu season. Journal of Pharmaceutical Health Care and Sciences. 2025 Mar 17;11(1):22.
18. Waters MD, Warren SG. A Tale of Two Drugs: Molnupiravir and Paxlovid. Mutation Research-Reviews in Mutation Research. 2025 Feb 6:108533.
19. Godwin PO, Polsonetti B, Caron MF, Oppelt TF. Remdesivir for the treatment of COVID-19: a narrative review. Infectious Diseases and Therapy. 2024 Jan;13(1):1-9.
20. Jogiraju V, Pawar P, Yager J, Ling J, Shen G, Chiu A, Hughes E, Palaparthy R, Carter C, Singh R. Pharmacokinetics and safety of once-yearly lenacapavir: a phase 1, open-label study. The Lancet. 2025 Apr 5;405(10485):1147-54.
21. Gillespie SW, Reddy AS, Burris DM, Naqvi SH, Byrareddy SN, Lorson CL, Singh K. Islatravir: evaluation of clinical development for HIV and HBV. Expert Opinion on Investigational Drugs. 2024 Feb 1;33(2):85-93.

Chapter 34

Recent Advances in the Management of Malaria

Author: Dr. Pranab Das

Introduction

Malaria continues to be a major global health issue, especially in sub-Saharan Africa, Southeast Asia, and certain regions of South America. Malaria, caused by Plasmodium parasites (particularly P. falciparum and P. vivax), results in hundreds of thousands of fatalities annually, primarily affecting young children. Despite enhanced initiatives in vector control (such as insecticide-treated nets and indoor residual spraying) and combination medicine therapy (particularly artemisinin-based combination therapies, ACTs), problems persist. This include drug-resistant parasite strains, notably P. falciparum resistant to artemisinin or its companion medications, as well as restricted access to therapeutic therapies in distant regions. This chapter succinctly examines established antimalarial protocols, investigates recent advancements in pharmacotherapy (including novel artemisinin derivatives, next-generation combination therapies, and non-artemisinin compounds), emphasises progress in malaria vaccination, and addresses emerging strategies for disease eradication. The global community aims to expedite progress towards complete eradication by integrating innovative interventions with comprehensive malaria surveillance and control methods.

Historical Perspective

The ongoing search for efficient antimalarial medications in the face of changing parasite resistance has influenced the fight against malaria. Quinine was first isolated in pure form by Pelletier and Caventou in 1820 after being taken from Cinchona bark by Jesuit missionaries in the 17th century, marking the beginning of the medicinal journey. Synthetic antimalarials were created in the 20th century to address quinine shortages during the war. Due to its effectiveness and tolerability, chloroquine—which was created by German scientists in 1934—became the mainstay of malaria treatment following World War II. However, by the late 1950s, chloroquine resistance had spread widely, especially in South America and Southeast Asia, which led to the 1970s introduction of mefloquine and sulfadoxine-pyrimethamine (SP).

The rediscovery of artemisinin, which Tu Youyou obtained from Artemisia annua in the 1970s as part of China's "Project 523," was a significant breakthrough. Her research produced artesunate and artemether, which provided quick parasite removal and served as the basis for contemporary artemisinin-based combination treatments (ACTs). Since the early 2000s, the WHO has approved ACTs like artemether-lumefantrine, dihydroartemisinin-piperaquine, and artesunate-amodiaquine as first-line treatments for Plasmodium falciparum malaria.

Development of next-generation antimalarials has been rekindled by the discovery of artemisinin partial resistance, which was initially documented in Cambodia in the early 2010s. Tafenoquine, a long-acting 8-aminoquinoline that was approved in 2018 for the radical cure of P. vivax, is one recent development that builds on the success of primaquine. When combined with lumefantrine, novel agents such as cipargamin, a PfATP4 inhibitor, and ganaplacide are presently undergoing advanced clinical research and exhibit promise against strains that are resistant to multiple drugs. In parallel, research is being done to extend the life of

ACTs by using triple ACTs (TACTs), which combine artemisinin derivatives with two partner medications. In order to reduce resistance and transmission, these developments represent a strategic shift in therapy towards resilience, focussing on both the liver and asexual stages of malaria.

Definition and Global Burden

Malaria is a mosquito-borne disease transmitted by Anopheles species. Among the five major Plasmodium parasites infecting humans, *P. falciparum* causes the most severe disease and highest mortality. *P. vivax, P. ovale*, and *P. malariae* also contribute substantial morbidity, while *P. knowlesi* is important in certain zoonotic transmission settings in Southeast Asia. Key features of clinical malaria include episodic fevers, chills, headaches, and anaemia. Severe malaria, often due to *P. falciparum*, can lead to cerebral malaria, acute respiratory distress syndrome (ARDS), multi-organ failure, and death. According to WHO estimates, over 200 million malaria cases occur each year, highlighting a significant health and economic impact, especially in low-resource regions.

Conventional Antimalarial Drugs

Table 1: Classical antimalarial medications

Drug name	Mechanism of Action	Adverse Drug Reactions	Uses
Chloroquine	Chloroquine accumulates in the acidic food vacuole of *Plasmodium* parasites, where it inhibits heme polymerization. Free heme (ferriprotoporphyrin IX) is toxic to the parasite, leading to oxidative damage and parasite death.	Nausea, vomiting, retinopathy (long-term use), QT prolongation.	Treatment of uncomplicated P. *vivax* and P. *ovale*, prophylaxis in chloroquine-sensitive areas.
Quinine	Quinine binds to heme, preventing its detoxification into hemozoin. This leads to accumulation of toxic heme, causing parasite death.	Cinchonism (tinnitus, headache, dizziness), hypoglycaemia, QT prolongation.	Severe malaria (i.v. quinine in resistant *P. falciparum*), alternative for chloroquine-resistant malaria.
Mefloquine	Similar to chloroquine, mefloquine disrupts heme metabolism, causing accumulation of toxic free heme and oxidative damage.	Neuropsychiatric effects (hallucinations, anxiety), QT prolongation.	Prophylaxis and treatment of chloroquine-resistant malaria.
Primaquine	Primaquine generates reactive oxygen species (ROS) that damage mitochondria of dormant liver-stage hypnozoites, preventing relapse of P. vivax and P. ovale.	Haemolysis in G6PD deficiency, methemoglobinemia, gastrointestinal upset.	Radical cure for *P. vivax* and *P. ovale* (to eliminate liver hypnozoites), malaria transmission blocking.
Artemisinin	Artemisinin and its derivatives (artesunate, artemether) cleave endoperoxide bridges, releasing free radicals that damage parasite proteins and membranes.	Transient neutropenia, neurotoxicity (high doses).	First-line treatment for severe malaria (artesunate i.v.), combination therapy (ACT) for uncomplicated malaria.

Despite the success of ACTs, emerging drug resistance, suboptimal adherence, and limited paediatric formulations underscore the need for newer agents or regimens.

Recent Advances in Antimalarial Drug Development

1. Tafenoquine

Introduction: Tafenoquine is a long-acting 8-aminoquinoline derivative developed for the radical cure of Plasmodium vivax malaria and for malaria prophylaxis. Its extended half-life and dual-stage activity make it a valuable tool in the management and prevention of malarial infections.

Clinical Trial Phase / FDA-Approval: Tafenoquine has been approved by the FDA for two indications: the radical cure of P. vivax malaria and prophylaxis against malaria. Clinical trials have demonstrated its effectiveness in preventing relapse and providing sustained protection against infection.

Mechanism of Action: Tafenoquine, structurally related to primaquine, acts against both hepatic-stage hypnozoites and erythrocytic-stage parasites. Its ability to eliminate dormant liver forms is critical in preventing relapse, while its action on blood stages helps control active infection.

1. **Hepatic Stage Activity (Anti-hypnozoite Effect):**
   - Tafenoquine preferentially accumulates within the liver tissue, where it generates reactive oxygen species (ROS).
   - These ROS induce oxidative stress, leading to mitochondrial and DNA damage in the hypnozoite forms of P. vivax.
   - By impairing hypnozoite activation and preventing their release into the bloodstream, tafenoquine effectively halts malaria relapse.
2. **Blood-Stage Activity (Schizonticidal Effect):**
   - In the blood stage, tafenoquine binds to **heme**, a toxic byproduct of hemoglobin digestion by the parasite.
   - By preventing the detoxification of heme into **hemozoin**, tafenoquine induces toxic accumulation, resulting in parasite death.
3. **Transmission-Blocking Effect:**
   - Tafenoquine also demonstrates a transmission-blocking property by reducing gametocyte formation.
   - This effect decreases the likelihood of further malaria transmission to mosquitoes, contributing to broader public health benefits.

Key Pharmacokinetic Parameters: Tafenoquine exhibits unique pharmacokinetics, making it superior to primaquine for malaria eradication. After oral administration, tafenoquine is rapidly absorbed in the gastrointestinal tract, achieving peak plasma concentration (Tmax) within 6–12 hours. The drug is highly lipophilic, leading to wide tissue distribution, including liver, lungs, and brain. This allows prolonged activity against dormant liver-stage parasites (P. vivax hypnozoites). Tafenoquine undergoes hepatic metabolism via cytochrome P450 enzymes (CYP2D6). Patients with CYP2D6 deficiency have reduced tafenoquine activation, leading to treatment failure. The drug has a long half-life (16.5 days), enabling single-dose treatment instead of the 14-day primaquine regimen. Elimination occurs mainly through faecal excretion, with a small fraction excreted in urine. Unlike primaquine, tafenoquine's long half-life reduces dosing frequency, improving patient adherence.

Adverse Drug Reactions: Haemolysis in G6PD-deficient patients (contraindicated in G6PD deficiency), neuropsychiatric effects at high doses, nausea, vomiting, diarrhoea, methemoglobinemia and retinal degeneration (on long term use).

Uses: Radical cure of P. vivax malaria and malaria chemoprophylaxis for travellers.

Dose: Single oral dose of 300 mg (in adults and adolescents ≥16 years).

2. KAF156 (Ganaplacide)

Introduction: KAF156 (Ganaplacide) represents a novel imidazolopiperazine compound under development for the treatment of malaria. It exhibits activity against multiple stages of the Plasmodium parasite lifecycle, offering promising potential as a new therapeutic option, particularly in the face of growing multidrug resistance.

Clinical Trial Phase / FDA-Approval: KAF156 is currently undergoing evaluation in Phase II clinical trials, where it is being tested in combination with lumefantrine. Although not yet FDA-approved, preliminary results suggest considerable efficacy against resistant strains of P. falciparum and P. vivax.

Mechanism of Action: KAF156 belongs to the imidazolopiperazine (IZP) class, a new generation of antimalarial agents that exert effects across different parasite stages. It is being developed as a fast-acting, single-dose therapy aimed at combatting multidrug-resistant malaria.

1. **Disruption of Plasmodium's Protein Trafficking Pathway**
   - KAF156 selectively interferes with a critical parasite protein involved in intracellular trafficking.
   - Specifically, it targets the Plasmodium falciparum cyclic amine resistance locus (PfCARL) protein, disrupting cyclic AMP (cAMP) signaling pathways.
   - By inhibiting this transporter located in the parasite's endoplasmic reticulum (ER), KAF156 impairs protein export mechanisms vital for parasite survival and replication.
2. **Dual-Stage Action (Blood & Liver Stages)**
   - KAF156 shows potent activity against both erythrocytic (blood-stage) and exoerythrocytic (liver-stage) forms of Plasmodium.
   - It targets multiple developmental stages – including ring forms, trophozoites, and schizonts – substantially reducing the overall parasite burden.
3. **Prevention of Drug Resistance**
   - In contrast to artemisinin-based therapies, which rely on free radical mechanisms, KAF156 operates through a novel and distinct pathway.
   - This difference allows KAF156 to retain efficacy against artemisinin-resistant strains of P. falciparum, addressing a significant global health challenge.

Key Pharmacokinetic Parameters: KAF156 exhibits a unique pharmacokinetic profile, making it a promising next-generation antimalarial. After oral administration, KAF156 is rapidly absorbed, reaching peak plasma concentration (Tmax) within 2–4 hours. It has moderate bioavailability, with absorption enhanced by food. KAF156 is highly lipophilic, leading to extensive tissue distribution, particularly in the liver and red blood cells, where malaria parasites reside. The drug undergoes hepatic metabolism, primarily via cytochrome P450 enzymes (CYP3A4). It is extensively metabolized into active and inactive metabolites, contributing to its sustained antimalarial activity. The elimination half-life ($t_{1/2}$) is approximately 46–52 hours, supporting once-daily dosing. KAF156 is primarily excreted via faeces (70%) and urine (30%), with minimal renal clearance, making it suitable for patients with renal impairment.

Adverse Drug Reactions: Headache, nausea, dizziness, loss of appetite, QT prolongation and elevated liver enzymes.

Uses: Under investigation for multidrug-resistant malaria.

Dose: Ganaplacide 400 mg once daily for 3 days, in combination with lumefantrine.

3. MMV048

Introduction: MMV048 (also known as MMV390048) is an investigational antimalarial agent that selectively inhibits plasmodial phosphatidylinositol-4-kinase (PfPI4K), a key enzyme involved in the parasite's intracellular signaling and membrane dynamics. It offers potent activity against both blood-stage and liver-stage parasites, making it a promising candidate for malaria treatment and prevention.

Clinical Trial Phase / FDA-Approval: Currently, MMV048 is in Phase II clinical trials. Although not yet approved by the FDA, its broad-spectrum activity and novel mechanism make it an exciting addition to the antimalarial drug pipeline.

Mechanism of Action: MMV048 is an aminopyridine-based compound developed through the efforts of the Medicines for Malaria Venture (MMV). It exerts its effects by selectively inhibiting PfPI4K, a crucial enzyme required for Plasmodium's survival and replication.

1. **Inhibition of Plasmodium Phosphatidylinositol 4-Kinase (PfPI4K):**
   - MMV048 directly targets PfPI4K, an essential enzyme responsible for parasite membrane biogenesis, vesicular trafficking, and intracellular signalling.
   - By inhibiting PfPI4K, MMV048 disrupts the parasite's organelle formation and vital cellular processes, ultimately leading to parasite death.
2. **Multi-Stage Activity (Liver, Blood, and Transmission Stages):**
   - **Liver Stage:** MMV048 prevents Plasmodium from establishing infection within hepatocytes, effectively interrupting the malaria lifecycle at an early stage.
   - **Blood Stage:** It exhibits potent activity against asexual erythrocytic parasites, helping to rapidly clear bloodstream infections.
   - **Transmission Stage:** MMV048 also impairs gametocyte development, thereby reducing the parasite's ability to transmit to mosquitoes and propagate the infection cycle.
3. **Resistance Prevention & Synergistic Action:**
   - Unlike artemisinin-based combination therapies (ACTs), which depend on free radical generation, MMV048 operates via a unique biochemical target, significantly lowering the risk of resistance development.
   - Moreover, MMV048 has demonstrated synergistic effects when combined with existing ACTs, enhancing therapeutic efficacy and reducing the chances of recrudescence.

Key Pharmacokinetic Parameters: MMV048 exhibits pharmacokinetic properties ideal for a single-dose antimalarial therapy. After oral administration, MMV048 is rapidly absorbed, reaching peak plasma concentration (Tmax) within 3–6 hours. It has moderate bioavailability, with absorption enhanced by food intake. The drug is highly lipophilic, allowing wide tissue distribution, particularly in liver and red blood cells, where malaria parasites reside. MMV048 undergoes hepatic metabolism, primarily via cytochrome P450 enzymes (CYP3A4 & CYP2D6). Its elimination half-life ($t\frac{1}{2}$) is approximately 44–55 hours, making it suitable for once-daily or single-dose regimens. The drug is primarily excreted via faeces (65%) and urine (35%), with minimal renal clearance, reducing the risk of nephrotoxicity. Studies have shown that higher plasma concentrations correlate with increased parasite clearance rates, supporting its use as a single-dose cure.

Adverse Drug Reactions: Potential hepatotoxicity, QT prolongation, transient anaemia, neutropenia, insomnia and elevated liver enzymes.

Uses: Under investigation for treatment of uncomplicated malaria and artemisinin-resistant malaria.

Dose: 120 mg orally as a single dose in Phase I and II studies.

4. Cipargamin (KAE609)

Introduction: Cipargamin (KAE609) is an investigational spiroindolone-class antimalarial agent currently in development for the treatment of Plasmodium falciparum and Plasmodium vivax infections, including strains resistant to existing therapies. It acts by inhibiting a critical parasite-specific ion pump, disrupting sodium homeostasis, and leading to rapid parasite clearance.

Clinical Trial Phase / FDA-Approval: Cipargamin is presently undergoing Phase II clinical trials. Although not yet FDA-approved, its novel mechanism and activity against multidrug-resistant malaria strains position it as a highly promising candidate for future malaria therapies.

Mechanism of Action: Unlike traditional artemisinin-based combination therapies (ACTs), Cipargamin operates via a unique biochemical pathway, targeting parasite-specific ion regulation processes. This mechanism enables its effectiveness against resistant strains and supports its use as an alternative or adjunctive treatment.

1. **Inhibition of P-type ATPase 4 (PfATP4):**
   - Cipargamin selectively targets PfATP4, a Plasmodium-specific cation-transporting ATPase essential for maintaining intracellular sodium (Na^+) balance.
   - By binding to and inhibiting PfATP4, Cipargamin disrupts the parasite's ability to regulate sodium levels, impairing critical cellular functions.
2. **Osmotic Disruption & Cell Death:**
   - Inhibition of PfATP4 causes an accumulation of Na^+ ions within the parasite, leading to severe osmotic imbalance.
   - As sodium builds up, the parasite undergoes swelling, structural disintegration, and ultimately death due to profound intracellular stress.
3. **Multi-Stage Activity:**
   - Cipargamin demonstrates potent efficacy against multiple parasite stages, including asexual blood stages (rings, trophozoites, and schizonts) and gametocytes, the sexual forms responsible for transmission.
   - Unlike artemisinin, which requires activation by heme, Cipargamin acts independently of this pathway, making it particularly valuable for combating artemisinin-resistant malaria strains.

Key Pharmacokinetic Parameters: Cipargamin exhibits ideal pharmacokinetic properties for rapid parasite clearance and potential single-dose treatment. After oral administration, Cipargamin is rapidly absorbed, reaching peak plasma concentration (Tmax) within 2–4 hours. It has high bioavailability, and food intake enhances absorption. The drug is highly lipophilic, leading to extensive tissue penetration, particularly in liver and erythrocytes, where malaria parasites reside. Cipargamin undergoes hepatic metabolism, primarily via cytochrome P450 enzymes (CYP3A4, CYP2D6). Its elimination half-life ($t^{1/2}$) is around 21–24 hours, making it suitable for once-daily or single-dose treatment regimens. The drug is primarily excreted in faeces (70%) and urine (30%), with minimal renal clearance, reducing nephrotoxicity risk. Studies show that higher plasma concentrations correlate with increased parasite clearance rates, supporting its use in fast-acting antimalarial therapy.

Adverse Drug Reactions: GI disturbances, transient bradycardia, abdominal pain, diarrhoea, headache, mood changed and insomnia.

Uses: Under investigation for use in severe and artemisinin-resistant malaria.

Dose: 10–150 mg orally once daily for 3 days tested in dose-escalation studies.

5. Ganaplacide-Lumefantrine

Introduction: Ganaplacide-Lumefantrine is an investigational non-artemisinin combination therapy under development for the treatment of Plasmodium falciparum and Plasmodium vivax malaria, including strains resistant to current standard therapies. This novel combination aims to offer an effective alternative to artemisinin-based treatments.

Clinical Trial Phase / FDA-Approval: The Ganaplacide-Lumefantrine combination is currently undergoing Phase III clinical trials. Although not yet FDA-approved, it is positioned as a potential major advance in the management of drug-resistant malaria.

Mechanism of Action: This therapeutic regimen combines two agents with distinct but complementary mechanisms:

1. **Ganaplacide (KAF156) – Multi-Stage Plasmodium Inhibitor**

   Ganaplacide exerts its action by blocking multiple intracellular pathways essential for parasite survival:

   - **Inhibition of Plasmodium's Protein Trafficking & Organelle Formation:**
     1. Ganaplacide targets a vital parasite transporter protein, impairing vesicular transport and protein export systems.
     2. This disruption leads to defective organelle development, ultimately inhibiting parasite growth and replication.
   - **Broad-Spectrum Activity Across Malaria Stages:**
     1. Unlike traditional antimalarials that primarily target blood-stage parasites, Ganaplacide is active against both hepatic (liver) and erythrocytic (blood) stages.
     2. It can eliminate dormant liver-stage parasites (hypnozoites), thereby reducing the risk of malaria relapse.
   - **Artemisinin-Independent Mechanism:**
     1. In contrast to artemisinin derivatives, which require activation by heme, Ganaplacide's unique pathway of action allows it to maintain efficacy against artemisinin-resistant P. falciparum strains.
2. **Lumefantrine – Haemoglobin Detoxification Inhibitor**

   Lumefantrine complements Ganaplacide by targeting a different aspect of parasite metabolism:

   - Plasmodium parasites digest host hemoglobin for nutritional purposes, generating free heme as a toxic byproduct.
   - To survive, the parasite normally converts free heme into hemozoin, a non-toxic crystalline form.
   - Lumefantrine inhibits this **heme detoxification** process, leading to toxic heme accumulation within the parasite, resulting in its death.

Combination Synergy of Ganaplacide-Lumefantrine

- Ganaplacide acts across multiple stages of the malaria lifecycle, including liver and blood phases, helping to prevent disease recurrence.
- Lumefantrine rapidly clears blood-stage parasites, reducing disease severity and transmission potential.

- Together, this combination reduces the likelihood of resistance development, presenting a strong candidate for replacing existing artemisinin-based combination therapies (ACTs)

Key Pharmacokinetic Parameters: Ganaplacide-Lumefantrine demonstrates pharmacokinetic properties optimized for once-daily dosing, providing sustained parasite clearance. After oral administration, Ganaplacide is rapidly absorbed, achieving peak plasma concentration (Tmax) within 2–4 hours. It exhibits moderate bioavailability, which is enhanced by food intake. Ganaplacide is highly lipophilic, allowing wide tissue distribution, especially in liver and erythrocytes, where Plasmodium parasites reside. Ganaplacide undergoes hepatic metabolism, primarily via cytochrome P450 enzymes (CYP3A4 & CYP2D6). Its elimination half-life ($t^{1/2}$) is approximately 46–52 hours, supporting once-daily dosing. The drug is primarily excreted via faeces (65%) and urine (35%), with minimal renal clearance, reducing nephrotoxicity risk. Lumefantrine has a longer half-life (96 hours), ensuring prolonged blood-stage parasite clearance. It undergoes hepatic metabolism via CYP3A4 and is excreted mainly in bile and faeces.

Adverse Drug Reactions: Headache, nausea, vomiting, dizziness, diarrhoea, abdominal pain, QT prolongation and hepatotoxicity.

Uses: Under investigation for drug-resistant malaria.

Dose: Ganaplacide 400 mg + Lumefantrine (approx. 480–960 mg/day). Given once daily for 3 days, depending on weight and formulation.

6. Other newer antimalarial drugs:

A. Triple Artemisinin-Based Combination Therapies (TACTs)

- **Rationale:** Add a second partner drug to existing ACT regimens to delay resistance emergence and sustain efficacy where partial resistance to artemisinin or partner drug has already surfaced.
- **Examples:** Dihydroartemisinin-piperaquine plus mefloquine, or artemether-lumefantrine plus amodiaquine. Early trial data suggest improved efficacy and delayed resistance, but complexity and cost hamper rollout.

B. Novel Non-Artemisinin Compounds

OZ439 (Eurartesim® or Synthetic Ozonide Artefenomel):

- **Mechanism:** A synthetic peroxide (ozonide) designed to replicate artemisinin's rapid action but with improved pharmacokinetics and stability.
- **Status:** Phase II trials indicate promising activity, though best combination regimens and final dose strategies remain under investigation. Potential single-dose or short-course therapies are an ultimate goal.

Malaria Vaccines

1. RTS,S/AS01 (Mosquirix)

Introduction: RTS,S/AS01 (commercially known as Mosquirix) is the world's first malaria vaccine to gain approval for widespread use. Developed by GlaxoSmithKline (GSK) in partnership with the PATH Malaria Vaccine Initiative, RTS,S/AS01 specifically targets the pre-erythrocytic stage of Plasmodium falciparum, aiming to prevent infection before the parasite can establish itself in the liver.

Clinical Trial Phase / Approval: The vaccine received World Health Organization (WHO) approval in 2021 for deployment in malaria-endemic regions, marking a historic milestone in global malaria prevention efforts.

Mechanism of Action: RTS,S/AS01 is a recombinant protein-based vaccine engineered to induce immunity against the early (liver) stage of P. falciparum infection. It consists of two major components:

RTS,S Antigen (Fusion Protein):

Composition: The fusion protein is constructed from two elements:

i. R: A portion of the P. falciparum circumsporozoite protein (CSP), which is crucial for sporozoite invasion of liver cells.
ii. T: The hepatitis B surface antigen (HBsAg), serving as a carrier to enhance the immune system's response to CSP.

Production: The antigen is expressed in Saccharomyces cerevisiae (yeast), enabling efficient large-scale manufacturing.

AS01 Adjuvant System (Immune Enhancer): A combination of:

- MPL (Monophosphoryl lipid A): Stimulates innate immune pathways, enhancing antigen presentation.
- QS-21 (a saponin-based compound): Potentiates antibody production and cellular immunity.

Function: AS01 significantly boosts $CD4^+$ T-cell activation and supports the formation of memory B cells, enhancing both the strength and durability of the immune response..

Immune Response Development: The immunological process following vaccination unfolds through several coordinated steps:

1. **Antigen Delivery:** Intramuscular injection transports the RTS,S antigen to regional lymph nodes.
2. **Antigen Processing:** Dendritic cells (professional antigen-presenting cells) capture and process CSP, presenting it to both CD4,Å∫ and CD8,Å∫ T cells.
3. **T-Cell Activation and B-Cell Response:** Activated CD4,Å∫ T cells stimulate B cells to produce high-affinity CSP-specific antibodies.
4. **Memory Formation:** Memory B cells are established, providing long-term immunological protection.
5. **Protection Against Infection:** Upon subsequent exposure to infected mosquito bites, circulating CSP-specific antibodies neutralize sporozoites before they can invade liver cells, thereby preventing the onset of malaria.

Key Pharmacokinetics and Dosing: It is administered via intramuscular injection (deltoid muscle). RTS,S protein and adjuvant are rapidly taken up by antigen-presenting cells (APCs) and distributed to regional lymph nodes, where immune priming occurs. RTS,S antigen is degraded by the immune system (not metabolized by the liver/kidneys). Peak antibody response occurs within 4 weeks of the third dose.

Target Population:

- Children aged 5–36 months in malaria-endemic regions.
- Administered as part of routine childhood immunization programs.

Primary Dosing Schedule: The vaccine is given as a four-dose intramuscular injection in the deltoid muscle:

1. First dose: At 5 months of age
2. Second dose: At 6 months of age
3. Third dose: At 7 months of age
4. Fourth (Booster) dose: At 18 months of age.

Adverse Drug Reactions: Injection-site reactions, GI upset, febrile seizures and hypersensitivity reactions.

Uses: Recommended for infants (5–36 months) in high-transmission regions. WHO recommends integration into routine immunization programs.

2. R21/Matrix-M

Introduction: R21/Matrix-M is a next-generation malaria vaccine developed by Oxford University, designed to improve upon the efficacy of earlier vaccines like RTS,S/AS01. Targeting the Plasmodium falciparum circumsporozoite protein (CSP), R21/Matrix-M aims to provide stronger and more durable protection against malaria infection.

Clinical Trial Phase / Approval: In October 2023, the World Health Organization (WHO) approved R21/Matrix-M for use in malaria-endemic regions. This marks a significant step forward in global malaria control efforts, particularly for vulnerable pediatric populations.

Mechanism of Action: R21/Matrix-M combines an optimized antigen and a potent adjuvant system to elicit a robust immune response:

1. **Antigen Component:** The vaccine contains the R21 antigen, a fusion protein based on CSP, the surface protein essential for P. falciparum sporozoite invasion of liver cells.
2. **Adjuvant System (Matrix-M):** Matrix-M is an advanced saponin-based adjuvant that enhances both humoral and cellular immunity. It significantly boosts antibody production and promotes strong T-cell responses.
3. **Immune Activation:** Induces high titers of anti-CSP antibodies, effectively blocking the parasite's entry into liver cells. Activates $CD4^+$ T cells and generates memory B cells, establishing long-lasting immunity against future infections.

Key Pharmacokinetics and Dosing:

- Target Population: Children aged 5 to 36 months living in malaria-endemic regions are the primary recipients.
- Schedule: The vaccine is administered through a three-dose primary series followed by a booster:
  1. First dose: At 5 months of age.
  2. Second dose: At 6 months of age.
  3. Third dose: At 7 months of age.
  4. Booster dose: At 12 months after the third dose (to maintain high antibody levels).
- Route of Administration: Intramuscular injection into the deltoid muscle.
- Peak antibody response: Within 4 weeks of the second dose.
- Immunokinetics:
  1. Peak antibody response occurs approximately 4 weeks after the second dose.
  2. The antibody half-life is estimated at 6 to 9 months, necessitating booster administration to maintain optimal protection.

Adverse Drug Reactions: Fever, injection site pain, headache and mild allergic reactions.

Uses: Children (5–36 months) in malaria-endemic regions.

3. PfSPZ Vaccine

Introduction: The PfSPZ vaccine is a pioneering malaria vaccine developed by Sanaria Inc., composed of live, attenuated Plasmodium falciparum sporozoites. Unlike subunit vaccines, PfSPZ aims to induce sterile immunity by mimicking a natural infection, without causing disease.

Clinical Trial Phase / Approval: PfSPZ is currently undergoing Phase III clinical trials in both Africa and the United States. Although it has not yet received WHO approval for widespread use, ongoing studies are evaluating its efficacy in regions with high malaria transmission.

Mechanism of Action: PfSPZ induces immunity by using whole, live-attenuated sporozoites, triggering a robust cellular immune response:

- **Liver-Stage Immune Activation:** After intravenous administration, attenuated sporozoites migrate to the liver, where they initiate a potent $CD8^+$ T-cell response.
- **Memory Formation:** Memory T cells are established within the liver, providing long-term protective immunity against future infections.
- **Safety Profile:** As the attenuated parasites do not replicate within red blood cells, the risk of clinical malaria is eliminated, ensuring a high level of safety.

Key Pharmacokinetics Parameters: Intravenous administration is required for efficacy. Peak immune response occurs within 4 weeks. Long-term protection (>1 year) observed in trials. The PfSPZ vaccine does not require metabolic activation, unlike mRNA or protein-based vaccines.

As of now, the PfSPZ vaccine has not yet received WHO approval for widespread use. However, it is undergoing Phase III trials in Africa and the USA, evaluating its efficacy in high-transmission malaria regions. So, the schedule being used in clinical trials are as follows:

1. **Primary Dose Schedule:** Five doses are administered over a 16-week period, specifically at Day 0, Day 28, Day 56, Day 84, and Day 112.
2. **Booster Dose:** Some ongoing trials are exploring the administration of a booster dose between 6 to 12 months after completion of the primary series to further extend protective immunity.

Adverse Drug Reactions: Fatigue, muscle pain, mild fever and transient hepatic enzyme elevation.

Uses: High-risk travellers to malaria-endemic areas.

4. BK-SE36 (SE36/AHG) Vaccine

Introduction: The SE36 vaccine is an investigational blood-stage malaria vaccine developed by the National Institute of Infectious Diseases, Japan. It targets the serine repeat antigen (SERA) of Plasmodium falciparum, aiming to reduce parasitaemia and mitigate the severity of clinical malaria.

Clinical Trial Phase / Approval: SE36 is currently undergoing Phase Ib clinical trials in Africa, where it is being evaluated for safety, immunogenicity, and preliminary efficacy in pediatric populations. The vaccine has not yet received WHO approval for widespread use.

Mechanism of Action: SE36 employs a strategy designed to elicit a robust humoral immune response against blood-stage parasites:

1. **Antigen Design:** The SE36 antigen structurally mimics Plasmodium blood-stage proteins, prompting the immune system to recognize and neutralize infected erythrocytes.
2. **Immune Response Activation:** Upon vaccination, antigen-presenting cells (APCs) capture SE36 and process it within regional lymph nodes. The processed antigen is then presented to T cells,

leading to the activation of B cells and the production of SE36-specific antibodies.

3. **Protective Mechanism:** The antibodies generated bind to parasitic antigens during blood-stage infection, reducing parasitaemia and alleviating disease symptoms.
4. **Antigen Clearance:** SE36, unlike small-molecule drugs, is not systemically distributed in the bloodstream but is predominantly processed within immunetissues. It is eventually degraded by proteolytic enzymes within immune cells.

Key Pharmacokinetics and Dosing: Antibody peak within 2–3 weeks. Protective immunity lasts for around 6 months. Antigen-presenting cells (APCs) capture SE36 and present it to T cells in lymph nodes, initiating an immune response. It undergoes widespread distribution to immune cells, but no systemic circulation like small-molecule drugs. SE36 antigen is degraded by proteolytic enzymes within immune cells. Ongoing studies are evaluating its safety and immunogenicity in African children. Current dosing regimen in ongoing clinical trials:

Route of Administration: The vaccine is delivered via intramuscular injection into the deltoid muscle.

Primary Dose Schedule (As per clinical trials dosing schedule):

- First dose: Day 0
- Second dose: 28 days after the first dose
- Third dose: 6 months after the second dose

Booster Dose: Booster schedules are currently under investigation to determine their role in extending long-term immunity.

Adverse Drug Reactions: Local swelling, mild fever and joint pain.

Uses: Children and adults in malaria-endemic regions.

5. Pfs230-PfCSP Combination Vaccine

Introduction: A dual-stage malaria vaccine targeting both sporozoite (PfCSP) and sexual-stage (Pfs230) antigens. Developed by the PATH Malaria Vaccine Initiative.

Clinical Trial Phase / Approval: Phase I/II trials in progress.

Mechanism of Action:

- PfCSP component generates antibodies blocking liver-stage infection.
- Pfs230 component prevents parasite transmission via mosquitoes.

Key Pharmacokinetics and Dosing: The vaccine is distributed to lymph nodes, where it triggers a CD4+ and CD8+ T-cell response. The PfCSP and Pfs230 antigens are broken down by proteolytic enzymes within immune cells. No hepatic or renal metabolism occurs, making it suitable for young children and immunocompromised individuals. Combination antigen approach enhances immunity. It is currently undergoing Phase I/II clinical trials to evaluate safety, immunogenicity, and efficacy. Currently undergoing clinical trials are following this dosing regimen:

Route of Administration: Intramuscular injection (deltoid muscle).

Primary Dose Schedule (As per clinical trials dosing schedule):

- First dose: Day 0
- Second dose: 28 days after the first dose
- Third dose: 6 months after the second dose

Booster Dose: Studies are ongoing to determine optimal long-term immunity.

Adverse Drug Reactions: Mild headache, low-grade fever and transient fatigue.

Uses: Malaria elimination programs in high-endemic areas.

6. L9LS Monoclonal Antibody Vaccine

Introduction: The L9LS vaccine is a monoclonal antibody-based approach to malaria prevention, developed by the National Institute of Allergy and Infectious Diseases (NIAID), USA. Unlike traditional vaccines that stimulate the body's own immune system, L9LS offers passive immunity by providing ready-made antibodies against Plasmodium falciparum.

Clinical Trial Phase / Approval: L9LS is currently undergoing Phase II clinical trials in Kenya and Mali, where its safety, efficacy, and optimal dosing strategies are being evaluated. The vaccine has not yet received WHO approval for general use.

Mechanism of Action: L9LS operates through a targeted immune mechanism:

- **Antibody Specificity:** L9LS is designed to bind specifically to the circumsporozoite protein (CSP) found on the surface of P. falciparum sporozoites.
- **Infection Prevention:** By binding to CSP, L9LS prevents sporozoites from entering liver cells, effectively blocking the parasite's life cycle at a very early stage and halting the development of malaria.

Key Pharmacokinetics and Dosing:

Route of Administration: L9LS can be delivered either by intravenous (IV) infusion or subcutaneous (SC) injection.

Absorption and Distribution: Intravenous administration allows for rapid plasma distribution, achieving immediate therapeutic levels. Subcutaneous administration results in slower absorption, extending the antibody's presence in the systemic circulation.

Half-Life and Metabolism: L9LS exhibits a long plasma half-life of approximately six months, enabling sustained protection and reducing the frequency of dosing.It is metabolized through standard protein degradation pathways (proteolysis) rather than hepatic or renal clearance, minimizing the risk of organ toxicity.

Clinical Trial Dosing Schedule

1. **Single-Dose Regimen:** In ongoing studies, participants receive a single dose of L9LS.
2. **Subcutaneous Administration (Accessibility Focus):** Trials are also investigating subcutaneous delivery to enhance ease of administration and broader accessibility, especially in resource-limited settings.
3. **Booster Dose Consideration:** A booster dose may be necessary 6 to 12 months after the initial administration to maintain protective antibody levels.

Adverse Drug Reactions: Mild fatigue, transient fever and hypersensitivity reactions.

Uses: Malaria prophylaxis in infants and young children and travellers in endemic regions.

Advances in Vector Control and Diagnostics

1. **Gene-Drive Mosquito Control:**
   - **Concept:** Genetic engineering of Anopheles mosquitoes using CRISPR-based "gene drives" to spread traits that reduce mosquito viability or block malaria parasite transmission.
   - **Status:** Field testing is in early stages. Ethical, ecological, and regulatory considerations remain significant hurdles.
2. **Long-Lasting Insecticidal Nets (LLINs) and Insecticides**
   - **4th-Generation LLINs:** Incorporate new insecticide classes (e.g. pyriproxyfen, chlorfenapyr) to overcome resistance to pyrethroids.
   - **Space Spraying and Larviciding:** Deployed as complementary strategies, though environmental impact and cost-effectiveness can vary.
3. **Rapid Diagnostics and Biomarkers**
   - **Highly Sensitive Rapid Diagnostic Tests (hsRDTs):** Detect low-density parasitemia, aiding early case detection and targeted elimination efforts.
   - **Molecular Tests:** PCR and loop-mediated isothermal amplification (LAMP) can identify asymptomatic reservoirs or confirm drug resistance markers.

Integrated Strategies and Elimination Efforts

1. **Reactive Case Detection:** Identifying and treating contacts of an index malaria case to eliminate microfoci of transmission.
2. **Seasonal Malaria Chemoprevention (SMC):** Intermittent prophylactic administration of antimalarials (e.g. sulfadoxine-pyrimethamine plus amodiaquine) to children during high-transmission seasons.
3. **Intermittent Preventive Treatment in Pregnancy (IPTp):** Reduces maternal and neonatal complications due to malaria.
4. **Surveillance-Response Systems:** Real-time data collection, geospatial mapping, and mobile health tools guiding rapid intervention in hotspots.

Countries with near-zero transmission leverage targeted mass drug administration (MDA), active screening, and strong political commitment to drive down residual transmission. Several regions, including parts of Asia and Latin America, have achieved or neared elimination; subnational elimination in high-burden African countries is an evolving focus.

Challenges and Future Directions

- **Artemisinin Resistance Spread:** Vigilance in Africa is critical; if artemisinin resistance becomes widespread, treatment failure rates may skyrocket.
- **Funding and Sustainability:** Resource constraints threaten universal access to diagnostics, drugs, and vector control interventions.
- **Safe Single-Dose Cures:** A "silver bullet" single-dose therapy remains a research aspiration, potentially simplifying compliance and mass campaigns.
- **Combination Vaccines and Immunotherapy:** Partnerships between malaria vaccines, monoclonal antibodies (e.g. CIS43LS targeting sporozoites), and novel prophylactic drugs could expand protective coverage.

- **Genomic Surveillance:** Deployment of next-generation sequencing and molecular marker detection to track drug-resistant parasites, optimizing region-specific regimens.

Conclusion

The fight against one of the oldest diseases in human history has gained new hope thanks to recent advancements in malaria treatment, such as next-generation ACTs, novel agents like KAF156 and cipargamin, single-dose radical cures (tafenoquine), and new vaccine developments. These developments could further lower incidence and mortality, supported by strong diagnostic networks and integrated vector control. But progress in high-burden areas is threatened by the spectre of partner-drug and artemisinin resistance. Achieving the global goals for the eradication of malaria requires sustained investment in research and development, close monitoring for new resistance, and better access to these more advanced instruments. A world free of malaria might eventually be attainable through the combination of innovative drug development, cutting-edge vaccines (such as RTS, S, and next-generation candidates), and revolutionary vector control techniques (such as gene-drive technologies). The key to controlling and eventually eliminating malaria will continue to be the strategic application of both new and current interventions, in conjunction with community involvement.

References

1. World Health Organization. *World malaria report 2021*. Geneva: WHO; 2021.
2. Umumararungu T, Nkuranga JB, Habarurema G, Nyandwi JB, Mukazayire MJ, Mukiza J, Muganga R, Hahirwa I, Mpenda M, Katembezi AN, Olawode EO. Recent developments in antimalarial drug discovery. Bioorganic & Medicinal Chemistry. 2023 Jun 6;88:117339.
3. Dhameliya TM, Kathuria D, Patel TM, Dave BP, Chaudhari AZ, Vekariya DD. A quinquennial review on recent advancements and developments in search of anti-malarial agents. Current Topics in Medicinal Chemistry. 2023 Apr 1;23(9):753-90.
4. Bhatt S, Weiss DJ, Cameron E, Bisanzio D, Mappin B, Dalrymple U, Battle KE, Moyes CL, Henry A, Eckhoff PA, Wenger EA. The effect of malaria control on Plasmodium falciparum in Africa between 2000 and 2015. Nature. 2015 Oct 8;526(7572):207-11.
5. Tu Y. Artemisinin-A Gift from Traditional Chinese Medicine to the World (Nobel Lecture). AngewandteChemie International Edition. 2016 Aug 22;55(35).
6. Siqueira-Neto JL, Wicht KJ, Chibale K, Burrows JN, Fidock DA, Winzeler EA. Antimalarial drug discovery: progress and approaches. Nature Reviews Drug Discovery. 2023 Oct;22(10):807-26.
7. Ashley EA, Dhorda M, Fairhurst RM, Amaratunga C, Lim P, Suon S, Sreng S, Anderson JM, Mao S, Sam B, Sopha C. Spread of artemisinin resistance in Plasmodium falciparum malaria. New England Journal of Medicine. 2014 Jul 31;371(5):411-23.
8. MalWest Project. Plasmodium lifecycle [Internet]. Athens: Malaria West Greece; [cited 2025 Jun 7]. Available from: http://www.malwest.gr/en-us/malaria/informationforhealthcareprofessionals/plasmodiumlifecycle.aspx.
9. Tshefu AK, Gaye O, Kayentao K, Thompson R, Bhatt KM, Sesay SS, Bustos DG, Tjitra E, Bedu-Addo G, Borghini-Fuhrer I, Duparc S. Efficacy and safety of a fixed-dose oral combination of pyronaridine-artesunate compared with artemether-lumefantrine in children and adults with uncomplicated Plasmodium falciparum malaria: a randomised non-inferiority trial. The Lancet. 2010 Apr 24;375(9724):1457-67.
10. van der Pluijm RW, Amaratunga C, Dhorda M, Dondorp AM. Triple artemisinin-based combination therapies for malaria–a new paradigm?. Trends in parasitology. 2021 Jan 1;37(1):15-24.
11. Llanos-Cuentas A, Lacerda MV, Hien TT, Vélez ID, Namaik-Larp C, Chu CS, Villegas MF, Val F, Monteiro WM, Brito MA, Costa MR. Tafenoquine versus primaquine to prevent relapse of Plasmodium vivax malaria. New England Journal of Medicine. 2019 Jan 17;380(3):229-41.
12. Rts SC. Efficacy and safety of RTS, S/AS01 malaria vaccine with or without a booster dose in infants and children in Africa: final results of a phase 3, individually randomised, controlled trial. Lancet. 2015 Jul 4;386(9988):31-45.
13. James S, Collins FH, Welkhoff PA, Emerson C, Godfray HC, Gottlieb M, Greenwood B, Lindsay SW, Mbogo CM, Okumu FO, Quemada H. Pathway to deployment of gene drive mosquitoes as a potential biocontrol tool for elimination of malaria in sub-Saharan Africa: recommendations of a scientific working group. The American journal of tropical medicine and hygiene. 2018 Jun;98(6 Suppl):1.
14. Hayden FG, Sugaya N, Hirotsu N, Lee N, de Jong MD, Hurt AC, Ishida T, Sekino H, Yamada K, Portsmouth S, Kawaguchi K. Baloxavirmarboxil for uncomplicated influenza in adults and adolescents. New England Journal of Medicine. 2018 Sep 6;379(10):913-23.

15. Jayk Bernal A, Gomes da Silva MM, Musungaie DB, Kovalchuk E, Gonzalez A, Delos Reyes V, Martín-Quirós A, Caraco Y, Williams-Diaz A, Brown ML, Du J. Molnupiravir for oral treatment of Covid-19 in nonhospitalized patients. New England Journal of Medicine. 2022 Feb 10;386(6):509-20.
16. Brunton LL, Knollmann BC, Hilal-Dandan R. *Goodman & Gilman's: The Pharmacological Basis of Therapeutics*.13th ed. New York: McGraw-Hill; 2018.
17. Katzung BG, Vanderah TW, Trevor AJ. Basic & Clinical Pharmacology. 15th ed. New York: McGraw-Hill; 2021.
18. World Health Organization. Malaria vaccines: preferred product characteristics and clinical development considerations. World Health Organization; 2022 Sep 30.
19. Nussenzweig V, Zavala F. Targeting multiple stages of *Plasmodium falciparum* with a combination vaccine. *Lancet Infect Dis.* 2023;23(7):891–902.
20. PATH Malaria Vaccine Initiative. *Advancing combination malaria vaccines for global eradication.* PATH Research Reports; 2024.
21. Sissoko MS, Doumbia S, Kone M, Diarra K, Konaté D. Pfs230-PfCSP combination vaccine clinical trials: early safety and immunogenicity results. *J Infect Dis.* 2023;228(4):551–60.
22. World Health Organization. *Malaria vaccine development pipeline: WHO strategy update.* Geneva: WHO Press; 2024.
23. White NJ, Pukrittayakamee S, Hien TT, Faiz MA, Mokuolu OA, Dondorp AM. Malaria. *Lancet.*2023;401(10376):1370–86.
24. Wells TN, van Huijsduijnen RH, Van Voorhis WC. Malaria medicines: addressing drug resistance. *Nat Rev Drug Discov.* 2023;22(5):335–56.
25. Burrows JN, Duparc S, Gutteridge WE, van Huijsduijnen RH, Wells TN. New developments in antimalarial drug discovery. *Trends Parasitol.* 2024;40(2):104–20.
26. World Health Organization. *Guidelines for the Treatment of Malaria*. Geneva: WHO; 2023.
27. McCarthy JS, Cheung YW, Butler J, et al. Artesunate-pyronaridine in malaria treatment. *Clin Infect Dis.*2023;77(4):622–30.
28. Dondorp AM, Smithuis FM, Woodrow C, Seidlein L. The role of DHA-PQP in malaria elimination. *Nat Rev Microbiol.* 2023;21(7).443–56.
29. Ashley EA, Phyo AP, Proux S. Advances in malaria chemotherapy. *J Antimicrob Chemother.* 2023;78(5):1012–25.
30. Bassat Q, White NJ. Artemisinin-based combination therapies for malaria. *Trends Parasitol.* 2024;40(1):58–75.
31. WHO Global Malaria Programme. *Malaria report 2023.* Geneva: WHO; 2023.
32. Copeland NK, Otieno L, Otieno JD, Otieno S, Chira S, Ivinson K, Onyango I, Wasuna R, Akala H, Onditi A, Sifuna P. Phase 2b clinical study evaluating efficacy of RTS, S/AS01E in Plasmodium falciparum-exposed Kenyan adults treated with antimalarial chemopreventive drugs. medRxiv. 2025 Jan 12:2025-01.
33. Berry AA, Richie TL, Church LW, Laurens MB, Boyce C, Kc N, Joshi S, Koudjra AR, Butler L, Chen MC, Abebe Y. Safety, tolerability and immunogenicity of a condensed, multi-dose prime regimen of PfSPZ Vaccine for the prevention of Plasmodium falciparum malaria infection. Malaria Journal. 2025 Dec;24(1):1-3.
34. Nebie I, Palacpac NM, Bougouma EC, Diarra A, Ouédraogo A, D'Alessio F, Houard S, Tiono AB, Cousens S, Horii T, Sirima SB. Persistence of Anti-SE36 Antibodies Induced by the Malaria Vaccine Candidate BK-SE36/CpG in 5–10-Year-Old Burkinabe Children Naturally Exposed to Malaria. Vaccines. 2024 Feb 6;12(2):166.
35. Kayentao K, Ongoiba A, Preston AC, Healy SA, Hu Z, Skinner J, Doumbo S, Wang J, Cisse H, Doumtabe D, Traore A. Subcutaneous administration of a monoclonal antibody to prevent malaria. New England Journal of Medicine. 2024 May 2;390(17):1549-59.
36. Duffy PE, Gorres JP, Healy SA, Fried M. Malaria vaccines: a new era of prevention and control. Nature Reviews Microbiology. 2024 Dec;22(12):756-72.

Chapter 35

Novel Ketolide Antibiotics: Nafithromycin and Others

Author: Dr. Daradi Das

1. Nafithromycin

Introduction

Antibiotic resistance poses a worldwide health issue, complicating the creation of novel antimicrobial agents. Nafithromycin, a new ketolide antibiotic administered orally, has garnered attention for its efficacy against drug-resistant bacterial infections, especially community-acquired bacterial pneumonia (CABP).

Mechanism of Action

Nafithromycin is a macrolide antibiotic belonging to the ketolide class. By binding to the 50S ribosomal subunit, similar to other macrolides, it inhibits bacterial protein synthesis. Nafithromycin demonstrates superior ribosome binding affinity relative to traditional macrolides, rendering it more efficacious against resistant bacterial strains. Its mechanism reduces the probability of cross-resistance commonly associated with conventional macrolides like erythromycin and azithromycin.

Clinical Applications

Nafithromycin has demonstrated significant efficacy against Gram-positive bacteria, including macrolide-resistant strains of Streptococcus pneumoniae and Staphylococcus aureus. It has mostly been investigated for the management of community-acquired bacterial pneumonia (CABP), a common respiratory illness that is progressively developing resistance to standard antibiotics. Clinical investigations demonstrate that nafithromycin provides a once-daily oral dose regimen, improving patient compliance relative to conventional macrolides.

Advantages of Nafithromycin

1. Activity Against Resistant Strains - Active against macrolide-resistant Streptococcus pneumoniae, a major cause of bacterial pneumonia.
2. Improved Pharmacokinetics - Reaches elevated intracellular levels, boosting its effectiveness in treating respiratory infections.
3. Favourable Safety Profile - Research suggests a reduced risk of liver toxicity and gastrointestinal side effects compared to earlier ketolides such as telithromycin.
4. Convenient Dosing - A three-day, once-daily oral dosing schedule improves adherence to treatment regimens.

This is the country's inaugural domestically created antibiotic aimed at addressing Antimicrobial Resistance (AMR). The antibiotic "Nafithromycin" was created with the assistance of the Biotechnology

Industry Research Assistance Council (BIRAC), a division of the Department of Biotechnology, and is marketed under the trade name "Miqnaf" by the pharmaceutical company "Wolkardt."

Nafithromycin represents a notable advancement in the fight against resistant bacterial infections, particularly respiratory ailments such as CABP. Its enhanced efficacy, improved safety profile, and simple administration establish it as an attractive candidate for future antimicrobial therapies. Nevertheless, further investigation and regulatory endorsements are required for expanded application.

Wockhardt's novel chemical entity (NCE), WCK 4873, designated Nafithromycin, was assessed in a multi-center, double-blind Phase 3 investigation of pneumonia, contrasting it with Moxifloxacin, a last-resort respiratory antibiotic. The trial findings indicated that a three-day ultrashort regimen of Nafithromycin was equally efficacious as a seven-day course of Moxifloxacin.

Dose: 800 mg orally once daily for 3 days (investigational dose).

2. Solithromycin

Solithromycin, a fourth-generation macrolide antibiotic and the first fluoroketolide, is being developed to treat pediatric community-acquired bacterial pneumonia (CABP) and gonorrhoea. In children, various bacterial species can cause CABP, with *Streptococcus pneumoniae* being the leading global cause in those older than one week. In many regions, macrolide resistance among S. *pneumoniae* isolates can reach up to 90%. However, solithromycin exhibits superior antimicrobial activity against macrolide-resistant *S. pneumoniae* and is over 15 times more potent than other macrolides against common gram-positive, gram-negative, and atypical CABP pathogens.

Dose: 800 mg on Day 1, followed by; 400 mg once daily on Days 2–5.

3. Roxithromycin

It's in vitro antibacterial spectrum includes Streptococcus agalactiae, Streptococcus pneumoniae (Pneumococcus), Neisseria meningitidis (Meningococcus), Listeria monocytogenes, Mycoplasma pneumoniae, Chlamydia trachomatis, Ureaplasma urealyticum, Legionella pneumophila, Helicobacter (Campylobacter), Gardnerella vaginalis, Bordetella pertussis, Moraxella catarrhalis (Branhamella catarrhalis), and Haemophilus ducreyi. Roxithromycin accumulates in polymorphonuclear leukocytes and macrophages, reaching intracellular concentrations higher than those in the extracellular environment. It enhances the adhesive and chemotactic functions of these immune cells, promoting phagocytosis and bacterial destruction in response to infection. Additionally, roxithromycin exhibits intracellular bactericidal activity.

Dose: 150 mg twice daily.

4. Telithromycin

Telithromycin, a semi-synthetic derivative of erythromycin, is part of a newly developed class of antibiotics known as ketolides. Ketolides have recently been incorporated into the macrolide-lincosamide-streptogramin antibiotic group. Like macrolide antibiotics, telithromycin inhibits bacterial growth by disrupting protein synthesis. It achieves this by binding to the 50S subunit of the 70S bacterial ribosome, thereby preventing further peptide elongation. Telithromycin is used to treat various bacterial infections, including pneumococcal infections, acute sinusitis, acute bacterial tonsillitis, acute bronchitis, bronchiolitis, lower respiratory tract infections, and pneumococcal (lobar) pneumonia.

Dose: 800 mg orally once daily for 5 days.

5. Dirithromycin

Dirithromycin is a prodrug that undergoes non-enzymatic conversion during intestinal absorption into its microbiologically active form, erythromycylamine. Erythromycylamine functions by binding to the 50S ribosomal subunit of susceptible bacteria, thereby inhibiting protein synthesis. Dirithromycin has favorable pharmacokinetic properties, including a long elimination half-life, which allows for once-daily dosing and results in higher and more sustained tissue concentrations compared to erythromycin. Its spectrum of activity, adverse effect profile, clinical effectiveness, and bacterial eradication rate are believed to be comparable to those of erythromycin. In addition, no drug interaction have been reported.

Dose: 500 mg orally once daily.

References

1. Press Information Bureau, Government of India. Successful completion of Phase 3 trial of Nafithromycin. 2024 Mar 20 [cited 2025 Apr 3]. Available from: https://pib.gov.in/PressReleasePage.aspx?PRID=2081506.
2. Wockhardt Ltd. Wockhardt announces successful completion of pivotal Phase 3 pneumonia study of its macrolide antibiotic Nafithromycin (WCK 4873). 2023 Dec [cited 2025 Apr 3]. Available from: https://www.wockhardt.com/wp-content/uploads/2023/12/wockhardt-announces-successful-completion-of-pivotal-phase-3-pneumonia-study-of-its-macrolide-antibiotic-nafithromycin-wck-4873.pdf.
3. Lang JE, Hornik CP, Elliott C, Silverstein A, Hornik C, Al-Uzri A, et al. Solithromycin in children and adolescents with community-acquired bacterial pneumonia. Pediatr Infect Dis J. 2022 Jul 1;41(7):556–62.
4. Gereige RS, Laufer PM. Pneumonia. Pediatr Rev. 2013 Oct;34(10):438–456; quiz 455–6.
5. Toda H, Satoh K, Komatsu M, Fukuda S, Nakamura T, Jikimoto T, et al. Laboratory surveillance of antimicrobial resistance and multidrug resistance among Streptococcus pneumoniae isolated in the Kinki region of Japan, 2001–2015. J Infect Chemother. 2018 Mar;24(3):171–6.
6. National Center for Biotechnology Information. PubChem Compound Summary for CID 6915744, Roxithromycin. Bethesda (MD): National Library of Medicine (US); 2004– [updated 2025 Apr 3; cited 2025 Apr 3]. Available from: https://pubchem.ncbi.nlm.nih.gov/compound/Rulide.
7. Clay KD, Hanson JS, Pope SD, Rissmiller RW, Purdum PP 3rd, Banks PM. Severe hepatotoxicity of telithromycin: three case reports and literature review. Ann Intern Med. 2006 Mar 21;144(6):415–20.
8. Wintermeyer SM, Abdel-Rahman SM, Nahata MC. Dirithromycin: a new macrolide. Ann Pharmacother. 1996 Oct;30(10):1141–9.
9. National Center for Biotechnology Information. PubChem Compound Summary for CID 6473883, Dirithromycin. Bethesda (MD): National Library of Medicine (US); 2004– [cited 2025 Apr 3]. Available from: https://pubchem.ncbi.nlm.nih.gov/compound/6473883.
10. Habiburrahman M, Soetikno V, Sirait WR, Savira M. Solithromycin as a potential novel antibiotic against Neisseria gonorrhoeae resistance. Indones J Pharm. 2020 Dec;31(4):335–53.
11. Adel K, Amor M, Alaeddine R, Emira N, Mousa A, Kaïss A, Siwar G, Jamal SA, Mohd A, De Feo V, Mejdi S. Comparative Computational Analysis of Dirithromycin and Azithromycin in Search for a Potent Drug against COVID-19 caused by SARS-CoV-2: Evidence from molecular docking and dynamic simulation. Cellular and Molecular Biology. 2021;67(5):371-86.

Section 10

Miscellaneous

Chapter 36

Newer Anticancer Drugs

Author: Dr. Pranab Das

Introduction

Cancer continues to be a leading cause of illness and mortality globally, imposing substantial economic, societal, and personal consequences. Conventional chemotherapeutic treatments, primarily cytotoxic medications aimed at rapidly proliferating cells, have enhanced survival rates for specific tumours; nevertheless, they frequently entail considerable toxicity and restricted selectivity. In the last twenty years, our increasing understanding of tumour biology has prompted a transition to more focused and personalised cancer treatments. This progression includes various creative strategies: small-molecule inhibitors that selectively target oncogenic pathways, immunotherapies that utilise the immune system to eliminate cancer cells, and sophisticated treatment modalities such as cell-based and gene therapies.

The justification for creating novel anticancer pharmaceuticals is to tackle the shortcomings of current treatments (toxicity, resistance, inadequate tumour control) as well as the molecular heterogeneity of cancers. The concurrent finding of predictive biomarkers and the implementation of new diagnostics, such as next-generation sequencing (NGS), are progressively facilitating precision oncology—treating patients according to the distinct molecular characteristics of their tumours. This chapter offers a succinct summary of traditional anticancer therapy and subsequently emphasises significant recent advancements, such as molecularly targeted medicines, immune checkpoint inhibitors, CAR T-cell therapies, antibody-drug conjugates (ADCs), and other novel modalities. This discussion of innovative approaches seeks to clarify the present advancements in cancer treatment and delineate the prospective future of cancer care.

Historical Perspective

Advances in molecular biology and genomics have led to a shift in the development of anticancer drugs from broad cytotoxic agents to targeted and immune-based therapies. The 1940s saw the invention of chemotherapy with Gilman and Goodman's use of nitrogen mustards, which ushered in the modern era of cancer pharmacotherapy. The development of antimetabolites, such as Sidney Farber's methotrexate, which brought childhood leukaemia into remission and demonstrated the promise of pharmacological cancer control, came next.

Targeted treatments first appeared in the latter half of the 20th century. The era of precision oncology began in 2001 when Druker and Lydon's imatinib was approved as the first tyrosine kinase inhibitor for chronic myeloid leukaemia (CML). It proved that by focussing on particular molecular drivers, like the BCR-ABL fusion protein, cancer could be successfully treated. Other targeted drugs, such as trastuzumab, a monoclonal antibody that targets HER2 in breast cancer and was created by Dennis Slamon, and erlotinib and gefitinib, which inhibit EGFR in lung cancer, were made possible by this discovery.

The introduction of immune checkpoint inhibitors in the 2010s signalled a paradigm shift. By enabling the immune system to fight cancer, ipilimumab, an anti-CTLA-4 antibody that was approved in 2011, and later PD-1/PD-L1 inhibitors like nivolumab and pembrolizumab transformed the treatment of melanoma, lung cancer, and other solid tumours. The 2018 Nobel Prize winners James Allison and Tasuku Honjo's groundbreaking work supported these discoveries.

While antibody-drug conjugates (ADCs) like trastuzumab deruxtecan provide precision cytotoxicity, new platforms like CAR-T cell therapies (e.g., tisagenlecleucel) have surfaced in recent years for haematologic malignancies. The next frontier consists of agents that take advantage of synthetic lethality, like PARP inhibitors (like olaparib) and small-molecule inhibitors that target KRAS G12C (like sotorasib). These advancements highlight a trend towards biomarker-driven and customised treatment, which improves outcomes for a range of cancer types and paves the way for further therapeutic advancements.

Definition

Cancer is characterized by uncontrolled proliferation and spread of abnormal cells, driven by genetic and epigenetic changes that endow malignant cells with growth advantages and escape mechanisms from host immune surveillance. Traditional definitions revolve around cellular hallmarks, such as sustained proliferative signalling, resistance to cell death, and the capacity to metastasize. Modern therapeutics seek to exploit vulnerabilities in these hallmarks or reinvigorate the immune system's capacity to eliminate cancer cells. In contemporary practice, "newer anticancer drugs" broadly refers to recently approved or investigational therapies that target specific molecular pathways, adopt novel delivery systems, or harness immunological mechanisms to improve efficacy and reduce toxicity compared to older chemotherapeutics.

Types

While there are many ways to categorize anticancer drugs, a practical overview includes:

1. **Conventional (Cytotoxic) Agents**
   - Examples include alkylating agents, antimetabolites, taxanes, and platinum-based compounds.
   - Typically disrupt DNA synthesis or cell division.
   - Broad impact on rapidly dividing cells, leading to significant side effects (e.g. myelosuppression, alopecia).
2. **Targeted Therapies**
   - Small-molecule inhibitors (e.g. kinase inhibitors) and monoclonal antibodies that specifically inhibit oncogenic proteins or pathways (e.g. EGFR, VEGF, BCR-ABL).
   - Often used in cancers with known driver mutations.
3. **Immunotherapies**
   - Immune checkpoint inhibitors (e.g. PD-1/PD-L1, CTLA-4 inhibitors) and adoptive cell therapies (e.g. CAR T-cells).
   - Potent but can have immune-related adverse effects.
4. **Others / Novel Emerging Modalities**
   - Antibody-drug conjugates, cancer vaccines, oncolytic viruses, and epigenetic modulators.

   This chapter concentrates on the recent and emerging therapies, with a focus on targeted drugs, immunotherapies, and specialized platforms that have shown promise in clinical trials or gained regulatory approval in recent years.

Brief Note on Conventional Medicines

Traditional cytotoxic chemotherapy has been the backbone of oncologic treatment for decades. Below is a succinct overview of these agents and their common side effects:

Table1: Concise overview of traditional anticancer pharmaceuticals

Drug Class / Drug Name	Mechanism of Action	Adverse Drug Reactions	Uses
Alkylating Agents (e.g. Cyclophosphamide)	Cyclophosphamide is a prodrug, activated by hepatic CYP450 enzymes to phosphoramide mustard, which cross-links DNA strands at the N7 position of guanine, leading to DNA damage, inhibition of replication, and apoptosis.	Common ADRs: Myelosuppression, nausea, vomiting, alopecia, haemorrhagic cystitis (due to acrolein production). Serious ADRs: Bone marrow suppression, secondary malignancies, infertility.	Non-Hodgkin's lymphoma, breast cancer, ovarian cancer, leukaemia, and immunosuppressive therapy in autoimmune diseases.
Platinum Compounds (e.g. Cisplatin, Carboplatin)	Cisplatin forms DNA cross-links by binding to guanine residues, leading to DNA damage, strand breaks, and apoptosis. Unlike classical alkylating agents, cisplatin induces platinum-DNA adduct formation.	Common ADRs: Nausea, vomiting (highly emetogenic), nephrotoxicity, ototoxicity, peripheral neuropathy. Serious ADRs: Acute kidney injury (AKI), irreversible hearing loss, severe nausea requiring aggressive antiemetic therapy (5-HT3 receptor antagonists).	Testicular cancer, ovarian cancer, bladder cancer, lung cancer, head and neck cancers.
Antimetabolites (e.g. Methotrexate, 5-FU)	Methotrexate inhibits dihydrofolate reductase (DHFR), preventing conversion of dihydrofolate (DHF) to tetrahydrofolate (THF), leading to depletion of thymidylate and purines, halting DNA and RNA synthesis in rapidly dividing cells.	Common ADRs: Mucositis, nausea, hepatotoxicity, myelosuppression. Serious ADRs: Pulmonary fibrosis, nephrotoxicity (due to precipitation in renal tubules). Leucovorin rescue is used to prevent toxicity.	Acute lymphoblastic leukaemia (ALL), choriocarcinoma, osteosarcoma, breast cancer, lung cancer. Also used for rheumatoid arthritis and psoriasis.
Topoisomerase Inhibitors (e.g. Doxorubicin, Etoposide)	Doxorubicin intercalates into DNA, inhibiting topoisomerase II, preventing DNA replication. It also generates reactive oxygen species (ROS), causing oxidative damage to cancer cells.	Common ADRs: Myelosuppression, nausea, alopecia. Serious ADRs: Cardiotoxicity (dose-dependent, leads to dilated cardiomyopathy), managed with dexrazoxane (iron chelator).	Breast cancer, Hodgkin's lymphoma, non-Hodgkin's lymphoma, sarcomas, solid tumours (lung, ovarian).
Antimicrotubule Agents (e.g. Paclitaxel, Vincristine)	Paclitaxel stabilizes microtubules, preventing their depolymerization, thereby inhibiting mitotic spindle function and blocking cell cycle progression at M-phase (mitotic arrest).	Common ADRs: Peripheral neuropathy, myelosuppression, alopecia. Serious ADRs: Hypersensitivity reactions (requires premedication with antihistamines/steroids), hepatotoxicity.	Ovarian cancer, breast cancer, non-small cell lung cancer (NSCLC), Kaposi's sarcoma.

Despite their broad cytotoxic effects, these agents remain foundational in many combination regimens, even when newer targeted or immunotherapeutic options are available. Nevertheless, cumulative toxicities and limited specificity underscore the need for novel treatments.

Newer Drugs / Recent Advances

The expansion of precision medicine has led to the development of a wide range of innovative cancer therapies. Below is a summary of some of the most influential and recent classes of newer anticancer drugs:

1. Dostarlimab (PD-1 Inhibitor – Immune Checkpoint Inhibitor)

Introduction: Dostarlimab is a fully humanized monoclonal antibody targeting the programmed death receptor-1 (PD-1), a critical immune checkpoint that tumours exploit to evade immune surveillance. By blocking PD-1, dostarlimab restores T-cell-mediated cytotoxicity, making it effective in tumours with mismatch repair deficiency (dMMR) and microsatellite instability-high (MSI-H) mutations.

Clinical Trial Phase / FDA-Approval: FDA-approved in 2021 for dMMR/MSI-H endometrial cancer. GARNET Trial (Phase 2) demonstrated an objective response rate (ORR) of 44% in dMMR tumours. Ongoing trials are evaluating its efficacy in colorectal, ovarian, and gastric cancers.

Mechanism of Action: Dostarlimab is a fully humanized monoclonal antibody that blocks the programmed death receptor-1 (PD-1), a key immune checkpoint receptor. By inhibiting PD-1, dostarlimab restores T-cell activation and enhances anti-tumour immune responses.

1. **Role of PD-1 in Immune Regulation**
   - PD-1 is an immune checkpoint receptor expressed on activated T-cells and B-cells.
   - It interacts with its ligands PD-L1 and PD-L2, which are overexpressed by cancer cells to evade immune destruction.
   - PD-1 activation by PD-L1 and PD-L2 inhibits T-cell proliferation and cytokine release, leading to immune tolerance and tumour progression.
2. **Dostarlimab's Binding to PD-1**
   - Dostarlimab binds with high affinity to PD-1, blocking its interaction with PD-L1 and PD-L2.
   - This prevents tumour cells from inactivating T-cells, thereby restoring T-cell-mediated cytotoxicity.
3. **Enhanced T-cell Cytotoxicity Against Cancer Cells**
   - The reactivation of T-cells leads to increased tumour infiltration by CD8+ cytotoxic T lymphocytes (CTLs).
   - Inflammatory cytokines (IFN-γ, TNF-α, IL-2) are released, promoting tumour cell apoptosis.
4. **Long-Term Immunological Memory**
   - Some patients experience durable responses as the immune system maintains an anti-tumour memory response, reducing recurrence risks.

Key Pharmacokinetic Parameters: It is administered as an intravenous infusion every 3 or 6 weeks, reaching peak plasma concentration 48 hours post-infusion. It shows large volume of distribution (8 L), suggesting wide tissue penetration. It is cleared via reticuloendothelial system (RES) and lysosomal degradation. It's terminal half-life is 23 days.

Adverse Drug Reactions: Immune-related adverse effects like pneumonitis, colitis, hepatitis, endocrinopathies and infusion-related reactions like fever, chills, hypotension.

Uses: FDA-approved for endometrial cancer and under investigation for colorectal, ovarian, and gastric cancers.

Dose: 500 mg IV every 3 weeks for 4 doses (induction), followed by 1000 mg IV every 6 weeks (maintenance phase).

2. Sotorasib (KRAS G12C Inhibitor – Targeted Therapy)

Introduction: Sotorasib is the first-in-class KRAS G12C inhibitor, a breakthrough therapy targeting a common driver mutation in lung cancer.

Clinical Trial Phase / FDA-Approval: FDA-approved in 2021 for KRAS G12C-mutant NSCLC. CodeBreaK 100 trial showed a 37% response rate in KRAS G12C-mutant lung cancer patients.

Mechanism of Action: Sotorasib is a first-in-class, irreversible inhibitor of KRAS G12C, a mutant form of KRAS frequently found in non-small cell lung cancer (NSCLC), colorectal cancer, and pancreatic cancer. The KRAS G12C mutation locks the KRAS protein in an active GTP-bound state, continuously driving oncogenic signalling. Sotorasib selectively and irreversibly binds to the mutant KRAS G12C protein, preventing its activation and leading to tumour cell apoptosis.

1. **KRAS G12C as an Oncogenic Driver**
   - KRAS is a GTPase that regulates cell proliferation and survival.
   - Mutations in KRAS G12C result in persistent activation of downstream pathways, promoting uncontrolled cancer cell growth.
   - Common pathways activated by mutant KRAS include:
     1. MAPK/ERK Pathway (promoting cell survival and proliferation).
     2. PI3K/AKT Pathway (enhancing metabolic adaptation and anti-apoptotic signalling).
2. **Selective Binding to KRAS G12C**
   - Sotorasib binds irreversibly to the cysteine residue at position 12 of mutant KRAS G12C.
   - This locks KRAS in its inactive GDP-bound state, preventing downstream oncogenic signalling.
   - Wild-type KRAS (KRAS WT) remains unaffected, reducing off-target toxicity.
3. **Inhibition of Oncogenic Signalling**
   - Shuts down ERK, MEK, and PI3K signalling, halting tumour proliferation.
   - Promotes cell-cycle arrest and apoptosis in KRAS G12C-mutated tumour cells.
4. **Synergy with Other Targeted Therapies**
   - KRAS inhibition leads to adaptive resistance via alternative pathways (e.g. EGFR reactivation).
   - Combination approaches with EGFR inhibitors (e.g. cetuximab), SHP2 inhibitors, or immune checkpoint inhibitors (ICIs) are under investigation to enhance Sotorasib's efficacy.

Key Pharmacokinetic Parameters: It is rapidly absorbed after oral administration, reaching peak plasma concentration (Tmax) in about 1-2 hours. Oral bioavailability is 73%, and food intake has minimal impact on oral absorption. It is highly plasma protein-bound (98%), resulting in a low volume of distribution. Selective penetration into tumour tissues expressing KRAS G12C. It is primarily metabolized by hepatic CYP3A4 enzymes. It is excreted primarily via faeces with minimal renal excretion.

Adverse Drug Reactions: Diarrhoea, nausea, fatigue, loss of appetite, hepatotoxicity and interstitial lung disease (ILD).

Uses: FDA-approved for KRAS G12C-mutant NSCLC and under investigation for use in colorectal and pancreatic cancers.

Dose: 960 mg orally once daily.

3. Tisagenlecleucel (CAR-T Cell Therapy - Immunotherapy)

Introduction: Tisagenlecleucel is a chimeric antigen receptor (CAR)-T cell therapy used for relapsed/refractory B-cell malignancies.

Clinical Trial Phase / FDA-Approval: FDA-approved for relapsed/refractory B-cell acute lymphoblastic leukaemia (ALL). ELIANA trial showed complete remission in 80% of paediatric ALL patients.

Mechanism of Action: Tisagenlecleucel is a chimeric antigen receptor (CAR) T-cell therapy specifically designed to target CD19-positive B-cell malignancies. It is an autologous cellular immunotherapy, where a patient's own T-cells are genetically modified to express a CD19-specific CAR, enabling direct tumour cell recognition and destruction.

1. **T-cell Collection and Genetic Modification**
   - Autologous T-cells are extracted from the patient through leukapheresis.
   - T-cells are genetically modified ex vivo using a lentiviral vector to encode a CAR construct.
2. **CAR Structure and Activation**
   - The CAR consists of an extracellular antigen-binding domain, a transmembrane domain, and intracellular signalling domains.
   - The extracellular single-chain variable fragment (scFv) specifically binds to CD19, a B-cell lineage antigen present in leukaemia and lymphoma cells.
   - The CD3 intracellular domain initiates T-cell activation, while co-stimulatory domains (4-1BB/CD137) enhance persistence and efficacy.
3. **Reinfusion into the Patient and Tumour Targeting**
   - The engineered CAR-T cells are expanded in vitro and re-infused into the patient.
   - These modified CAR-T cells circulate in the body and recognize CD19-positive tumour cells.
4. **Direct Cytotoxicity and Tumour Eradication**
   - Upon binding to CD19, CAR-T cells undergo activation, releasing perforin and granzyme, which induce tumour cell apoptosis.
   - Cytokine release (IL-2, IFN-γ, TNF-α) amplifies the immune response, recruiting additional immune cells for sustained tumour clearance.
5. **Long-Term Immune Surveillance**
   - CAR-T cells persist in circulation for months to years, maintaining long-term protection against tumour relapse.

Key Pharmacokinetic Parameters: Tisagenlecleucel, as a cellular treatment, demonstrates pharmacokinetics that are unusual compared to conventional medications.

- **Expansion Phase:** Following infusion, CAR-T cells have swift in vivo proliferation, reaching a zenith between 7 to 14 days post-infusion. The extent of growth is associated with anti-tumor effectiveness.
- **Persistence:** CAR-T cells can endure in circulation for months to years, facilitating prolonged remission. Certain studies indicate the presence of detectable CAR-T cells for up to two years following infusion.
- **Clearance:** Over time, CAR-T cells experience immune-mediated elimination, resulting in a progressive reduction in circulating cells.
- **Determinants Affecting Pharmacokinetics:**

Tumour burden: Increased tumour load facilitates enhanced CAR-T growth.

Lymphodepleting chemotherapy (fludarabine and cyclophosphamide) promotes CAR-T growth by establishing a conducive immunological milieu.

Adverse Drug Reactions: Cytokine release syndrome (CRS): it can be managed with tocilizumab (IL-6 inhibitor) with or without steroids and neurotoxicity: Confusion, encephalopathy.

Uses: FDA-approved for B-ALL and diffuse large B-cell lymphoma (DLBCL).

Dose: Weight-based dosing:

1. ≤50 kg: 0.2–5 × 10^6 CAR-positive T cells/kg
2. 50 kg: 0.1–2.5 × 10^8 CAR-positive T cells total (single IV infusion)

4. Belantamab Mafodotin (Antibody-Drug Conjugate – Multiple Myeloma)

Introduction: Belantamab mafodotin (BLENREP) is a first-in-class antibody-drug conjugate (ADC) targeting B-cell maturation antigen (BCMA), a crucial protein highly expressed in multiple myeloma cells. It consists of an anti-BCMA monoclonal antibody linked to monomethyl auristatin F (MMAF), a potent microtubule-disrupting agent. By selectively binding BCMA-expressing plasma cells, belantamab mafodotin induces apoptosis and inhibits tumour growth.

Clinical trial phase / FDA-Approval: FDA-approved for relapsed/refractory multiple myeloma (RRMM).

Mechanism of action:

1. **Targeting BCMA:**
   - BCMA is highly expressed on multiple myeloma cells but has limited expression on normal tissues, making it an ideal therapeutic target.
   - The anti-BCMA monoclonal antibody selectively binds to BCMA, facilitating internalization into tumour cells.
2. **Intracellular Delivery of MMAF (Cytotoxic Agent):**
   - Upon internalization, lysosomal enzymes cleave the linker, releasing MMAF into the cytoplasm.
   - MMAF inhibits tubulin polymerization, leading to mitotic arrest and apoptosis.
3. **Induction of Antibody-Dependent Cellular Cytotoxicity (ADCC) and Phagocytosis (ADCP):**
   - Macrophages and natural killer (NK) cells recognize Fcγ receptor-expressing tumour cells, enhancing immune-mediated tumour cell destruction.

Key Pharmacokinetic Parameters: Belantamab mafodotin exhibits non-linear pharmacokinetics due to target-mediated drug disposition (TMDD). It is administered intravenously every 3 weeks at 2.5 mg/kg. It exhibits a large volume of distribution (11 L), indicating broad tissue penetration. Cleaved by lysosomal proteases into inactive metabolites. It shows minimal hepatic CYP450 metabolism, thereby reducing drug-drug interactions. Half-life is about 12 days.

Adverse Drug Reactions: Ocular toxicity, thrombocytopenia, hepatotoxicity and infusion reactions.

Uses: Indicated for relapsed/refractory multiple myeloma (RRMM) patients post multiple prior lines of therapy. Under investigation for BCMA-positive hematologic malignancies.

Dose: 2.5 mg/kg IV once every 3 weeks.

5. Tebentafusp (Bispecific T-cell Engager - Uveal Melanoma)

Introduction: Tebentafusp is a first-in-class bispecific T-cell receptor (TCR) fusion protein approved for metastatic uveal melanoma (mUM). It is a dual-specific molecule that bridges tumour cells and T-cells, facilitating immune-mediated tumour destruction.

Clinical Trial Phase/FDA-Approval: FDA-Approval for HLA-A*02:01-positive metastatic uveal melanoma. IMCgp100-202 Trial (Phase 3): Showed a significant overall survival (OS) benefit over pembrolizumab or ipilimumab in HLA-A*02:01 patients.

Mechanism of Action:

1. **Recognition of Tumour Cells via TCR Binding to gp100 Antigen**
   - Tebentafusp's engineered TCR specifically binds to gp100, a melanoma-associated antigen.
   - gp100 is present on melanoma cells but not on normal tissues, ensuring high tumour specificity.
2. **Recruitment of Cytotoxic T-cells via CD3 Engagement**
   - The anti-CD3 domain binds CD3 receptors on cytotoxic T-cells, activating the immune response.
   - T-cell activation leads to granzyme-mediated apoptosis of gp100-expressing melanoma cells.
3. **Cytokine Release and Immune Cell Expansion**
   - Activated T-cells release IFN-γ, TNF-α, and IL-2, enhancing systemic anti-tumour immunity.

Key Pharmacokinetic Parameters: Tebentafusp follows linear pharmacokinetics with dose-dependent plasma concentrations. It is administered via i.v. infusion over 15-30 minutes once weekly. It shows moderate volume of distribution. It exhibits rapid tumour infiltration due to high affinity for gp100-expressing melanoma cells. It is metabolised via proteolytic degradation by reticuloendothelial system with minimal CYP450 involvement. Plasma half-life is about 6-7 hours.

Adverse Drug Reactions: Cytokine Release Syndrome (CRS): fever, hypotension, and tachycardia due to massive cytokine release which is managed with corticosteroids and IL-6 inhibitors (tocilizumab). Skin rash, vitiligo, hepatotoxicity and hypotension are the other ADRs.

Uses: First-line treatment for HLA-A*02:01-positive metastatic uveal melanoma. Ongoing trials in cutaneous melanoma and other gp100-expressing tumours.

Dose: Initial step-up dosing:

1. Day 1: 20 mcg IV
2. Day 8: 30 mcg IV
3. Day 15 and onward: 68 mcg IV weekly.

6. Other recent advances in cancer chemotherapy

Table 2: Modern advances in chemotherapy for cancer

Drug Class / Drug Name	Mechanism of Action	Clinical Trial Phase / Approval	Adverse Drug Reactions	Distinctive / Salient Features
Small-Molecule Kinase Inhibitors (e.g. Osimertinib, Larotrectinib)	Inhibit specific mutated or overactive kinases (EGFR, ALK, TRK, etc.), blocking oncogenic signalling pathways.	FDA-Approved for various malignancies (NSCLC, solid tumours)	Rash, diarrhoea, hepatotoxicity, QT prolongation (varies by agent).	High specificity for driver oncogenes; improved outcomes in biomarker-selected patients.
Antibody-Drug Conjugates (ADCs) (e.g. Ado-trastuzumab Emtansine, Sacituzumab Govitecan)	Monoclonal antibodies linked to cytotoxic payloads, delivering chemotherapy specifically to tumour cells expressing the target antigen.	FDA-Approved for breast cancer, other solid tumours; multiple ADCs in trials	Myelosuppression, neuropathy, GI toxicity, infusion reactions.	Enhanced specificity and potency; can overcome resistance to conventional antibodies alone.
PARP Inhibitors (e.g. Olaparib, Niraparib)	Inhibit poly (ADP-ribose) polymerase, impairing DNA repair in BRCA-mutated or HR-deficient cancer cells.	FDA-Approved for ovarian, breast, prostate cancers with BRCA/HRD	Nausea, fatigue, anaemia, thrombocytopenia, potential for MDS/AML (rare).	Synthetic lethality approach; personalized therapy in DNA repair-deficient tumours.

Key Therapeutic Targets & Strategies

1. **Molecularly Targeted Kinase Inhibitors:** The identification of driver mutations in genes like EGFR, ALK, ROS1, and BRAF has paved the way for small-molecule inhibitors that selectively block aberrant signalling. The success of osimertinib (EGFR T790M mutation in non-small cell lung cancer) and larotrectinib (TRK fusion-positive cancers) exemplifies how precise molecular targeting can yield durable responses with relatively fewer off-target effects. Ongoing research continually identifies new actionable mutations, expanding treatment possibilities.

2. **Immune Checkpoint Modulation:** Immune checkpoint inhibitors, by blocking PD-1, PD-L1, or CTLA-4, have revolutionized oncology, especially in melanoma, non-small cell lung cancer, and renal cell carcinoma. Long-lasting remissions have been observed, though only a fraction of patients benefit. Current efforts focus on predictive biomarkers (e.g. PD-L1 expression, tumor mutational burden), combination regimens with chemotherapy or other immunotherapies, and management of immune-related toxicities.

3. **Adoptive Cell Therapies (CAR T):** By genetically engineering T-cells to express chimeric antigen receptors specific to tumour antigens, CAR T therapy can induce deep remissions in refractory hematologic malignancies. As research evolves, investigators are exploring allogeneic (off-the-shelf) CAR T products, new antigen targets (e.g. BCMA in multiple myeloma), and technologies to reduce life-threatening toxicities such as cytokine release syndrome and neurotoxicity.

4. **Antibody-Drug Conjugates (ADCs):** Traditional monoclonal antibodies sometimes fail to eradicate tumours completely, partly due to modest cytotoxic potency. ADCs link a powerful cytotoxic drug to a tumour-specific antibody, selectively delivering chemotherapy to the malignant cell. Examples include ado-trastuzumab emtansine (T-DM1) in HER2-positive breast cancer and sacituzumabgovitecan

in triple-negative breast cancer. Current research focuses on optimizing linker technology, antigen selection, and combination strategies.

5. **DNA Repair Inhibition / Synthetic Lethality:** The concept of synthetic lethality underlies PARP inhibitors, which are particularly effective in tumours with defective homologous recombination (e.g. BRCA1/2 mutations). By inhibiting alternative DNA repair pathways, cancer cells accumulate lethal DNA damage. This precision approach underscores the synergy between genetic testing and targeted therapy, laying the groundwork for future drug development aimed at other DNA repair pathways.

6. **Next-Generation Strategies:**
   - Epigenetic Modulators: Agents targeting histone deacetylases (HDAC), DNA methyltransferases (DNMT), or bromodomain proteins (BET) to restore normal gene expression patterns in cancer cells.
   - Oncolytic Viruses: Viruses engineered to selectively infect and kill cancer cells while activating anti-tumour immunity.
   - Cancer Vaccines: Personalized mRNA or peptide-based vaccines that stimulate an immune response against tumour-specific neoantigens.
   - Bispecific T-Cell Engagers (BiTEs): Engineered antibodies that simultaneously bind a tumour antigen and a T-cell antigen (e.g. CD3), bringing immune cells in direct contact with tumour cells.

Conclusion

The cancer therapy paradigm has significantly altered, transitioning from non-selective cytotoxic agents to sophisticated, biology-based therapies. These breakthroughs, including as targeted kinase inhibitors, immune checkpoint inhibitors, CAR T-cell treatments, and antibody-drug conjugates (ADCs), have markedly enhanced outcomes in various cancers formerly deemed untreatable. Nonetheless, obstacles remain: resistance mechanisms frequently develop, drug-related toxicities may constrain treatment, and only particular patient subgroups (with specific biomarkers or molecular profiles) get sustained benefit. Financial and accessibility obstacles persist as significant concerns, given that these innovative therapies can be excessively costly. Future endeavours in oncology will probably persist in prioritising precision and personalization—creating therapies that target specific tumour weaknesses and integrating them with effective biomarker methodologies. Combination strategies, such as integrating immunotherapy with targeted therapy or employing various immune-modulatory drugs, are being optimised to address treatment resistance. Moreover, the emergence of sophisticated methodologies such as single-cell genomics, CRISPR-based functional assays, and artificial intelligence-enhanced drug discovery is poised to expedite the advancement of novel anticancer therapeutics. Despite considerable obstacles, the continuous advancement of knowledge in tumour biology and immunology suggests a future in which numerous cancer types may become either curable or manageable over the long term.

References

1. Siegel RL, Miller KD, Fuchs HE, Jemal A. Cancer statistics, 2022. *CA Cancer J Clin.* 2022;72(1):7–33.
2. Farber S, Diamond LK, Mercer RD, et al. Temporary remissions in acute leukemia in children produced by folic acid antagonist, 4-aminopteroyl-glutamic acid. N Engl J Med. 1948;238(23):787–793.
3. Goodman LS, Wintrobe MM, Dameshek W, et al. Nitrogen mustard therapy: use of methyl-bis(beta-chloroethyl)amine hydrochloride for Hodgkin's disease, lymphosarcoma, leukemia, and certain allied and miscellaneous disorders. JAMA. 1946;132(3):126–132.
4. Tsimberidou AM, Iskander NG, Hong DS, Wheler JJ, Falchook GS, Fu S, Piha-Paul S, Naing A, Janku F, Luthra R, Ye Y. Personalized medicine in a phase I clinical trials program: the MD Anderson Cancer Center initiative. Clinical cancer research. 2012 Nov 15;18(22):6373-83.
5. Hanahan D, Weinberg RA. Hallmarks of cancer: the next generation. cell. 2011 Mar 4;144(5):646-74.

6. Subramanian J, Govindan R. Molecular profile of lung cancer in never smokers. European Journal of Cancer Supplements. 2013 Sep 1;11(2):248-53.
7. DeVita VT, Lawrence TS, Rosenberg SA, editors. DeVita, Hellman, and Rosenberg's cancer: principles & practice of oncology. Lippincott Williams & Wilkins; 2008.
8. Drilon A, Laetsch TW, Kummar S, DuBois SG, Lassen UN, Demetri GD, Nathenson M, Doebele RC, Farago AF, Pappo AS, Turpin B. Efficacy of larotrectinib in TRK fusion–positive cancers in adults and children. New England Journal of Medicine. 2018 Feb 22;378(8):731-9.
9. Ribas A, Wolchok JD. Cancer immunotherapy using checkpoint blockade. Science. 2018 Mar 23;359(6382):1350-5.
10. Neelapu SS, Locke FL, Bartlett NL, Lekakis LJ, Miklos DB, Jacobson CA, Braunschweig I, Oluwole OO, Siddiqi T, Lin Y, Timmerman JM. Axicabtageneciloleucel CAR T-cell therapy in refractory large B-cell lymphoma. New England Journal of Medicine. 2017 Dec 28;377(26):2531-44.
11. Lin J, Jin L, Ma L, Sun L, Li Y, Shi J, et al. Harnessing gut microbiota for drug delivery and improving oral drug bioavailability. Drug Discov Today. 2023 Aug;28(8):103710.
12. Bardia A, Mayer IA, Vahdat LT, Tolaney SM, Isakoff SJ, Diamond JR, O'Shaughnessy J, Moroose RL, Santin AD, Abramson VG, Shah NC. Sacituzumab govitecan-hziy in refractory metastatic triple-negative breast cancer. New England Journal of Medicine. 2019 Feb 21;380(8):741-51.
13. Lord CJ, Ashworth A. PARP inhibitors: Synthetic lethality in the clinic. Science. 2017 Mar 17;355(6330):1152-8.\
14. Katzung BG, Masters SB, Trevor AJ. *Basic and Clinical Pharmacology*. 15th ed. McGraw-Hill; 2021.
15. Albini A, Pennesi G, Donatelli F, Cammarota R, De Flora S, Noonan DM. Cardiotoxicity of anticancer drugs: the need for cardio-oncology and cardio-oncological prevention. Journal of the National Cancer Institute. 2010 Jan 6;102(1):14-25.
16. Liang Z, He Y, Hu X. Cardio-oncology: mechanisms, drug combinations, and reverse cardio-oncology. International journal of molecular sciences. 2022 Sep 13;23(18):10617.
17. Xie P, Wang Y, Wei D, Zhang L, Zhang B, Xiao H, Song H, Mao X. Nanoparticle-based drug delivery systems with platinum drugs for overcoming cancer drug resistance. Journal of Materials Chemistry B. 2021;9(26):5173-94.
18. *Goodman & Gilman's: The Pharmacological Basis of Therapeutics*. 14th ed. New York: McGraw-Hill; 2022.
19. Sharma P, Allison JP. The future of immune checkpoint therapy. Science. 2015 Apr 3;348(6230):56-61.
20. Wang J, Zhang B, Peng L, Liu X, Sun J, Su C, Wang H, Zhao Z, Si L, Duan J, Zhang H. Chinese expert consensus recommendations for the administration of immune checkpoint inhibitors to special cancer patient populations. Therapeutic Advances in Medical Oncology. 2023 Jul;15:17588359231187205.
21. Janjigian YY, Shitara K, Moehler M, et al. First-line nivolumab plus chemotherapy in advanced gastric cancer. *N Engl J Med*. 2021;384(22):2187–2200.
22. Hong DS, Fakih MG, Strickler JH, Desai J, Durm GA, Shapiro GI, Falchook GS, Price TJ, Sacher A, Denlinger CS, Bang YJ. KRASG12C inhibition with sotorasib in advanced solid tumors. New England Journal of Medicine. 2020 Sep 24;383(13):1207-17.
23. Porter DL, Levine BL, Kalos M, Bagg A, June CH. Chimeric antigen receptor–modified T cells in chronic lymphoid leukemia. New England Journal of Medicine. 2011 Aug 25;365(8):725-33.
24. Garon EB, Hellmann MD, Rizvi NA, Carcereny E, Leighl NB, Ahn MJ, Eder JP, Balmanoukian AS, Aggarwal C, Horn L, Patnaik A. Five-year overall survival for patients with advanced non–small-cell lung cancer treated with pembrolizumab: results from the phase I KEYNOTE-001 study. Journal of Clinical Oncology. 2019 Oct 1;37(28):2518-27.
25. Nathan P, Hassel JC, Rutkowski P, Baurain JF, Butler MO, Schlaak M, Sullivan RJ, Ochsenreither S, Dummer R, Kirkwood JM, Joshua AM. Overall survival benefit with tebentafusp in metastatic uveal melanoma. New England Journal of Medicine. 2021 Sep 23;385(13):1196-206.

Chapter 37

Recent Advances in the Management of Obesity

Author: Dr. Pranab Das

Introduction

Excessive accumulation of adipose tissue is a hallmark of obesity, a chronic, relapsing disease that raises the risk of type 2 diabetes, heart disease, and some types of cancer. Due to genetic, environmental, and lifestyle factors, its prevalence has increased dramatically worldwide in recent decades, raising serious concerns about public health. Obesity has an effect on mental health in addition to physical health, which lowers quality of life and causes stigma. The obesity epidemic is still spreading despite increased awareness, which emphasises the need for more long-term and efficient treatment approaches.

Though they have advantages, traditional management strategies like diet, exercise, behavioural therapy, and medication frequently have trouble maintaining weight and long-term adherence. Along with novel endoscopic and surgical techniques, recent developments have brought promising new pharmacologic agents, such as GLP-1 receptor agonists and other neuroendocrine-targeting therapies. An overview of obesity classification and traditional treatments is given at the beginning of this chapter, which then focusses on new interventions that promote customised, multidisciplinary care for long-lasting weight loss results.

Historical Perspective

The management of obesity has significantly evolved, prompted by the acknowledgement of obesity as a chronic metabolic disorder rather than merely a lifestyle choice. Initial pharmacological treatments in the mid-20th century were amphetamine-derived anorectics, including desoxyephedrine, which were subsequently retracted due to cardiovascular and addiction hazards. The 1959 endorsement of phentermine, a sympathomimetic appetite suppressant, established the basis for pharmacological weight management. Nonetheless, the amalgamation of fenfluramine and phentermine (fen-phen) in the 1990s achieved significant popularity before its withdrawal in 1997 following allegations of valvular heart disease, as investigated by Connolly and associates.

In 1999, the FDA sanctioned orlistat, a gastrointestinal lipase inhibitor created by Roche, as the inaugural long-term anti-obesity medication with a unique mechanism that focusses on fat absorption rather than hunger suppression. Over the subsequent two decades, other combination medications were approved, including phentermine/topiramate and naltrexone/bupropion, designed to regulate central appetite pathways via various neurochemical methods.

A significant breakthrough occurred with the emergence of glucagon-like peptide-1 (GLP-1) receptor agonists, initially employed in the therapy of diabetes. Liraglutide, created by Novo Nordisk, obtained FDA clearance in 2014 for the management of chronic weight after exhibiting substantial weight reduction in the SCALE trials. Subsequently, semaglutide, a weekly GLP-1 agonist, demonstrated enhanced efficacy in the STEP trials and received approval for obesity in 2021 under the brand name Wegovy. Recently, dual agonists such as tirzepatide, which target both GLP-1 and glucose-dependent insulinotropic polypeptide (GIP) receptors, have demonstrated remarkable weight loss outcomes in clinical studies like SURMOUNT-1, indicating a new phase in metabolic illness management. These findings indicate a paradigm change from appetite suppression to hormonal and neuroendocrine control, facilitating the development of more sustainable, effective, and personalised obesity treatments.

Definition

Obesity is defined by an excess of body fat that negatively impacts health. The commonly used metric to assess overweight and obesity in adults is the Body Mass Index (BMI), calculated as weight in kilograms divided by the square of height in meters (kg/m2). The World Health Organization (WHO) classifies adults with a body mass index (BMI) of 25 kg/m^2 or higher as overweight, and those with a BMI of 30 kg/m^2 or higher as obese. While BMI offers a convenient estimate of body fat based on height and weight, it has important limitations. It does not differentiate between fat and lean mass, nor does it capture the distribution of body fat — factors that significantly influence metabolic health. As a result, individuals with similar BMIs may have vastly different cardiometabolic profiles. To achieve a more accurate assessment of health risks, additional measures such as waist circumference, waist-to-hip ratio, and body composition analysis are increasingly used. These tools help identify central adiposity and provide deeper insights into an individual's overall metabolic risk, offering a more nuanced perspective than BMI alone.

Types

Obesity can be categorized in multiple ways, although the following classifications are commonly used in clinical and research settings:

1. **BMI-Based Classification**
   - Class I (Mild Obesity): BMI 30.0–34.9.
   - Class II (Moderate Obesity): BMI 35.0–39.9.
   - Class III (Severe Obesity): BMI ≥40.0.
2. **Central (Visceral) vs. Peripheral (Subcutaneous) Obesity**
   - Central Obesity: Excess fat around the abdomen and trunk, generally associated with insulin resistance and higher cardiometabolic risk.
   - Peripheral Obesity: Excess fat distributed over the hips, thighs, and buttocks; may be relatively less harmful metabolically.
3. **Phenotypic or Metabolic Classifications**
   - Metabolically Healthy Obesity (MHO): Individuals with obesity who maintain normal glucose tolerance, lipid profiles, and blood pressure.
   - Metabolically Unhealthy Obesity (MUO): Individuals with obesity who display metabolic syndrome components (e.g. insulin resistance, hypertension, dyslipidaemia) and elevated cardiovascular risk.

Understanding the distinct pathophysiological underpinnings of different obesity phenotypes can guide treatment choices and improve long-term outcomes.

Brief Note on Conventional Medicines

Traditional pharmacotherapies for obesity aim to suppress appetite, enhance satiety, or reduce nutrient absorption. Below is a concise summary of some commonly used agents:

Table 1: Concise overview of conventional pharmaceuticals utilized in obesity management.

Drug Name / Drug Class	Mechanism of Action	Adverse Drug Reactions	Uses
Orlistat	Inhibits gastric and pancreatic lipase, preventing hydrolysis of dietary fats into absorbable free fatty acids and monoglycerides. Reduces fat absorption by 30%, leading to reduced caloric intake and weight loss.	Gastrointestinal (GI) side effects: steatorrhea, flatulence, faecal incontinence, diarrhoea. Fat-soluble vitamin deficiency (A, D, E, K). Rare cases of hepatotoxicity and kidney stones.	Approved for long-term obesity treatment in adults and adolescents ≥12 years.
Phentermine (sympathomimetic) + Topiramate (anticonvulsant) combination	Phentermine: Releases norepinephrine in the hypothalamus, activating the sympathetic nervous system and suppressing appetite. Topiramate: Modulates GABA receptors, voltage-gated sodium channels, and AMPA/kainate receptors, leading to decreased appetite and food cravings.	CNS effects: Insomnia, dizziness, paresthesia. Cardiovascular effects: Increased heart rate, hypertension. Teratogenicity: Risk of cleft lip/palate in newborns.	FDA-approved for chronic weight management. Indicated in patients with BMI ≥30 kg/m² or BMI ≥27 kg/m² with comorbidities (diabetes, hypertension).
Naltrexone (opioid antagonist) + Bupropion (dopamine/ norepinephrine reuptake inhibitor)	Naltrexone: Blocks opioid receptors, enhancing POMC (pro-opiomelanocortin) neuron activity, reducing appetite. Bupropion: Increases dopamine and norepinephrine, further stimulating POMC neurons for appetite suppression.	GI effects: Nausea, vomiting, constipation. CNS effects: Insomnia, anxiety, increased risk of seizures. CVS effects: Hypertension (due to norepinephrine effects).	Approved for long-term weight management in patients with BMI ≥30 kg/m² or BMI ≥27 kg/m² with comorbidities. Effective in patients with binge-eating disorders or emotional eating. Contraindicated in patients with seizure disorders.
Liraglutide (GLP-1 receptor agonist)*	Mimics glucagon-like peptide-1 (GLP-1), leading to delayed gastric emptying, appetite suppression, and increased insulin secretion. Enhances satiety, reducing caloric intake.	GI effects: Nausea, vomiting, diarrhoea. Pancreatitis risk (rare but serious).	Approved for chronic weight management. Used in obese or overweight patients with metabolic disorders (diabetes, dyslipidaemia).

* At higher doses (e.g. 3 mg daily), liraglutide is specifically indicated for chronic weight management.

While these medications can yield modest to moderate weight loss, patient response varies, and long-term adherence may be difficult due to side effects or cost.

Newer Drugs / Recent Advances

Recent advances in the understanding of neuroendocrine regulation in obesity have paved the way for the development of innovative therapies that target multiple biological pathways simultaneously. This evolving knowledge has spurred the creation of novel pharmacologic agents and interventions designed to achieve more effective and sustained weight management. The following provides a summary of some of the most promising breakthroughs in this rapidly advancing field.

1. Semaglutide (GLP-1 Receptor Agonist)

Introduction: Semaglutide is a glucagon-like peptide-1 (GLP-1) receptor agonist that mimics the action of endogenous GLP-1, a hormone crucial for appetite regulation, glucose metabolism, and gastric motility. Originally developed for the treatment of type 2 diabetes mellitus, semaglutide later demonstrated significant weight loss benefits in clinical trials, leading to its FDA approval for obesity management in 2021. Its once-weekly dosing regimen and potent satiety-enhancing effects have positioned it as a cornerstone therapy in the modern treatment of obesity.

Clinical Trial Phase / FDA-Approval: Semaglutide received FDA approval in 2021 for chronic weight management, marketed under a specific brand name. Its efficacy was notably demonstrated in the STEP (Semaglutide Treatment Effect in People with obesity) clinical trials, where participants achieved an average weight loss of approximately 15% over 68 weeks.

Mechanism of Action: Semaglutide exerts its therapeutic effects by mimicking endogenous GLP-1, engaging multiple physiological pathways that regulate appetite, glucose homeostasis, and energy balance:

1. **GLP-1 Receptor Activation in the Pancreas:**
   - Semaglutide binds to GLP-1 receptors located on pancreatic beta cells, stimulating glucose-dependent insulin secretion.
   - This action improves postprandial glucose control and helps prevent hyperglycemia.
2. **Suppression of Glucagon Secretion:**
   - In the context of elevated blood glucose, semaglutide inhibits glucagon release from pancreatic alpha cells.
   - This suppression reduces hepatic glucose production, further contributing to blood glucose regulation.
3. **Delayed Gastric Emptying and Enhancement of Satiety:**
   - By activating GLP-1 receptors in the gastrointestinal tract, semaglutide delays gastric emptying, helping to blunt postprandial glucose excursions.
   - Additionally, activation of GLP-1 receptors in the hypothalamus enhances satiety signals, leading to reduced caloric intake.
4. **Weight Reduction and Regulation of Energy Balance:**
   - Semaglutide acts centrally within the hypothalamus to decrease appetite and suppress food cravings.
   - It also reduces hedonic eating behaviors (reward-driven eating), thereby supporting sustained weight loss over time.
5. **Cardiovascular and Metabolic Effects:**
   - Treatment with semaglutide is associated with a modest reduction in systolic blood pressure (approximately 4–5 mmHg).

- It improves lipid metabolism by lowering LDL cholesterol and triglyceride levels.
- Furthermore, semaglutide may provide cardiovascular protection through mechanisms involving reduction of systemic inflammation and oxidative stress.

Key Pharmacokinetic Parameters: It is available in both subcutaneous injection and oral formulation. Oral formulation shows low bioavailability (0.8%), requiring gastric absorption enhancers. It is highly protein-bound (98-99%), ensuring slow systemic clearance. It is degraded by enzymatic proteolysis, not significantly metabolized by CYP450 enzymes. Plasma half-life: approximately 7 days, allowing once-weekly dosing. It is primarily excreted via urine and faeces in metabolized form.

Adverse Drug Reactions: Nausea, vomiting, diarrhoea, pancreatitis (rare but serious), gallstones, hypoglycaemia and potential thyroid C-cell tumours (seen in animal studies).

Uses: Approved for BMI ≥30 kg/m^2 or BMI ≥27 kg/m^2 with obesity-related conditions. Also used in type 2 diabetes.

Dose: 2.4 mg subcutaneously once weekly.

2. Tirzepatide (Dual GLP-1/GIP Receptor Agonist)

Introduction: Tirzepatide is a novel dual agonist that targets both the glucagon-like peptide-1 (GLP-1) and glucose-dependent insulinotropic polypeptide (GIP) receptors. It is designed to enhance glucose-dependent insulin secretion, suppress appetite, and improve overall metabolic function. Initially approved by the FDA in 2022 for the management of type 2 diabetes mellitus, tirzepatide has shown significant promise in early clinical trials for the treatment of obesity, and studies are ongoing to evaluate its efficacy in this broader population.

Clinical Trial Phase / FDA-Approval: FDA-approved (2022) for type 2 diabetes and also FDA approved (2023) for chronic weight management in adults with obesity. The SURMOUNT trials demonstrated unprecedented weight loss (about 20%), making it one of the most promising next-generation anti-obesity drugs.

Mechanism of Action:

Tirzepatide is a first-in-class dual agonist targeting both the glucose-dependent insulinotropic polypeptide (GIP) and glucagon-like peptide-1 (GLP-1) receptors. This innovative approach distinguishes it from traditional GLP-1 receptor agonists by delivering enhanced glycemic control, appetite regulation, and broader metabolic improvements.

1. **GLP-1 Receptor Activation (Pancreas and Brain)**
    - Tirzepatide mimics the action of endogenous GLP-1, stimulating glucose-dependent insulin secretion from pancreatic beta cells.
    - It concurrently suppresses glucagon secretion from alpha cells, leading to reductions in both fasting and postprandial glucose levels.
    - By slowing gastric emptying, tirzepatide further helps to minimize postprandial glucose excursions.
    - In the central nervous system, activation of hypothalamic GLP-1 receptors reduces appetite and caloric intake, supporting weight loss.
2. **GIP Receptor Activation (Adipose Tissue and Muscle)**
    - Through GIP receptor activation, tirzepatide enhances insulin sensitivity in both adipose tissue and skeletal muscle, promoting more efficient glucose uptake.

- It also stimulates fat oxidation and lipolysis, contributing to meaningful reductions in fat mass and supporting overall metabolic health.
- Unlike GLP-1 receptor agonists alone, GIP activity is closely associated with direct modulation of lipid metabolism.

3. **Synergistic Action of GLP-1 and GIP Pathways**
   - The simultaneous activation of GLP-1 and GIP receptors produces a synergistic effect that enhances the therapeutic impact beyond that of GLP-1 agonism alone.
   - Clinical trials have demonstrated that tirzepatide achieves greater weight reduction—approximately 20% of baseline body weight—compared to the ~15% typically observed with semaglutide.
   - Additionally, tirzepatide improves lipid profiles, leading to reductions in low-density lipoprotein (LDL)cholesterol and triglyceride levels, further contributing to cardiovascular risk reduction.

Key Pharmacokinetic Parameters: It is administered subcutaneously with peak plasma concentration (Tmax) is achieved within 48 hours. It is highly protein-bound (approximately 99%), allowing slow systemic clearance. It penetrates the central nervous system (CNS), contributing to appetite suppression. It is not metabolized by CYP450 enzymes and is degraded by enzymatic proteolysis. It thereby shows minimal risk of drug interactions. Plasma half-life is about 5 days, allowing once-weekly dosing. It is excreted primarily via urine.

Adverse Drug Reactions: Common adverse effects associated with tirzepatide include nausea, diarrhoea, injection-site reactions, and an increased risk of hypoglycaemia, particularly when used alongside insulin or insulin secretagogues. Rare but serious adverse events, such as acute pancreatitis, have also been reported, necessitating careful patient monitoring during therapy.

Uses: Tirzepatide has received FDA approval for the management of type 2 diabetes mellitus and is also approved for the treatment of obesity and overweight in individuals with associated comorbidities.

Dose: The recommended starting dose of tirzepatide is 2.5 mg, administered subcutaneously once weekly. Dose escalation may be considered based on patient tolerance and therapeutic response, following clinical guidelines.

3. Cagrilintide

Introduction: Cagrilintide is a first-in-class amylin receptor agonist developed for the treatment of obesity and related metabolic conditions. Amylin, a peptide hormone co-secreted with insulin by pancreatic beta cells, plays a pivotal role in appetite regulation, gastric motility, and energy balance. Early clinical trials have shown that cagrilintide can achieve substantial weight loss—approximately 11% of baseline body weight—making it a promising therapeutic candidate. Additionally, combination therapy with semaglutide is being explored to harness complementary mechanisms for enhanced weight reduction.

Clinical Trial Phase / FDA-Approval: Cagrilintide is currently in Phase III clinical trials, where it continues to demonstrate significant efficacy, including about 11% weight loss over 26 weeks. While not yet FDA-approved, its progress through late-stage development suggests strong potential for future regulatory approval.

Mechanism of Action: Cagrilintide is a synthetic, long-acting analogue of amylin, designed to mimic the actions of endogenous amylin and target multiple regulatory pathways involved in energy homeostasis:

1. **Amylin Receptor Activation in the Brain**
   - Cagrilintide binds to amylin receptors (AMY1, AMY2, and AMY3) located in the hypothalamus and brainstem, regions critical for appetite control.
   - This activation enhances satiety signaling, leading to reduced food intake and lower caloric consumption.
2. **Delayed Gastric Emptying**
   - By slowing gastric emptying, cagrilintide prolongs feelings of fullness and helps to attenuate postprandial glucose spikes.
   - This mechanism is similar to that of GLP-1 receptor agonists, supporting its use either alone or as a complementary therapy alongside GLP-1 agents..
3. **Inhibition of Glucagon Secretion**
   - Cagrilintide suppresses glucagon release from pancreatic alpha cells, leading to decreased hepatic glucose production and contributing to improved glycaemic control..
4. **Weight Loss and Regulation of Energy Expenditure**
   - Clinical studies have shown that cagrilintide promotes a weight loss of approximately 10–11% over 26 weeks, a magnitude comparable to that achieved with semaglutide and tirzepatide.
   - Unlike GLP-1 receptor agonists, cagrilintide does not stimulate insulin secretion directly, making it particularly suitable for non-diabetic patients seeking weight management interventions.

Key Pharmacokinetic Parameters: Cagrilintide is a long-acting peptide drug designed for prolonged amylin receptor activation, allowing once-weekly administration. It is widely distributed, with strong binding to albumin (99%), allowing slow systemic clearance. It crosses the blood-brain barrier, acting on hypothalamic satiety centres. It is degraded by proteolytic enzymes and is not metabolized by CYP450 enzymes.

Adverse Drug Reactions: Mild GI symptoms (nausea, constipation) and injection-site reactions.

Uses: In development for obesity and diabetes.

Dose: 0.3 mg to 4.5 mg subcutaneously once weekly (as per clinical trial dose).

4. Bimagrumab (Activin Type II Receptor Antagonist)

Introduction: Bimagrumab is a monoclonal antibody that targets the activin type II receptor, which regulates muscle growth and fat metabolism. Unlike other anti-obesity drugs, it reduces fat mass while increasing lean muscle mass, making it particularly beneficial for obese patients with metabolic dysfunction or sarcopenia. Although not yet FDA-approved, Phase II trials demonstrated significant reductions in body fat percentage, making it a unique metabolically favourable obesity treatment.

Clinical Trial Phase / FDA-Approval: Bimagrumab has demonstrated promising results in Phase II clinical trials, achieving nearly 6.5% reduction in body fat among participants. Although not yet FDA-approved, it is under active investigation for metabolic disorders involving obesity and muscle loss.

Mechanism of Action: Bimagrumab is a monoclonal antibody (IgG1) that functions as an antagonist to activin type II receptors (ActRIIA and ActRIIB). These receptors regulate muscle growth, fat metabolism, and insulin sensitivity by interacting with myostatin and other transforming growth factor-beta (TGF-β) family proteins.

1. **Blocking Myostatin and Activin Signalling**
   - Myostatin and activin A are natural inhibitors of skeletal muscle growth.

   Bimagrumab binds to ActRIIA and ActRIIB receptors, blocking their interaction with myostatin and activins, thereby enhancing muscle protein synthesis and promoting muscle hypertrophy.
2. **Enhancing Muscle Growth and Strength**
   - By relieving myostatin-mediated inhibition, bimagrumab stimulates muscle stem cells (satellite cells), supporting muscle regeneration and increased lean muscle mass.
   - Clinical trials have shown a 5–8% increase in lean mass among sarcopenic and obese patients.
3. **Promoting Fat Reduction via Energy Expenditure**
   - Bimagrumab boosts energy metabolism, enhancing lipolysis and fat oxidation.

   It facilitates free fatty acid uptake by muscles, resulting in a significant 20% reduction in body fat in obese individuals.
4. **Improving Insulin Sensitivity and Glucose Homeostasis**
   - The simultaneous increase in muscle mass and decrease in fat mass improves glucose uptake by skeletal muscle, thereby reducing insulin resistance.
   - These effects are particularly beneficial in patients with obesity and type 2 diabetes.

Key Pharmacokinetic Parameters: It is administered intravenously (i.v.) as a single infusion or repeated dosing every 4 weeks. It is widely distributed across muscle and adipose tissue. It is degraded by proteolysis via reticuloendothelial system and is not metabolized by CYP450 enzymes. It is cleared primarily via hepatic and lymphatic degradation pathways.

Adverse Drug Reactions: Reported side effects include injection-site reactions, gastrointestinal disturbances, and occasional cases of hypercalcemia.

Uses: Bimagrumab is being explored primarily for the treatment of obesity-associated muscle loss and sarcopenic obesity.

Dose: 30 mg/kg IV every 4 weeks, for 48 weeks (trial dosing).

5. Setmelanotide (MC4 Receptor Agonist)

Introduction: Setmelanotide is a melanocortin-4 receptor (MC4R) agonist designed specifically for genetic obesity disorders, such as pro-opiomelanocortin (POMC) deficiency and leptin receptor mutations. It is FDA-approved (2020) for rare obesity syndromes and works by restoring normal hunger signalling in the hypothalamus. While its use is currently limited to genetic obesity, it represents a breakthrough in precision obesity medicine.

Clinical Trial Phase / FDA-Approval: Setmelanotide received FDA approval in 2020 for the treatment of rare genetic obesity syndromes such as pro-opiomelanocortin (POMC) deficiency, leptin receptor (LEPR) deficiency, and Bardet-Biedl syndrome (BBS). It represents a major breakthrough in precision medicine targeting monogenic obesity.

Mechanism of Action: Setmelanotide is a selective melanocortin-4 receptor (MC4R) agonist, crucial for the regulation of appetite, energy expenditure, and metabolism.

1. **MC4R Activation in the Hypothalamus (Appetite Suppression)**
   a. Setmelanotide binds to and activates MC4R in the hypothalamus, restoring defective hunger signaling in patients with MC4R pathway mutations.

b. This activation promotes satiety, reduces caloric intake, and supports sustained weight loss.

2. **Enhancement of Energy Expenditure (Thermogenesis)**
   - Setmelanotide stimulates brown adipose tissue (BAT), increasing thermogenesis (heat production).
   - By boosting energy expenditure, it contributes to fat loss while preserving lean body mass.
3. **Regulation of Glucose and Lipid Metabolism**
   - MC4R activation improves insulin sensitivity, reduces fasting glucose, and lowers lipid levels, helping to manage the metabolic complications often associated with obesity.
4. **Reduction in Hyperphagia (Excessive Hunger) in Genetic Obesity Syndromes**
   - Setmelanotide effectively diminishes hyperphagia (excessive hunger), a hallmark of disorders like POMC and LEPR deficiencies.
   - Clinical studies report significant reductions in hunger episodes and caloric consumption, leading to clinically meaningful weight loss.

Key Pharmacokinetic Parameters: It is administered as a subcutaneous injection, reaching peak plasma concentration (Tmax) in about 8-12 hours. Widely distributed in the central nervous system (CNS), particularly the hypothalamus, where it exerts its appetite-suppressing effects. It is primarily degraded by proteolytic enzymes, with minimal hepatic metabolism. It is cleared primarily via renal excretion in metabolized form.

Adverse Drug Reactions: Skin hyperpigmentation, nausea, diarrhoea and injection-site reactions.

Uses: Approved for genetic obesity syndromes (e.g. POMC deficiency).

Dose: For individuals aged 2 years and older: administer 1 mcg/kg/day subcutaneously. For adults, the treatment begins at a dosage of 2 mg per day, which may be adjusted to a maximum of 3 mg per day depending on weight loss and individual tolerance.

6. Other recent advances in the treatment of obesity:

Table 2: Additional recent advancements in obesity therapy

Drug / Intervention	Mechanism of Action	Clinical Trial Phase	Adverse Reactions	Distinctive / Salient Features
Endoscopic Bariatric Therapies (e.g. Endoscopic Sleeve Gastroplasty, Intragastric Balloons)	Reduce stomach volume or slow gastric emptying via minimally invasive endoscopic procedures, promoting early satiety.	FDA-approved.	Nausea, vomiting, abdominal pain, risk of balloon deflation or migration.	Offer less invasive alternative to surgical interventions, shorter recovery time.
TransPyloric Shuttle / Duodenal-Jejunal Bypass Liner	Endoscopic devices that delay nutrient passage and/ or reduce calorie absorption in the proximal gut.	Limited approvals in some countries and under investigation in others.	GI discomfort, device migration, possible GI bleeding.	Potential bridging therapy for patients who are not surgical candidates or awaiting surgery.

Key Therapeutic Targets & Strategies

1. **Incretin-Based Therapies:** Building on the success of GLP-1 receptor agonists, multi-agonists such as tirzepatide—which targets both GLP-1 and GIP receptors—are gaining considerable attention. These

agents simultaneously engage multiple satiety and metabolic pathways, leading to superior weight loss outcomes and improved glycaemic control, without significantly increasing adverse effects.

2. **Amylin and Other Gut Hormones:** Amylin analogues, such as cagrilintide, offer complementary benefits when used alongside GLP-1 agonists by further enhancing satiety signals. In addition, ongoing research is investigating the therapeutic potential of other gut-derived peptides, including peptide YY (PYY) and oxyntomodulin (OXM), for their possible synergistic effects in weight management strategies.

3. **Myostatin/Activin Pathway:** Targeting the myostatin/activin signaling pathway represents a novel approach aimed at preserving muscle mass while simultaneously reducing adipose tissue. Agents such as bimagrumab have demonstrated encouraging results, increasing lean body mass and reducing fat mass. However, more robust, long-term data are needed to fully validate this strategy.

4. **Endoscopic and Minimally Invasive Interventions:** Advances in endoscopic bariatric therapies and the development of minimally invasive devices offer alternatives to traditional surgical interventions. Techniques that reduce gastric volume or bypass portions of the small intestine have shown significant weight loss outcomes with fewer complications, reduced costs, and greater reversibility or adjustability, providing flexibility in long-term obesity management.

5. **Combination Approaches:** Given the multifactorial nature of obesity, it has become increasingly evident that a "one-size-fits-all" model is insufficient. Current research is exploring combinatorial strategies, such as pairing pharmacologic agents with endoscopic devices or using multiple drug classes concurrently to optimize weight loss while minimizing side effects. Personalizing treatment based on genetic, metabolic, and behavioral profiles is poised to further improve long-term outcomes.

Conclusion

The emergence of novel anti-obesity therapies has fundamentally transformed the landscape of obesity management. These new agents offer enhanced efficacy, improved safety profiles, and innovative mechanisms of action compared to traditional weight-loss interventions. Semaglutide and tirzepatide, both GLP-1-based therapies, have demonstrated remarkable weight reduction by enhancing satiety, delaying gastric emptying, and improving metabolic function. Cagrilintide, an amylin analogue, shows strong potential as an adjunct to GLP-1 agonists, amplifying appetite suppression and weight loss effects. Bimagrumab, an activin receptor antagonist, offers a unique advantage by simultaneously reducing fat mass while preserving lean muscle, making it particularly beneficial for patients affected by obesity-related sarcopenia. Meanwhile, setmelanotide represents a breakthrough in precision medicine, effectively addressing rare genetic obesity syndromes through selective MC4R activation. These advancements mark a significant paradigm shift—moving beyond simple appetite suppression toward multi-pathway, individualized interventions that better address the complex biology of obesity. As research evolves, combination therapies and personalized treatment approaches are expected to become foundational pillars of long-term obesity management, offering solutions that encompass both weight reduction and cardiometabolic health. Future studies will focus on optimizing these therapies for sustained efficacy, cardiovascular protection, and long-term safety, paving the way for a new era in obesity pharmacotherapy.

References

1. Blüher M, Aras M, Aronne LJ, Batterham RL, Giorgino F, Ji L, Pietiläinen KH, Schnell O, Tonchevska E, Wilding JP. New insights into the treatment of obesity. Diabetes, Obesity and Metabolism. 2023 Aug;25(8):2058-72.
2. Cornier MA. A review of current guidelines for the treatment of obesity. American Journal of Managed Care. 2022 Dec 2;28.
3. Bray GA. Historical framework for the development of obesity therapies. Obes Res. 1992;1(1):9–22.
4. Connolly HM, Crary JL, McGoon MD, et al. Valvular heart disease associated with fenfluramine-phentermine. N Engl J Med. 1997;337(9):581–588.

5. Zeng Q, Li N, Pan XF, Chen L, Pan A. Clinical management and treatment of obesity in China. The lancet Diabetes & endocrinology. 2021 Jun 1;9(6):393-405.
6. Jastreboff AM, Aronne LJ, Ahmad NN, Wharton S, Connery L, Alves B, Kiyosue A, Zhang S, Liu B, Bunck MC, Stefanski A. Tirzepatide once weekly for the treatment of obesity. New England Journal of Medicine. 2022 Jul 21;387(3):205-16.
7. Ng M, Fleming T, Robinson M, Thomson B, Graetz N, Margono C, Mullany EC, Biryukov S, Abbafati C, Abera SF, Abraham JP. Global, regional, and national prevalence of overweight and obesity in children and adults during 1980–2013: a systematic analysis for the Global Burden of Disease Study 2013. The lancet. 2014 Aug 30;384(9945):766-81.
8. Corrao S, Pollicino C, Maggio D, Torres A, Argano C. Tirzepatide against obesity and insulin-resistance: pathophysiological aspects and clinical evidence. Front Endocrinol (Lausanne). 2024;15:1402583.
9. Hruby A, Hu FB. The epidemiology of obesity: a big picture. Pharmacoeconomics. 2015 Jul;33:673-89.
10. MacLean PS, Wing RR, Davidson T, Epstein L, Goodpaster B, Hall KD, Levin BE, Perri MG, Rolls BJ, Rosenbaum M, Rothman AJ. NIH working group report: innovative research to improve maintenance of weight loss. Obesity. 2015 Jan;23(1):7-15.
11. Puzziferri N, Roshek TB, Mayo HG, Gallagher R, Belle SH, Livingston EH. Long-term follow-up after bariatric surgery: a systematic review. Jama. 2014 Sep 3;312(9):934-42.
12. World Health Organization. Obesity and Overweight Fact Sheet. WHO; 2021. Available from: https://www.who.int/news-room/fact-sheets/detail/obesity-and-overweight.
13. Pi-Sunyer X, Astrup A, Fujioka K, Greenway F, Halpern A, Krempf M, Lau DC, Le Roux CW, Violante Ortiz R, Jensen CB, Wilding JP. A randomized, controlled trial of 3.0 mg of liraglutide in weight management. New England Journal of Medicine. 2015 Jul 2;373(1):11-22.
14. Wilding JP, Batterham RL, Calanna S, Davies M, Van Gaal LF, Lingvay I, McGowan BM, Rosenstock J, Tran MT, Wadden TA, Wharton S. Once-weeklysemaglutide in adults with overweight or obesity. New England Journal of Medicine. 2021 Mar 18;384(11):989-1002.
15. Elmaleh-Sachs A, Schwartz JL, Bramante CT, Nicklas JM, Gudzune KA, Jay M. Obesity management in adults: a review. Jama. 2023 Nov 28;330(20):2000-15.
16. Katzung BG, Trevor AJ. *Basic & Clinical Pharmacology.* 15th ed. McGraw-Hill Education; 2021.
17. Brunton LL, Hilal-Dandan R, Knollmann BC, editors. *Goodman & Gilman's: The Pharmacological Basis of Therapeutics.* 14th ed. McGraw-Hill Education; 2022.
18. Jensen MD, Ryan DH, Apovian CM, Ard JD, Comuzzie AG, Donato KA, Hu FB, Hubbard VS, Jakicic JM, Kushner RF, Loria CM. Reprint: 2013 AHA/ACC/TOS guideline for the management of overweight and obesity in adults. J Am Pharm Assoc. 2014;54(1):e3.
19. Garvey WT, Mechanick JI, Brett EM, Garber AJ, Hurley DL, Jastreboff AM, Nadolsky K, Pessah-Pollack R, Plodkowski R. American Association of Clinical Endocrinologists and American College of Endocrinology comprehensive clinical practice guidelines for medical care of patients with obesity. Endocrine Practice. 2016 Jul 1;22:1-203.
20. Srivastava G, Apovian CM. Current pharmacotherapy for obesity. Nature Reviews Endocrinology. 2018 Jan;14(1):12-24.
21. Wadden TA, Tronieri JS, Butryn ML. Lifestyle modification approaches for the treatment of obesity in adults. American psychologist. 2020 Feb;75(2):235.
22. Yanovski SZ, Yanovski JA. Long-term drug treatment for obesity: a systematic and clinical review. Jama. 2014 Jan 1;311(1):74-86.
23. Kosmalski M, Deska K, Bąk B, Różycka-Kosmalska M, Pietras T. Pharmacological support for the treatment of obesity—present and future. InHealthcare 2023 Feb 2 (Vol. 11, No. 3, p. 433). MDPI.
24. Yanovski SZ, Yanovski JA. Approach to obesity treatment in primary care: a review. JAMA internal medicine. 2024 Jul 1;184(7):818-29.
25. Beshir SA, Elnour AA, Soorya A, Mohamed AP, Goh SS, Hussain N, Al Haddad AH, Hussain F, Khidir IY, Abdelnassir Z. A narrative review of approved and emerging anti-obesity medications. Saudi Pharmaceutical Journal. 2023 Oct 1;31(10):101757.
26. Friedman JM. The discovery and development of GLP-1 based drugs that have revolutionized the treatment of obesity. Proceedings of the National Academy of Sciences. 2024 Sep 24;121(39):e2415550121.

Chapter 38

Role of Artificial Intelligence in Pharmacology

Author: Dr. Pranab Das

Introduction

Artificial Intelligence (AI) has experienced significant growth over the past decade, revolutionising various industries and swiftly broadening its presence in biomedical research. In pharmacology, AI-driven techniques—such as machine learning (ML) and deep learning (DL)—are progressively employed to expedite drug discovery, enhance drug design, tailor patient treatment, and augment clinical trial efficiencies. With the increasing complexity and amount of biochemical, genetic, and clinical data, AI provides robust tools to derive significant insights, discover new targets, and forecast therapeutic efficacy or toxicity profiles at unparalleled speeds. The historical trajectory from preclinical medication discovery to regulatory approval is protracted, costly, and characterised by elevated failure rates.

AI-driven methodologies offer potential solutions to these difficulties by utilising algorithms trained on extensive datasets to identify interesting chemical scaffolds, predict pharmacokinetic properties (ADME), and propose possible adverse events (ADRs) prior to expensive clinical trials. In addition to drug development, AI is revolutionising routine clinical practice by facilitating precision dosing and personalised medicine approaches, assisting doctors with evidence-based decision-making tools. This chapter offers a comprehensive overview of AI applications in pharmacology, examines the diverse subtypes and tools of AI pertinent to drug research and clinical application, and analyses the benefits and drawbacks of these developing technologies. Despite considerable challenges, the continuous advancement of understanding in tumour biology and immunology suggests a future in which numerous cancer types may become either curable or manageable over the long term.

Definition

Artificial Intelligence is an umbrella term encompassing computer systems or algorithms designed to perform tasks that typically require human intelligence—such as pattern recognition, problem-solving, and decision-making. In pharmacology, AI entails leveraging data-driven models to simulate or predict biological phenomena, optimize drug molecules, and derive insights into disease mechanisms, therapeutic targets, and clinical outcomes. Some core facets of AI relevant to pharmacology include:

1. **Machine Learning (ML):** Algorithms that learn from data without being explicitly programmed, adapting or improving their performance as they ingest more information.
2. **Deep Learning (DL):** A subset of ML that uses multi-layered neural networks to automatically extract complex features and patterns from high-dimensional data.
3. **Natural Language Processing (NLP):** A field of AI focusing on the understanding, interpretation, and generation of human language; useful for mining clinical notes or scientific literature.
4. **Reinforcement Learning (RL):** A paradigm where algorithms learn optimal actions through trial and error in a simulated or real-world environment, often used for drug design or robotic automation.

Types and Subsets of AI in Pharmacology

The discipline of "AI in pharmacology" spans multiple approaches, each addressing a distinct set of problems:

1. **AI in Drug Discovery and Design**
   - Ligand-based Virtual Screening: Employs ML algorithms trained on known active and inactive compounds to predict whether new molecules might bind a given target.
   - Structure-based Drug Design (SBDD): Incorporates 3D structures of protein targets to identify or design compounds using molecular docking and AI-driven scoring functions.
   - Generative Modelling: Deep generative models create novel chemical structures likely to possess the desired biological properties.
2. **AI in Preclinical Research**
   - Omics Data Analysis: Utilizes ML to analyse genomic, transcriptomic, proteomic, and metabolomic data, identifying biomarkers or novel drug targets.
   - Toxicity and ADMET Predictions: Predicts absorption, distribution, metabolism, excretion, and toxicity profiles from chemical structure and in vitro screening data.
3. **AI in Clinical Pharmacology**
   - Patient Stratification: Identifies subpopulations likely to respond better to a therapy, facilitating precision medicine.
   - Dose Optimization: Uses AI models to calculate individualized dosing regimens based on pharmacokinetic and pharmacodynamic variables.
   - Adverse Drug Reaction (ADR) Monitoring: NLP algorithms can scan electronic health records (EHRs), social media, and other sources to flag potential side effects in real-time.
4. **AI in Post-Marketing Surveillance**
   - Pharmacovigilance: Automated systems that monitor spontaneous reporting databases, literature, and patient forums to detect emerging safety signals quickly.
   - Real-World Evidence (RWE): Analyses large-scale EHRs and claims data to evaluate drug effectiveness, adherence, and long-term outcomes outside of clinical trial settings.

Brief Note on Conventional (Non-AI) Approaches

Traditionally, pharmacological R&D has relied on a stepwise pipeline:

Table 1: Concise overview of traditional (Non-AI) methodologies

Stage	Typical Methods	Limitations
Target Identification & Validation	Basic science research, high-throughput screening of protein function, knockout models.	Time-intensive, may yield many false positives, limited by existing biological knowledge.
Lead Compound Discovery	Combinatorial chemistry, structure-activity relationship (SAR) studies, manual or automated screening.	Large libraries require extensive wet-lab screening, high costs, slower hit identification.
Pre-clinical Testing	In vitro assays, animal models, ADMET profiling.	Translation to humans remains uncertain, ethical and regulatory constraints.
Clinical Trials	Phase I–III randomized controlled trials (RCTs).	High failure rate (over 90%), expensive, lengthy (10–15 years to approval).
Post-Marketing Surveillance	Spontaneous ADR reports, periodic safety updates, observational studies.	Underreporting, time delays in detecting rare or long-term side effects.

While these methodologies have led to numerous breakthrough drugs, they are resource-intensive. Incorporating AI can streamline each step by pinpointing the most promising leads, optimizing candidate selection, and detecting toxicity signals earlier.

Newer Developments / Recent Advances

AI innovations are reshaping multiple aspects of pharmacology and drug development. Below is a table summarizing notable applications:

Table 2: Recent innovations in artificial intelligence within the pharmacology sector

AI Application	Mechanism / Approach	Clinical Trial Phase / Real-World Usage	Advantages	Examples / Distinctive Features
Generative Adversarial Networks (GANs) for De Novo Drug Design	Uses two neural networks in competition: one generates new molecules, and another evaluates their plausibility or "drug-likeness."	Preclinical lead generation, used by biotech start-ups.	Rapidly proposes unique molecular structures; reduces screening libraries.	Many novel scaffolds discovered; start-ups like In-silico Medicine & Benevolent AI harness GANs to expedite drug discovery.
AI-Driven Molecular Docking	Integrates deep learning with classical physics-based docking to predict ligand-protein binding more accurately.	In vitro validation of top hits, bridging to early clinical phases.	Speeds up screening, enhances specificity of docking scores.	Improved docking performance in GPCRs, kinases; synergy with high-performance computing clusters.

Reinforcement Learning in Drug Synthesis	Algorithms "rewarded" for producing compounds with specific ADMET properties or strong binding affinity, refining lead molecules iteratively.	Research usage in pharma labs, platform expansions.	Minimizes labour-intensive synthetic steps, helps in multi-parameter optimization (MPO).	Demonstrated for creating molecules with balanced potency and solubility, advanced by Atomwise, DeepMind-based prototypes.
AI-Enhanced Clinical Trial Design	Machine learning models identify biomarkers or predict patient subgroups likely to respond, guiding trial inclusion criteria and endpoints.	Phase I–III optimization, some real-world applications.	Potentially reduces trial size, cost, and increases success rates.	AstraZeneca & Merck using AI for adaptive trial designs; predictive analytics to ensure balanced cohorts.
Real-Time Pharmacovigilance	NLP algorithms monitor online health forums, EHRs, and social media for patient-reported ADRs or drug inefficacy.	Increasing adoption post-approval; complements traditional safety data.	Early signal detection, more comprehensive patient feedback, faster regulatory response.	Regulatory bodies (e.g. FDA, EMA) exploring AI-based systems to supplement adverse event reporting in real-time.
Personalized Dosing and Digital Therapeutics	ML-based tools analyse patient-specific data – genetics, comorbidities, lifestyle – to optimize dosage or combine with digital health interventions.	Some FDA-cleared software (e.g. for insulin dosing).	Reduces adverse effects, improves adherence, supports precision medicine.	AI-based insulin titration apps, warfarin dosing calculators integrated with EHR, wearable data integration.

Key Breakthroughs and Strategies

1. **De Novo Drug Design:** Traditional drug design has largely relied on incremental changes to known scaffolds. Deep learning techniques, especially Generative Adversarial Networks (GANs) and Variational Autoencoders (VAEs), have flipped this paradigm by creating new chemical entities from scratch, guided by objectives such as potency, selectivity, or favourable pharmacokinetic properties. This approach substantially reduces the number of compounds requiring synthesis and experimental testing.

2. **Predictive ADMET Modelling:** The largest cause of late-stage drug failures is poor toxicity and pharmacokinetic profiles. AI-based QSAR (Quantitative Structure-Activity Relationship) models combine chemical structure descriptors with experimental data to predict ADMET properties early. Early removal of molecules with high toxicity risk can save millions in R&D costs.

3. **Biomarker Discovery for Precision Medicine:** Integrative AI-driven analyses of multi-omics datasets (genomics, proteomics, metabolomics) identify patient subgroups more likely to benefit from certain drugs. This not only improves response rates in clinical trials but also paves the way for truly personalized therapies, reducing adverse events and improving cost-effectiveness.
4. **Clinical Decision Support:** AI algorithms embedded in clinical workflows can provide clinicians with evidence-based dosing suggestions, warnings about potential drug interactions, and prognostic insights. For instance, leveraging EHR data and real-time labs can help AI systems recommend dose adjustments before toxicity thresholds are reached.
5. **Post-Marketing Surveillance and Real-World Evidence:** Traditional pharmacovigilance heavily relies on spontaneous reporting, which often underestimates the true incidence of ADRs. AI tools can scan voluminous data sources—electronic health records, social media, wearable device data—to detect early signals of adverse effects or off-label benefits. Such proactive monitoring enhances patient safety and may guide label expansions or additional warnings.

Advantages of AI in Pharmacology

1. **Speed and Efficiency:** By rapidly processing vast data sets—ranging from chemical libraries to patient records—AI accelerates target identification, lead optimization, and clinical trial design.
2. **Cost Reduction:** Early elimination of poor drug candidates can slash development costs, while more targeted clinical trials can reduce enrolment expenses and time to market.
3. **Improved Accuracy:** ML models often outperform traditional statistical methods in pattern recognition, especially for nonlinear relationships in complex biological data.
4. **Personalization:** AI can integrate multiple data streams (genomic, proteomic, clinical, lifestyle) to tailor drug regimens, potentially boosting efficacy and reducing toxicity.
5. **Continuous Learning:** AI-driven systems continually refine their algorithms as new data becomes available, offering dynamic adaptation to emerging evidence and shifting paradigms.

Limitations and Challenges

Despite its promise, AI adoption in pharmacology faces several barriers:

1. **Data Quality and Quantity:** AI algorithms depend on large, well-curated datasets. Inadequate or biased data can yield misleading models or perpetuate inequalities.
2. **Interpretability:** Many deep learning models operate as "black boxes," making it difficult for regulators and clinicians to trust predictions without clear explanations.
3. **Regulatory Hurdles:** Regulatory frameworks around AI-based drug discovery, digital therapeutics, and adaptive trials are still evolving. Demonstrating safety, efficacy, and robustness remains crucial.
4. **Computational Resources:** Training large models, especially for de novo design or multi-omics analysis, requires significant computational power and expertise.
5. **Integration into Clinical Practice:** Adoption by clinicians depends on user-friendly interfaces, minimal workflow disruptions, and demonstrable improvements in patient outcomes.

Conclusion

Artificial Intelligence is transforming pharmacology by incorporating extensive data streams to accelerate drug discovery, optimise clinical trials, and enhance personalised patient care. Although conventional research and development is essential, artificial intelligence offers the potential to decrease time and expenses, enhance safety, and explore new avenues in precision medicine. AI-driven de novo chemical creation, real-time pharmacovigilance, and personalised dosage tactics signify a future where we can expedite the development of more effective medications and customise therapy to each patient's distinct profile. The forthcoming path entails addressing technical obstacles, ethical and regulatory factors, and barriers to clinical implementation. As computer power increases and data-driven approaches advance, the use of AI in pharmacology is expected to rise, resulting in significant enhancements in the discovery, development, and deployment of drugs.

References

1. Schneider G. Automating drug discovery. Nature reviews drug discovery. 2018 Feb;17(2):97-113.
2. Mak KK, Pichika MR. Artificial intelligence in drug development: present status and future prospects. Drug Discov Today. 2019;24(3):773–780.
3. LeCun Y, Bengio Y, Hinton G. Deep learning. nature. 2015 May 28;521(7553):436-44.
4. Hughes JP, Rees S, Kalindjian SB, Philpott KL. Principles of early drug discovery. *Br J Pharmacol.*2011;162(6):1239–1249.
5. Jumper J, Evans R, Pritzel A, Green T, Figurnov M, Ronneberger O, Tunyasuvunakool K, Bates R, Žídek A, Potapenko A, Bridgland A. Highly accurate protein structure prediction with AlphaFold. nature. 2021 Aug;596(7873):583-9.
6. Harpaz R, Callahan A, Tamang S, Low Y, Odgers D, Finlayson S, Jung K, LePendu P, Shah NH. Text mining for adverse drug events: the promise, challenges, and state of the art. Drug safety. 2014 Oct;37:777-90.
7. Deng S, Li C, Cao J, Cui Z, Du J, Fu Z, Yang H, Chen P. Organ-on-a-chip meets artificial intelligence in drug evaluation. Theranostics. 2023 Aug 15;13(13):4526.
8. Schneider P, Walters WP, Plowright AT, Sieroka N, Listgarten J, Goodnow Jr RA, Fisher J, Jansen JM, Duca JS, Rush TS, Zentgraf M. Rethinking drug design in the artificial intelligence era. Nature reviews drug discovery. 2020 May;19(5):353-64.
9. Iglesias A, Gálvez A, Suárez P. The role of artificial intelligence and machine learning for the fight against COVID-19. InMathematicalModeling and Intelligent Control for Combating Pandemics 2023 May 12 (pp. 111-128). Cham: Springer Nature Switzerland.
10. Crisafulli S, Ciccimarra F, Bellitto C, Carollo M, Carrara E, Stagi L, Triola R, Capuano A, Chiamulera C, Moretti U, Santoro E. Artificial intelligence for optimizing benefits and minimizing risks of pharmacological therapies: challenges and opportunities. Frontiers in Drug Safety and Regulation. 2024 Mar 18;4:1356405.
11. Ajmal CS, Yerram S, Abishek V, Nizam VM, Aglave G, Patnam JD, Raghuvanshi RS, Srivastava S. Innovative Approaches in Regulatory Affairs: Leveraging Artificial Intelligence and Machine Learning for Efficient Compliance and Decision-Making. The AAPS Journal. 2025 Jan 7;27(1):22.
12. Allam H. Prescribing the Future: The Role of Artificial Intelligence in Pharmacy. Information. 2025 Feb 11;16(2):131.
13. Pathak M. Role of AI in Advancing Pharmacology. InAI-Powered Advances in Pharmacology 2025 (pp. 1-14). IGI Global.

Chapter 39

Computer-Assisted Learning (CAL) In Pharmacology

Author: Dr. Pranab Das

Introduction

Pharmacology, a cornerstone of medical and pharmaceutical education, encompasses the study of drug action, pharmacodynamics, pharmacokinetics, and therapeutic applications. Historically taught through lectures, textbooks, and laboratory demonstrations, pharmacology education has faced numerous challenges in the modern era, including expanding curricula, diverse learning styles, and the need for interactive, experiential learning.

Computer-Assisted Learning (CAL)—an umbrella term for technology-based instructional tools—has emerged as a transformative approach to address these challenges. From virtual simulations to adaptive learning platforms, CAL is reshaping how students, educators, and professionals acquire pharmacological knowledge. This chapter explores the role of CAL in pharmacology education, offering definitions, types, and conventional versus modern perspectives. It also delves into recent advances, highlighting the integration of CAL with emerging technologies like artificial intelligence (AI), virtual reality (VR), and online interactive resources. Finally, the chapter discusses key advantages and limitations, aiming to provide a comprehensive perspective on how CAL can optimize teaching and learning in pharmacology.

Definition

Computer-Assisted Learning (CAL), in broad terms, refers to the use of computer technology to augment or replace traditional instructional methods. Rather than relying solely on lectures or textbooks, CAL leverages multimedia, interactive tutorials, games, simulations, and other digital platforms to enhance students' engagement, retention, and mastery of subject matter. In pharmacology, CAL may focus on:

1. Drug Mechanisms and Interactions - Simulations that visualize molecular pathways, receptor binding, or drug-drug interactions.
2. Clinical Case Scenarios - Virtual patients that present specific symptoms, requiring learners to apply pharmacological principles and make treatment decisions.
3. Assessment and Feedback - Online quizzes and adaptive tests that provide real-time feedback, customizing the learning path based on student performance.

   While CAL does not necessarily replace traditional methods, it complements them by providing learner-centric, flexible, and often more engaging experiences.

Types of Computer-Assisted Learning in Pharmacology

CAL can take many forms, each tailored to specific educational objectives and learner needs. Below is an overview of common CAL modalities in pharmacology:

1. **Interactive Tutorials**
   - Web-based modules presenting structured content in a self-paced manner.
   - Include embedded questions and multimedia (videos, animations, graphics) to illustrate complex pharmacological concepts such as receptor-ligand interactions.
2. **Virtual and Augmented Reality (VR/AR) Simulations**
   - Immersive environments where students can "explore" drug mechanisms at the molecular level or practice administering treatments in a simulated clinical setting.
   - AR overlays additional information on physical objects, aiding hands-on training (e.g. scanning a medication vial to see interactive dosing instructions).
3. **Computerized Case-Based Learning**
   - Realistic scenarios prompting critical thinking about drug selection, dose calculation, and therapeutic monitoring.
   - May integrate branching logic, wherein learner choices alter subsequent case progression.
4. **Adaptive Learning Platforms**
   - Use algorithms to track student performance and adjust difficulty levels or topic emphasis accordingly.
   - Provide targeted remediation where needed, optimizing study efficiency.
5. **Serious Games and Gamification**
   - Educational games that incorporate competition, storytelling, and rewards to motivate learners.
   - Commonly used to memorize drug classifications, indications, or side effects.
6. **Online Discussion Forums and Collaborative Tools**
   - Encourage peer-to-peer learning, group projects, and instructor-led discussions on complex topics like new drug approvals or clinical trial results.

   Each modality can be utilized alone or in combination, forming a blended learning environment that aligns with contemporary instructional best practices.

Brief Note on Conventional Approaches

Before the widespread adoption of CAL, pharmacology was predominantly taught using traditional methods that still hold significance in many institutions. Below is a concise overview of these conventional approaches:

Table 1: Concise overview of traditional methods of learning in Pharmacology.

Method	Typical Features	Limitations
Lectures & Didactic Sessions	Organized presentations by faculty, often accompanied by slides or overheads.	Passive learning environment, limited real-time interaction or feedback.
Textbooks & Reference Materials	Core reading for theory, updated editions for new drug information.	Can become outdated quickly in a rapidly evolving discipline; reading volumes may be overwhelming.
Wet-Lab Demonstrations	Practical sessions involving animal experiments or in vitro drug assays.	Ethical concerns, logistical constraints, and limited interactivity for large class sizes.
Group Discussions & Tutorials	Small-group problem-solving and question-answer sessions guided by instructors.	Scope and depth may vary based on instructor expertise; time constraints can limit practice.
Clinical Rotations (for advanced learners)	Observational or participatory clinical experience, applying pharmacological principles to patient care.	Highly dependent on patient availability, instructor oversight, and time resources.

These methods remain core elements of pharmacology education. However, they are increasingly supplemented—or partially replaced—by computer-based interventions to cater to diverse learning needs and the dynamic nature of drug knowledge.

Newer / Advanced Approaches (CAL)

Below is a table summarizing key advanced CAL tools that have recently gained traction in pharmacology education:

Table 2: Contemporary / Sophisticated methodologies (CAL) in Pharmacology

CAL Tool / Approach	Mechanism / Approach	Implementation Stage	Advantages	Examples / Distinctive Features
Virtual Reality (VR) Environments	Immersive 3D simulations that allow learners to manipulate molecular structures or clinical scenarios.	Pilot programs and selected institutions worldwide	High engagement; can simulate rare or complex scenarios safely; immediate feedback.	VR-based drug mechanism tours; VR labs for dose preparation and safe injection practice.
Augmented Reality (AR) Apps	Overlay virtual drug info or patient data on real-world objects (tablets, mannequins, medication vials).	Early adopters in pharm programs, growing research interest	Enhances spatial awareness; user-friendly for practical demonstrations.	AR drug labelling apps that show mechanism-of-action videos upon scanning QR codes.
AI-Driven Simulators	Adaptive algorithms generate individualized case challenges based on student performance metrics.	Experimental to early integration in some e-learning platforms	Scalable, personalized learning paths; continuous improvement as data grows.	AI-based tutoring systems, predictive modelling of student errors to remediate knowledge gaps.

Serious Games & Gamification	Utilize game mechanics like point scoring, levels, and storylines to teach drug categories and interactions.	Commercially available educational game software; pilot studies in some universities	Encourages competition and motivation; can enhance retention of large knowledge sets.	Examples include "PharmaQuest" or custom gamified quizzes integrated into LMS.
Online Interactive Platforms (e.g. MOOCs, e-Learning Modules)	On-demand lectures, self-assessment quizzes, discussion boards, and guided learning paths.	Widely used; expanded during remote learning phases	Flexible, cost-effective, can incorporate multimedia content; suits blended learning.	Coursera, edX courses on pharmacology; institution-specific Moodle or Blackboard modules.

Emerging Trends in CAL

1. **Immersive Learning:** Enhanced realism in VR/AR provides experiential opportunities to practice drug administration or dissect molecular pathways that are otherwise abstract in textbooks.
2. **Adaptive Assessments:** AI-driven analytics can monitor a learner's progression and knowledge gaps, automatically adjusting the difficulty or content focus to tailor individualized learning paths.
3. **Remote and Hybrid Models:** The COVID-19 pandemic accelerated the shift toward online learning, boosting reliance on digital platforms for delivering simulations, tutorials, and exams.
4. **Collaborative Environments:** Interactive whiteboards, shared digital notes, and virtual lab spaces foster teamwork, critical thinking, and instructor feedback—even across geographical distances.

Advantages of CAL in Pharmacology

1. **Enhanced Engagement and Motivation:** Interactive simulations and gamification can make learning pharmacology more compelling compared to didactic lectures. Higher engagement often translates to better comprehension and long-term retention of core concepts.
2. **Flexibility and Personalization:** Students can learn at their own pace, revisiting difficult topics as needed. CAL platforms often allow for customized learning paths, catering to individual strengths and weaknesses.
3. **Immediate Feedback:** Online assessments, quizzes, and simulations provide prompt feedback, enabling learners to quickly identify mistakes and correct misconceptions before they become ingrained.
4. **Efficient Resource Utilization:** CAL can complement or even replace certain animal labs, addressing ethical concerns while also reducing costs associated with maintaining wet-lab facilities. Virtual experiments in pharmacology eliminate the need for animal sacrifice and complex lab protocols.
5. **Scalability and Accessibility:** Once developed, CAL modules can be accessed by an unlimited number of learners worldwide, offering equitable education opportunities. This is especially valuable in regions with limited faculty or physical infrastructure.
6. **Data-Driven Improvements:** Digital platforms generate analytics on usage, quiz performance, and engagement metrics, allowing educators to refine instructional materials and identify widespread knowledge gaps within a cohort.

Limitations and Challenges

Despite the advantages, CAL is not without challenges:

1. **Development Costs and Technical Barriers:** Creating high-quality CAL resources—especially VR/AR simulations—can be expensive, requiring interdisciplinary teams of programmers, designers, and subject-matter experts.
2. **Faculty Training and Acceptance:** Successful implementation depends on educators' willingness and ability to integrate CAL into their teaching. Some faculty may lack technical expertise or remain skeptical of e-learning's efficacy.
3. **Over-Reliance on Technology:** Students may become dependent on interactive tools, potentially undermining their ability to learn through traditional critical reading or problem-solving exercises.
4. **Infrastructure Requirements:** Institutions need reliable internet access, sufficient hardware (VR headsets, computer labs), and IT support, which can be challenging in resource-constrained settings.
5. **Quality Control and Accreditation:** Not all CAL modules are created equal; some may lack scientific rigor or consistent updates. Ensuring quality and alignment with curricular standards is crucial.
6. **Limited Hands-On Experience:** While simulations offer a safe environment, they cannot fully replicate the tactile feedback and unpredictability of real-world labs or clinical encounters. Thus, CAL should complement, not entirely replace, practical training where possible.

Conclusion

Computer-Assisted Learning (CAL) has emerged as a pivotal tool in the modern pharmacology educational landscape. From interactive tutorials that cover fundamental principles to advanced VR/AR simulations that allow exploration of molecular pathways, CAL addresses diverse learning preferences while promoting engagement, retention, and practical application. Its flexibility and scalability suit today's fast-evolving academic environments, particularly where learners have varying levels of access to instructors and laboratory resources. Nevertheless, the successful incorporation of CAL requires careful planning, robust instructional design, and ongoing faculty development. Challenges related to cost, infrastructure, and ensuring pedagogical quality must be navigated thoughtfully. Moreover, CAL should serve as a supplement to, rather than a complete replacement for, crucial hands-on or face-to-face experiences—particularly in clinical pharmacology where real-life patient interaction is essential.

In the long term, the continued intersection of CAL with other educational technologies—including artificial intelligence, adaptive learning algorithms, and wearable devices—offers an exciting trajectory for further innovation. As educators gain experience and confidence in implementing digital tools, and as development costs potentially decrease with broader adoption, CAL is poised to become an integral, if not dominant, component of pharmacology instruction worldwide.

References

1. Bélanger M, Potvin P, Horstis S, Shtulman A, Mortimer EF. Multidisciplinary perspectives on representational pluralism in human cognition. Routledge; 2023.
2. Das P, Roy D, Saha N. Online Medical Education During the COVID-19 Pandemic: Experience and Perception of Second-Year Bachelor of Medicine and Bachelor of Surgery (MBBS) Students in a Tertiary Care Hospital in Assam, India. Cureus. 2024 Jul 25;16(7).
3. Ruiz JG, Mintzer MJ, Leipzig RM. The impact of e-learning in medical education. Academic medicine. 2006 Mar 1;81(3):207-12.
4. Reisoğlu I, Topu B, Yılmaz R, Karakuş Yılmaz T, Göktaş Y. 3D virtual learning environments in education: A meta-review. Asia Pacific Education Review. 2017 Mar;18:81-100.
5. Niu W, Zhang W, Zhang C, Chen X. The role of artificial intelligence autonomy in higher education: A uses and gratification perspective. Sustainability. 2024 Feb 2;16(3):1276.

6. Hattie J. Visible learning: A synthesis of over 800 meta-analyses relating to achievement. Routledge; 2008 Nov 19.
7. Dailah HG, Koriri M, Sabei A, Kriry T, Zakri M. Artificial intelligence in nursing: technological benefits to Nurse's mental health and patient care quality. InHealthcare 2024 Dec 18 (Vol. 12, No. 24, p. 2555). MDPI.
8. Kara M, Abuelizz HA, Er-rahmani S, Elhallaoui M. In silico insights into the design of novel NR2B-selective NMDA receptor antagonists: QSAR odelling, ADME-toxicity predictions, molecular docking, and molecular dynamics investigations.
9. Mergen M, Graf N, Meyerheim M. Reviewing the current state of virtual reality integration in medical education-a scoping review. BMC Medical Education. 2024 Jul 23;24(1):788.
10. Abou Ghayda R, Cannarella R, Calogero AE, Shah R, Rambhatla A, Zohdy W, Kavoussi P, Avidor-Reiss T, Boitrelle F, Mostafa T, Saleh R. Artificial intelligence in andrology: from semen analysis to image diagnostics. The World Journal of Men's Health. 2023 Jun 15;42(1):39.
11. Brunton LL, Hilal-Dandan R, Knollmann BC, editors. *Goodman & Gilman's The Pharmacological Basis of Therapeutics*. 14th ed. New York: McGraw-Hill; 2022.
12. Katzung BG. Basic & Clinical Pharmacology. 15th ed. New York: McGraw-Hill; 2021.
13. Salas M, Petracek J, Yalamanchili P, Aimer O, Kasthuril D, Dhingra S, Junaid T, Bostic T. The use of artificial intelligence in pharmacovigilance: a systematic review of the literature. Pharmaceutical medicine. 2022 Oct;36(5):295-306.
14. D'Apice C, Guasconi M. International Partnerships in Health Education: Adapting E-Learning Models for Conflict-Affected Myanmar. InHealthcare 2025 Jan 31 (Vol. 13, No. 3, p. 285). MDPI.

Chapter 40

Clustered Regularly Interspaced Short Palindromic Repeats (CRISPR)

Author: Dr. Daradi Das

Introduction

CRISPR, abbreviated for Clustered Regularly Interspaced Short Palindromic Repeats, is an advanced gene-editing method that enables scientist to precisely modify the DNA of living organisms.

When a virus or other invader enters a bacterial cell, the bacterium integrates some of the trespasser virus's DNA into its own genome. This allows it to identify and destroy the virus if it attacks again in the future.

This process is similar to the human immune system. When a virus infects us, we generate an immune memory in the form of antibodies. Then, when the same virus infects us again, these antibodies quickly recognize the invaders and eliminate them.

When a virus infects a bacterial cell, CRISPR helps establish a memory - a genetic one. The bacterium takes a piece of the virus's genome and inserts the DNA into its own genome. From that newly acquired DNA sequence, CRISPR creates a new "guide RNA," a sequence that helps CRISPR find the invader via sequence complementarity (i.e., A binds to T and C binds to G). So, the next time when the virus infects that bacteria cell, the guide RNA rapidly recognizes the virus DNA sequence, binds to it, and destroys it.

History and Discovery

The beginnings of CRISPR date to the 1980s, when researchers observed atypical repeating sequences in bacterial DNA. Researchers did not recognise until 2005 that these patterns constituted a bacterial defence mechanism against viruses. The innovative advancement of a gene-editing method utilising CRISPR–Cas9 was awarded the Nobel Prize in Chemistry in 2020, over a decade after the identification of all the chemical components of the system. This award represented a significant milestone, being the inaugural occasion on which the Nobel Prize in Chemistry was jointly conferred upon two women—Emmanuelle Charpentier and Jennifer Doudna—for their crucial contributions to CRISPR–Cas9 technology, commonly known as "genetic scissors."

Mechanism of CRISPR-Cas9

CRISPR functions through the CRISPR-associated protein 9 (Cas9) enzyme, which acts as molecular scissors (Figure 1). The process involves three main steps:

1. **Target Identification:** A guide RNA (gRNA) is designed to match the DNA sequence that needs modification.
2. **DNA Cutting:** Cas9, directed by the gRNA, locates and cuts the target DNA at a precise location.
3. **Gene Editing:** The cell repairs the cut, either disabling a gene or inserting a new genetic sequence.

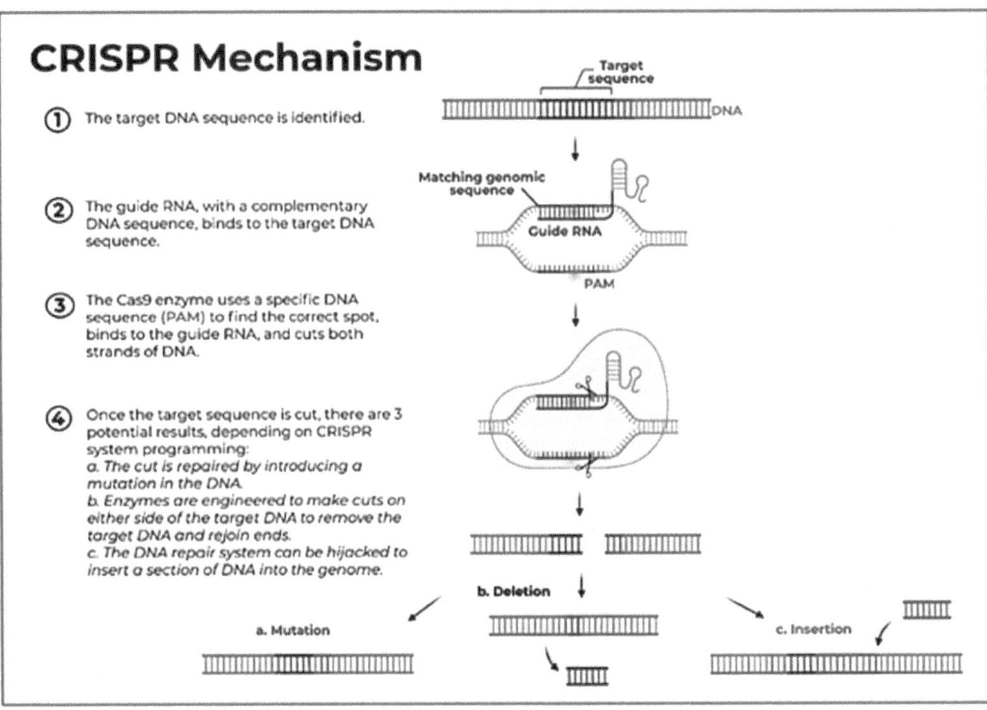

Figure 1: CRISPR Mechanism (Source: Edra et al.).

Attempts to Treat Diseases

1. **Cancer:** The CRISPR/Cas9 system is being delivered to target conditions such as cancer, liver fibrosis, obesity, and cardiovascular diseases. In experimental studies, APACPs, exosomes, PICASSO, and CHO-PEGA were administered to mice via intravenous injection, while AAV9 was given intraperitoneally. APACPs travel through the bloodstream to reach tumor sites, where low-oxygen (hypoxic) environments enhance their uptake into tumor cells.

2. **Liver diseases:**
   - Phenylketonuria: Correcting mutated bases with a single-base editor that changes C-G base pairs to T-A base pairs restores PAH gene expression and helps lower elevated phenylalanine levels in the blood.
   - Hepatitis B virus (HBV): Wang ET AL. developed a bionanoparticle activated by infrared light to deliver the CRISPR/Cas9 system to cells infected with HBV. This approach successfully disabled the HBV cccDNA.

3. **Cardiovascular diseases:** Delivering CRISPRa (CRISPR activation) systems directly into cardiomyocytes poses challenges due to limited efficiency and the potential for widespread off-target effects. To address this, Schoger et al. created a transgenic mouse model expressing dCas9/VPR, with the sequence placed downstream of the myosin heavy chain (Myh6) promoter, ensuring it is transcribed alongside Myh6

4. **SARS-CoV-2 detection:** SHERLOCK is an RNA detection tool previously constructed by Zhang Feng et al. based on Cas13a.

5. **Sickle cell disease and β-thalassemia:** Wu et al. used CRISPR/Cas9 to cleave the BCL11A enhancer sequence in HSCs and successfully downregulated its expression without inducing significant side effects.

Ethical and Safety Concerns

Despite its potential, CRISPR raises several ethical and safety issues. The primary concerns include:

- Off-Target Effects: Unintended changes to the genome could lead to harmful mutations.
- Germline Editing: Altering genes in human embryos poses long-term risks and ethical dilemmas regarding designer babies.
- Bioterrorism Risks: The accessibility of CRISPR raises concerns about its misuse in biological warfare.

Conclusion

In 2019, Victoria Grey became the inaugural individual in the U.S. to undergo a CRISPR-based therapy for the genetic disorder sickle cell anaemia. Since that time, CRISPR medicines have received approval in both the United States and the United Kingdom. Initially, there were considerable apprehensions over the safety of employing these bacterial molecules in humans, especially the hazards linked to the manipulation and alteration of human DNA. Although the long-term implications beyond clinical trial durations are still being studied, the current results indicates that CRISPR can be both safe and effective.

The subsequent challenge is to expand the spectrum of disorders that CRISPR-based therapeutics can target. Formulating therapies requires time, particularly when various diseases stem from distinct biological systems. Numerous CRISPR clinical trials are under underway, focussing on diverse tissues like the liver, immune system, eyes, and muscles. Moreover, CRISPR-based epigenetic editing is broadening the horizons, presenting prospective therapies for muscle dystrophies, retinal abnormalities, and neurological illnesses.

References

1. Stanford University. What is CRISPR? A bioengineer explains. Stanford Report. 2024 Jun [cited 2025 Apr 7]. Available from: https://news.stanford.edu/stories/2024/06/stanford-explainer-crispr-gene-editing-and-beyond.
2. Mojica FJM, Juez G, Rodriguez-Valera F. Transcription at different salinities of *Haloferaxmediterranei* sequences adjacent to partially modified PstI sites. Mol Microbiol. 1993;9(3):613–21. Doi:10.1111/j.1365-2958.1993.tb01721.x.
3. Horvath P, Barrangou R, Fremaux C, Boyaval P, Romero D. Use of a Cas Gene in Combination with CRISPR Repeats for Modulating Resistance in a Cell. US Patent Application No. PCT/US2006/033167. 2007.
4. Masepohl B, Görlitz K, Böhme H. Long tandemly repeated repetitive (LTRR) sequences in the filamentous cyanobacterium *Anabaena sp.* PCC 7120. BiochimBiophys Acta Gene Struct Expr. 1996;1307(1):26–30. Doi:10.1016/0167-4781(96)00040-1.
5. Mir A, Edraki A, Lee J, Sontheimer EJ. Type II-C CRISPR-Cas9 biology, mechanism and application. ACS Chem Biol. 2018;13(2):357–65. Doi:10.1021/acschembio.7b00688.
6. Jiang C, Meng L, Yang B, Luo X. Application of CRISPR/Cas9 gene editing technique in the study of cancer treatment. Clin Genet. 2020;97(1):73–88. Doi:10.1111/cge.13632.
7. Manghwar H, Lindsey K, Zhang X, Jin S. CRISPR/Cas system: recent advances and future prospects for genome editing. Trends Plant Sci. 2019;24(12):1102–25. Doi:10.1016/j.tplants.2019.09.006.
8. Wang D, Zhang H, Li M, Francy CA, Guo Y, Chen Y, et al. CRISPR/Cas9 delivery by NIR-responsive biomimetic nanoparticles for targeted HBV therapy. J Nanobiotechnol. 2022;20:27. Doi:10.1186/s12951-021-01179-z.
9. Schoger E, Li X, Holley CL, et al. CRISPR-mediated activation of endogenous gene expression in the postnatal heart. Circ Res. 2020;126(1):6–24. Doi:10.1161/CIRCRESAHA.119.314736
10. Gootenberg JS, Abudayyeh OO, Kellner MJ, Joung J, Collins JJ, Zhang F. Nucleic acid detection with CRISPR-Cas13a/C2c2. Science. 2017;356(6336):438–42. Doi:10.1126/science.aam9321.
11. Wu Y, Zeng J, Roscoe BP, Liu P, Yao Q, Lazzarotto CR, et al. Highly efficient therapeutic gene editing of human hematopoietic stem cells. Nat Med. 2019;25(5):776–83. Doi:10.1038/s41591-019-0410-8.

Chapter 41

Novel FDA Drug Approvals for 2025

Table 1: Latest FDA Pharmaceutical authorizations for 2025 (Up to 12/06/2025).

Sl. No.	Brand Name	Generic Drug	Date of Approval (DD/MM/YYY)	FDA-Approved Indication
1.	Datroway	Datopotamabderuxtecan-dlnk	17/01/2025	To treat unresectable or metastatic, Hormone Receptor-positive, HER2-negative breast cancer who have received prior endocrine-based therapy and chemotherapy for unresectable or metastatic disease.
2.	Grafapex	Treosulfan	21/01/2025	To be utilized in combination with fludarabine as a preparative regimen for allogeneic hematopoietic stem cell transplantation in cases of acute myeloid leukaemia (AML) and myelodysplastic syndrome.
3.	Journavx	Suzetrigine	30/01/2025	To treat moderate to severe acute pain.
4.	Gomekli	Mirdametinib	11/02/2025	To treat Neurofibromatosis type 1 in patients with symptomatic plexiform neurofibromas not amenable to complete resection.
5.	Romvimza	Vimseltinib	14/02/2025	To treat symptomatic tenosynovial giant cell tumour when surgical excision may exacerbate functional limitations or result in significant morbidity.
6.	Blujepa	Gepotidacin	25/03/2025	To treat uncomplicated urinary tract infections.
7.	Qfitlia	Fitusiran	28/03/2025	To prevent or reduce the frequency of bleeding episodes in haemophilia A or B.
8.	Vanrafia	Atrasentan	02/04/2025	To diminish proteinuria in people with primary immunoglobulin A nephropathy susceptible to fast disease advancement.
9.	Penpulimab-kcqx	Penpulimab-kcqx	23/04/2025	Administered in conjunction with either cisplatin or carboplatin and gemcitabine for the treatment of people with recurrent or metastatic non-keratinizing nasopharyngeal carcinoma (NPC), or as a monotherapy following platinum-based chemotherapy and at least one additional prior line of treatment.
10.	Imaavy	Nipocalimab-aahu	29/04/2025	Therapy for generalised myasthenia gravis.

11.	Avmapki Fakzynja Co-Pack	Avutometinib and defactinib	08/05/2025	To treat KRAS-mutated recurrent low-grade serous ovarian cancer (LGSOC) after prior systemic therapy
12.	Emrelis	Telisotuzumabvedotin-tllv	14/05/2025	To address locally progressed or metastatic, non-squamous non-small cell lung cancer (NSCLC) exhibiting elevated c-Met protein overexpression following previous systemic treatment.
13.	Tryptyr	Acoltremon	28/05/2025	To address the manifestations of dry eye illness.
14.	Enflonsia	Clesrovimab-cfor	09/06/2025	To avert respiratory syncytial virus (RSV) lower respiratory tract illness in neonates and children born during or approaching their inaugural RSV season.

References:

1. U.S. Food and Drug Administration. Novel Drug Approvals for 2025 [Internet]. Silver Spring (MD): FDA; 2025 [cited 2025 Jun12]. Available from: https://www.fda.gov/drugs/novel-drug-approvals-fda/novel-drug-approvals-2025.

Chapter 42

Novel FDA Drug Approvals for 2024

Table 1: Latest FDA Pharmaceutical authorizations for 2024.

Sl. No.	Brand Name	Generic Drug	Date of Approval (DD/MM/YYY)	FDA-Approved Indication
1.	Zelsuvmi	Berdazimer	05/01/2024	To treat Molluscum contagiosum.
2.	Exblifep	Cefepime, enmetazobactam	22/02/2024	To treat complicated urinary tract infections.
3.	Letybo	LetibotulinumtoxinA-wlbg	29/02/2024	To temporarily improve the appearance of moderate-to-severe glabellar lines.
4.	Tevimbra	Tislelizumab-jsgr	13/03/2024	To treat unresectable or metastatic oesophageal squamous cell carcinoma.
5.	Rezdiffra	Resmetirom	14/03/2024	To treat non-cirrhotic non-alcoholic steatohepatitis with moderate to advanced liver scarring.
6.	Tryvio	Aprocitentan	19/03/2024	Treatment of hypertension.
7.	Duvyzat	Givinostat	21/03/2024	To treat Duchenne Muscular Dystrophy in individuals aged 6 years and older.
8.	Winrevair	Sotatercept-csrk	26/03/2024	To treat Pulmonary arterial hypertension.
9.	Vafseo	Vadadustat	27/03/2024	Treatment of anaemia due to chronic kidney disease.
10.	Voydeya	Danicopan	29/03/2024	To treat extravascular haemolysis with paroxysmal nocturnal haemoglobinuria.
11.	Zevtera	Ceftobiprole medocaril sodium	03/04/2024	Treatment of bloodstream infections, bacterial skin and associated tissue infections, and community-acquired bacterial pneumonia.
12.	Lumisight	Pegulicianine	17/04/2024	As an optical imaging agent for the detection of cancerous tissue.
13.	Anktiva	Nogapendekin alfa inbakicept-pmln	22/04/2024	Bladder cancer management.
14.	Ojemda	Tovorafenib	23/04/2024	Medical management of relapsed or refractory paediatric low-grade glioma.
15.	Xolremdi	Mavorixafor	26/04/2024	Treatment of WHIM syndrome (warts, hypogammaglobulinemia, infections and myelokathexis).
16.	Imdelltra	Tarlatamab-dlle	16/05/2024	To treat extensive stage small cell lung cancer.
17.	Rytelo	Imetelstat	06/06/2024	Treatment of low to intermediate risk myelodysplastic syndromes.

18.	Iqirvo	Elafibranor	10/06/2024	To treat primary biliary cholangitis in combination with ursodeoxycholic acid.
19.	Sofdra	Sofpironium	18/06/2024	Primary axillary hyperhidrosis management.
20.	Piasky	Crovalimab-akkz	20/06/2024	Medical management of Paroxysmal Nocturnal Haemoglobinuria.
21.	Ohtuvayre	Ensifentrine	26/06/2024	Treatment of Chronic obstructive pulmonary disease.
22.	Kisunla	Donanemab-azbt	02/07/2024	Alzheimer's disease management.
23.	Leqselvi	Deuruxolitinib	25/07/2024	Treatment of severe alopecia areata.
24.	Voranigo	Vorasidenib	06/08/2024	Medical management of grade 2 astrocytoma or oligodendroglioma.
25.	Yorvipath	Palopegteriparatide	09/08/2024	Hypoparathyroidism treatment.
26.	Nemluvio	Nemolizumab-ilto	12/08/2024	To treat Prurigo nodularis.
27.	Niktimvo	Axatilimab-csfr	14/08/2024	To treat Chronic graft-versus-host disease (cGVHD).
28.	Livdelzi	Seladelpar	14/08/2024	To treat Primary biliary cholangitis (PBC).
29.	Lazcluze	Lazertinib	19/08/2024	Non-small cell lung cancer management.
30.	Ebglyss	Lebrikizumab-lbkz	13/09/2024	To treat moderate-to-severe atopic dermatitis.
31.	Miplyffa	Arimoclomol	20/09/2024	Medical management of Niemann-pick disease type c.
32.	Aqneursa	Levacetylleucine	24/09/2024	To treat Niemann-pick disease type c.
33.	Cobenfy	Xanomeline and trospium chloride	26/09/2024	To treat Schizophrenia.
34.	Flyrcado	FlurpiridazF 18	27/09/2024	A radioactive diagnostic drug to evaluate for myocardial ischemia and infarction.
35.	Itovebi	Inavolisib	10/10/2024	To treat locally advanced or metastatic breast cancer.
36.	Hympavzi	Marstacimab-hncq	11/10/2024	Prevention or reducing bleeding episodes related to haemophilia A or B.
37.	Vyloy	Zolbetuximab-clzb	18/10/2024	Gastric or gastroesophageal junction adenocarcinoma treatment.
38.	Orlynvah	Sulopenemetzadroxil, probenecid	25/10/2024	To treat uncomplicated urinary tract infections.
39.	Revuforj	Revumenib	15/11/2024	To treat relapsed or refractory acute leukaemia.
40.	Ziihera	Zanidatamab-hrii	20/11/2024	To treat unresectable or metastatic HER2-positive (IHC 3+) biliary tract cancer.
41.	Rapiblyk	Landiolol	22/11/2024	Supraventricular tachycardia treatment.
42.	Attruby	Acoramidis	22/11/2024	Medical management of cardiomyopathy of wild-type or variant transthyretin-mediated amyloidosis.

43.	Iomervu	Iomeprol	27/11/2024	Radiographic contrast agent.
44.	Bizengri	Zenocutuzumab-zbco	04/12/2024	Medical management of non-small cell lung cancer and pancreatic adenocarcinoma.
45.	Crenessity	Crinecerfont	13/12/2024	Classical congenital adrenal hyperplasia treatment.
46.	Unloxcyt	Cosibelimab-ipdl	13/12/2024	Medical management of cutaneous squamous cell carcinoma treatment.
47.	Ensacove	Ensartinib	18/12/2024	Non-small cell lung cancer treatment.
48.	Tryngolza	Olezarsen	19/12/2024	To treat Familial chylomicronaemia syndrome.
49.	Alhemo	Concizumab-mtci	20/12/2024	For routine prophylaxis to prevent bleeding episodes in haemophilia A and B.
50.	Alyftrek	Vanzacaftor, tezacaftor, and deutivacaftor	20/12/2024	To treat Cystic fibrosis.

References:

1. U.S. Food and Drug Administration. Novel Drug Approvals for 2024 [Internet]. Silver Spring (MD): FDA; 2024 [cited 2025 Jun 12]. Available from: https://www.fda.gov/drugs/novel-drug-approvals-fda/novel-drug-approvals-2024.

Chapter 43

Novel FDA Drug Approvals for 2023

Table 1: Latest FDA Pharmaceutical authorizations for 2023.

Sl. No.	Brand Name	Generic Drug	Date of Approval (DD/MM/YYY)	FDA-Approved Indication
1.	Leqembi	Lecanemab-irmb	06/01/2023	To treat Alzheimer's disease.
2.	Brenzavvy	Bexagliflozin	20/01/2023	To treat Type 2 diabetes mellitus as an adjunct to diet and exercise.
3.	Jaypirca	Pirtobrutinib	27/01/2023	To treat relapsed or refractory mantle cell lymphoma in adults who have had at least two lines of systemic therapy, including a BTK inhibitor.
4.	Orserdu	Elacestrant	27/01/2023	To treat oestrogen receptor-positive, human epidermal growth factor receptor 2-negative, ESR1-mutated, advanced or metastatic breast cancer with disease progression following at least one line of endocrine therapy.
5.	Jesduvroq	Daprodustat	01/02/2023	To treat anaemia caused by chronic kidney disease for adults on dialysis for at least four months.
6.	Lamzede	Velmanase alfa-tycv	16/02/2023	To managenon-central nervous system manifestations of alpha-mannosidosis.
7.	Filspari	Sparsentan	17/02/2023	To reduce proteinuria in adults with primary immunoglobulin A nephropathy at risk of rapid disease progression.
8.	Skyclarys	Omaveloxolone	28/02/2023	To treat Friedrich's ataxia.
9.	Zavzpret	Zavegepant	09/03/2023	To treat migraine treatment.
10.	Daybue	Trofinetide	10/03/2023	To treat Rett syndrome.
11.	Zynyz	Retifanlimab-dlwr	22/03/2023	To treat metastatic or recurrent locally advanced Merkel cell carcinoma.
12.	Rezzayo	Rezafungin	22/03/2023	Candidemia and invasive candidiasis treatment.
13.	Joenja	Leniolisib	24/03/2023	Medical management activated phosphoinositide 3-kinase delta syndrome.
14.	Qalsody	Tofersen	25/04/2023	To treat Amyotrophic lateral sclerosis in adults who have a SOD1 gene mutation.
15.	Elfabrio	Pegunigalsidase alfa-iwxj	09/05/2023	Fabry disease management.

16.	Veozah	Fezolinetant	12/05/2023	To treat moderate to severe hot flashes caused by menopause.
17.	Miebo	Perfluorhexyloctane	18/05/2023	Dry eye disease treatment.
18.	Epkinly	Epcoritamab-bysp	19/05/2023	Medical management of relapsed or refractory diffuse large B-cell lymphoma (not otherwise specified) and high-grade B-cell lymphoma after two or more lines of systemic therapy.
19.	Xacduro	Sulbactam, durlobactam	23/05/2023	Treatment of Hospital-acquired bacterial pneumonia and ventilator-associated bacterial pneumonia caused by susceptible isolates of *Acinetobacter baumannii-calcoaceticus complex*.
20.	Paxlovid	Nirmatrelvir, ritonavir	25/05/2023	Mild-to-moderate COVID-19 management in adults at high risk for progression to severe COVID-19.
21.	Posluma	Flotufolastat F 18	25/05/2023	To be used with positron emission tomography imaging in certain patients with prostate cancer.
22.	Inpefa	Sotagliflozin	26/05/2023	Medical management heart failure.
23.	Columvi	Glofitamab-gxbm	15/06/2023	Medical management of diffuse large B-cell lymphoma, not otherwise specified, or large B-cell lymphoma arising from follicular lymphoma after two or more lines of systemic therapy.
24.	Litfulo	Ritlecitinib	23/06/2023	Medical management of severely patchy hair loss.
25.	Rystiggo	Rozanolixizumab-noli	26/06/2023	To treat generalized myasthenia gravis in adults who are anti-acetylcholine receptor- or anti-muscle-specific tyrosine kinase antibody-positive.
26.	Ngenla	Somatrogon-ghla	27/06/2023	Medical management of growth failure due to inadequate secretion of endogenous growth hormone.
27.	Beyfortus	Nirsevimab-alip	17/07/2023	Prevention of respiratory syncytial virus (RSV) lower respiratory tract disease.
28.	Vanflyta	Quizartinib	20/07/2023	To be used as part of a treatment regimen for newly diagnosed acute myeloid leukaemia.
29.	Xdemvy	Lotilaner	25/07/2023	Demodex blepharitis treatment.
30.	Zurzuvae	Zuranolone	04/08/2023	To treat postpartum depression.
31.	Izervay	Avacincaptad pegol	04/08/2023	To treat geographic atrophy secondary to age-related macular degeneration.
32.	Talvey	Talquetamab-tgvs	09/08/2023	Medical management of adults with relapsed or refractory multiple myeloma who have received at least four prior therapies.

33.	Elrexfio	Elranatamab-bcmm	14/08/2023	Medical management of adults with relapsed or refractory multiple myeloma who have received at least four prior lines of therapy.
34.	Sohonos	Palovarotene	16/08/2023	To reduce the volume of new heterotopic ossification in adults and paediatric patients (aged 8 years and older for females and 10 years and older for males) with fibro dysplasia ossificans progressive.
35.	Veopoz	Pozelimab-bbfg	18/08/2023	Medical management of patients 1 year old and older with CD55-deficient protein-losing enteropathy (PLE), also known as CHAPLE disease.
36.	Aphexda	Motixafortide	08/09/2023	To be used with filgrastim (G-CSF) to mobilize hematopoietic stem cells to the peripheral blood for collection and subsequent autologous transplantation in patients with multiple myeloma.
37.	Ojjaara	Momelotinib	15/09/2023	To treat intermediate or high-risk myelofibrosis in adults with anaemia.
38.	Exxua	Gepirone	22/09/2023	Major depressive disorder treatment.
39.	Pombiliti	Cipaglucosidase alfa-atga	28/09/2023	To treat late-onset Pompe disease.
40.	Rivfloza	Nedosiran	29/09/2023	To reduce urinary oxalate levels in patients 9 years and older with primary hyperoxaluria type 1 and relatively preserved kidney function.
41.	Velsipity	Etrasimod	12/10/2023	To treat moderate to severe ulcerative colitis in adults.
42.	Zilbrysq	Zilucoplan	17/10/2023	To treat generalized myasthenia gravis in adults who are anti-acetylcholine receptor (AchR) antibody positive.
43.	Bimzelx	Bimekizumab	17/10/2023	To treat moderate to severe plaque psoriasis in adults who are candidates for systemic therapy or phototherapy.
44.	Agamree	Vamorolone	26/10/2023	Duchenne muscular dystrophy management.
45.	Omvoh	Mirikizumab-mrkz	26/10/2023	Medical management of Ulcerative colitis.
46.	Loqtorzi	Toripalimab-tpzi	27/10/2023	To treat recurrent or metastatic nasopharyngeal carcinoma when used together with or following other therapies.
47.	Fruzaqla	Fruquintinib	08/11/2023	To treat refractory, metastatic colorectal cancer.
48.	Defencath	Taurolidine, heparin	15/11/2023	To reduce the incidence of catheter-related bloodstream infections in adults with kidney failure receiving chronic haemodialysis through a central venous catheter.

49.	Augtyro	Repotrectinib	15/11/2023	ROS1-positive non-small cell lung cancer management.
50.	Ryzneuta	Efbemalenograstim alfa-vuxw	16/11/2023	Neutropenia treatment.
51.	Truqap	Capivasertib	16/11/2023	To treat breast cancer that meets certain disease criteria.
52.	Ogsiveo	Nirogacestat	27/11/2023	To treat adults with progressing desmoid tumours who require systemic treatment.
53.	Fabhalta	Iptacopan	05/12/2023	Paroxysmal nocturnal haemoglobinuria treatment.
54.	Filsuvez	Birch triterpenes	18/12/2023	Management of wounds associated with dystrophic and junctional epidermolysis bullosa.
55.	Wainua	Eplontersen	21/12/2023	Polyneuropathy of hereditary transthyretin-mediated amyloidosis management.

References:

1. U.S. Food and Drug Administration. Novel Drug Approvals for 2023 [Internet]. Silver Spring (MD): FDA; 2023 [cited 2025 Jun 12]. Available from: https://www.fda.gov/drugs/novel-drug-approvals-fda/novel-drug-approvals-2023.

Chapter 44

Novel FDA Drug Approvals for 2022

Table 1: Latest FDA Pharmaceutical authorizations for 2022

Sl. No.	Brand Name	Generic Drug	Date of Approval (DD/MM/YYY)	FDA-Approved Indication
1.	Quviviq	Daridorexant	07/01/2022	Insomnia treatment.
2.	Cibinqo	Abrocitinib	14/01/2022	Medical management of refractory, moderate-to-severe atopic dermatitis.
3.	Kimmtrak	Tebentafusp-tebn	25/01/2022	To treat unresectable or metastatic uveal melanoma.
4.	Vabysmo	Faricimab-svoa	28/01/2022	To treat neovascular (Wet) aged-related macular degeneration and diabetic macular oedema.
5.	Enjaymo	Sutimlimab-jome	04/02/2022	To decrease the need for red blood cell transfusion due to haemolysis in cold agglutinin disease.
6.	Pyrukynd	Mitapivat	17/02/2022	To treat haemolytic anaemia in pyruvate kinase deficiency.
7.	Vonjo	Pacritinib	28/02/2022	To treat intermediate or high-risk primary or secondary myelofibrosis in adults with low platelets.
8.	Ztalmy	Ganaxolone	18/03/2022	To treat seizures in cyclin-dependent kinase-like 5 deficiency disorder.
9.	Opdualag	Nivolumab and relatlimab-rmbw	18/03/2022	To treat unresectable or metastatic melanoma management.
10.	Pluvicto	Lutetium (177Lu) vipivotide tetraxetan	23/03/2022	To treat prostate-specific membrane antigen-positive metastatic castration-resistant prostate cancer following other therapies.
11.	Vivjoa	Oteseconazole	26/04/2022	To reduce the incidence of recurrent vulvovaginal candidiasis (RVVC) in females with a history of RVVC who are not of reproductive potential.
12.	Camzyos	Mavacamten	28/04/2022	Obstructive hypertrophic cardiomyopathy management.
13.	Voquezna	Vonoprazan, amoxicillin, and clarithromycin	03/05/2022	To treat *Helicobacter pylori infection.*
14.	Mounjaro	Tirzepatide	13/05/2022	To manage Type-2 Diabetes Mellitus.
15.	Vtama	Tapinarof	23/05/2022	Plaque psoriasis management.

16.	Amvuttra	Vutrisiran	13/06/2022	Polyneuropathy of hereditary transthyretin-mediated amyloidosis management.
17.	Xenpozyme	Olipudase alfa	31/08/2022	Medical management of acid sphingomyelinase deficiency.
18.	Spevigo	Spesolimab-sbzo	01/09/2022	Generalized pustular psoriasis flares treatment.
19.	Daxxify	DaxibotulinumtoixnA-lanm	07/09/2022	Medical management of moderate-to-severe glabellar lines associated with corrugator and/or procerus muscle activity.
20.	Sotyktu	Deucravacitinib	09/09/2022	Moderate-to-severe plaque psoriasis treatment.
21.	Rolvedon	Eflapegrastim	09/09/2022	To decrease the incidence of infection in patients with non-myeloid malignancies receiving myelosuppressive anti-cancer drugs associated with clinically significant incidence of febrile neutropenia.
22.	Terlivaz	Terlipressin	14/09/2022	To treat adults with hepatorenal syndrome with rapid reduction in kidney function.
23.	Elucirem	Gadopiclenol	21/09/2022	To detect and visualize lesions, together with MRI, with abnormal vascularity in the central nervous system and the body.
24.	Omlonti	Oomidenepag isopropyl ophthalmic solution	22/09/2022	To treat open angle glaucoma or ocular hypertension.
25.	Relyvrio	Sodium phenylbutyrate/ taurursodiol	29/09/2022	To treat Amyotrophic lateral sclerosis (ALS).
26.	Lytgobi	Futibatinib	30/09/2022	To manage intrahepatic cholangiocarcinoma harbouring fibroblast growth factor receptor 2 (FGFR2) gene fusions or other rearrangements.
27.	Imjudo	Tremelimumab	21/10/2022	Unresectable hepatocellular carcinoma management.
28.	Tecvayli	Teclistamab-cqyv	25/10/2022	Medical management of relapsed or refractory multiple myeloma among adults who have received at least four specific lines of therapy.
29.	Elahere	Mirvetuximabsoravtansine-gynx	14/11/2022	Medical management of recurrent ovarian cancer that is resistant to platinum therapy.

30.	Tzield	Teplizumab-mzwv	18/11/2022	To delay the onset of stage 3 type 1 diabetes.
31.	Rezlidhia	Olutasidenib	01/12/2022	To treat relapsed or refractory acute myeloid leukaemia with a susceptible isocitrate dehydrogenase-1 (IDH1) mutation.
32.	Krazati	Adagrasib	12/12/2022	To manage KRAS G12C-mutated locally advanced or metastatic non-small cell lung cancer in adults who have received at least one prior systemic therapy.
33.	Sunlenca	Lenacapavir	22/12/2022	To treat adults with HIV whose HIV infections cannot be successfully treated with other available treatments due to resistance, intolerance, or safety considerations.
34.	Lunsumio	Mosunetuzumab-axgb	22/12/2022	To manage adults with relapsed or refractory follicular lymphoma, a type of non-Hodgkin lymphoma.
35.	Xenoview	Hyperpolarized xe-129	23/12/2022	Evaluation of pulmonary function and imaging.
36.	Briumvi	Ublituximab-xiiy	28/12/2022	To treat relapsing forms of multiple sclerosis.
37.	Nexobrid	Anacaulase-bcdb	28/12/2022	To remove eschar in adults with deep partial thickness or full thickness thermal burns.

References:

1. U.S. Food and Drug Administration. Novel Drug Approvals for 2022 [Internet]. Silver Spring (MD): FDA; 2022 [cited 2025 Jun 12]. Available from: https://www.fda.gov/drugs/novel-drug-approvals-fda/novel-drug-approvals-2022.

Chapter 45

Novel FDA Drug Approvals for 2021

Table 1: Latest FDA Pharmaceutical authorizations for 2021.

Sl. No.	Brand Name	Generic Drug	Date of Approval (DD/MM/YYY)	FDA-Approved Indication
1.	Verquvo	Vericiguat	19/01/2021	To mitigate the risk of cardiovascular death and hospitalization for chronic heart failure.
2.	Cabenuva	Cabotegravir and rilpivirine (co-packaged)	21/01/2021	HIV treatment.
3.	Lupkynis	Voclosporin	22/01/2021	To treat Lupus nephritis.
4.	Tepmetko	Tepotinib	03/02/2021	Medical management of non-small cell lung cancer.
5.	Ukoniq	Umbralisib	05/02/2021	Marginal zone lymphoma and follicular lymphoma management.
6.	Evkeeza	Evinacumab-dgnb	11/02/2021	Homozygous familial hypercholesterolemia management.
7.	Cosela	Trilacicilib	12/02/2021	Medical management of chemotherapy-induced myelosuppression in small cell lung cancer.
8.	Amondys 45	Casimersen	25/02/2021	Duchenne muscular dystrophy treatment.
9.	Nulibry	Fosdenopterin	2/26/2021	To treat Molybdenum cofactor deficiency Type A.
10.	Pepaxto	Melphalan flufenamide	26/02/2021	To treat relapsed or refractory multiple myeloma
11.	Azstarys	Serdexmethylphenidate and dexmethylphenidate	02/03/2021	To manage attention deficit hyperactivity disorder.
12.	Fotivda	Tivozanib	10/03/2021	To treat renal cell carcinoma.
13.	Ponvory	Ponesimod	18/03/2021	Medical management of relapsing forms of multiple sclerosis.
14.	Zegalogue	Dasiglucagon	22/03/2021	Severe hypoglycaemia treatment.
15.	Qelbree	Viloxazine	02/04/2021	To treat attention deficit hyperactivity disorder (ADHD).
16.	Nextstellis	Drospirenone and estetrol	15/04/2021	Contraception.
17.	Jemperli	Dostarlimab-gxly	22/04/2021	Endometrial cancertreatment.
18.	Zynlonta	Loncastuximabtesirine-lpyl	23/04/2021	Relapsed or refractory large B-cell lymphoma management.

19.	Empaveli	Pegcetacoplan	14/05/2021	Paroxysmal nocturnal haemoglobinuria treatment.
20.	Rybrevant	Amivantamab-vmjw	21/05/2021	Non-small cell lung cancer treatment.
21.	Pylarify	Piflufolastat F 18	26/05/2021	To identify prostate-specific membrane antigen-positive lesions in prostate cancer.
22.	Lumakras	Sotorasib	28/05/2021	To treat non-small cell lung cancer.
23.	Truseltiq	Infigratinib	28/05/2021	Cholangiocarcinoma treatment.
24.	Lybalvi	Olanzapine and samidorphan	28/05/2021	To treat Schizophrenia and certain aspects of bipolar I disorder.
25.	Brexafemme	Ibrexafungerp	01/06/2021	To manage Vulvovaginal candidiasis.
26.	Aduhelm	Aducanumab-avwa	07/06/2021	To treat Alzheimer's disease.
27.	Rylaze	Asparaginase erwiniachrysanthemi (recombinant)-rywn	30/06/2021	To treat acute lymphoblastic leukaemia and lymphoblastic lymphoma in patients who are allergic to E. Coli-derived asparaginase products, as a component of a chemotherapy regimen.
28.	Kerendia	Finerenone	09/07/2021	To reduce the risk of kidney and heart complications in chronic kidney disease associated with type 2 diabetes.
29.	Fexinidazole	Fexinidazole	16/07/2021	To treat human African trypanosomiasis caused by the parasite Trypanosoma brucei gambiense.
30.	Rezurock	Belumosudil	16/07/2021	Management of chronic graft-versus-host disease after failure of at least two prior lines of systemic therapy.
31.	Bylvay	Odevixibat	20/07/2021	Pruritus management.
32.	Saphnelo	Anifrolumab-fnia	30/07/2021	Medical management of moderate-to severe systemic lupus erythematousus along with standard therapy.
33.	Nexviazyme	Avalglucosidase alfa-ngpt	06/08/2021	Late-onset Pompe disease management.
34.	Welireg	Belzutifan	13/08/2021	To treat Von Hippel-Lindau disease under certain conditions.
35.	Korsuva	Difelikefalin	23/08/2021	To treat moderate-to-severe pruritus associated with chronic kidney disease in certain populations.
36.	Skytrofa	Lonapegsomatropin-tcgd	25/08/2021	To treat short stature due to inadequate secretion of endogenous growth hormone.

37.	Exkivity	Mobocertinib	15/09/2021	To manage locally advanced or metastatic non-small cell lung cancer with epidermal growth factor receptor exon 20 insertion mutations.
38.	Tivdak	Tisotumabvedotin-tftv	20/09/2021	To treat recurrent or metastatic cervical cancer with disease progression on or after chemotherapy.
39.	Qulipta	Atogepant	28/09/2021	Migraine prophylaxis.
40.	Livmarli	Maralixibat	29/09/2021	To treat cholestatic pruritus associated with Alagille syndrome.
41.	Tavneos	Avacopan	07/10/2021	Medical management of severe active anti-neutrophil cytoplasmic autoantibody-associated vasculitis (granulomatosis with polyangiitis and microscopic polyangiitis) in combination with standard therapy, including glucocorticoids.
42.	Scemblix	Asciminib	29/10/2021	To treat Philadelphia chromosome-positive chronic myeloid leukaemia with disease that meets certain criteria.
43.	Besremi	Ropeginterferon alfa-2b-njft	12/11/2021	To manage Polycythaemia vera, a blood disease that causes the overproduction of red blood cells.
44.	Voxzogo	Vosoritide	19/11/2021	To improve growth in children five years of age and older with achondroplasia and open epiphyses.
45.	Livtencity	Maribavir	23/11/2021	To treat post-transplant cytomegalovirus (CMV) infection/ disease that does not respond (with or without genetic mutations that cause resistance) to available antiviral treatment for CMV.
46.	Cytalux	Pafolacianine	29/11/2021	Identification of ovarian cancer lesions.
47.	Tezspire	Tezepelumab-ekko	17/12/2021	To treat severe asthma as an add-on maintenance therapy.
48.	Vyvgart	Efgartigimod alfa-fcab	17/12/2021	Generalized myasthenia gravis treatment.
49.	Leqvio	Inclisiran	22/12/2021	To treat heterozygous familial hypercholesterolemia or clinical atherosclerotic cardiovascular disease as an add-on therapy.
50.	Adbry	Tralokinumab-ldrm	27/12/2021	To manage moderate-to-severe atopic dermatitis.

References:

1. U.S. Food and Drug Administration. Novel Drug Approvals for 2021 [Internet]. Silver Spring (MD): FDA; 2024 May 22 [cited 2025 Apr 21]. Available from: https://www.fda.gov/drugs/novel-drug-approvals-fda/novel-drug-approvals-2021.

Chapter 46

Novel CDSCO Drug Approvals for 2025

Table 1: Latest CDSCO Pharmaceutical authorizations for 2025 (Up to 12/06/2025).

Sl. No.	Drug Name	Date of Approval (DD/MM/YYYY)	Indication
1.	Tafamidis	16/01/2025	To treat wild-type or inherited transthyretin amyloidosis in adult patients exhibiting cardiomyopathy (ATTR-CM).
2.	Letermovir	17/01/2025	Prophylaxis of cytomegalovirus (CMV) infection and illness in adult CMV-seropositive recipients of an allogeneic haematopoietic stem cell transplant. Prophylaxis of CMV illness in adult kidney transplant recipients at elevated risk (Donor CMV seropositive/Recipient CMV seronegative [D+/R-]).
3.	Fexuprazan hydrochloride	10/02/2025	Medical management of Erosive esophagitis(EE).
4.	Edoxaban Tosylate	20/02/2025	Prevention of stroke and systemic embolism in adult patients with non-valvular atrial fibrillation (NVAF) who possess one or more risk factors, including congestive heart failure, hypertension, age ≥ 75 years, diabetes mellitus, or a history of stroke or transient ischaemic attack (TIA). Management of deep vein thrombosis (DVT) and pulmonary embolism (PE), as well as for the prophylaxis of recurrent DVT and PE in adults.
5.	Sodium Zirconium Cyclosilicate	05/03/2025	Treatment of hyperkalaemia in adult patients.
6.	Rimegepant	27/03/2025	Acute management of migraine, with or without aura, in individuals who have previously demonstrated an inadequate response to triptans.
7.	Doravirine	28/03/2025	To be used in conjunction with other antiretroviral medicines for the management of HIV-1 infection in adults and paediatric patients weighing a minimum of 35 kg with no previous history of antiretroviral treatment (treatment naïve).

8.	Zanubrutinib	08/04/2025	This treatment is suggested for adult patients with mantle cell lymphoma (MCL) who have undergone at least one prior therapy. Waldenström's macroglobulinemia (WM). Patients with relapsed or refractory marginal zone lymphoma (MZL) who have undergone at least one anti-CD20-based treatment regimen. Chronic lymphocytic leukaemia (CLL) or small lymphocytic lymphoma (SLL). Relapsed or refractory follicular lymphoma (FL), in conjunction with obinutuzumab, following two or more courses of systemic therapy.
9.	Tucatinib	08/04/2025	Recommended in conjunction with trastuzumab and capecitabine for the treatment of adult patients with advanced unresectable or metastatic HER2-positive breast cancer, including those with brain metastases, who have undergone one or more previous anti-HER2-based therapies in the metastatic context.
10.	Linaclotide	21/04/2025	Indicated for adults in the management of chronic idiopathic constipation.
11.	Siponimod	09/05/2025	For the management of individuals with secondary progressive multiple sclerosis (SPMS) exhibiting active disease, as indicated by relapses or imaging characteristics of inflammatory activity.
12.	Ivosidenib	14/05/2025	It is suggested in conjunction with Azacitidine for the treatment of adult patients with newly diagnosed acute myeloid leukaemia (AML) possessing an isocitrate dehydrogenase-1 (IDH1) R132 mutation who are ineligible for routine induction chemotherapy. As a monotherapy for the treatment of adult patients with locally advanced or metastatic cholangiocarcinoma exhibiting an IDH1 R132 mutation, who have previously undergone at least one line of systemic therapy.
13.	Tegoprazan	28/05/2025	Recommended for: Erosive gastroesophageal reflux disease, non-erosive gastroesophageal reflux disease, and gastric ulcer.

References:

1. Central Drugs Standard Control Organization. List of new drugs approved in the year 2025 till date [Internet]. New Delhi (IN): CDSCO; 2025 [cited 2025 Jun 12]. Available from: https://cdsco.gov.in/opencms/opencms/system/modules/CDSCO.WEB/elements/download_file_division.jsp?num_id=MTI2NDQ=.

Chapter 47

Novel CDSCO Drug Approvals for 2024

Table 1: Latest CDSCO Pharmaceutical authorizations for 2024.

Sl. No.	Drug Name	Date of Approval (DD/MM/YYYY)	Indication
1.	Tirzepatide	19/01/2024	Type 2 diabetes mellitus management.
2.	Plazomicin	02/02/2024	To treat adult patients for the treatment of complex urinary tract infections (cUTI), including pyelonephritis, caused by the following susceptible microorganisms: Escherichia coli, Klebsiella pneumoniae, Proteus mirabilis, and Enterobacter cloacae.
3.	Etifoxine Hydrochloride	21/03/2024	To treat psychosomatic anxiety manifestations.
4.	Vonoprazan fumarate	08/05/2024	To treat reflux oesophagitis (RE), gastric ulcer (GU), duodenal ulcer (DU), prevention of gastric or duodenal ulcer recurrence with low-dose aspirin therapy. Prevention of recurrence of gastric or duodenal ulcers following NSAID use. Used as an adjunct to Helicobacter pylori eradication associated, with gastric ulcer, duodenal ulcer, gastric MALT lymphoma, idiopathic thrombocytopenic purpura, the stomach post-endoscopic resection of early-stage malignancy, or Helicobacter pylori gastritis.
5.	rdESAT-6 and rCFP-10 (Cy-Tb) injection	16/05/2024	Detection of latent tuberculosis in individuals aged one year and older and also in detection of Latent TB for populations under one year of age in implementation research mode just inside the National program.
6.	Selpercatinib	16/05/2024	To treat adult patients with metastatic RET fusion-positive non-small cell lung carcinoma (NSCLC). To manage adult and paediatric patients aged 12 years and older with advanced or metastatic RET mutant medullary thyroid carcinoma (MTC) necessitating systemic therapy. To treat adult and paediatric patients aged 12 years and older with advanced or metastatic RET fusion-positive thyroid cancer necessitating systemic therapy and who are resistive to radioactive iodine, if applicable.
7.	Nelarabine	31/05/2024	To treat T-cell Lymphoblastic leukaemia and T-cell Lymphoblastic lymphoma in both adult and paediatric patients aged 1 year and older, whose condition has either not responded to or has recurred after undergoing at least two chemotherapy regimens.

8.	Enmetazobactam & Cefipime	31/05/2024	Indicated for the treatment of adult patients for: • Complicated urinary tract infections (CUTI), including acute pyelonephritis. • Hospital-acquired pneumonia (HAP), including ventilator-associated pneumonia (VAP). • Bacteraemia associated with severe urinary tract infection or nosocomial pneumonia.
9.	Methenamine	09/07/2024	Prevention and management of urinary tract infections. Prevention of urinary tract infections, particularly in individuals with catheters. Asymptomatic bacteriuria, long-term treatment for the prevention of recurrent cystitis.
10.	Sodium Phenylbutyrate	09/07/2024	Designated as supplementary therapy for the chronic care of patients with urea cycle diseases characterised by deficits in carbamyl phosphate synthetase (CPS), ornithine transcarbamylase (OTC), or argininosuccinic acid synthetase (AS). It is indicated for all individuals with neonatal-onset insufficiency (complete enzymatic impairment occurring within the first 28 days of life). It is also indicated for patients with late-onset illnesses (partial enzymatic impairment, manifesting after the first month of birth) who have a history of hyperammonemic encephalopathy.
11.	Elobixibat	15/07/2024	To treat chronic constipation, excluding cases linked to organic illnesses.
12.	Tedizolid Phosphate	19/07/2024	To treat acute bacterial skin and skin structure infections (ABSSSI) in adults and adolescents aged 12 years and older.
13.	Remifentanil	31/07/2024	Opioid analgesic used in anaesthesia.
14.	Pimavanserin	02/08/2024	Medical management of hallucinations and delusions related to Parkinson's disease psychosis.
15.	Elagolix Sodium	09/08/2024	To treat moderate to severe pain related to endometriosis.
16.	Brigatinib	18/09/2024	Designated as monotherapy for the management of adult patients with anaplastic lymphoma kinase (ALK)-positive advanced non-small cell lung cancer (NSCLC) who have not previously received treatment with an ALK inhibitor. Brigatinib is approved as monotherapy for adult patients with ALK-positive advanced non-small cell lung cancer (NSCLC) who have previously had treatment with crizotinib.
17.	Mavacamten	08/10/2024	To treat symptomatic obstructive hypertrophic cardiomyopathy (oHCM) classified as New York Heart Association (NYHA) class II-III in adult patients.

18.	Ferumoxytol	08/10/2024	Iron replacement product suggested for the treatment of iron deficiency anaemia (IDA) in adult patients: • who exhibit resistance to oral iron or have seen an inadequate response to oral iron, or • who suffer from chronic kidney disease (CKD).
19.	Belumosudil	22/11/2024	To treat patients aged 12 years and older with chronic Graft-versus-Host Disease (cGvHD) following the ineffectiveness of at least two previous systemic therapies.
20.	Lumateperone	26/12/2024	To treat depressive episodes linked to bipolar I or II disorder (bipolar depression) in adults, both as monotherapy and as supplementary therapy with lithium or valproate.
21.	Trelagliptin	26/12/2024	Type 2 diabetes mellitus management.

References:

1. Central Drugs Standard Control Organization. List of new drugs approved in the year 2024 [Internet]. New Delhi (IN): CDSCO; 2024 Nov 26 [cited 2025 Apr 21]. Available from: https://cdsco.gov.in/opencms/opencms/system/modules/CDSCO.WEB/elements/download_file_division.jsp?num_id=MTI2NDQ=.

Chapter 48

Novel CDSCO Drug Approvals for 2023

Table 2: Latest CDSCO Pharmaceutical authorizations for 2023.

Sl. No.	Drug Name	Date of Approval (DD/MM/YYYY)	Indication
1.	Fesoterodine	06/01/2023	Treatment of overactive bladder with symptoms of urge urinary incontinence, urgency and frequency.
2.	Trifarotene	13/01/2023	Medical management of Acne Vulgaris of the face and /or trunk in patients 12 years of age and older.
3.	Crisaborole	20/01/2023	To treat mild to moderate atopic dermatitis in adults and paediatric patients aged 2 years and older.
4.	Prussian Blue & Magnesium Hydroxide	20/01/2023	The decorporation agent is approved for the treatment of patients with confirmed or suspected internal contamination by radioactive caesium and/ or radioactive or non-radioactive thallium to enhance their removal rates.
5.	Prussian Blue	27/01/2023	In order to improve the rates of elimination of patients with known or suspected internal contamination with radioactive caesium and/ or radioactive or non-radioactive thallium, this decorporation agent is recommended.
6.	Imeglimin	06/01/2023	Type-2 Diabetes mellitus management.
7.	Crisaborole	10/02/2023	To treat mild to moderate atopic dermatitis in adults and paediatric patients aged 2 years and older.
8.	Remifentanil	15/02/2023	As an analgesic for induction and maintenance of general anaesthesia in both inpatient and outpatient procedures. To maintain analgesia during the immediate postoperative phase in adult patients under the direct supervision of an anaesthesia practitioner in a postoperative anaesthesia care unit or intensive care environment. As an analgesic element of supervised anaesthesia management in adult patients.
9.	Cannabidiol	06/04/2023	Treatment of seizures associated with Lennox-Gastaut syndrome, Dravet Syndrome, or tuberous sclerosis complex in patients 1 year of age and older.

10.	3-(trimethoxysilyl) propyl dimethyl octadecylammonumchloride, Benzalkonium chloride, & Didecyl Dimethyl ammonium chloride	24/04/2023	Surface disinfectant and hand sanitizer.
11.	Ibuprofen	26/04/2023	For the alleviation of mild to moderate pain, including headache, backache, dysmenorrhea, tooth pain, neuralgia, rheumatic and muscular pain, migraine, cold and flu symptoms, sore throat, and fever.
12.	Niraparib	01/05/2023	Monotherapy for the maintenance treatment of adult patients with advanced epithelial (FIGO stage III and IV) high-grade ovarian, fallopian tube, or primary peritoneal cancer who exhibit a response (complete or partial) after completing first-line platinum-based chemotherapy. Monotherapy for the maintenance treatment of adult patients with platinum-sensitive relapsed high-grade serous epithelial ovarian, fallopian tube, or primary peritoneal cancer who exhibit a response (complete or partial) to platinum-based chemotherapy.
13.	Polmacoxib	01/05/2023	To manage idiopathic (primary) osteoarthritis of the hip/knee.
14.	Amines, N- C10-16-alkyl trimethylenedi-, reaction products with chloro acetic acid 1.0000%	04/05/2023	Surface disinfectant, aerial misting, hand sanitisation (not for COVID-19 use).
15.	Squaric Acid	04/05/2023	Disinfection of inanimate surface like floor, toilet, garbage areas only.
16.	Dalbavancin	23/05/2023	Adult patients with acute bacterial skin and skin structure infections (ABSSSI) should be treated with dalabavancin injection. These infections are brought on by susceptible isolates of the following Gram-positive microorganisms: Enterococcus faecalis (vancomycin susceptible strains), Staphylococcus aureus (including methicillin susceptible and methicillin resistant strains), Streptococcus pyogenes, Streptococcus agalactiae, Streptococcus dysgalactiae, and Streptococcus angiosus group (including S. anginosus, S. intermedius, and S. constellatus).
17.	Lobeglitazone Sulfate + Glimepiride	23/05/2023	Recommended as an addition to diet and exercise to enhance glycaemic control in individuals with type 2 diabetes mellitus who are currently receiving treatment with a thiazolidinedione and sulfonylurea, or who exhibit insufficient glycaemic control on either a thiazolidinedione or a sulfonylurea alone.
18.	Sovateltide	31/05/2023	Medical management of cerebral ischemic stroke.

19.	Lifitegrast	05/06/2023	To treat Dry eye disease (DED).
20.	Plecanatide	08/06/2023	Treatment of chronic idiopathic constipation (CIC) and irritable bowel syndrome with constipation (IBS-C).
21.	Treprostinil	27/07/2023	To treat idiopathic or hereditary pulmonary arterial hypertension (PAH) to enhance exercise capacity and alleviate illness symptoms in patients categorised as New York Heart Association (NYHA) functional class III.
22.	Icaridin	19/09/2023	Used as mosquito and insectrepellent.
23.	Inclisiran	22/09/2023	Inclisiran is intended for adults with primary hypercholesterolaemia (both heterozygous familial and non-familial) or mixed dyslipidaemia, as an addition to dietary management: in conjunction with a statin or a statin combined with other lipid-lowering therapies for patients who cannot achieve LDL-C targets with the maximum tolerated dose of a statin, or either independently or in combination with other lipid-lowering therapies for patients who are intolerant to statins or for whom statins are contraindicated.
24.	Relugolix	16/10/2023	To treat advance prostate cancer in adult patients.
25.	Asciminib	20/10/2023	To treat adult patients with Philadelphia chromosome-positive chronic myeloid leukaemia (Ph+CML) in the chronic phase (CP), who have previously received two or more tyrosine kinase inhibitors (TKIs). Also used in Philadelphia chromosome-positive chronic myeloid leukaemia with the T315I mutation.
26.	Lasmiditan	29/11/2023	Migraine treatment with or without aura in adult.
27.	Abrocitinib	29/11/2023	To treat adults with refractory, moderate-to-severe atopic dermatitis that is inadequately managed by other systemic medications, including biologics, or when the use of such therapies is contraindicated.

References:

1. Central Drugs Standard Control Organization. List of new drugs approved in the year 2023 till date [Internet]. New Delhi (IN): CDSCO; 2023 [cited 2025 Apr 21]. Available from: https://cdsco.gov.in/opencms/opencms/system/modules/CDSCO.WEB/elements/download_file_division.jsp?num_id=MTI2NDQ=.

Chapter 49

Novel CDSCO Drug Approvals for 2022

Table 1: Latest CDSCO Pharmaceutical authorizations for 2022.

Sl. No.	Drug Name	Date of Approval (DD/MM/YYYY)	Indication
1.	Triamcinolone	20/01/2022	For intraarticular, intra-synovial, or periarticular administration in adults and adolescents for the symptomatic management of subacute and chronic inflammatory joint disorders, including rheumatoid arthritis, Juvenile Idiopathic Arthritis (JIA), osteoarthritis, post-traumatic arthritis, synovitis, tendinitis, bursitis, and epicondylitis.
2.	Gimeracil, Oteracil potassium & Tegafur	01/02/2022	Advanced gastric cancer management when administered in conjunction with cisplatin.
3.	Topiroxostat	04/02/2022	Gout, hyperuricemia treatment.
4.	Nitric oxide nasal spray	08/02/2022	To treat adult high-risk patients with mild Covid-19 having risk of progression of the disease.
5.	Vericiguat	25/02/2022	To reduce the risk ofcardiovascular death and heart failure(HF) hospitalization following ahospitalization for heart failure or needforoutpatient IV diuretics, in adults with symptomatic chronic HF and ejectionfraction less than 45%.
6.	Inosine	02/03/2022	As add on therapy for treatment of mildCovid-19 patients with co-morbidities andmoderate Covid-19 patients, in light of Covid 19 outbreak for restrictedemergency use in the country.
7.	Desidustat	03/03/2022	Medical management of anaemia in adult patients with chronic kidney disease (CKD) not ondialysis and on dialysis.
8.	Lumacaftor & Ivacaftor	11/03/2022	Cystic fibrosis (CF) treatment in patient aged 2 years and older who are homozygous for the F508del mutation in the CFTR gene.
9.	Liothyronine	04/04/2022	To treat some of the more severe conditions in which the thyroiddoes notproduce enough thyroxine and balance the effect of medicines used to treat an overactive thyroid.
10.	Polyhexamethylene guanidine hydrochloride	06/04/2022	Surface disinfectant.

11.	Finerenone	11/04/2022	Recommended to mitigate the risk of persistent eGFR decline, end-stage renal disease, cardiovascular mortality, non-fatal myocardial infarction, and hospitalization due to heart failure in adult patients with chronic kidney disease (CKD) linked to type 2 diabetes (T2D).
12.	Sugammadex	18/04/2022	Reversal of neuromuscular blockadeinduced by rocuronium or vecuronium in adults undergoing surgery.
13.	Nirmatrelvir & Ritonavir	21/04/2022	To treat adult patients withCOVID-19, with SpO2 >93% and who have high risk of progression of the disease including hospitalization or death,in light of Covid 19 outbreak for restricted emergency use in the country.
14.	Aviptadil	29/04/2022	Treatment of patients with severe COVID-19 with Acute Respiratory Distress Syndrome (ARDS), in light of COVID 19 outbreak for restricted emergency use in the country.
15.	Bempedoic acid	09/05/2022	Adjunct to diet and maximally toleratedstatin therapy for the treatment of adults with heterozygous familial hypercholesterolemia or established atherosclerotic cardiovasculardisease who require additional lowering of LDL-C.
16.	rdESAT-6; rCFP-10 and rdESAT-6 and rCFP-10 (Cy-Tb) injection	09/05/2022	For detection of Latent TB for population of 18 years and above.
17.	Pralsetinib	26/05/2022	To treat adult patients with metastatic rearranged during transfection (RET) fusion-positive non- small cell lung cancer. To manage adult and paediatric patients 12 years of age and older with advanced or metastatic RET-mutant medullary thyroid cancer who require systemic therapy. Treatment of adult and paediatric patients 12 years of age and older with advanced or metastatic RET-fusion positive thyroid cancer who require systemic therapy and who are radioactive iodine-refractory (if radioactive iodine is appropriate).
18.	Nitisinone	09/06/2022	To treat Hereditary tyrosinemia type 1 (HT 1) in combination with dietary restriction of tyrosine and phenylalanine and treatment of adult patients with Alkaptonuria (AKU).
19.	Tepotinibe	12/08/2022	Management of adult patients with metastatic non-small cell lung cancer (NSCLC) who have mesenchymal-epithelial transition (MET) exon 14 skipping alterations.

20.	Lobeglitazone Sulfate	16/09/2022	Adult type 2 diabetes mellitus patients as monotherapy: • who are inadequately controlled by diet & exercise, for whom metformin is inappropriate because of contraindications or intoleranceor as dual oral therapy in combination with. • who are inadequately controlled by diet& exercise and taking metformin despitemaximal tolerated dose of metformin monotherapy. • who are inadequately controlled by diet& exercise and taking a sulphonylurea atmaximal tolerated dose of sulphonylurea monotherapy in which metformin is inappropriate because of contraindications or intolerance.
21.	Idelalisib	14/10/2022	To manage relapsed chronic lymphocytic leukaemia (CLL), in combination with rituximab, in patients for whom rituximab alone would be considered appropriate therapy due to other co-morbidities. Relapsed follicular B-cell non-Hodgkin lymphoma (FL) in patients who have received at least two prior systemic therapies. Relapsed small lymphocytic lymphoma (SLL) in patients who have received at least two prior systemic therapies.
22.	Bempedoic acid + Ezetimbe	07/11/2022	Indicated as an adjunct to diet andmaximally tolerated statin therapy for the treatment of adults with heterozygousfamilial hypercholesterolemia or established atherosclerotic cardiovascular disease who require additional lowering of LDL-C.
23.	Naftifine HCL	09/11/2022	Superficial fungal infection of the skin (tinea corporisand Tinea cruris) treatment.
24.	Entrectinib	18/11/2022	To treat adult patients with metastatic non-smallcell lung cancer (NSCLC) whose tumoursare ROS1-positive. Adult and paediatric patients 12 years of age and older with solid tumours that: 1. Have a neurotrophictyrosine receptor kinase (NTRK) genefusion without a known acquiredresistance mutation. 2. Are metastatic or where surgical resection is likely to resultin severe morbidity and 3. Have progressed following treatment or have nosatisfactory alternative therapy.
25.	Sitagliptin Fentanil Phaohate	29/11/2022	Type-2 Diabetes Mellitus management.
26.	Imeglimin	06/10/2022	Type-2 Diabetes Mellitus management.

27.	Apalutamide	18/11/2022	Metastatic castration-resistant prostate cancer (M-CRPC) and non-metastatic, castration resistant prostate cancer (NM-CRPC) treatment.
28.	Icatibant	02/12/2022	Treatment of acute attacks of hereditary angioedema (HAE) in adults 18 years of age and older.
29.	Lobeglitazone & Metformin	30/12/2022	As an adjunct to diet and exercise– inpatients who have inadequate glycaemic control with maximum tolerated dose of metformin alone or in patients who are already receiving combination therapy of lobeglitazone and metformin.
30.	Sodium Glycerophosphate	30/12/2022	Medical management of hypophosphatemia due to refeeding syndrome.
31.	Gilteritinib	30/12/2022	To manage adult patients who have relapsed or refractory acute myeloid leukaemia (AML) with as FLT3 mutation.

References:

1. Central Drugs Standard Control Organization. List of new drugs approved in the year 2022 till date [Internet]. New Delhi (IN): CDSCO; 2022 [cited 2025 Apr 21]. Available from: https://cdsco.gov.in/opencms/opencms/system/modules/CDSCO.WEB/elements/download_file_division.jsp?num_id=MTI2NDQ=.

Chapter 50

Novel CDSCO Drug Approvals for 2021

Table 1: Latest CDSCO Pharmaceutical authorizations for 2021.

Sl. No.	Drug Name	Date of Approval (DD/MM/YYYY)	Indication
1.	Avanafil	26/02/2021	To treat erectile dysfunction.
2.	Omidenepag	12/03/2021	Glaucoma and ocularhypertension management.
3.	Ozenoxacin	15/04/2021	Topical management of impetigo due to staphylococcus aureus or streptococcus pyogenes in adult andpaediatric patients 2 months of age andolder.
4.	2-Deoxy-D-Glucose	01/05/2021	As an adjunct therapy in moderate tosevere COVID-19 patients.
5.	Capmatinib	12/05/2021	Medical management of adult patient withmetastatic non-small cell lung cancer(NSCLC) whose tumours have a mutationthat leads to mesenchymal epithelialtransition (MET) exon 14 skipping.
6.	Rucaparib	12/05/2021	Ovarian cancer & Prostate cancer management.
7.	Trientine	08/06/2021	Medical management of Wilson's disease (hepatolenticular degeneration) in patientsintolerant to Penicillamine. It should beused when continued treatment withPenicillamine is no longer possible because of intolerable or life endangering side effects.
8.	Vigabatrin	18/06/2021	For the treatment of 1) Refractory Complex Partial seizures asadjunctive therapy in patients 2 years ofage and older who have respondedinadequately to several alternative treatments. 2) Infantile Spasms - monotherapy ininfants 1 month to 2 years of age for whom the potential benefits outweigh thepotential risk of vision loss.
10.	Cangrelor	21/06/2021	As an adjunct to percutaneous coronary intervention (PCI) to reduce therisk of periprocedural myocardial infarction (MI), repeat coronary revascularization, and stent thrombosis (ST) in patients who have not been treated with a P2Y12 platelet inhibitor and are not being given a glycoprotein IIb/IIIa inhibitor.
11.	Rifapentine	28/06/2021	Treatment of latent tuberculosis, caused by Mycobacterium tuberculosis (For use in NTEP only).
12.	Lemborexant	01/07/2021	Medical management of insomnia.
13.	Cetilistat	09/07/2021	Treatment of obesity (limited to patients with both type 2 diabetes mellitus and dyslipidaemia, and with a BMI ≥ 25 kg/m2 inspite of dietary treatment and /or exercise therapy).

14.	Benzonatate	15/07/2021	Refractory cough management.
15.	Cariprazine	16/07/2021	For the treatment of Schizophrenia inadults. Acute treatment of manic or mixedepisodes associated with bipolar I disorder in adults.
16.	Gadoteridol	29/07/2021	For intravenous use in magnetic resonance imaging (MRI) in adults andpaediatric patients over 2 years of age forwhole body MRI including the head, neck, liver, breast, musculoskeletal system and soft tissue pathologies.
17.	Darolutamide	13/08/2021	Non-metastatic castration resistant prostate cancer (nmCRPC) management.
18.	Tetracosactide	13/08/2021	Diagnostic test for the investigation ofadrenocortical insufficiency.
19.	Cabozantinib	10/09/2021	Management of advanced renal cell carcinoma (RCC) & Hepatocellular Carcinoma (HCC) who have been previously treated with sorafenib.
20.	Tipiracil& FDC of Trifluridine + Tipiracil	16/09/2021	Treatment of adult patients with metastatic colorectalcancer who have been previously treatedwith fluoropyrimidine, oxaliplatin andirinotecan-based chemotherapy, an anti-VEGF biological therapy, and RAS wild-type, an anti-EGFR therapy.
21.	Selumetinib	17/09/2021	Medical management of adult patients with metastatic gastric orgastroesophageal junctionadenocarcinoma previously treated with at least two prior lines of chemotherapy that included a fluoropyrimidine, a platinum, either a taxane or irinotecan, and if appropriate, HER2/ neu-targeted therapy. Management of paediatric patients 3 years of age and older with neurofibromatosis type 1 (NF1) and who have symptomatic, inoperable plexiform neurofibromas (PN).
22.	Biapenem	17/09/2021	Medical management of complicated urinary tract infections.
23.	Tafamidis	30/11/2021	To treat wild-type or hereditary transthyretin amyloidosis in adult patients with cardiomyopathy (ATTR-CM).
24.	Molnupiravir	28/12/2021	Adult patients with COVID-19, with SpO2 >93% and who havehigh risk of progression of the disease including hospitalization or death, in lightof COVID-19 outbreak for restrictedemergency use in the country.
25.	Selexipag	31/12/2021	Treatment of Pulmonary Arterial Hypertension (PAH, WHO Group I) to delay disease progression and reduce the risk of hospitalization for PAH.

References:

1. Central Drugs Standard Control Organization. List of new drugs approved in the year 2021 till date [Internet]. New Delhi (IN): CDSCO; 2021 Dec [cited 2025 Apr 25]. Available from: https://cdsco.gov.in/opencms/opencms/system/modules/CDSCO.WEB/elements/download_file_division.jsp?num_id=MTI2NDQ=.

Quick Bites

Newer Drug Delivery System

Nanoparticles

Tiny carriers (10–1000 nm) that deliver drugs in a targeted and controlled manner, often coated with ligands to bind specific receptors. Improve bioavailability and efficacy but involve complex manufacturing and possible toxicity risks.

Examples: Abraxane (FDA-approved for cancers), Onivyde (FDA-approved for metastatic pancreatic cancer).

Liposomes

Spherical vesicles made of lipid bilayers, encapsulating hydrophilic and lipophilic drugs. They merge with cell membranes for drug delivery, offering biocompatibility and reduced toxicity but face stability and cost challenges.

Examples: Doxil (FDA-approved for cancer), AmBisome (FDA-approved for fungal infections).

Microneedles

Micron-sized painless needles create micro-channels in the skin to deliver drugs directly into capillaries. They bypass first-pass metabolism but allow only limited dosing.

Examples: Qtrypta (FDA-approved for migraine), MicronJet (under trials for insulin).

Implantable Devices

Devices surgically implanted for controlled, long-term drug release through diffusion or degradation. They boost compliance but require surgery and carry infection risks.

Examples: Norplant (FDA-approved for contraception), Gliadel Wafer (FDA-approved for glioblastoma).

Hydrogels

Three-dimensional, water-retaining polymer networks that release drugs via swelling and diffusion. Highly biocompatible, though mechanically fragile with limited loading capacity.

Examples: HemCon bandage (FDA-approved for wound healing), ReGel (under trials for cancer therapy).

Other Emerging Systems

1. **Occusert:** Ocular inserts releasing drugs over time, FDA-approved for glaucoma and dry eye (Lacrisert).
2. **Transdermal Patches:** Nicoderm and Duragesic patches provide steady systemic delivery through skin diffusion.
3. **Erythrosomes:** Drugs loaded into red blood cells for prolonged circulation; currently investigational.
4. **Micelles:** Amphiphilic structures improving solubility and targeting through enhanced permeability (e.g., Genexol-PM, SP1049C under trials).

Future Directions

Gene Therapy with Nanocarriers: Merging gene therapy and nanoparticles for treating genetic disorders.

Personalized Drug Delivery: Tailoring delivery systems based on genomics and proteomics profiles.

AI-Driven Drug Delivery: Machine learning is optimizing drug design, targeting, and release strategies, potentially reducing costs and development time.

Gene Therapy

Definition

Gene therapy is a medical technique aimed at treating or preventing diseases by modifying genetic information within a patient's cells. It works by replacing, inactivating, or introducing new genes to correct underlying conditions.

Vectors in Gene Therapy

- Plasmid DNA: Engineered circular DNA for gene transfer.
- Viral Vectors: Modified viruses (AAV, Lentivirus, Retrovirus) deliver therapeutic genes.
- Bacterial Vectors: Non-pathogenic bacteria used for gene delivery.
- Gene Editing Tools: CRISPR-Cas9 and others directly modify DNA.
- Patient-derived Cells: Modified ex vivo and reintroduced.

Principles of Action

- Gene Replacement: Substituting defective genes with functional ones.
- Gene Inactivation: Silencing malfunctioning genes.
- Gene Addition: Introducing new therapeutic genes.

Types of Gene Therapy

- Germline Gene Therapy: Modifies reproductive cells; experimental use.
- Somatic Gene Therapy: Alters non-reproductive cells; clinically approved use.

Modification Methods

- Ex Vivo: Genetic modification outside the body (e.g., CAR-T therapy).
- In Vivo: Direct delivery into the body (e.g., AAV-based treatments).

Procedure Overview

- Target gene identification
- Selection of viral or non-viral delivery method
- Gene insertion or editing
- Monitoring therapeutic effects and immune responses
- Long-term follow-up for safety

Applications of Gene Therapy

- Genetic Disorders: SMA (Zolgensma), Haemophilia, Sickle Cell Disease (Casgevy, Lyfgenia)
- Cancer: CAR-T cell therapy (Kymriah, Yescarta), Oncolytic virus therapy (T-VEC)
- Neurological Diseases: Huntington's, Parkinson's (early-stage trials)
- Eye Disorders: Inherited retinal dystrophy (Luxturna)
- Infectious Diseases: HIV gene editing under research

Advantages

- Potential curative approach for genetic diseases
- Possibility of one-time treatment
- Reduces lifelong medication burden
- Enables personalized medicine
- Lower systemic side effects compared to traditional treatments

Limitations

- Extremely high costs
- Risk of immune rejection
- Lack of extensive long-term safety data
- Ethical debates, particularly around germline editing
- Limited global access.

Stem Cell Therapy

Definition

Stem cell treatment utilizes stem cells to regenerate, repair, or replace damaged tissues and organs. Stem cells are obtained either autologously (from the patient) or allogeneically (from a donor).

Types of Stem Cells

- Embryonic Stem Cells (ESCs) are pluripotent and can differentiate into any cell type; however, their application is restricted due to ethical considerations.
- Adult Stem Cells (ASCs): Multipotent cells located in tissues such as bone marrow and adipose tissue; utilized in the treatment of leukemia and cardiovascular disorders.
- Induced Pluripotent Stem Cells (iPSCs): Reprogrammed somatic cells that circumvent ethical problems and facilitate personalized treatment.

Mode of Action

- Differentiate into specialized cells to regenerate damaged tissues.
- Secrete bioactive compounds that enhance cell viability and facilitate tissue regeneration.
- Regulate immune responses to diminish inflammation and autoimmune.

Summary of Procedure

- Assessment of the patient by medical history, imaging studies, and laboratory analyses.
- Stem cell procurement (autologous, allogeneic, embryonic stem cells, or induced pluripotent stem cells), succeeded by processing and amplification.
- Administration through intravenous infusion, intra-arterial delivery, intrathecal injection, direct tissue injection, or scaffold implantation.
- Post-treatment surveillance utilizing imaging and biomarker analysis.

Benefits

- Restores injured tissues and organs.
- Minimally invasive alternatives decrease surgical risks.
- Beneficially modulates the immunological system.
- Facilitates individualized therapies with enduring advantages.

Recent Developments

- Mesenchymal Stem Cells (MSCs): Therapeutic applications in graft-versus-host disease, Crohn's disease, and myocardial infarction.
- Induced pluripotent stem cells: Personalized treatments for amyotrophic lateral sclerosis, Parkinson's disease, and pharmacological evaluation.
- Neural Stem Cells (NSCs): Potential for neuronal replacement in neurodegenerative disorders.
- Hematopoietic Stem Cells (HSCs): Essential for hematological illnesses and increasing applications in gene therapy.

FDA-Approved Treatments

- HSCT: Conventional therapy for hematological malignancies and hereditary hematological conditions.
- Strimvelis and Zynteglo: Gene-modified autologous stem cell treatments.
- Remestemcel-L (Ryoncil): Mesenchymal stem cell treatment for pediatric graft-versus-host disease.

Challenges

- Ethical discussions over the utilization of embryonic stem cells continue.
- Risk of immunological rejection in allogeneic transplants.
- Concerns with tumorigenicity, especially in relation to embryonic stem cells (ESCs) and induced pluripotent stem cells (iPSCs).
- Regulatory intricacies impede the approval and widespread implementation of therapies.

Prospective Trajectories

- CRISPR-utilized gene-edited stem cells for the treatment of genetic disorders.
- Incorporation of bioengineering techniques (3D scaffolds, bioprinting) for the fabrication of transplantable tissues.
- Stem cell therapy to mitigate aging and prolong healthy lifespan.

Recent Advances in the Treatment of Glaucoma

Drug Name	Clinical Trial Phase	Mechanism of Action	Adverse Drug Reaction	Uses	Dose
Netarsudil	FDA-approved (Rhopressa); evaluated in ROCKET-1 & ROCKET-2 trials.	Inhibits Rho kinase (ROCK), enhancing trabecular meshwork outflow, reducing episcleral venous pressure (EVP), and decreasing aqueous humour production via NET inhibition.	Conjunctival hyperaemia, corneal verticillata, mild irritation, blurred vision.	First-line or adjunct treatment in primary open-angle glaucoma (POAG) and ocular hypertension (OHT).	0.02% ophthalmic solution, one drop daily in the evening (topical).
Latanoprostene Bunod	FDA-approved (Vyzulta); studied in VOYAGER and APOLLO trials.	Dual mechanism—prostaglandin F2α analog increases uveoscleral outflow; nitric oxide (NO) enhances trabecular outflow and reduces EVP.	Conjunctival hyperaemia, eyelash growth, iris pigmentation changes, macular oedema.	First-line IOP-lowering therapy for POAG and OHT.	0.024% ophthalmic solution, one drop daily in the evening (topical).
Bimatoprost SR (Sustained-Release Implant)	FDA-approved (Durysta); studied in ARTEMIS trials.	PGF2α analog increases uveoscleral outflow via ECM remodeling. Implant provides sustained drug release over 4–6 months.	Conjunctival hyperaemia, mild eye irritation, foreign body sensation, corneal endothelial cell loss.	Long-term management of POAG and OHT.	10 mcg intracameral implant, administered once every 4–6 months.
Travoprost Punctal Plug Delivery	Phase III trials ongoing.	PGF2α analog increases uveoscleral outflow. Delivered via biodegradable punctal plug for sustained release.	Conjunctival hyperaemia, punctal plug displacement, mild irritation, corneal epithelial defects.	Long-term IOP control in non-adherent POAG patients.	500–1000 mcg twice daily via topical punctal plug delivery.
Trabodenoson	Phase III trials completed; further approval pending.	Selective A1 adenosine receptor agonist. Increases trabecular meshwork outflow, remodels ECM, and shows potential neuroprotection.	Mild conjunctival hyperaemia, foreign body sensation, blurred vision.	Investigational for POAG and OHT.	15 mcg per plug inserted in lower punctum; sustained release for up to 90 days.

Recent Advances in the Treatment of Myasthenia Gravis

Drug Name	Clinical Trial Phase	Mechanism of Action	Adverse Drug Reaction	Uses	Dose
Rozanolixi-zumab	FDA approved in 2023 for generalized myasthenia gravis (gMG) in adults with AChR or MuSK antibodies.	Targets and blocks FcRn receptors, preventing IgG recycling. This reduces circulating pathogenic autoantibodies and improves neuromuscular transmission.	Headache, injection site reactions, nausea, infections, hypersensitivity.	Approved for gMG; under evaluation for CIDP.	7 mg/kg subcutaneously, once weekly for 6 weeks.
Zilucoplan	FDA approved in 2023 for AChR-positive gMG.	Inhibits complement C5 to block membrane attack complex (MAC) formation, reducing neuromuscular inflammation and tissue damage.	Injection site reactions, headache, fatigue, nausea, infections.	Approved for gMG; under investigation for NMOSD.	0.3 mg/kg subcutaneously, once daily.
Efgartigimod	FDA approved in 2021 for gMG; 2024 for CIDP.	Binds FcRn to prevent IgG autoantibody recycling. This lowers pathogenic IgG levels and reduces autoimmune attack at the neuromuscular junction.	Headache, site reactions, infections, hypersensitivity.	Approved for AChR-positive gMG and CIDP.	10 mg/kg IV once weekly for 4 weeks (1 cycle).
Ravulizumab	FDA approved for gMG (2022), NMOSD (2024), PNH, and aHUS.	Long-acting C5 inhibitor that prevents MAC formation, reducing complement-mediated neuromuscular injury with extended dosing intervals.	Meningococcal infections, infusion reactions, URTIs, headache.	Approved for gMG, NMOSD, PNH, aHUS.	Weight-based IV loading dose - maintenance every 8 weeks.
Batoclimab	Phase III for gMG and CIDP.	Inhibits FcRn, leading to rapid breakdown of IgG autoantibodies while sparing other immune components.	Dyslipidaemia, headache, mild GI symptoms, injection-site reactions.	Under investigation for gMG, CIDP, thyroid eye disease.	680 mg subcutaneously once weekly (clinical trial).

Recent Advances in General Anaesthesia

Drug Name	Clinical Trial Phase	Mechanism of Action	Adverse Drug Reaction	Uses	Dose
Ciprofol	Approved in China in 2020 for sedation during GI endoscopy; later expanded to bronchoscopy, general anaesthesia, and ICU sedation.	Acts as a GABA-A receptor agonist and positive allosteric modulator, enhancing chloride influx into neurons. This hyperpolarizes cell membranes and produces sedative and anaesthetic effects.	Respiratory depression, bradycardia, hypotension, arrhythmias.	Sedation and anaesthesia in procedural settings, ICU, and general induction.	0.4–0.5 mg/kg IV (induction); 0.2–0.3 mg/kg/h IV (maintenance).
Remimazolam	FDA approved in 2020 for procedural sedation; also approved in China and Japan.	Binds benzodiazepine sites on GABA-A receptors, increasing chloride influx and neuronal inhibition. Acts rapidly and is metabolised by non-specific esterases.	Headache, drowsiness, hypotension, involuntary movements.	General anaesthesia, ICU sedation, and procedural sedation (e.g., endoscopy).	6–12 mg/kg/h IV (induction); 1–2 mg/kg/h (maintenance).
Sugammadex	FDA approved for rapid reversal of neuromuscular blockade.	Encapsulates rocuronium and vecuronium in plasma, forming stable inclusion complexes that are renally excreted. This rapidly reverses neuromuscular blockade.	Nausea, headache, bradycardia, QT prolongation, dysgeusia.	Reversal of non-depolarizing neuromuscular blockade after surgery.	2 mg/kg IV (moderate block), 4 mg/kg IV (deep block), 16 mg/kg IV (rapid reversal).

Dexmedeto-midine	FDA approved for ICU and peri-procedural sedation.	Selective alpha-2 agonist that reduces norepinephrine release and sympathetic tone, producing sedation, analgesia, and anxiolysis without respiratory depression.	Bradycardia, hypotension, hypertension.	ICU sedation, procedural sedation, adjunctive analgesia, off-label uses include delirium, alcohol withdrawal, and insomnia.	1 μg/kg over 10 min (loading); 0.2–0.7 μg/kg/h (maintenance).
Cyclopropyl-Methoxycarbonyl Metomidate (CPMM)	Currently in Phase I trials.	Positive modulator of GABA-A receptors, enhancing GABA activity and producing rapid sedation. Designed to minimize adrenal suppression seen with etomidate.	Involuntary movements, hypotension, injection-site pain, nausea, vomiting.	Investigational agent for anaesthetic induction and maintenance.	Under evaluation.

Newer Sedatives and Hypnotics

Drug Name	Clinical Trial Phase	Mechanism of Action	Adverse Drug Reaction	Uses	Dose
Dual Orexin Receptor Antagonists (DORAs)	Suvorexant – FDA approved in 2014 (Belsomra). Lemborexant – FDA approved in 2019 (Dayvigo). Daridorexant – FDA approved in 2022 (Quviviq)	Blocks orexin receptors OX1R and OX2R in the brain's arousal pathways, reducing histamine release and promoting sleep without next-day sedation.	Somnolence, abnormal dreams, hallucinations, sleep paralysis, headache.	Approved for chronic insomnia management.	Lemborexant: 5–10 mg orally at bedtime. Daridorexant: 25–50 mg orally at bedtime. Suvorexant: 10–20 mg orally at bedtime
Remimazolam	FDA approved in 2020 for procedural sedation; Phase 3 trials ongoing for insomnia.	Binds to GABA-A receptors at benzodiazepine sites, increasing chloride influx and neuronal inhibition. Rapid onset with short duration via tissue esterase metabolism.	Headache, drowsiness, hypotension, involuntary movements.	Sedation for ICU, procedural use, and investigational in sleep disorders.	Initial 5 mg IV over 1 minute; then 2.5 mg every 2 minutes as needed.
Zuranolone	FDA approved in 2023 for postpartum depression (Zurzuvae); under study for sedative use.	A neuroactive steroid that modulates both synaptic and extrasynaptic GABA-A receptors (non-benzodiazepine binding site), enhancing chloride conductance and neuronal inhibition.	Drowsiness, dizziness, diarrhoea, fatigue, mild cognitive impairment.	Approved for postpartum depression; under trial as sedative.	30–50 mg orally once daily.
Agomelatine	EMA approved; Phase III trials ongoing in other regions.	Acts as an MT1/MT2 agonist to regulate circadian rhythm and induce sleep; also antagonizes 5-HT2C receptors to enhance dopamine and norepinephrine release in the prefrontal cortex.	Headache, dizziness, nausea, potential hepatotoxicity.	Used for major depressive episodes with insomnia in adults.	25–50 mg orally at bedtime.
Tasimelteon	FDA approved for Non-24-Hour Sleep-Wake Disorder (N24HSWD).	Melatonin receptor agonist (MT1/MT2) in the suprachiasmatic nucleus, resynchronizing circadian rhythms and inducing sleep.	Headache, liver enzyme elevation, nightmares, insomnia.	Approved for N24HSWD, Smith-Magenis syndrome sleep disturbance (age-specific formulations).	20 mg orally once daily at the same time every night.

Newer Antiepileptics

Drug Name	Clinical Trial Phase	Mechanism of Action	Adverse Drug Reaction	Uses	Dose
Brivaracetam	FDA-approved (Briviact) for partial-onset seizures.	Binds selectively to SV2A protein on synaptic vesicles, modulating neurotransmitter release. Also inhibits voltage-gated sodium channels, reducing excitatory neuronal firing.	Mood changes, dizziness, fatigue, poor coordination, drowsiness.	Adjunct therapy for partial-onset seizures in patients ≥16 years.	50 mg/day (25 mg BID or 50 mg once daily).
Perampanel	FDA-approved (Fycompa) for focal and tonic-clonic seizures.	Non-competitive antagonist of AMPA glutamate receptors, reducing excitatory neurotransmission and seizure spread.	Dizziness, fatigue, somnolence, ataxia, irritability, falls (especially in elderly).	Monotherapy or adjunct for focal seizures in patients ≥4 years, and tonic-clonic seizures in those ≥12 years.	2 mg once daily at bedtime.
Eslicarba-zepine Acetate	FDA-approved (Aptiom) for partial-onset seizures.	Enhancesslow inactivation of voltage-gated sodium channels in overactive neurons and inhibits Cav3.2 T-type calcium channels. Enhances seizure control with fewer cognitive side effects.	Dizziness, diplopia, headache, nausea, vision disturbances, fatigue.	Monotherapy or adjunctive therapy for focal seizures.	400 mg once daily.
Lacosamide	FDA-approved (Vimpat) for focal seizures.	Enhances slow inactivation of voltage-gated sodium channels, stabilizing hyperexcitable neurons without affecting fast currents.	Dizziness, nausea, blurred vision, tremors, cardiac conduction issues.	Treatment of partial-onset seizures & GTCS in adults and children ≥4 years; used in both IR and extended-release forms.	50 mg BID.
Ganaxolone	FDA approved (Ztalmy, 2022) for CDKL5 deficiency disorder.	Positive allosteric modulator of synaptic and extrasynaptic GABA-A receptors. Enhances tonic inhibition without hormonal effects.	Drowsiness, fatigue, dizziness, diarrhoea, gait instability.	Seizure control in CDKL5 deficiency syndrome; being explored for other genetic epilepsies.	63 mg/kg/day (divided doses).

Recent Advances in the Management of Parkinsonism

Drug Name	Clinical Trial Phase	Mechanism of Action	Adverse Drug Reaction	Uses	Dose
Liposome-Based Targeting of Dopamine to the Brain	Preclinical stage.	APP-targeted liposomes cross the blood-brain barrier to deliver dopamine directly into the brain, increasing striatal dopamine levels with significantly lower doses than levodopa.	Not yet established.	Investigational approach for targeted dopamine delivery in Parkinson's disease.	Not yet standardized.
Safinamide	FDA-approved (Xadago) as an adjunct in advanced Parkinson's disease.	Reversible MAO-B inhibitor that enhances dopamine levels. Also modulates sodium and N-type calcium channels, reducing glutamate release and possibly aiding non-motor symptoms.	Nausea, insomnia, dyskinesia, orthostatic hypotension.	Add-on to levodopa in managing motor fluctuations. Also used in advanced Parkinsonism.	50–100 mg orally once daily.
IRX4204	In Phase I/II trials.	Activates the RXR-Nurr1 pathway, promoting dopaminergic neuron survival, reducing neuroinflammation, and improving mitochondrial function.	Nausea, diarrhoea, hypersensitivity, potential hepatotoxicity.	Investigational neuroprotective therapy for Parkinson's disease.	1–5 mg/day (trial dosing).
Prasinezumab	Phase IIb trials (PASADENA).	Humanised monoclonal antibody targeting aggregated alpha-synuclein; inhibits its spread and reduces neurodegeneration.	Under investigation.	Investigational disease-modifying agent in early Parkinson's disease.	1500–4500 mg IV every 4 weeks.

Istradefylline	FDA-approved (Nourianz).	A2A adenosine receptor antagonist that reduces GABA release in the indirect motor pathway, enhancing movement and reducing "off" episodes.	Dyskinesia, hallucinations, nausea, insomnia, constipation.	Add-on to levodopa to reduce "off" time.	20–40 mg orally once daily.

Additional FDA-Approved Therapies & Phase IV Advances

- **Inhaled Levodopa:** Rapid-onset levodopa powder for "off" periods.
  1. **Dose:** 84 mg up to 5× daily
  2. **ADR:** Cough, URTI, nausea.
- **Scored Levodopa/Carbidopa Tablets:** Flexible-dose segmented tablets for precision titration.
  1. **Dose:** 1 pill (25/100 mg) three times daily
- **Sublingual Apomorphine:** Dopamine agonist for acute "off" episodes.
  1. **Dose:** 10–30 mg, up to 5× daily (>2 hrs apart)
  2. **ADR:** Nausea, site reactions; anti-emetic recommended prior to initiation.
- **Opicapone:** Once-daily COMT inhibitor to extend levodopa effect.
  1. **Dose:** 50 mg daily (25 mg if hepatic impairment)
  2. **ADR:** Dyskinesia, hypotension, diarrhea.
- **Extended-Release Amantadine:** NMDA receptor antagonist for levodopa-induced dyskinesia.
  1. **Dose:** 129 mg daily
  2. **ADR:** Hallucinations, dizziness, dry mouth, constipation.

Newer Antipsychotics

Drug Name	Clinical Trial Phase	Mechanism of Action	Adverse Drug Reaction	Uses	Dose
Cariprazine	FDA-approved (Vraylar); also approved in Canada.	Partial agonist at dopamine D2/D3 and serotonin 5-HT1A receptors; antagonist at 5-HT2A receptors. Offers dopamine-serotonin modulation for mood and psychosis.	Akathisia, nausea, insomnia, minimal weight gain, mild sedation.	Schizophrenia, bipolar I disorder, and adjunct for major depressive disorder.	1.5–6 mg once daily orally.
Lumateperone	FDA-approved (Caplyta) for schizophrenia.	Antagonist at 5-HT2A receptors, partial agonist at presynaptic D2 receptors, antagonist at postsynaptic D2 receptors. Also modulates glutamatergic pathways.	Drowsiness, dizziness, nausea, seizures, hypotension.	Positive and negative symptoms in schizophrenia; being studied in bipolar depression.	42 mg once daily orally.
Brexpiprazole	FDA-approved (Rexulti).	Partial agonist at dopamine D2 and serotonin 5-HT1A receptors; antagonist at 5-HT2A receptors. Lower D2 activity reduces EPS risk.	Akathisia, somnolence, constipation, fatigue, weight gain.	Schizophrenia, adjunct for major depressive disorder, agitation in Alzheimer's.	1–4 mg/day orally.
Pimavanserin	FDA-approved (Nuplazid)	Selective inverse agonist at 5-HT2A receptors without dopaminergic activity – ideal for psychosis in Parkinson's without worsening motor symptoms.	Confusion, oedema, constipation, gait issues, nausea.	Hallucinations and delusions in Parkinson's disease psychosis; being studied in Alzheimer's and schizophrenia.	34 mg once daily orally.
Aripiprazole Lauroxil	FDA-approved (Aristada).	Long-acting injectable prodrug of aripiprazole – partial dopamine D2 agonist with serotonin modulation. Improves adherence and reduces relapse risk in schizophrenia.	Akathisia, weight gain, injection-site reactions, sedation.	Long-term management of schizophrenia.	441–1064 mg IM every 4–8 weeks.

Newer Antidepressants

Drug Name	Clinical Trial Phase	Mechanism of Action	Adverse Drug Reaction	Uses	Dose
Esketamine	FDA-approved nasal spray (Spravato) for treatment-resistant depression (TRD).	NMDA receptor antagonist – ↓ GABAergic inhibition in PFC – ↑ glutamate release – AMPA receptor activation – ↑ BDNF & synaptic growth – rapid antidepressant effect.	Dissociation, sleepiness, dizziness, nausea.	TRD (with oral antidepressant); MDD with acute suicidal ideation.	56–84 mg intranasally twice/ week for 4 weeks, then weekly/ biweekly.
Brexanolone	FDA-approved in 2019 (Zulresso) for postpartum depression.	Neuroactive steroid that enhances tonic inhibition at extrasynaptic GABA-A receptors – ↑ chloride channel activity – ↓ neuronal hyperexcitability – rapid mood stabilization.	Sedation, dry mouth, hot flashes, confusion, syncope.	Postpartum depression (hospital-monitored).	90 μg/kg/hr continuous IV infusion over 60 hours.
Agomelatine	Approved in Europe and Australia; not FDA-approved.	Agonist at MT1/MT2 melatonin receptors (↑ sleep and circadian alignment); antagonist at 5-HT2C receptors – ↓ GABAergic inhibition – ↑ DA & NA release in prefrontal cortex.	Headache, dizziness, nausea, hepatotoxicity.	Major depressive episodes (especially with circadian dysregulation).	25–50 mg orally at bedtime.
Vortioxetine	FDA-approved (Brintellix/ Trintellix).	Inhibits SERT – ↑ synaptic 5-HT; partial agonist at 5-HT1A/1B – modulates serotonin release; 5-HT3/7 antagonist – may improve cognition and reduce nausea.	Nausea, headache, dry mouth, dizziness; rare: suicidality, pancreatitis.	Major depressive disorder (including cognitive dysfunction).	10–20 mg once daily.
Vilazodone	FDA-approved (Viibryd) for major depressive disorder.	SERT inhibition – ↑ 5-HT release; partial 5-HT1A agonist - desensitizes autoreceptors - sustained 5-HT↑; also facilitates faster tolerance to serotonin-related side effects.	Headache, nausea, diarrhoea, mild GI upset; lower sexual side effect risk than SSRIs.	Major depressive disorder.	Start at 10 mg/day (7 days), then 20–40 mg/ day.

Recent Advances in the Management of Alzheimer's Disease

Drug Name	Clinical Trial Phase	Mechanism of Action	Adverse Drug Reaction	Uses	Dose
Lecanemab	FDA-approved (2023, CLARITY-AD).	Binds soluble Aβ protofibrils – prevents aggregation – promotes microglial clearance – ↓ plaque formation & neuroinflammation – slows cognitive decline.	ARIA (oedema, microhae-morrhage), headache, infusion reactions.	Early Alzheimer's disease.	10 mg/kg IV every 2 weeks.
Donanemab	Phase III (TRAILBLAZER-ALZ 2); not FDA-approved yet.	Targets pyroglutamate-modified Aβ – microglial phagocytosis – plaque clearance – ↓ tau hyperphosphorylation – slows neurodegeneration.	ARIA, infusion reactions, flu-like symptoms.	Mild to moderate Alzheimer's disease.	700 mg IV Q2W (x3 doses), then 1400 mg IV Q4W.
Blarcamesine (ANAVEX 2-73)	Phase IIb/III completed.	Sigma-1 receptor agonist – regulates ER-mitochondria crosstalk – ↓ oxidative stress & tau phosphorylation – ↑ synaptic plasticity.	Dizziness, fatigue, GI issues, neuropsychiatric effects.	Alzheimer's disease, cognitive impairment in Parkinson's.	30–50 mg/day orally.
GV-971 (Sodium Oligomannate)	Approved in China; Phase III global trials ongoing.	Modulates gut microbiota – ↓ systemic/CNS inflammation – inhibits Aβ aggregation – neuroprotection via gut-brain axis.	Diarrhoea, nausea, allergic reactions.	Mild to moderate Alzheimer's disease.	450 mg orally BID.
Simufilam	Phase III trials ongoing.	Restores filamin A structure – blocks Aβ-FLNA interaction – ↓ inflammation – improves NMDA receptor signalling & cognition.	Fatigue, headache, QT prolongation.	Mild to moderate Alzheimer's disease.	100–300 mg orally BID.

Gantenerumab	Phase III (Graduate 1 & 2); failed primary endpoints but under analysis.	Binds fibrillar Aβ - microglial-mediated clearance - ↓ plaque growth - indirect tau suppression.	ARIA-H & ARIA-E, injection-site reactions, flu-like symptoms.	Investigational (early Alzheimer's).	1,020 mg SC monthly.
Zagotenemab	Phase II (Tau NextGen, TRAILBLAZER-ALZ).	Binds misfolded tau - prevents tau propagation - microglial phagocytosis - ↓ tangle formation & neurotoxicity.	Injection reactions, fatigue, rare ARIA.	Investigational for AD & tauopathies (e.g. FTD).	70–210 mg SC every 4 weeks.

Recent Advances in the Management of Bipolar Mood Disorder

Drug Name	Clinical Trial Phase	Mechanism of Action	Adverse Drug Reaction	Uses	Dose
Cariprazine	FDA-approved under Vraylar; Health Canada approved (2022).	5-HT2A antagonism – ↓ glutamate from PFC - ↓ DA in emotional striatum - relieves mania. D2 partial agonism – antipsychotic effects with minimal extrapyramidal symptoms or prolactin rise. 5-HT1A partial agonism – stabilises DA in motor striatum & PFC - reduces depressive symptoms & extrapyramidal side effects.	Akathisia, nausea, insomnia, sedation.	Manic, depressive & mixed episodes in bipolar disorder; schizophrenia.	1.5–6 mg once daily orally.
Lumateperone	FDA-approved (2021) for Bipolar I/II depression.	Presynaptic D2 partial agonist – ↓ dopamine overactivity. Postsynaptic D2 antagonist – stabilises dopaminergic tone. 5-HT2A antagonism – ↑ glutamate transmission - mood elevation. NMDA/ AMPA modulation & GABAergic enhancement – improves neuroplasticity and calmness.	Drowsiness, hypotension, dizziness, nausea.	Bipolar depression (monotherapy or adjunct); schizophrenia.	42 mg once daily orally.

KarXT (Xanomeline-Trospium)	Phase III trials ongoing for bipolar psychosis.	Xanomeline (M1/ M4 agonist): Restores cholinergic tone in limbic system - improves mania, mood regulation. Trospium (peripheral antagonist): Blocks unwanted cholinergic side effects peripherally - reduces GI/cardiac issues.	Dry mouth, nausea; minimal metabolic & no EPS risk.	Investigational for bipolar mania and schizophrenia.	30–50 mg/day 125–150 mg xanomeline / 30–40 mg trospiumBID..
Seltorexant	Phase III for bipolar depression.	Selective orexin-2 antagonist: ↓ histamine release - ↓ arousal - improves sleep & emotional control. ↓ Cortisol release: Reduces stress axis hyperactivity - stabilises mood.	Mild sedation, cognitive fog, nausea, hypotension.	Bipolar depression with insomnia.	20 mg orally at bedtime (trial phase dosing).
Esketamine	FDA-approved for TRD; Phase III ongoing for bipolar depression.	NMDA receptor blockade: ↓ GABA release in PFC - ↑ glutamate - AMPA receptor activation - ↑ BDNF - rapid synaptic growth. Rapid mood elevation & antidepressant effect within hours.	Sedation, dissociation, hypertension, nausea.	TRD; under trial for bipolar depression.	56–84 mg intranasally twice/week × 4 weeks.

Recent Advances in the Management of Migraine

Drug Name	Clinical Trial Phase	Mechanism of Action	Adverse Drug Reaction	Uses	Dose
Ubrogepant	FDA-approved for acute migraine; ongoing trials for prophylaxis.	CGRP antagonist – blocks CGRP receptors in trigeminal system – prevents CGRP-induced vasodilation & neurogenic inflammation – inhibits nociceptor sensitisation – reduces migraine pain and associated symptoms like nausea, photophobia & phonophobia.	Nausea, dizziness, dry mouth, hepatotoxicity, hypersensitivity.	Acute migraine attacks in adults.	50–100 mg orally; second dose after 2 hours if needed.
Rimegepant	FDA-approved for both acute & preventive migraine therapy.	CGRP receptor antagonist – blocks CGRP binding in trigeminal ganglion & dura – prevents vasodilation & mast-cell mediated inflammation – inhibits nociceptive transmission – provides acute relief & prophylaxis.	Nausea, somnolence, elevated liver enzymes, rare anaphylaxis.	Acute and preventive treatment of migraine in adults.	75 mg orally once daily (acute); not more than 1 dose per 24 hours.
Eptinezumab (CGRP Monoclonal Antibody)	FDA-approved (2020) for episodic/ chronic migraine prevention.	Humanised IgG1 mAb – binds circulating CGRP ligand – blocks CGRP activation at meningeal vessels & trigeminal nociceptors – reduces vasodilation, inflammation, and central sensitisation – rapid onset due to IV route – long half-life ensures prolonged effect.	Hypersensitivity, dizziness, fatigue, nasopharyngitis, liver enzyme elevation.	Preventive treatment of frequent migraines	100 mg IV every 3 months.
Lasmiditan (Selective 5-HT1F Agonist)	FDA-approved for acute migraine with/ without aura.	Selective 5-HT1F agonist – acts on trigeminal neurons without affecting blood vessels – inhibits CGRP & glutamate release – reduces trigeminal pain signalling & central sensitisation.	Dizziness, drowsiness, nausea, serotonin syndrome.	Acute migraine attacks, especially for patients at risk of cardiovascular complications.	50, 100, or 200 mg orally as needed (max 200 mg/day).

Zavegepant (Intranasal CGRP Antagonist)	FDA-approved (2023) for acute migraine.	Nasal CGRP receptor antagonist – binds CGRP receptors in trigeminal ganglion & dura – blocks vasodilation & inflammation – inhibits trigeminal pain signalling – nasal route - rapid absorption – effective in migraine with nausea.	Nasal congestion, altered taste, nausea, hypersensitivity.	Fast relief of acute migraine attacks.	10 mg intranasally, single dose per episode.

Recent Advances in the Management of Shock

Drug Name	Clinical Trial Phase	Mechanism of Action	Adverse Drug Reaction	Uses	Dose
Angiotensin II	FDA-approved for distributive and septic shock; Phase IV safety evaluations ongoing.	Activates AT1 receptors - vasoconstriction via Gq–PLC–IP3/DAG cascade - ↑ intracellular Ca^{2+} - smooth muscle contraction. Stimulates aldosterone release - Na^{+}/water retention - ↑ intravascular volume. Enhances sympathetic NE release - ↑ HR & contractility. Maintains GFR by constricting efferent arterioles and reduces AKI risk. Also reduces pro-inflammatory cytokines and improves endothelial tone.	Hypertension, thrombosis, tachyarrhythmia, renal impairment.	Catecholamine-resistant septic and distributive shock.	Start at 20 ng/kg/min IV; titrate up to 80 ng/kg/min.
Selepressin	Phase III (SEPSIS-ACT trial) for septic shock.	Selective V1A receptor agonist - Gq-PLC pathway - ↑ intracellular Ca^{2+} - vasoconstriction - ↑ MAP without activating V2 receptors - avoids water retention, hyponatremia & oedema. Reduces pro-inflammatory cytokines (TNF-α, IL-6), stabilizes capillaries, limits fluid leakage and pulmonary congestion.	Hypertension, peripheral ischemia, reduced cardiac output.	Septic shock with hypotension unresponsive to standard vasopressors.	2.5 ng/kg/min IV infusion.

Methylene Blue	Phase III trials for vasoplegic and septic shock.	Inhibits sGC - blocks NO-mediated cGMP production - reverses vasodilation. Scavenges excess NO and enhances systemic vascular resistance. Supports mitochondrial ETC - improved ATP production & reduced ROS. Stabilizes endothelium - ↓ permeability & capillary leak. Functions without acting on adrenergic receptors - suitable for catecholamine-resistant shock.	Methemoglobinemia, serotonin syndrome (with SSRIs), thrombosis, cardiac arrhythmia.	Vasoplegic and septic shock unresponsive to catecholamines.	1–2 mg/kg IV over 30 min; may follow with 0.25–2 mg/kg/h infusion.
Ularitide	Phase III for cardiogenic shock and acute heart failure.	Activates NPR-A - ↑ cGMP - vasodilation (arterial + venous) - ↓ preload, afterload & myocardial oxygen demand. Promotes natriuresis - ↓ fluid overload. Enhances renal perfusion & diuresis - ↑ GFR. Suppresses RAAS - ↓ Ang II & aldosterone.	Hypotension, nausea, electrolyte imbalance.	Acute decompensated heart failure and cardiogenic shock.	15–30 ng/kg/min IV infusion.
Landiolol	Approved in Japan/Europe; Phase III for cardiogenic shock.	Selective β1-blocker - ↓ HR & AV node conduction (chronotropic & dromotropic effects) - stabilizes arrhythmias (AF, SVT). Maintains contractility with minimal inotropic depression - safe in shock. Lowers myocardial O_2 demand & reduces sympathetic overdrive - protects heart, improves perfusion.	Bradycardia, hypotension.	Cardiogenic shock with concurrent tachyarrhythmia.	1–10 µg/kg/min IV infusion, titrated as per response.

Recent Advances in the Management of Myocardial Infarction

Drug Name	Clinical Trial Phase	Mechanism of Action	Adverse Drug Reaction	Uses	Dose
Zalunfiban	In Phase III trials for STEMI during PCI.	Zalunfiban binds selectively to integrin αIIbβ3, blocking **fibrinogen** and **vWF** binding hyper inhibits **platelet aggregation** hyper reduces **thrombus formation**. Its **short half-life and reversibility** make it ideal for acute PCI settings, especially in STEMI.	Bleeding, thrombocytopenia, nausea, hypotension.	Acute STEMI/ NSTEMI and adjunct in PCI.	3–6 µg/kg IV bolus, then infusion.
Finerenone	FDA-approved for CKD-related cardiovascular risk; Phase II for MI.	Blocks **mineralocorticoid receptors (MR)** in cardiac fibroblasts hyper reduces **TGF-β** and **collagen synthesis** hyper prevents **fibrosis.** Inhibits **NF-κB** and **M1 macrophage infiltration,** preserving microvascular and endothelial function. Mitigates **LV hypertrophy and apoptosis** post-MI hyper prevents adverse cardiac remodelling.	Hyperkalaemia, hypotension, fatigue.	Post-MI heart failure prevention; CV risk in diabetic CKD.	10–20 mg orally daily.

Semaglutide	Phase III trials for MI prevention in diabetics/obese patients.	Activates **GLP-1R** in the heart and endothelium hyper increases **NO** and mitochondrial protection hyper reduces **inflammation,** macrophage infiltration, and **oxidative stress**. Prevents **fibrosis** and **cardiac remodelling** post-MI. Improves **glucose uptake,** energy efficiency, and **lipid profiles**, reducing atherosclerosis risk.	Nausea, cholelithiasis, hypoglycemia.	CV protection in T2DM, obesity; MI prevention.	0.25 mg SC weekly, titrated up to 1–2 mg weekly.
Selatogrel	Phase III for acute MI (self-administered).	Reversibly blocks **P2Y12 receptors** on platelets hyper inhibits **ADP-induced** aggregation hyper prevents GP **IIb/ IIIa activation** and thrombus formation. Rapid-onset and SC delivery make it ideal for **pre-hospital MI treatment.**	Injection site reactions, bradycardia, bleeding.	Emergency antiplatelet therapy during MI.	16 mg SC single dose.
Inclisiran	FDA-approved for hyperlipidemia; Phase II trials for MI.	Silences **PCSK9 mRNA** via siRNA in hepatocytes hyper prevents **LDLR degradation** hyper reduces **LDL-C levels by 50–60%.** Stabilizes atherosclerotic plaques, reduces **macrophage inflammation,** and improves **NO bioavailability.** Long-acting and dosed biannually.	Myalgia, liver enzyme elevation, injection reactions.	Recurrent MI prevention in atherosclerosis patients.	284 mg SC on Day 1, 90, then every 6 months.

Recent Advances in the Management of Hypertension

Drug Name	Clinical Trial Phase	Mechanism of Action	Adverse Drug Reaction	Uses	Dose
Aprocitentan	FDA Approved (March 2024)	Selectively blocks both ETA and ETB endothelin receptors – inhibits vasoconstriction driven by endothelin-1 – enhances vasodilation – reduces peripheral vascular resistance and maintains blood pressure control through sustained activity due to a long half-life.	Peripheral oedema, headache, anaemia, fatigue, nasal congestion, hepatic dysfunction	Approved for resistant hypertension; off-label use in pulmonary arterial hypertension	12.5 mg to 25 mg once daily (oral)
Baxdrostat	Phase III Clinical Trials	Selectively inhibits aldosterone synthase (CYP11B2) – reduces aldosterone synthesis without affecting cortisol – diminishes sodium retention, vascular inflammation and fibrosis – lowers blood pressure in treatment-resistant cases	Headache, nausea, fatigue, hyperkalaemia, hypotension, mild adrenal insufficiency	Resistant hypertension and primary aldosteronism (under investigation)	2 mg to 5 mg once daily (oral)
Sacubitril/ Valsartan (ARNI)	FDA Approved	Sacubitril inhibits neprilysin – increases natriuretic peptides and bradykinin – promotes vasodilation, diuresis, and antifibrotic effects – Valsartan blocks angiotensin II receptors, reducing vasoconstriction and sodium retention – synergistic hemodynamic benefit.	Headache, nausea, hypokalaemia, hypotension, fatigue	Approved for heart failure with reduced ejection fraction and hypertension	100 mg twice daily (sacubitril 49 mg / valsartan 51 mg)
Zilebesiran	Phase II Clinical Trials	RNA interference targets AGT mRNA in hepatocytes – reduces angiotensinogen production – decreases levels of angiotensin I and II – leads to long-lasting vasodilation and blood pressure control	Injection site reactions, fatigue, hypotension, hyperkalaemia, potential hepatotoxicity	Hypertension (investigational, long-term control)	300 mg to 600 mg subcutaneously every 6 months

Firibastat	Phase II Clinical Trials	Brain-penetrant prodrug converted to EC33 – inhibits aminopeptidase A in the brain – prevents conversion of Ang II to Ang III – reduces sympathetic activity, aldosterone release and blood pressure – neurogenic target with cardiovascular protection	Headache, fatigue, nausea, hypotension, mild cognitive changes	Resistant hypertension (under investigation)	250 mg twice daily (oral, trial dose)
Esaxerenone	Approved in Japan, Phase III globally	Selective mineralocorticoid receptor antagonist - blocks aldosterone effects - reduces sodium retention, inflammation and cardiac fibrosis.	Hyperkalaemia, hypotension, renal impairment.	Primary hypertension, Diabetic nephropathy (investigational)	1.25 mg to 2.5 mg once daily (oral)
Cicletanine	Phase II Clinical Trials	Phosphodiesterase-9 inhibitor - increases cGMP - promotes vasodilation and natriuresis - reduces oxidative stress and vascular stiffness.	Headache, dizziness, nausea, hypotension, QT prolongation	Resistant hypertension (investigational)	50 mg to 100 mg once daily (oral, trial dose)

Recent Advances in the Management of Heart Failure

Drug Name	Clinical Trial Phase	Mechanism of Action	Adverse Drug Reaction	Uses	Dose
Empagliflozin	FDA approved (2021) for HFrEF and HFpEF	Empagliflozin inhibits SGLT2 in the renal proximal tubules, reducing glucose and sodium reabsorption. This leads to glucosuria and natriuresis, which lowers plasma volume, preload, and blood pressure. It also exerts pleiotropic effects including inhibition of cardiac fibrosis through NF-κB and HIF-1α pathways, improvement in renal hemodynamics, and modulation of lipid profile and weight.	Urinary tract infections, polyuria, dehydration, mild hypoglycaemia, hypotension, acute kidney injury, diabetic ketoacidosis (rare)	Heart failure (HFrEF and HFpEF), Type 2 diabetes mellitus	10 mg once daily (oral)
Vericiguat	FDA approved for HFrEF	Vericiguat stimulates soluble guanylate cyclase (sGC), enhancing cGMP production even with diminished NO. This activates protein kinase G, leading to vascular relaxation, decreased calcium influx, and inhibition of cardiac fibrosis. It reduces systemic vascular resistance and improves renal perfusion.	Hypotension, syncope, anaemia, headache, dizziness, fatigue, teratogenicity	HFrEF with high risk of hospitalization	2.5–5 mg once daily
Omecamtiv Mecarbil	Phase III trials (GALACTIC-HF completed)	A cardiac myosin activator that enhances cross-bridge formation between actin and myosin, prolongs systolic ejection time, and increases stroke volume without raising oxygen demand. It avoids β-adrenergic receptor activation, preventing increases in heart rate or arrhythmogenicity.	Arrhythmias, myocardial ischaemia, headache, dizziness, fatigue	Systolic heart failure (HFrEF)	25 mg or 50 mg twice daily (oral)

Tirzepatide	Phase III (SUMMIT and SURPASS-HF)	Dual GLP-1 and GIP receptor agonist that improves cardiac contractility, reduces inflammation and fibrosis, and enhances metabolic efficiency. It promotes natriuresis, inhibits Na^+/H^+ exchanger, increases nitric oxide, and decreases pro-inflammatory cytokines and oxidative stress.	Nausea, vomiting, diarrhoea, hypoglycaemia, pancreatitis	FDA-approved for Type 2 diabetes and obesity; under investigation for heart failure	2.5 mg once weekly (subcu-taneous)
Dapagliflozin	FDA approved for HFrEF and HFpEF	SGLT2 inhibitor that induces natriuresis and diuresis, lowering preload and afterload. Enhances myocardial efficiency by shifting energy metabolism, reduces cytokine-driven inflammation, and limits cardiac fibrosis through TGF-β inhibition.	Dehydration, urinary tract infections, polyuria, mild hypoglycaemia, diabetic ketoacidosis, Fournier's gangrene (rare)	Type 2 diabetes mellitus, HFrEF, HFpEF	10 mg once daily (oral)

Newer Anti-Arrhythmic Drugs

Drug Name	Clinical Trial Phase	Mechanism of Action	Adverse Drug Reaction	Uses	Dose
Flecainide	FDA-approved for paroxysmal AF, SVT, and ventricular tachycardia	Flecainide inhibits fast sodium channels (NaV1.5), slowing Phase 0 depolarization and conduction velocity. It prolongs PR and QRS intervals and exhibits use-dependent blockade, making it effective at high heart rates. Additionally, it has minor potassium channel inhibition and uniquely blocks RyR2-mediated calcium release, preventing arrhythmias in CPVT.	Dizziness, blurred vision, worsening of heart failure in structural disease, ventricular proarrhythmia	Atrial fibrillation, supraventricular tachycardia, ventricular tachycardia, CPVT	50–100 mg twice daily
Vernakalant	Approved in Europe and Canada for acute AF; not FDA-approved	Vernakalant blocks atrial-specific potassium (IKur) and sodium currents, prolonging atrial refractoriness while preserving ventricular repolarization. It selectively slows atrial conduction, suppresses re-entry circuits, and demonstrates rate-dependent blockade, making it effective for cardioversion in rapid AF.	Dysgeusia, hypotension, nausea, dizziness, bradycardia	Rapid conversion of recent-onset atrial fibrillation	3 mg/kg IV over 10 minutes
Ranolazine	Approved for chronic angina; under Phase II/III trials for AF and VT	Ranolazine inhibits late sodium current (INa-Late), reducing intracellular sodium and calcium overload. This stabilizes cardiac repolarization and prevents early and delayed afterdepolarizations. It weakly inhibits IKr and has minimal QT prolongation, offering antiarrhythmic effects particularly in ischemic and heart failure-related AF.	Dizziness, nausea, constipation, QT prolongation, hypotension, renal impairment	Chronic stable angina, under investigation for AF and VT	500–1000 mg twice daily

AZD7009	Phase II trials	AZD7009 blocks INa, IKr, and IKur, prolonging atrial action potentials and refractory periods without affecting ventricular tissue significantly. It mildly inhibits ICa-L, suppressing ectopic activity. Atrial selectivity and use-dependent blockade make it effective for AF termination with low proarrhythmic risk.	Mild QT prolongation, GI upset, bradycardia, AV block	Under investigation for AF and atrial flutter	0.5 to 2.5 mg/kg IV over 10–20 minutes
Mexiletine	FDA-approved for ventricular arrhythmias	Mexiletine blocks voltage-gated sodium channels, reducing conduction velocity in depolarized tissue. It shortens APD and ERP, suppressing re-entrant ventricular circuits. Use-dependent blockade enhances selectivity during tachyarrhythmias. It has minimal potassium current effect, limiting proarrhythmic risk.	CNS disturbances (dizziness, tremors), nausea, hepatotoxicity, QT prolongation	Ventricular arrhythmias, LQT3 (investigational), off-label in neuropathic pain and myotonia	200–300 mg every 8 hours

Newer Anti-Thrombotic Agents

Drug Name	Clinical Trial Phase	Mechanism of Action	Adverse Drug Reaction	Uses	Dose
Rivaroxaban	FDA-approved for stroke prevention in atrial fibrillation (AF), treatment and prevention of venous thromboembolism (VTE), and acute coronary syndrome	Rivaroxaban is a direct oral inhibitor of Factor Xa, binding to both free and clot-bound Factor Xa. This prevents the conversion of prothrombin to thrombin, thereby inhibiting fibrin formation and platelet activation. Its mechanism allows anticoagulation without the need for antithrombin III and provides stable pharmacokinetics.	Bleeding events including gastrointestinal and intracranial haemorrhage, anaemia, dyspepsia, liver enzyme elevation	Prevention of stroke in non-valvular AF, treatment and prophylaxis of DVT and PE, post-operative (orthopaedic) thromboprophylaxis	15 mg twice daily for 21 days, followed by 20 mg once daily
Dabigatran	FDA-approved for stroke prevention in AF and treatment of VTE	Dabigatran is a direct thrombin (Factor IIa) inhibitor that binds reversibly to its active site. It blocks the conversion of fibrinogen to fibrin and inhibits thrombin-induced platelet aggregation. It acts independently of antithrombin III and is rapidly activated from its prodrug form. A key safety advantage is its dedicated reversal agent, idarucizumab.	Major bleeding, especially gastrointestinal, dyspepsia, nausea, headache, hepatotoxicity (rare)	Stroke prevention in AF, DVT and PE treatment and prophylaxis	150 mg twice daily
Milvexian	In Phase III clinical trials for post-operative thromboprophylaxis and stroke prevention	Milvexian selectively inhibits activated Factor XI (FXIa), an upstream mediator in the intrinsic coagulation cascade. This reduces thrombin formation without directly impacting platelet function or primary haemostasis, resulting in lower bleeding risk compared to conventional anticoagulants. It does not require antithrombin III.	Gastrointestinal disturbances, dizziness, elevated liver enzymes, minimal bleeding events	Under investigation for stroke prevention in AF, post-surgical VTE prevention, secondary prevention after ACS or MI	25 mg to 200 mg once or twice daily (oral, trial-based)

Vorapaxar	FDA-approved for secondary prevention in patients with prior myocardial infarction or peripheral artery disease	Vorapaxar is a PAR-1 receptor antagonist that inhibits thrombin-induced platelet aggregation without significantly disrupting primary haemostasis. It specifically blocks thrombin's interaction with platelets, distinguishing it from ADP-based antiplatelet drugs. Its long half-life sustains effect for weeks after cessation, though no specific reversal agent exists.	Intracranial haemorrhage in high-risk patients, fatigue, hypotension, headache	Prevention of thrombotic cardiovascular events post-MI or in peripheral artery disease	2.08 mg once daily (equivalent to 2.5 mg vorapaxar sulfate)
Bentracimab	Under FDA priority review for reversal of ticagrelor-induced bleeding	Bentracimab is a monoclonal antibody that binds with high affinity to ticagrelor and its active metabolite. It immediately neutralizes ticagrelor's antiplatelet effects within minutes, restoring platelet function without affecting baseline haemostasis. Its effect is sustained for 12–24 hours and does not interfere with other coagulation pathways.	Injection-site reactions, dizziness, headache, allergic responses	Emergency reversal of ticagrelor in life-threatening bleeding or urgent surgical settings	6 g IV bolus followed by 6 g infusion over 4 hours

Newer Hypolipidemic Drugs

Drug Name	Clinical Trial Phase	Mechanism of Action	Adverse Drug Reaction	Uses	Dose
Evolocumab	FDA-approved for familial hypercholesterolemia (FH) and ASCVD prevention	Evolocumab is a monoclonal antibody that inhibits PCSK9 — a protein that normally binds LDL receptors and marks them for degradation. By neutralizing PCSK9, more LDL receptors recycle to the hepatocyte surface — leading to enhanced LDL clearance and a 50–60% reduction in LDL-C. When combined with statins, the LDL-lowering effect is further amplified due to PCSK9 counteraction.	Injection-site reactions, myalgias, flu-like symptoms, cognitive impairment, risk of diabetes	Familial hypercholesterolemia, primary hyperlipidaemia, ASCVD prevention	140 mg every 2 weeks or 420 mg monthly, subcutaneously
Inclisiran	FDA-approved; ORION trials confirm efficacy	Inclisiran is an siRNA therapy that targets PCSK9 mRNA in hepatocytes — reducing PCSK9 protein synthesis at the genetic level. It uses GalNAc for liver-specific delivery and acts via RNA-induced silencing complex (RISC), resulting in prolonged LDL receptor availability and sustained LDL clearance.	Mild injection-site reactions, transient flu-like symptoms, slight liver enzyme elevations	Hypercholesterolemia, familial hypercholesterolemia, ASCVD prevention	284 mg subcutaneously on Day 0, at 3 months, then every 6 months

Bempedoic Acid	FDA-approved; supported by CLEAR trials	Bempedoic acid is a prodrug activated in hepatocytes — inhibits ATP-citrate lyase, a precursor enzyme in cholesterol biosynthesis upstream of HMG-CoA reductase. This reduces hepatic cholesterol, upregulates LDL receptors, and enhances LDL clearance. Activation in the liver alone avoids muscle-related side effects.	Hyperuricemia, mild myalgias, elevated liver enzymes, rare tendon rupture	Statin-intolerant patients, ASCVD prevention, primary hypercholesterolemia	180 mg orally once daily
Evinacumab	FDA-approved; ELIPSE-HoFH trial	Evinacumab is a monoclonal antibody that blocks ANGPTL3 — a key inhibitor of lipoprotein and endothelial lipase. Inhibition of ANGPTL3 leads to enhanced lipolysis and LDL clearance, independent of LDL receptor activity — making it suitable for HoFH patients with defective LDLR function.	Flu-like symptoms, nasopharyngitis, rare hypersensitivity	Homozygous familial hypercholesterolemia, severe hypertriglyceridemia, resistant dyslipidemia	15 mg/kg IV over 1 hour every 4 weeks
Pemafibrate	Phase 3 ongoing (PROMINENT trial); approved in Japan	Pemafibrate selectively activates PPAR-α in liver and muscle — enhances β-oxidation, stimulates lipoprotein lipase, reduces triglyceride synthesis, and promotes HDL maturation via ApoA-I upregulation. It also reduces inflammatory cytokines and endothelial dysfunction.	Mild gastrointestinal symptoms, increased liver enzymes, minimal renal toxicity	Hypertriglyceridemia, NAFLD, metabolic syndrome-related dyslipidemia	0.2 mg orally twice daily

Recent Advances in the Management of Bronchial Asthma

Drug Name	Clinical Trial Phase	Mechanism of Action	Adverse Drug Reaction	Uses	Dose
Benralizumab	FDA-approved; SIROCCO & CALIMA trials	Benralizumab targets IL-5Rα on eosinophils and basophils – blocks IL-5 signalling – induces antibody-dependent cell-mediated cytotoxicity (ADCC) via NK cells – leads to rapid eosinophil depletion – reduces mucus hypersecretion and airway inflammation – prevents airway remodelling.	Headache, sore throat, hypersensitivity reactions, herpes zoster infections	Severe eosinophilic asthma (≥12 years)	30 mg subcutaneously every 4 weeks (first 3 doses), then every 8 weeks
Tezepelumab	FDA-approved; PATHWAY & NAVIGATOR trials	Tezepelumab binds TSLP – blocks activation of dendritic and Th2 cells – suppresses IL-4, IL-5, IL-13, IL-17 – reduces both eosinophilic and neutrophilic inflammation – inhibits goblet cell hyperplasia – prevents airway remodelling and smooth muscle contraction.	Nasopharyngitis, arthralgia, fatigue, injection-site reactions	Severe asthma, including non-eosinophilic phenotypes	210 mg subcutaneously every 4 weeks
Dupilumab	FDA-approved; QUEST & VENTURE trials	Dupilumab blocks IL-4Rα – inhibits IL-4 and IL-13 signalling – reduces eosinophilic airway inflammation – suppresses mucus hypersecretion – prevents airway fibrosis and remodelling – lowers corticosteroid dependence in severe asthma.	Conjunctivitis, eosinophilic pneumonia, injection reactions	Moderate-to-severe asthma, steroid-dependent asthma (≥12 years)	400/600 mg loading, then 200/300 mg subcutaneously every 2 weeks

Rilzabrutinib	Phase III trials ongoing	Rilzabrutinib inhibits Bruton's Tyrosine Kinase – blocks IgE-mediated and non-IgE mast cell activation – suppresses histamine and cytokine release – modulates B cell-driven IL-4, IL-5, IL-13 secretion – reduces both allergic and T2-low inflammation.	Headache, nausea, infection risk, neutropenia	Under investigation for asthma and chronic urticaria	200 mg orally twice daily (trial dosing)
Fevipiprant	Phase III completed; not FDA-approved	Fevipiprant antagonizes DP2 (CRTh2) receptor – blocks prostaglandin D2-mediated eosinophil and Th2 recruitment – reduces IL-4, IL-5, IL-13 secretion – promotes eosinophil apoptosis – prevents airway remodelling and smooth muscle hypertrophy.	Diarrhoea, nausea, QT prolongation, liver enzyme elevation	Investigational use in severe asthma	150–450 mg once daily (oral)

Recent Advances in the Management of Pulmonary Hypertension

Drug Name	Clinical Trial Phase	Mechanism of Action	Adverse Drug Reaction	Uses	Dose
Sotatercept	FDA-approved (2024); STELLAR trial	Sotatercept acts as a ligand trap for activin and other TGF-β ligands – reduces smooth muscle proliferation and fibrosis – restores BMPR2 signalling – improves pulmonary vascular tone – lowers pulmonary vascular resistance and right ventricular strain.	Fatigue, headache, elevated haemoglobin, GI upset	Add-on therapy in PAH (WHO Group 1) to improve exercise capacity	0.3–0.7 mg/kg subcutaneously every 3 weeks
Selexipag	FDA-approved; GRIPHON trial	Selexipag selectively activates IP receptors – increases cAMP in pulmonary arterial smooth muscle – promotes vasodilation – inhibits vascular proliferation – reduces platelet aggregation and pulmonary vascular resistance.	Flushing, jaw pain, headache, hepatic dysfunction	Oral therapy for PAH to slow progression and improve symptoms	200 mcg orally twice daily
Riociguat	FDA-approved for PAH and CTEPH; PATENT & CHEST trials	Riociguat stimulates sGC independently and sensitizes it to NO – boosts cGMP – promotes smooth muscle relaxation – reduces pulmonary arterial pressure – inhibits arterial remodelling and improves cardiac output.	Hypo-tension, oedema, dizziness, bleeding risk	PAH and inoperable or recurrent CTEPH (WHO Groups 1 and 4)	1 mg orally three times daily
Macitentan	FDA-approved; SERAPHIN trial	Macitentan blocks both ETA and ETB receptors – prevents endothelin-1-mediated vasoconstriction, proliferation, and fibrosis – reduces PVR – delays disease progression and right heart overload.	Hepato-toxicity, anaemia, oedema, nasal congestion	First-line oral therapy for long-term PAH management	10 mg orally once daily
Treprostinil	FDA-approved; FREEDOM trials	Treprostinil activates IP receptors – increases cAMP – causes pulmonary vasodilation – inhibits platelet aggregation – reduces vascular smooth muscle proliferation and fibrosis.	Flushing, nausea, diarrhoea, hypotension, injection pain	Advanced PAH, especially as an alternative to intravenous prostacyclin	1.25 ng/kg/min via SC or IV infusion

Recent Advances in the Management of Rheumatoid Arthritis

Drug Name	Clinical Trial Phase	Mechanism of Action	Adverse Drug Reaction	Uses	Dose
Otilimab	Phase III completed; not FDA-approved	Otilimab binds GM-CSF – blocks its receptor-mediated activation of macrophages and neutrophils – inhibits downstream JAK-STAT and MAPK signalling – reduces TNF-α, IL-6, IL-1β – suppresses joint inflammation and osteoclast-driven bone erosion.	Injection site reactions, URTIs, mild liver enzyme elevation, leukopenia	Investigational in RA (DMARD-resistant) and osteoarthritis	180 mg subcutaneous weekly (trial dose)
Upadacitinib	FDA-approved; SELECT trials	Upadacitinib selectively inhibits JAK1 – blocks cytokine-triggered STAT activation – reduces expression of pro-inflammatory cytokines (TNF-α, IL-6, IFN-γ) – suppresses T-cell and macrophage activation – decreases joint inflammation and destruction.	Headache, infections, liver enzyme elevation, dyslipidaemia	Moderate-to-severe RA unresponsive to methotrexate	15 mg orally once daily
Filgotinib	Approved in EU and Japan; not FDA-approved	Filgotinib inhibits JAK1 – blocks IL-6, IL-23, IFN-γ pathways – reduces inflammatory gene transcription – suppresses macrophage and neutrophil activity – improves joint function with fewer off-target effects.	URTIs, headache, VTE risk, mild GI upset	RA (moderate-to-severe)	200 mg orally once daily
Abrocitinib	Phase III ongoing	Abrocitinib selectively inhibits JAK1 – disrupts cytokine-driven STAT signalling – suppresses IL-6, TNF-α, IL-23 activity – reduces synovial inflammation and joint damage – spares JAK2/JAK3, reducing haematologic toxicity.	URTIs, nausea, diarrhoea, mild LFT elevations	Under investigation for RA, IBD, osteoporosis	100–200 mg orally once daily (trial dosing)

Bimekizumab	Phase III trials ongoing	Bimekizumab neutralizes IL-17A and IL-17F – suppresses synovial fibroblast activation – reduces matrix metalloproteinase release – blocks osteoclast activation – inhibits Th17-driven inflammation and joint destruction.	Fungal infections, fatigue, nasopha-ryngitis, GI upset	Investigational for RA and other Th17-driven diseases	160–320 mg subcuta-neously every 4 weeks

Recent Advances in the Management of Osteoporosis

Drug Name	Clinical Trial Phase	Mechanism of Action	Adverse Drug Reaction	Uses	Dose
Romosozumab (Anti-Sclerostin Monoclonal Antibody)	FDA-approved (FRAME, ARCH trials)	Inhibits sclerostin - enhances Wnt/β-catenin signaling - increases osteoblast activity - reduces osteoclast formation	Arthralgia, myalgia, injection site reactions, hypocalcaemia, osteonecrosis of jaw	Osteoporosis in postmenopausal women at high fracture risk	210 mg s.c. once monthly (for 12 months)
Abaloparatide	FDA-approved (ACTIVE, ACTIVExtend)	Binds to PTH1R RG conformation - stimulates osteoblasts - reduces osteoclast activity	Hypercalcaemia, dizziness, hypotension, palpitations	Severe osteoporosis with high fracture risk	80 mcg s.c. once daily
Odanacatib	Discontinued after Phase III (LOFT)	Selectively inhibits cathepsin K - reduces collagen degradation - maintains osteoclast viability	Increased risk of stroke, atrial fibrillation, musculoskeletal pain, diarrhoea	Previously under investigation for postmenopausal osteoporosis (development discontinued)	50 mg orally once weekly (investi-gational)
Denosumab + Teriparatide	Phase IV (DATA & DATA-HD)	Denosumab blocks RANKL - suppresses osteoclasts; Teriparatide activates PTH1R - enhances osteoblasts	Denosumab: Hypocalcaemia, infections, ONJ; Teriparatide: Hypercalcaemia, dizziness, headache	High-risk osteoporosis, especially with multiple fractures or severe BMD loss	Denosumab: 60 mg s.c. every 6 months; Teriparatide: 20–40 mcg s.c. daily
TransCon PTH	Phase III (ongoing)	Sustained PTH1R activation - enhances osteoblast activity - stabilizes calcium metabolism	Hypercalcaemia, hypercalciuria, nausea, dizziness, injection-site pain	Osteoporosis and hypopara-thyroidism under investigation	18–20 µg s.c. once daily

Recent Advances in the Management of Diabetes Mellitus

Drug Name	Clinical Trial Phase	Mechanism of Action	Adverse Drug Reaction	Uses	Dose
Dapagliflozin (SGLT2 Inhibitor)	FDA-approved – Evaluated in DECLARE-TIMI 58 trial.	Dapagliflozin selectively inhibits the SGLT2 transporter in the proximal renal tubule, reducing glucose reabsorption and promoting glucosuria. This leads to lower blood glucose, modest weight loss, and improvements in insulin sensitivity. It also reduces blood pressure and albuminuria, offering cardiovascular and renal protection.	UTIs, genital infections, hypotension, dehydration, acute kidney injury.	Type 2 diabetes, heart failure (HFrEF), chronic kidney disease.	10 mg orally once daily.
Canagliflozin	FDA-approved – Evaluated in CANVAS trial	Canagliflozin blocks SGLT2 in the renal proximal tubule, decreasing glucose reabsorption and enhancing urinary glucose excretion. This improves glycemic control, insulin sensitivity, and reduces glucotoxic stress. Cardiovascular and renal protection occurs through natriuresis and hemodynamic effects.	UTIs, polyuria, hypotension, dehydration, rare Fournier's gangrene.	Type 2 diabetes with cardiovascular or renal risk.	100 mg orally once daily before breakfast.

Teplizumab	FDA-approved (2022)	Teplizumab is a monoclonal antibody that binds to the CD3ε subunit on T lymphocytes. This interaction prevents full T-cell activation, promotes immune tolerance, and expands regulatory T-cell populations. As a result, it delays autoimmune destruction of pancreatic β-cells and preserves endogenous insulin secretion in at-risk individuals, effectively delaying the clinical onset of type 1 diabetes.	Lymphopenia, rash, upper respiratory infections, cytokine release syndrome, viral reactivation.	Delaying the onset of type 1 diabetes in genetically or immunologically predisposed individuals.	IV infusion for 14 days, titrated from 65 μg/m^2 to 1,030 μg/m^2/day.
Tirzepatide	FDA-approved (2022) – SURPASS Trial	Tirzepatide activates both GLP-1 and GIP receptors, leading to glucose-dependent insulin secretion, reduced glucagon levels, delayed gastric emptying, and appetite suppression. It improves insulin sensitivity and promotes significant weight loss. The dual receptor action offers superior glycemic and metabolic control compared to GLP-1 alone.	Nausea, vomiting, hypoglycemia (with insulin/ sulfonylureas), pancreatitis, appetite reduction, weight loss.	Type 2 diabetes, with additional benefits in weight management.	2.5 mg subcutaneously once weekly.
Retatrutide	Phase III trials ongoing	Retatrutide is a triple agonist targeting GLP-1, GIP, and glucagon receptors. It enhances insulin secretion, reduces glucagon, increases energy expenditure, and significantly promotes weight loss. Its effect on hepatic lipid metabolism offers promise for NAFLD and broader cardiometabolic benefits.	Nausea, vomiting, diarrhea, dizziness, hypoglycemia, pancreatitis, thyroid C-cell hyperplasia.	Investigational use for type 2 diabetes and obesity.	1–12 mg subcutaneously once weekly (trial-dependent).

Ultra-Rapid Lispro (URLi)	FDA-approved (2020) – PRONTO-T1D/T2D Trial	This formulation contains absorption enhancers that accelerate insulin lispro activity, mimicking physiological insulin response to meals. It reduces postprandial glucose spikes more effectively than standard rapid-acting insulin.	Hypoglycemia, injection site reactions.	Type 1 and type 2 diabetes for mealtime glucose control.	Individualized; given immediately before or up to 20 minutes after meals.
Insulin Icodec	Phase III trials ongoing – ONWARDS Trial	A once-weekly basal insulin analog with slow and consistent release due to high albumin binding. It maintains stable glucose levels across the week and reduces injection frequency.	Hypoglycemia (less frequent), injection site reactions.	Investigational therapy for diabetes.	70 units subcutaneously once weekly (in trials).
Insulin Glargine U-300	FDA-approved	Concentrated insulin formulation that forms microprecipitates post-injection, providing flat and prolonged basal insulin release for over 36 hours.	Hypoglycemia, weight gain.	Basal insulin therapy in type 1 and type 2 diabetes.	0.2 units/kg once daily, titrated to clinical response.
Insulin Degludec	FDA-approved	Forms multi-hexamers at the injection site, ensuring an ultra-long basal insulin profile with a duration exceeding 42 hours and reduced glucose variability.	Hypoglycemia, lipodystrophy, injection site reactions.	Long-acting basal insulin for type 1 and 2 diabetes.	0.2–0.4 units/kg/day.
Insulin AspartFiasp	FDA-approved	Contains niacinamide to speed absorption of insulin aspart, allowing quicker onset for postprandial glucose control.	Hypoglycemia, peripheral edema, injection-site reactions.	Mealtime insulin in type 1 and 2 diabetes.	Dosed before or shortly after meals; unit-for-unit conversion with other rapid insulins.

Newer Contraceptives

Drug Name	Clinical Trial Phase	Mechanism of Action	Adverse Drug Reaction	Uses	Dose
Norgestrel (Opill)	FDA-approved (2023)	Norgestrel acts primarily by suppressing ovulation through inhibition of gonadotropin release, particularly luteinizing hormone. It increases cervical mucus viscosity, impeding sperm penetration and motility. It also induces endometrial atrophy, reducing the likelihood of implantation, and delays ovum transport by altering tubal motility. Additionally, it diminishes sperm capacitation, further decreasing the chances of fertilization.	Irregular bleeding, breast tenderness, headache, mood changes, mild acne.	Over-the-counter oral contraceptive for reproductive-age women.	0.075 mg (75 mcg) once daily at the same time each day.
Dapivirine-Levonorgestrel Vaginal Ring	Phase III - MTN-044, DREAM trials.	Levonorgestrel suppresses ovulation, thickens cervical mucus, and thins the endometrial lining, creating a hostile environment for fertilization and implantation. Dapivirine, an NNRTI, inhibits HIV reverse transcriptase locally within the vaginal environment, blocking viral replication. The ring maintains high local concentrations with minimal systemic exposure, offering dual protection.	Menstrual irregularities, headache, nausea, acne, mood disturbances, breast tenderness.	Under investigation for dual protection: contraception and HIV prevention.	Releases 4 mg/day dapivirine and 20 mcg/day levonorgestrel over 90 days.

Segesterone Acetate + Ethinyl Oestradiol (Annovera)	FDA-approved	Segesterone acetate inhibits FSH and LH secretion, suppressing ovulation, while also thickening cervical mucus and thinning the endometrial lining. The ring provides continuous, low-dose hormonal release through vaginal absorption without daily administration. Ethinyl estradiol stabilizes the endometrium and supports cycle control.	Vaginal discharge, breast tenderness, nausea, headache, irregular bleeding.	Long-acting reversible contraception (1-year use).	Releases 150 mcg/day segesterone acetate and 13 mcg/day ethinyl oestradiol; used in 21/7-day cycles for 13 cycles per ring.,
17α-Ethynylestradiol + Levonorgestrel Transdermal Patch (Twirla)	FDA-approved	Twirla combines levonorgestrel and ethinyl estradiol to inhibit the HPO axis, suppressing ovulation. It also increases cervical mucus viscosity and induces endometrial thinning. The transdermal system ensures consistent hormone levels, avoiding hepatic first-pass metabolism and minimizing hormonal fluctuations.	Skin irritation, breakthrough bleeding, weight gain, rare hepatic dysfunction.	Weekly contraceptive patch.	Delivers 30 mcg/day ethinyl estradiol and 120 mcg/day levonorgestrel; applied weekly for 3 weeks, followed by 1 patch-free week.
Drospirenone-Only Pill (Slynd)	FDA-approved	Drospirenone suppresses ovulation by inhibiting FSH and LH secretion. It thickens cervical mucus and causes endometrial thinning, reducing fertilization and implantation. Additionally, its anti-mineralocorticoid action helps reduce water retention, while anti-androgenic effects can benefit women with hormonal imbalances such as PCOS.	Irregular bleeding, nausea, bloating, breast tenderness, mood swings, hyperkalaemia.	Oral contraception, especially beneficial in estrogen-sensitive women.	4 mg once daily in a 24 active + 4 inert pill cycle.

Recent Advances in the Management of Peptic Ulcer

Drug Name	Clinical Trial Phase	Mechanism of Action	Adverse Drug Reaction	Uses	Dose
Vonoprazan	FDA-approved (2022) – PHALCON-EE, PHALCON-HP	Vonoprazan is a potassium-competitive acid blocker that directly inhibits the H^+/K^+-ATPase in gastric parietal cells. It binds reversibly at the potassium site, leading to rapid and prolonged suppression of gastric acid without requiring activation in acidic conditions. Its acid stability allows for consistent acid suppression within 2 hours of dosing, improving healing rates in peptic ulcers and enhancing the efficacy of H. pylori eradication therapies.	Headache, nausea, diarrhoea, hypergastrinemia, increased risk of C. difficile infection.	Peptic ulcer disease, H. pylori eradication, gastroesophageal reflux disease (GERD).	20 mg orally once daily.
Tegoprazan	Approved in South Korea & China; Phase III (U.S.)	Tegoprazan inhibits the gastric H^+/K^+-ATPase through potassium-competitive binding, offering immediate and reversible suppression of acid secretion. Unlike PPIs, it does not require acid activation and achieves a faster onset of action with sustained acid control, enhancing ulcer healing and H. pylori therapy efficacy.	Diarrhoea, nausea, dizziness, hypomagnesemia, hypergastrinemia, C. difficile risk.	Peptic ulcer disease, GERD, H. pylori therapy.	50 mg orally once daily.
Rebamipide	Approved in Japan, China, and South Korea	Rebamipide enhances gastric mucosal defense by stimulating prostaglandin synthesis, increasing mucus and bicarbonate secretion, and promoting mucosal repair. It also reduces oxidative stress and inflammation through cytokine suppression and antioxidant activity, protecting against NSAID-induced and H. pylori-associated damage.	Mild nausea, constipation, elevated liver enzymes, hypersensitivity.	NSAID-induced ulcers, peptic ulcers, mucosal protection.	100 mg orally three times daily.

Lafutidine	Approved in Japan	Lafutidine is a second-generation H_2 receptor antagonist that blocks histamine-mediated acid secretion and activates capsaicin-sensitive sensory neurons. It stimulates mucus, bicarbonate secretion, and blood flow, enhancing mucosal healing. Its anti-inflammatory and antioxidant properties provide added protection against NSAIDs and H. pylori-associated gastritis.	Dizziness, mild nausea, hepatotoxicity, hyperse-nsitivity.	Peptic ulcer disease, GERD.	10 mg orally twice daily.
Ilaprazole	Approved in China and South Korea	Ilaprazole is a long-acting proton pump inhibitor that irreversibly binds to gastric H^+/K^+-ATPase via acid activation in parietal cells. It forms stable bonds with cysteine residues on the pump, leading to prolonged suppression of acid secretion. It also promotes mucosal healing and has more predictable metabolism across populations due to reduced CYP2C19 dependence.	Nausea, dizziness, fracture risk, rare interstitial nephritis.	Peptic ulcer disease, GERD.	10–20 mg orally once daily.

Recent Advances in the Management of Irritable Bowel Syndrome (IBS)

Drug Name	Clinical Trial Phase	Mechanism of Action	Adverse Drug Reaction	Uses	Dose
Linaclotide	FDA-approved – Linzess IBS-C Trials.	Linaclotide binds to guanylate cyclase-C receptors on intestinal epithelial cells, increasing intracellular and extracellular cyclic GMP. This enhances chloride and bicarbonate secretion via CFTR channels, inhibits sodium absorption, and hydrates stool to promote bowel movements. Extracellular cyclic GMP also modulates sensory neuron activity, reducing visceral pain.	Diarrhoea, abdominal pain, bloating, allergic reactions.	IBS-C, chronic idiopathic constipation (CIC).	290 mcg once daily, 30 minutes before the first meal.
Lubiprostone	FDA-approved – Amitiza IBS-C Trials	Lubiprostone activates type-2 chloride channels (ClC-2) on intestinal epithelial cells, promoting chloride-rich fluid secretion and inhibiting sodium absorption. It also acts on prostaglandin EP4 receptors to enhance secretion and motility, and may reduce inflammation and visceral hypersensitivity, aiding in symptom relief for IBS-C.	Nausea, diarrhoea, headache, abdominal distension.	IBS-C, opioid-induced constipation, chronic idiopathic constipation.	8 mcg twice daily with food and water.
Tegaserod	FDA-approved for IBS-C in women under 65	Tegaserod is a selective 5-HT4 receptor agonist that enhances acetylcholine and CGRP release in the gut, promoting peristalsis, fluid secretion, and improving bowel transit. It reduces visceral hypersensitivity and may exhibit anti-inflammatory properties, without significant action on 5-HT3 receptors, minimizing nausea and diarrhoea.	Diarrhoea, abdominal pain, nausea, allergic reactions.	IBS-C, chronic idiopathic constipation.	6 mg twice daily before meals.

Eluxadoline	FDA-approved for IBS-D	Eluxadoline acts as a mixed μ-opioid receptor agonist, δ-opioid receptor antagonist, and κ-opioid receptor agonist. It decreases colonic motility and secretion while providing visceral analgesia without significant central opioid effects. It reduces stool frequency, improves consistency, and alleviates abdominal pain.	Nausea, abdominal pain, constipation, pancreatitis (rare).	IBS-D.	100 mg twice daily with food; 75 mg twice daily in special populations.
Rifaximin	FDA-approved for IBS-D	Rifaximin is a minimally absorbed antibiotic that binds to bacterial RNA polymerase, reducing bacterial overgrowth and modulating gut microbiota without disturbing beneficial flora. It reduces intestinal inflammation, normalizes motility, and improves gut-brain axis signalling, offering symptom relief in IBS-D.	Nausea, flatulence, headache, abdominal pain, risk of C. difficile infection.	IBS-D, traveller's diarrhoea, hepatic encephalopathy.	400–550 mg three times daily for 14 days.
Alosetron	Phase II ongoing (restricted FDA approval)	Alosetron selectively inhibits 5-HT3 receptors on enteric neurons, reducing colonic motility, slowing transit, and inhibiting excessive intestinal secretion. It modulates visceral pain signaling to the brain and enhances stool consistency. Its use is restricted due to the rare risk of ischemic colitis.	Constipation, nausea, abdominal pain, flatulence, headache, dry mouth, ischaemic colitis (rare).	Severe IBS-D in women unresponsive to conventional therapy.	0.5 mg twice daily; may increase to 1 mg twice daily after 4 weeks.

Recent Advances in the Management of Inflammatory Bowel Disease (IBD)

Drug Name	Clinical Trial Phase	Mechanism of Action	Adverse Drug Reaction	Uses	Dose
Vedolizumab	FDA-approved - GEMINI I & II Trials	Vedolizumab is a gut-selective IgG1 monoclonal antibody that binds α4β7 integrin, blocking lymphocyte interaction with MAdCAM-1 on gut endothelial cells. This prevents T-cell migration into intestinal mucosa, reducing local inflammation without systemic immunosuppression. Inhibition of pro-inflammatory cytokine release promotes mucosal healing and lowers infection risks compared to systemic biologics.	Nasopharyngitis, headache, joint pain, rare risk of progressive multifocal leukoencephalopathy.	Moderate-to-severe ulcerative colitis (UC) and Crohn's disease (CD), particularly post anti-TNF failure.	300 mg IV at weeks 0, 2, and 6, then every 8 weeks thereafter.
Ustekinumab	FDA-approved - Amitiza IBS-C Trials	Ustekinumab inhibits the shared p40 subunit of IL-12 and IL-23 cytokines, suppressing Th1 and Th17 immune responses central to IBD pathology. It decreases production of IFN-γ, TNF-α, IL-17, and IL-22, reducing intestinal inflammation, restoring epithelial barrier integrity, and minimizing systemic immunosuppression compared to TNF inhibitors.	Nasopharyngitis, arthralgia, headache, upper respiratory tract infections.	Moderate-to-severe ulcerative colitis and Crohn's disease.	IV induction (260 mg, 390 mg, or 520 mg based on weight); then 90 mg subcutaneously every 8 weeks.

Risankizumab	FDA-approved (2022) – ADVANCE and MOTIVATE Trials	Risankizumab selectively targets the p19 subunit of IL-23, preventing Th17 cell survival and reducing secretion of IL-17, IL-22, and TNF-α. It promotes mucosal healing by decreasing neutrophilic infiltration, restoring gut barrier function, and downregulating chronic intestinal inflammation.	Nasopharyngitis, headache, arthralgia, elevated liver enzymes, hypersensitivity reactions.	Moderate-to-severe Crohn's disease; trials ongoing for ulcerative colitis.	600 mg IV at weeks 0, 4, and 8; maintenance 360 mg subcutaneously every 8 weeks.
Upadacitinib	FDA-approved (2022) – U-ACHIEVE and U-ACCOMPLISH Trials	Upadacitinib is a selective JAK1 inhibitor that blocks pro-inflammatory cytokine signaling via the JAK-STAT pathway, particularly suppressing IL-6, IL-12, IL-23, and IFN-γ. By targeting gut-specific inflammation while preserving hematopoietic pathways, it supports mucosal healing and restores epithelial integrity with a lower hematologic risk than non-selective JAK inhibitors.	Nasopharyngitis, headache, dyslipidaemia, thrombotic risk, opportunistic infections.	Moderate-to-severe ulcerative colitis; trials ongoing for Crohn's disease.	Induction 45 mg orally once daily for 8 weeks; maintenance 15–30 mg orally once daily.
Ozanimod	FDA-approved – TRUE NORTH Trial	Ozanimod selectively modulates S1P1 and S1P5 receptors, trapping lymphocytes within lymphoid tissues and reducing their infiltration into gut mucosa. This localizes immune suppression to the intestine, minimizes systemic immune deficits, and supports mucosal healing with fewer cardiovascular and systemic side effects than earlier S1P modulators.	Bradycardia, hypertension, nasopharyngitis, elevated liver enzymes.	Moderate-to-severe ulcerative colitis; trials ongoing for Crohn's disease.	Initiation titration: 0.23 mg daily (Days 1–4), 0.46 mg (Days 5–7), then 0.92 mg daily thereafter.

Newer Beta-Lactam Antibiotics

Drug Name	Clinical Trial Phase	Mechanism of Action	Adverse Drug Reaction	Uses	Dose
Ceftazidime-Avibactam	FDA-approved – complicated IAI, UTI, and HAP.	Ceftazidime inhibits PBP3-mediated bacterial cell wall synthesis in Gram-negative organisms, causing cell death. Avibactam, a novel β-lactamase inhibitor, binds and inactivates Class A, C, and some D β-lactamases, restoring ceftazidime efficacy against resistant strains. This combination covers CRE and MDR Pseudomonas but not Acinetobacter.	Hypersensitivity, diarrhoea, headache, nausea, hypokalaemia, elevated liver enzymes.	CRE and MDR Gram-negative infections.	2.5 g (ceftazidime 2 g + avibactam 0.5 g) IV over 2 hours every 8 hours.
Meropenem-Vaborbactam	FDA-approved – complicated UTI, HAP, bloodstream infections.	Meropenem inhibits bacterial cell wall synthesis by targeting PBPs. Vaborbactam, a boronic acid derivative, inactivates KPC and other Class A β-lactamases. It restores meropenem activity against CRE, offering superior potency compared to older combinations.	Hypokalaemia, diarrhoea, seizures (rare), elevated liver enzymes.	CRE infections and complicated UTI.	4 g (meropenem 2 g + vaborbactam 2 g) IV over 3 hours every 8 hours.
Imipenem-Cilastatin-Relebactam	FDA-approved – complicated UTI, cIAI, HAP/VAP.	Imipenem inhibits cell wall synthesis; cilastatin prevents renal degradation of imipenem; relebactam inhibits β-lactamases restoring imipenem activity against KPC-producing Enterobacterales and MDR Pseudomonas.	CNS toxicity (seizures), nephrotoxicity, elevated liver enzymes.	CRE infections, MDR Pseudomonas, complicated UTI, cIAI, HAP/VAP.	1.25 g (imipenem 500 mg + cilastatin 500 mg + relebactam 250 mg) IV over 30 minutes every 6 hours.

Cefepime-Enmeta-zobactam	FDA-approved (2024) – complicated UTI.	Cefepime binds PBPs disrupting cell wall synthesis. Enmetazobactam, a potent β-lactamase inhibitor, restores cefepime activity against ESBL-producing and some carbapenemase-producing bacteria.	Hypersensitivity, gastrointestinal upset, C. difficile infection, elevated liver enzymes.	Complicated UTIs due to ESBL-producing bacteria.	2 g cefepime + 0.5 g enmeta-zobactam IV over 2 hours every 8 hours.
Cefiderocol	FDA-approved – complicated UTI, HAP, VAP.	Cefiderocol uses siderophore-mediated transport to actively enter Gram-negative bacteria, bypassing porin resistance. It inhibits PBPs, achieving potent bactericidal activity against CRE, MDR Pseudomonas, Acinetobacter, and Stenotrophomonas.	Neurotoxicity, nausea, injection-site reactions.	MDR Gram-negative infections including CRE and Acinetobacter.	2 g IV every 8 hours (infused over 3 hours).
Ceftobiprole	FDA-approved – CAP and HAP (not VAP).	Ceftobiprole inhibits PBPs, including PBP2a in MRSA and PBP2x in penicillin-resistant S. pneumoniae, offering broad Gram-positive and Gram-negative coverage. Limited against ESBL and carbapenemase producers.	Hypersensitivity, C. difficile infection, hepatotoxicity.	Community-acquired pneumonia (CAP), hospital-acquired pneumonia (HAP), MRSA infections.	500 mg IV every 8 hours (infused over 2 hours).
Razupenem	Completed Phase II trials.	Razupenem is a carbapenem that binds PBPs (especially PBP2 and PBP3), inhibiting peptidoglycan cross-linking. It shows stability against ESBLs and MRSA but limited against MBL-producing strains.	Seizures (rare), hypokalaemia, nephrotoxicity, nausea.	Investigational use for MDR Gram-negative infections, MRSA, HAP/VAP.	Phase II trials – 500 mg to 1 g IV every 8 hours.

Newer Antifungals

Drug Name	Clinical Trial Phase	Mechanism of Action	Adverse Drug Reaction	Uses	Dose
Ibrexafungerp	FDA-approved – Vulvovaginal Candidiasis (VVC); investigational for invasive candidiasis.	Ibrexafungerp inhibits (1,3)-β-D-glucan synthase, disrupting fungal cell wall biosynthesis, leading to cell death. It is fungicidal against Candida and fungistatic against Aspergillus. It covers fluconazole-resistant and some echinocandin-resistant Candida strains.	GI disturbances, headache, dizziness, hepatotoxicity.	FDA-approved for VVC; under investigation for invasive Candida infections.	300 mg orally twice daily for 1 day (total 600 mg).
Meropenem-Vaborbactam	FDA-approved – complicated UTI, HAP, bloodstream infections.	Meropenem inhibits bacterial cell wall synthesis by targeting PBPs. Vaborbactam, a boronic acid derivative, inactivates KPC and other Class A β-lactamases. It restores meropenem activity against CRE, offering superior potency compared to older combinations.	Hypokalaemia, diarrhoea, seizures (rare), elevated liver enzymes.	CRE infections and complicated UTI.	4 g (meropenem 2 g + vaborbactam 2 g) IV over 3 hours every 8 hours.
Oteseconazole	FDA-approved – recurrent vulvovaginal candidiasis (RVVC).	Oteseconazole selectively inhibits fungal CYP51, impairing ergosterol biosynthesis and leading to membrane dysfunction. It shows potent activity against fluconazole-resistant Candida species, with reduced toxicity compared to earlier azoles.	Headache, nausea, QT prolongation, hepatotoxicity.	FDA-approved for RVVC; investigational for resistant Candida infections.	Loading: 600 mg Day 1, 450 mg Day 2; Maintenance: 150 mg weekly for 11 weeks.

Rezafungin	FDA-approved – candidemia and invasive candidiasis.	Rezafungin inhibits (1,3)-β-D-glucan synthase, compromising fungal cell wall integrity. Its long half-life allows once-weekly dosing, offering an advantage over traditional echinocandins. It retains potency against azole- and echinocandin-resistant Candida strains.	Infusion reactions, hepatic enzyme elevation, hypokalaemia.	Candidemia and invasive candidiasis; under study for invasive aspergillosis.	400 mg IV on Day 1, then 200 mg IV weekly.
Olorofim	Phase III trials – invasive aspergillosis and mould infections.	Olorofim inhibits fungal dihydroorotate dehydrogenase (DHODH), disrupting pyrimidine biosynthesis and causing fungal cell death. It is highly selective for fungal DHODH, offering a novel mechanism of action distinct from existing antifungals.	Infusion reactions, headache, GI upset, hepatic toxicity.	Investigational for invasive Aspergillus and rare mould infections.	150 mg orally twice daily (clinical trial dose).
Fosmanogepix	Phase III trials – invasive Candida and mould infections.	Fosmanogepix inhibits Gwt1 enzyme required for GPI-anchor biosynthesis, impairing fungal cell wall integrity and leading to cell death. It shows activity against resistant Candida and Aspergillus strains.	GI disturbances, hepatic enzyme elevation, hypersensitivity reactions.	Investigational for invasive Candida and Aspergillus infections.	1000 mg IV twice on Day 1 (loading), then 600 mg IV daily or oral 700 mg twice daily.

Newer Antiviral Drugs

Drug Name	Clinical Trial Phase	Mechanism of Action	Adverse Drug Reaction	Uses	Dose
Baloxavir Marboxil (Newer Anti-Influenza Drug)	FDA-approved for acute influenza.	Baloxavir inhibits the cap-dependent endonuclease (CEN) activity of the influenza viral polymerase, blocking viral mRNA transcription at an early stage. This prevents cap-snatching, halting replication of both influenza A and B viruses, including oseltamivir-resistant strains.	Diarrhoea, nasopharyngitis, headache, neuropsychiatric symptoms.	Influenza A & B infection (within 48 hours of symptom onset).	40 mg (body weight 40–<80 kg) or 80 mg (≥80 kg) as a single oral dose.
Molnupiravir (Newer Anti-COVID Drug)	FDA Emergency Use Authorization (2021).	Molnupiravir induces lethal mutagenesis by incorporating itself into viral RNA through its active form (NHC-TP), causing error catastrophe and collapse of SARS-CoV-2 replication.	Nausea, diarrhoea, headache, potential teratogenicity.	Mild to moderate COVID-19 in high-risk patients.	800 mg orally every 12 hours for 5 days.
Remdesivir (Newer Anti-COVID Drug)	FDA-approved (2020) for hospitalized COVID-19 patients.	Remdesivir is an adenosine analogue that terminates RNA synthesis by the SARS-CoV-2 RNA-dependent RNA polymerase (RdRp), causing delayed chain termination and halting viral replication.	Hepatotoxicity, nausea, nephrotoxicity, bradycardia.	Severe COVID-19 requiring hospitalization.	Day 1: 200 mg IV; Days 2–5: 100 mg IV daily.
Besifovir (Newer Anti-HBV Drug)	Phase III trials completed, nearing approval.	Besifovir is a nucleotide reverse transcriptase inhibitor (NtRTI) that causes premature termination of HBV DNA chain elongation by HBV polymerase, selectively inhibiting viral replication with minimal renal toxicity compared to tenofovir.	Fatigue, hepatotoxicity, lactic acidosis.	Chronic Hepatitis B infection.	150 mg orally once daily.
Lenacapavir (Newer Anti-HIV Drug)	FDA-approved (2022) for multidrug-resistant HIV-1.	Lenacapavir binds to the HIV-1 capsid protein, inhibiting uncoating, nuclear import, and assembly, disrupting the HIV life cycle at multiple stages and showing efficacy against resistant strains.	Injection site reactions, weight gain, hepatic dysfunction.	Multidrug-resistant HIV-1.	600 mg orally on Day 1 and Day 2 (loading) followed by subcutaneous injections.

Islatravir (Newer Anti-HIV Drug)	Phase III trials for HIV-1 treatment and prevention (PrEP).	Islatravir inhibits reverse transcriptase by immediate chain termination and translocation inhibition, displaying potent activity even against drug-resistant HIV strains.	Lymphopenia, headache, nausea, hypersensitivity.	HIV-1 PrEP and treatment (investigational).	0.75 mg oral daily combined with other antiretrovirals.

Recent Advances in the Management of Malaria

Drug Name	Clinical Trial Phase	Mechanism of Action	Adverse Drug Reaction	Uses	Dose
Tafenoquine	FDA-approved for radical cure of P. vivax malaria and prophylaxis.	Tafenoquine eliminates dormant P. vivax hypnozoites by generating reactive oxygen species (ROS) in hepatocytes and inhibits heme detoxification during blood stages. It also blocks gametocyte transmission.	Hemolysis (G6PD deficiency), neuropsy-chiatric effects, nausea, diarrhoea, methemog-lobinemia.	Radical cure of P. vivax malaria and malaria chemopro-phylaxis.	300 mg orally as a single dose (≥16 years of age).
KAF156 (Ganaplacide)	Phase II trials ongoing (with lumefantrine).	Ganaplacide disrupts Plasmodium intracellular trafficking by targeting PfCARL, impairing protein export and killing liver and blood-stage parasites.	Headache, nausea, QT prolongation, elevated liver enzymes.	Under investigation for multidrug-resistant malaria.	400 mg orally once daily for 3 days with lumefantrine.
Remdesivir (Newer Anti-COVID Drug)	FDA-approved (2020) for hospitalized COVID-19 patients.	Remdesivir is an adenosine analogue that terminates RNA synthesis by the SARS-CoV-2 RNA-dependent RNA polymerase (RdRp), causing delayed chain termination and halting viral replication.	Hepatotoxicity, nausea, nephrotoxicity, bradycardia.	Severe COVID-19 requiring hospitalization.	Day 1: 200 mg IV; Days 2–5: 100 mg IV daily.
MMV048	Phase II trials ongoing.	MMV048 inhibits Plasmodium phosphatidylinositol-4-kinase (PfPI4K), disrupting parasite membrane biogenesis and blocking liver, blood, and transmission stages.	Hepatotoxicity, anaemia, QT prolongation.	Investigational for uncomplicated and artemisinin-resistant malaria.	120 mg orally as a single dose.

Cipargamin (KAE609)	Phase II trials ongoing.	Cipargamin inhibits PfATP4, a parasite Na^+/H^+ pump, causing osmotic lysis of the parasite, effective against blood stages and gametocytes, including drug-resistant strains.	GI disturbances, headache, bradycardia, insomnia.	Severe and artemisinin-resistant malaria (investi-gational).	10–150 mg orally once daily for 3 days in studies.
Ganaplacide-Lumefantrine (Non-Artemisinin Combination)	Phase III trials ongoing.	Ganaplacide disrupts parasite organelle formation; lumefantrine blocks heme detoxification, leading to parasite death. Together, they offer broad activity against liver and blood stages.	Headache, nausea, diarrhoea, QT prolongation, hepatotoxicity.	Under investigation for multidrug-resistant malaria.	Ganaplacide 400 mg + Lumefantrine (480–960 mg/ day) orally once daily for 3 days.

Malaria Vaccines

Vaccine Name	Clinical Trial Phase / Approval	Mechanism of Action	Adverse Drug Reaction	Uses	Dosing schedule
RTS,S/AS01 (Mosquirix)	WHO-approved (2021) for endemic regions.	Fusion protein vaccine (CSP + HBsAg) triggers anti-sporozoite antibodies and T-cell responses, blocking liver-stage P. falciparum infection.	Injection-site reactions, febrile seizures, GI upset.	Malaria prevention in children aged 5–36 months.	Four-dose IM schedule: 5, 6, 7, and 18 months.
R21/ Matrix-M	WHO-approved (October 2023).	Next-generation CSP-based vaccine with Matrix-M adjuvant enhances humoral and cellular immunity, improving protection over RTS,S.	Fever, injection site pain, headache.	Malaria prevention in children aged 5–36 months.	Three primary IM doses + booster at 12 months post-primary series.
PfSPZ Vaccine	Phase III trials ongoing.	Live attenuated sporozoite vaccine induces robust CD8+ T-cell liver immunity without blood-stage replication.	Fatigue, mild fever, transient hepatic enzyme rise.	High-risk travellers (investi-gational).	Five IV doses over 16 weeks; boosters under study.
BK-SE36 (SE36/AHG) Vaccine	Phase Ib trials ongoing.	SE36 antigen generates strong antibody responses against blood-stage Plasmodium, reducing parasitemia and disease severity.	Local swelling, joint pain, mild fever.	Malaria control in endemic children and adults.	IM at Day 0, Day 28, and 6 months.
Pfs230-PfCSP Combination Vaccine	Phase I/ II trials underway.	Dual antigen vaccine: PfCSP blocks liver invasion; Pfs230 prevents mosquito transmission.	Headache, low-grade fever, fatigue.	Malaria elimination programs (investi-gational).	IM at Day 0, Day 28, and 6 months; boosters under evaluation.
L9LS Monoclonal Antibody Vaccine	Phase II trials underway.	Passive immunity via monoclonal antibody neutralizing sporozoites before liver infection.	Fatigue, fever, mild hyperse-nsitivity.	Malaria prophylaxis for young children and travellers.	Single IV or SC dose; booster considered at 6–12 months.

Novel Ketolide Antibiotics: Nafithromycin and Others

Drug Name	Introduction	Mechanism of Action	Adverse Drug Reaction	Uses	Dose
Nafithromycin	First oral ketolide active against drug-resistant respiratory pathogens, especially Streptococcus pneumoniae.	Binds strongly to 50S ribosomal subunit, inhibiting protein synthesis even in macrolide-resistant strains.	GI upset, mild hepatotoxicity (lower than telithromycin).	Community-acquired bacterial pneumonia (CABP).	800 mg orally once daily for 3 days.
Solithromycin	Fourth-generation fluoroketolide developed for CABP and gonorrhoea; superior potency against macrolide-resistant S. pneumoniae.	Inhibits 50S ribosomal protein synthesis; retains activity against resistant Gram-positive and atypical bacteria.	Liver enzyme elevation, GI disturbances.	CABP, gonorrhoea (investi-gational).	800 mg on Day 1, followed by 400 mg once daily on Days 2–5.
Roxithromycin	Macrolide with high intracellular accumulation, promoting enhanced phagocyte-mediated bacterial killing.	Inhibits bacterial protein synthesis at 50S ribosomal subunit; boosts immune cell bacterial clearance.	GI upset, rash, mild liver enzyme elevations.	Respiratory infections, STIs, atypical bacterial infections.	150 mg twice daily.
Telithromycin	First-generation ketolide developed for respiratory infections; semi-synthetic derivative of erythromycin.	Binds to domain II and V of 23S rRNA within the 50S subunit, overcoming traditional macrolide resistance.	Hepatotoxicity, blurred vision, QT prolongation (black box warning).	CABP, sinusitis, bronchitis (restricted use).	800 mg orally once daily for 5 days.
Dirithromycin	Macrolide prodrug converted to erythromy-cylamine, offering better pharmacokinetics and fewer GI side effects.	Inhibits bacterial 50S ribosomal protein synthesis post-activation to erythromycylamine.	Minimal GI upset, rare hepatotoxicity; no major drug interactions reported.	Mild-to-moderate respiratory and skin infections.	500 mg orally once daily.

Newer Anticancer Drugs

Drug Name	Clinical Trial Phase	Mechanism of Action	Adverse Drug Reaction	Uses	Dose
Dostarlimab (PD-1 Inhibitor)	DA-Approved (2021) for dMMR/ MSI-H Endometrial Cancer.	PD-1 inhibitor - Restores T-cell activation - Enhances anti-tumour immunity.	Immune-mediated toxicities (pneumonitis, colitis, hepatitis, endocrinopathies), infusion reactions.	Endometrial cancer (dMMR/ MSI-H); ongoing trials in colorectal, ovarian, gastric cancers.	500 mg IV every 3 weeks × 4 doses; then 1000 mg IV every 6 weeks.
Sotorasib	FDA-Approved (2021) for KRAS G12C-mutant NSCLC.	Irreversible inhibitor of KRAS G12C - Blocks MAPK/ ERK and PI3K/ AKT pathways - Inhibits tumour proliferation.	Diarrhoea, hepatotoxicity, fatigue, interstitial lung disease (ILD).	KRAS G12C-mutant NSCLC; trials ongoing for colorectal and pancreatic cancer.	960 mg orally once daily.
Tisagenlecleucel	FDA-Approved (2017) for B-ALL.	CD19-specific CAR-T therapy - Direct tumour lysis via cytotoxic T-cell activation.	Cytokine Release Syndrome (CRS), neurotoxicity (encephalopathy, confusion).	Relapsed/ refractory B-ALL, DLBCL.	≤50 kg: 0.2–5 × 10^6 CAR+ T cells/kg; 50 kg: 0.1–2.5 × 10^8 CAR+ T cells total (single IV infusion).
Belantamab Mafodotin	FDA-Approved (2020) for relapsed/ refractory multiple myeloma (RRMM).	Anti-BCMA antibody-drug conjugate (ADC) - Delivers MMAF cytotoxin - Inhibits tubulin polymerization - Apoptosis.	Ocular toxicity (keratopathy), thrombocytopenia, hepatotoxicity, infusion reactions.	Relapsed/ refractory multiple myeloma post multiple prior therapies.	2.5 mg/kg IV every 3 weeks.
Tebentafusp	FDA-Approved (2022) for HLA-A*02:01-positive metastatic uveal melanoma.	Bispecific T-cell engager - TCR binding to gp100 antigen + CD3 activation - T-cell-mediated melanoma cell lysis.	Cytokine Release Syndrome (CRS), skin rash, hypotension, hepatotoxicity.	Metastatic uveal melanoma (HLA-A*02:01-positive).	Day 1: 20 mcg IV; Day 8: 30 mcg IV; Day 15 onwards: 68 mcg IV weekly.

Recent Advances in the Management of Obesity

Drug Name	Clinical Trial Phase	Mechanism of Action	Adverse Drug Reaction	Uses	Dose
Semaglutide	FDA-approved (2021) for chronic weight management – STEP Trials	Semaglutide is a glucagon-like peptide-1 (GLP-1) receptor agonist that mimics endogenous GLP-1, stimulating insulin secretion, inhibiting glucagon release, and delaying gastric emptying.	Nausea, vomiting, diarrhoea, pancreatitis, gallstones, hypoglycaemia, potential thyroid C-cell tumours.	Management of obesity in adults with BMI ≥30 kg/m² or BMI ≥27 kg/m² with comorbidities; also used in type 2 diabetes.	2.4 mg subcutaneously once weekly.
Tirzepatide	FDA-approved (2023) for chronic weight management – SURMOUNT Trials	Tirzepatide is a dual agonist of the GLP-1 and glucose-dependent insulinotropic polypeptide (GIP) receptors, enhancing glucose-dependent insulin secretion, reducing glucagon levels, delaying gastric emptying, and suppressing appetite. GIP activation also promotes fat oxidation and improves insulin sensitivity, synergistically resulting in profound weight loss and metabolic improvement.	Nausea, diarrhoea, pancreatitis, hypoglycaemia, injection site reactions.	Treatment of obesity and type 2 diabetes.	2.5 mg subcutaneously once weekly.

Cagrilintide	Phase III clinical trials ongoing.	Cagrilintide is a long-acting amylin receptor agonist that enhances satiety by activating amylin receptors in the hypothalamus and brainstem, leading to appetite suppression. It delays gastric emptying, reduces postprandial glucose spikes, inhibits glucagon secretion, and promotes sustained weight loss without directly stimulating insulin release.	Mild gastrointestinal symptoms such as nausea and constipation, and injection-site reactions.	Being investigated for obesity and diabetes.	0.3 mg to 4.5 mg subcutaneously once weekly (clinical trial dose).
Bimagrumab	Phase II trials demonstrated significant body fat reduction.	Bimagrumab is a monoclonal antibody that blocks activin type II receptors, antagonizing myostatin and activin A signalling. This promotes skeletal muscle growth while reducing adipose tissue through enhanced energy metabolism and fat oxidation, offering simultaneous muscle mass gain and fat loss.	Injection-site reactions, gastrointestinal upset, hypercalcaemia.	Being investigated for obesity-related muscle loss and sarcopenic obesity.	30 mg/kg intravenous infusion every 4 weeks for 48 weeks.
Setmelanotide	FDA-approved (2020) for genetic obesity disorders.	Setmelanotide selectively activates the melanocortin-4 receptor (MC4R) in the hypothalamus, restoring appetite regulation in individuals with genetic defects in the MC4R pathway. It suppresses hyperphagia, enhances energy expenditure through brown adipose tissue activation, and improves metabolic parameters like glucose and lipid levels.	Skin hyperpigmentation, nausea, diarrhoea, injection-site reactions.	Approved for rare genetic obesity syndromes including POMC deficiency and leptin receptor mutations.	1 mcg/kg/day subcutaneously for children; adults start with 2 mg/day subcutaneously, adjustable up to 3 mg/day.

Role of Artificial Intelligence in Pharmacology

Definition

Artificial Intelligence (AI) denotes computer systems engineered to execute activities necessitating human intelligence, including pattern recognition, problem-solving, and decision-making. In pharmacology, artificial intelligence use data-driven models to replicate biological processes, enhance drug design, and forecast clinical outcomes.

Principal Categories and Subcategories of Artificial Intelligence

- Machine Learning (ML): Algorithms that evolve by acquiring knowledge from data.
- Deep Learning (DL): Multi-layered neural networks that manage intricate patterns.
- Natural Language Processing (NLP): Artificial Intelligence comprehending human language to facilitate clinical note analysis.
- Reinforcement Learning (RL): Algorithms that acquire optimal tactics by trial and error.

Utilization of Artificial Intelligence in Pharmacology

- Pharmaceutical Discovery and Development: Virtual screening, structure-based drug design, generative modeling of novel molecules.
- Preclinical Research: Analysis of omics data, preliminary ADMET assessment, and toxicity prediction. Clinical Pharmacology: Patient stratification, personalized dose, adverse event surveillance.
- Post-Marketing Surveillance: Immediate pharmacovigilance and evaluation of real-world evidence.

Recent Advancements

- Generative Adversarial Networks (GANs): Generate innovative drug-like compounds.
- AI-Enhanced Molecular Docking: Improves predictions of drug-target interactions.
- Reinforcement Drug Synthesis Education: Enhances chemicals according to specified characteristics.
- AI-Optimized Clinical Trial Design: Discerns biomarkers and responding subpopulations.
- Real-Time Pharmacovigilance: Oversees internet platforms for the prompt identification of hazardous medication reactions.
- Customized Dosing & Digital Therapeutics: Adapts treatment according to individual patient characteristics.

Significant Advancements

- Novel medication design utilizing deep learning methods.
- Predictive ADMET modeling mitigates late-stage medication failures.
- Identification of biomarkers for precision medicine methodologies.
- AI-enhanced clinical decision support systems optimizing patient management.
- Proactive post-marketing surveillance with real-world data analysis.

Benefits of Artificial Intelligence in Pharmacology

- Enhances the efficiency of drug research and clinical trials.
- Decreases total research and development expenditures.
- Improves the precision of predictions regarding drug efficacy and toxicity.
- Facilitates genuinely individualized treatment.
- Perpetually enhances by the assimilation of novel data.

Constraints and Obstacles

- Data quality deficiencies may skew results.
- Numerous AI models have a deficiency in interpretability, raising concerns regarding their "black box" nature.
- Regulatory frameworks for AI applications are still being developed.
- Elevated computational requirements may restrict accessibility.
- Incorporation into therapeutic environments necessitates accessible, dependable instruments.

Computer-Assisted Learning (CAL) In Pharmacology

Definition

Computer-Assisted Learning (CAL) denotes the utilization of digital resources such as tutorials, simulations, and interactive platforms to enhance or substitute conventional pharmacological instructional techniques. CAL prioritizes learner-centered, adaptable, and stimulating education.

Types of CAL in Pharmacology

- Interactive Tutorials: Autonomous modules include videos and assessments.
- Virtual Reality (VR) and Augmented Reality (AR): Three-dimensional simulations for viewing pharmacological activities and clinical situations.
- Computerized Case-Based Learning: Virtual patients necessitating pharmaceutical decision-making.
- Adaptive Learning Platforms: Modify content complexity according to student performance.
- Serious Games and Gamification: Educational games that enhance engagement and facilitate information retention.
- Online Discussion Forums: Collaborative platforms for peer-to-peer and instructor-student engagement.

Traditional (Non-CAL) Methods

Traditional means of education, like as lectures, manuals, wet-lab demonstrations, group discussions, and clinical rotations, were frequently constrained by passive learning, ethical dilemmas, and logistical challenges.

Sophisticated CAL Methodologies

- VR Labs: Engaging three-dimensional settings for the practice of drug administration.
- Augmented Reality Applications: Immediate information superimposition on tangible items.
- AI Simulators: Customized case-based tasks that adjust according to student achievement.
- Gamified Platforms: Engaging quizzes and narratives for the acquisition of medication categorization.
- MOOCs and e-Learning Modules: Versatile, multimedia-rich courses available worldwide.

Emerging Trends

- Engaging education with virtual and augmented reality.
- Adaptive assessments with artificial intelligence.
- Acceleration of remote and hybrid learning following the COVID-19 pandemic.
- Collaborative virtual laboratory environments promoting teamwork.

Benefits of CAL

- Increased engagement and motivation.
- Adaptable, individualized educational trajectories.
- Prompt feedback mechanisms for rapid rectification.

- Ethical and economically viable alternatives to animal experimentation.
- Enhanced accessibility within international institutions.
- Improvements to the course based on analytics.

Constraints and Obstacles

- Elevated development expenses and intricate technicalities.
- Faculty reluctance and deficiency in digital competencies.
- Peril of excessive reliance on technology.
- Infrastructure limitations in resource-poor environments.
- Inconsistent quality and accreditation issues.
- Incapability of completely substituting authentic clinical or laboratory exposure.

Clustered Regularly Interspaced Short Palindromic Repeats (CRISPR)

Definition

CRISPR is a ground-breaking gene-editing technique derived from bacterial immune defense mechanisms. It enables precise modification of DNA in living organisms by using guide RNAs and the Cas9 enzyme to locate and cut target genetic sequences.

History and Discovery

First observed as peculiar DNA repeats in the 1980s, the defensive function of CRISPR in bacteria was identified in 2005. In 2020, Emmanuelle Charpentier and Jennifer Doudna received the Nobel Prize in Chemistry for developing CRISPR–Cas9 as a powerful gene-editing tool, often referred to as "genetic scissors."

Mechanism of CRISPR-Cas9

A specifically designed guide RNA (gRNA) directs the Cas9 enzyme to the target DNA sequence. Cas9 makes a precise double-strand cut at the selected site, enabling gene disruption or insertion of new genetic material through the cell's natural repair processes.

Applications in Disease Treatment

- Cancer: CRISPR systems are delivered using nanoparticles and exosomes to tumor cells, exploiting hypoxic environments for targeted therapy.
- Liver Diseases: Phenylketonuria corrected by single-base editing; HBV infections managed by disabling viral DNA using infrared-activated nanoparticles.
- Cardiovascular Diseases: CRISPRa systems selectively activated in cardiomyocytes to overcome delivery challenges.
- SARS-CoV-2 Detection: SHERLOCK, a CRISPR-Cas13a-based RNA detection method, enables rapid viral diagnosis.
- Sickle Cell Disease and β-Thalassemia: CRISPR used to edit hematopoietic stem cells, reducing disease-causing gene expression with minimal side effects.

Ethical and Safety Concerns

CRISPR's promise is tempered by concerns about unintended off-target mutations, risks linked to germline editing, and potential misuse for bioterrorism.